Advances in Organic Chemistry
Methods and Results

VOLUME 6

Advisory Board

D. H. R. BARTON
Imperial College of Science and Technology, London, England

K. W. BENTLEY
J. F. Macfarlan and Co., Edinburgh, Scotland

A. J. BIRCH
University of Manchester, England

J. W. COOK
University of Exeter, England

CARL DJERASSI
Stanford University, California

A. ESCHENMOSER
Eidg. Technische Hochschule, Zürich, Switzerland

R. GREWE
Universität Kiel, Germany

R. HUISGEN
Ludwig-Maximilians-Universität, Munich, Germany

E. C. KOOYMAN
Rijksuniversiteit, Leiden, The Netherlands

E. LEDERER
Institut de Chimie des Substances Naturelles, Gif-sur-Yvette, France

G. OURISSON
Université de Strasbourg, France

A. QUILICO
Instituto de Chimica Generale del Politecnico, Milan, Italy

S. STÄLLBERG-STENHAGEN
University of Gothenberg, Sweden

G. STORK
Columbia University, New York

LORD TODD
University Chemical Laboratory, Cambridge, England

M. VISCONTINI
University of Zürich, Switzerland

A. WEISSBERGER
Eastman Kodak Company, Rochester, New York

K. WIESNER
Ayerst, McKenna and Harrison, Ltd., Montreal, Canada

F. Y. WISELOGLE
Squibb Institute for Medical Research, New Brunswick, New Jersey

R. B. WOODWARD
Harvard University, Cambridge, Massachusetts

Advances in
Organic Chemistry
Methods and Results

VOLUME 6

Editors

EDWARD C. TAYLOR, *Princeton University, Princeton, New Jersey*
HANS WYNBERG, *The University, Groningen, The Netherlands*

1969
Interscience Publishers
a division of John Wiley & Sons, New York · London · Sydney · Toronto

Copyright © 1969 by John Wiley & Sons, Inc.

All rights reserved. No part of this book may be reproduced by any means, nor transmitted, nor translated into a machine language without the written permission of the publisher.

LIBRARY OF CONGRESS CATALOG CARD NUMBER 59-13036
SBN 470   846402

PRINTED IN THE UNITED STATES OF AMERICA

Contents

Nonbenzenoid Conjugated Cyclic Hydrocarbons
  By P. J. Garratt and M. V. Sargent, Department of Chemistry, University College, London, England ... 1

Organic Syntheses by Means of Noble Metal Compounds
  By Jiro Tsuji, Basic Research Laboratories, Toyo Rayon Company, Kamakura, Japan ... 109

Electrochemical Preparation of Cyclic Compounds
  By J. D. Anderson, J. P. Petrovich, and M. M. Baizer, Central Research Department, Monsanto Company, St. Louis, Missouri ... 257

Dimethylsulfoxide (DMSO) in Organic Synthesis
  By T. Durst, Department of Chemistry, University of Ottawa, Ottawa, Canada ... 285

Author Index ... 389

Subject Index ... 413

Cumulative Index, Volumes 1–6 ... 431

NONBENZENOID CONJUGATED CYCLIC HYDROCARBONS

By P. J. GARRATT* AND M. V. SARGENT,† *University Chemical Laboratory, Cambridge, England*

CONTENTS

I. Introduction	1
II. Monocyclic Systems	2
A. $n = 0$	2
B. $n = 1$	12
C. $n = 2$	28
D. $n > 2$	38
1. $n = 3$	38
2. $n = 4$	45
3. $n > 4$	51
III. Polycyclic Systems	54
A. Systems with 3-Membered Rings	55
B. Systems with 4-Membered Rings	57
C. Systems with 5-Membered Rings	62
D. Systems with 6-Membered Rings	75
E. Systems with Rings Greater than 6-Membered	77
IV. Conclusion	79
V. Addendum	80
References	94

I. Introduction

Aromatic compounds have intrigued both the experimental and theoretical chemist since their discovery as a class of highly unsaturated compounds with anomalous chemical behavior. Kekulé's (1) classical formulation of benzene was generalized by Bamberger (2) into a hexacentric theory, which was later formulated by Armit and Robinson (3) in electronic terms as the "aromatic sextet." The demonstration by Willstätter and his co-workers (4) that cyclooctatetraene was not a

* Present address: William Ramsey and Ralph Forster Laboratories, University College, London, England.

† Present address: University Chemical Laboratory, University of Kent, Canterbury, England.

"super" benzene supported the sextet hypothesis, but the difference between 6 π and 8 π electron systems had no theoretical foundation. The necessary theoretical basis was provided by Hückel (5) in the early 1930's in terms of the molecular orbital (MO) theory. His conclusions have been summarized in the now familiar Hückel rule, which states that monocyclic systems with $(4n + 2)$ π electrons will be aromatic, whereas those with $4n$ π electrons will not.

The MO theory accounted for the acidity of cyclopentadiene and predicted that the cycloheptatrienyl cation (tropylium cation) would be a stable system. Little attention was paid to this prediction by experimental chemists until Dewar (6), in 1945, postulated that stipitatic acid and colchicine both contained a seven-membered aromatic ring, derived from Hückel's tropylium cation. The synthesis of the tropylium cation by Doering and Knox (7) placed the Hückel theory on a sound experimental basis and encouraged interest in the synthesis of systems predicted by the theory to be stable. The dramatic success attained in the preparation of these stable systems has recently led to an investigation of the $4n$ series, which have zero or negative delocalization energy (DE). Examples of both types of system have been reported (8).

The present review deals with mono- and polycarbocycles of both the $4n$ and $(4n + 2)$ π electron series, excluding benzene. The last exhaustive account of work in this area appeared in 1959 (9), although aspects of the more recent work have been reviewed (10). A text has appeared (11).

Those systems which are exhaustively treated elsewhere will not be covered in detail here. The monocyclic hydrocarbons, to which the Hückel theory strictly applies, will be considered first, primarily in order of increasing value of n, and secondarily in order of increasing ring size. The polycyclic hydrocarbons will then be considered in order of increasing size of the smallest ring.

II. Monocyclic Systems

A. $n=0$

This group consists of aromatic systems with 2 π electrons and the simplest member of the series is the cyclopropenyl cation **(1)**, which was predicted to have 2.0β DE (12). The first derivative of this system was prepared by Breslow (13) in 1957. Phenyl diazoacetonitrile was reacted with phenyl acetylene to yield 1,2,3-triphenyl-3-cyanocyclopropene (2). The cyclopropene (2) with boron trifluoride etherate in water gave the *sym*-triphenyl cyclopropenyl cation (3a) as the mixed fluoroborate, hydrofluoroborate salt. The cation 3a reacted with methanol to give

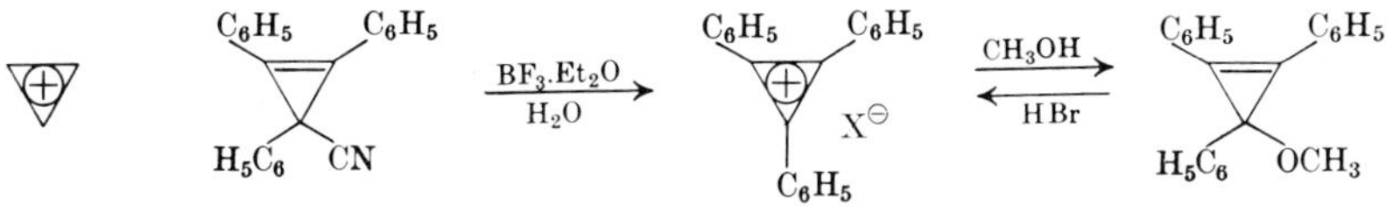

(1) (2) (3a) X = BF_4, HBF_4 (3b) X = Br (4)

the methyl ether 4, which can be converted to the cation 3b with hydrogen bromide. An x-ray determination (14) of the mixed salt of 3a confirmed the symmetrical nature of the cation and indicated that the phenyl groups are twisted by 21° out of the plane of the cyclopropenyl ring.

Subsequent syntheses of the cyclopropenyl cation with alkyl substituents have been reported. 1,2-Di-*n*-propyl-3-carboxycyclopropene (5) reacted with perchloric acid or fluoroboric acid in acetic anhydride to give the 1,2-di-*n*-propylcyclopropenyl cation (6a, 6b) (15). The NMR spectrum revealed a proton at very low field, τ −0.31 (in 5% CF_3CO_2H) (16), and two equivalent *n*-propyl groups [τ 6.84 (4H), τ 8.11 (4H), τ 8.98 (6H)], consistent with a symmetrical species with one-third of a positive charge on each cyclopropenyl carbon atom. The chemical shifts were still lower in sulfuric acid (15a). The 1,2-diphenylcyclopropenyl cation (7a) (17,18) the 1,2-diphenyl-3-*n*-propylcyclopropenyl cation (7b) (15b), the tri-*n*-propylcyclopropenyl cation (8) (15b), and

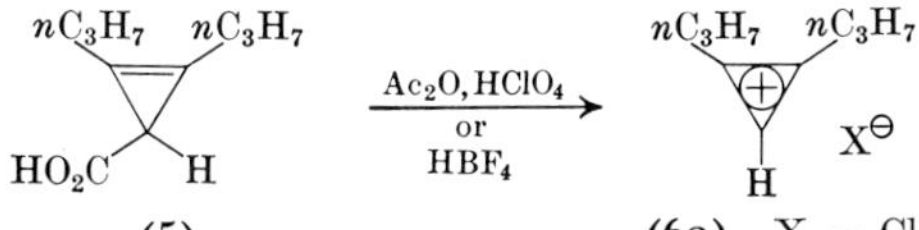

(5) (6a) X = ClO_4 (6b) X = BF_4

substituted triarylcyclopropenyl ions (9) (19) have been synthesized. The pK_{R+} values for a series of compounds (19) have shown that the inductive effect of the alkyl group increases the stability of the ion more than the mesomeric effect of the phenyl substituents. Little charge separation into the phenyl ring occurs, contrary to the simple MO calculation (20). The variation of pK in the triaryl series agrees with a simple MO treatment (19).

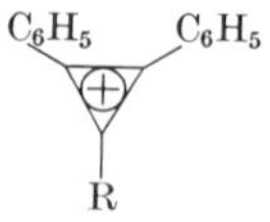

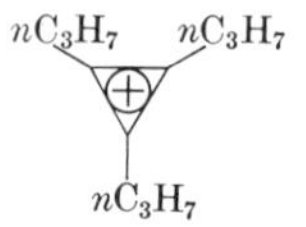

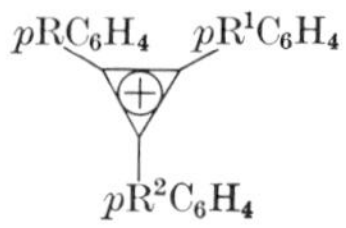

(7a) R = H		(8)		(9a) R = R¹ = R² = H	
(7b) R = nC₃H₇				(9b) R = R¹ = H, R² = OCH₃	
				(9c) R = H, R¹ = R² = OCH₃	
				(9d) R = R¹ = R² = OCH₃	

Substituents on the cyclopropenyl rings (as shown in the structures above): **(7a)** C₆H₅, C₆H₅, R; **(7b)** same with R = nC₃H₇; **(8)** nC₃H₇, nC₃H₇, nC₃H₇; **(9a–d)** pRC₆H₄, pR¹C₆H₄, pR²C₆H₄.

Alternating current polarography (21) of **9a** to the cyclopropenyl radical **10** gave a value for the reverse reduction potential of -1.132 eV. Higher values were obtained with **9b** and **9d** $[-1.24$ eV, -1.49 eV]. Comparison with the reverse reduction potential of the triphenylmethyl cation **(11)**, -0.09 eV, for which simple MO theory predicts no loss of DE, gave a value of -1.04 eV (24 kcal mole^{-1}) for the loss in DE on addition of an electron to the cyclopropenyl cation. This agrees well with the predicted value of -0.504β, β in such cases having been suggested to be of the order of 2 eV (10a). Attempted chemical reduction of **9a** gave only the dimer **12**, which did not dissociate to **10**, but rearranged to hexaphenyl benzene (22).

$$\mathbf{9a} \underset{-e}{\overset{+e}{\rightleftarrows}} \mathbf{(10)} \quad \mathbf{(11)} \quad \mathbf{(12)}$$

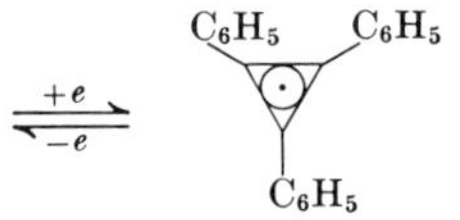

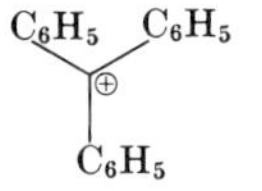

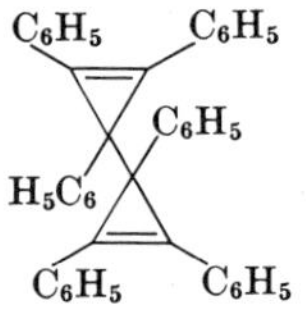

where **(10)** is the triphenylcyclopropenyl radical, **(11)** the triphenylmethyl cation, and **(12)** the hexaphenyl dimer.

The simple trichlorocyclopropenyl cation **(14)** has been synthesized by the reaction of tetrachlorocyclopropene **(13)** with Lewis acids (23).

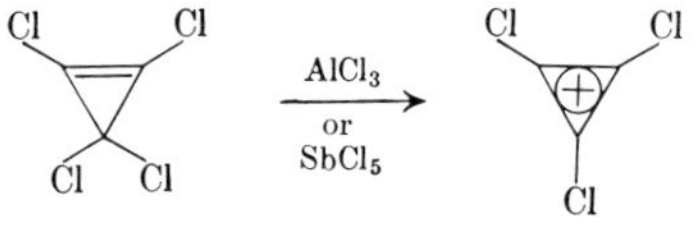

$$\mathbf{(13)} \xrightarrow[\text{or SbCl}_5]{\text{AlCl}_3} \mathbf{(14)}$$

The IR spectrum has three bands, and the Raman spectrum shows a band attributed to AlCl$_4^-$; the data agree well with those calculated for a species of D_{3h} symmetry. The C—C stretching force constant was calculated to be unusually large. The trimethylcyclopropenyl cation **(16)** has recently been prepared by the photolysis and subsequent acidification of **15**.

The parent cyclopropenylium ion, **(1)**, has been reported to be the primary product in the oxidation of acetylene (25a) and the thermal dissociation of iodoform (25b). A $C_3H_3^+$ fragment has also been observed in the mass spectra of furans (26) and of photo-2-pyrone (27).

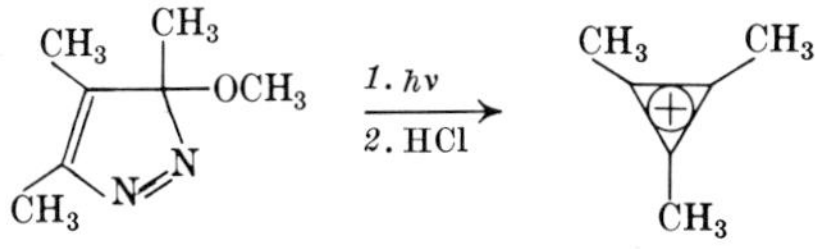

Cyclopropenone (17) is the lower homolog of tropolone, and the dipolar structure 17a should enhance its stability. Cyclopropenone would be expected to be more stable than cyclopropanone, which is only isolable as the ketal (28). Although the parent compound is unknown a number of substituted cyclopropenones have been obtained.

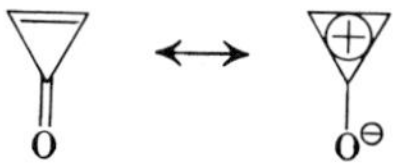

The first, diphenylcyclopropenone (19), was synthesized independently by Vol'pin and Breslow and their respective co-workers in 1959 (29,30). A number of synthetic methods have since been described and these have recently been reviewed (31,32). The best method is reported to be the Favorski elimination of hydrogen bromide from α,α'-dibromodibenzyl ketone (18). The infrared spectrum of 19 shows two strong bands at 1850 and 1640 cm^{-1}. Although assignments have been made to these bands (31), it seems probable that they are so strongly coupled that a unique assignment is not possible (33). (However see Sec. V., Addendum.) The high dipole moment (5.1 D) (29,31) is indicative of a large contribution from the dipolar form. Diphenylcyclopropene is also strongly basic and forms salts (29). Photolysis of 19 gives diphenyl acetylene and carbon monoxide (34).

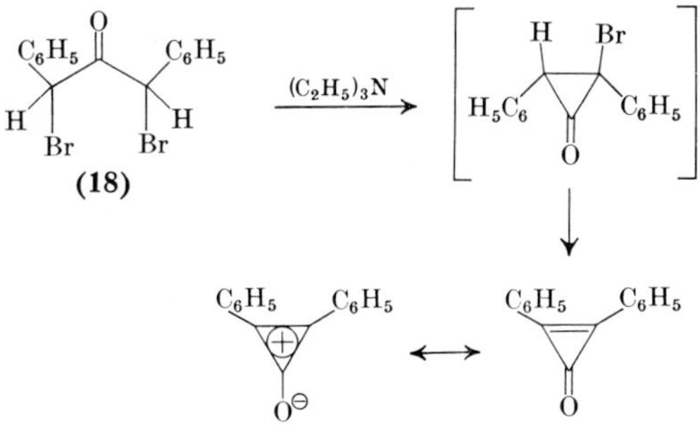

A number of alkylcyclopropenones have been synthesized (35). Di-n-propylacetylene reacts with sodium trichloroacetate to yield 1,2-di-n-propylcyclopropenone (20), together with some dichloro-di-n-propylcyclobutenone (21) (36). The alkylcyclopropenone 20 is more

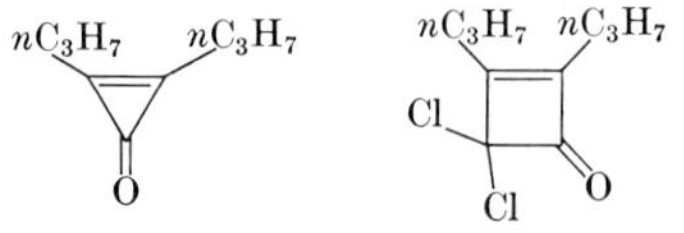

(20) (21)

basic than 19, which again indicates the lack of charge delocalization into the phenyl rings. Favorski elimination is a versatile synthetic method and yields a number of interesting cyclopropenones, e.g., 22a,b.

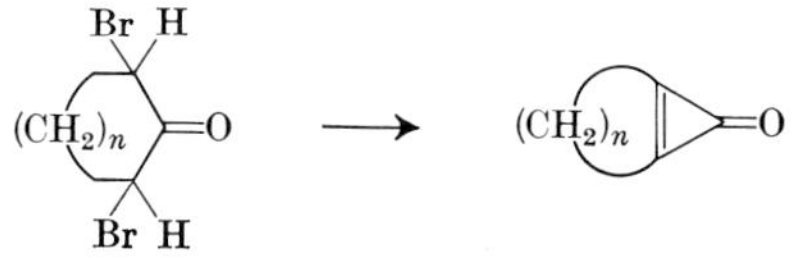

(22a) $n = 5$
(22b) $n = 9$

Dehmlow (36) has reported that the addition of dichlorocarbene to diacetylenes or vinylacetylenes followed by subsequent hydrolysis yields cyclopropenones with unsaturated side chains, e.g., 23. Monosubstituted cyclopropenones, e.g., 24a–24d, have recently been synthesized by two methods (33,37). The reaction of lithium trichloro-

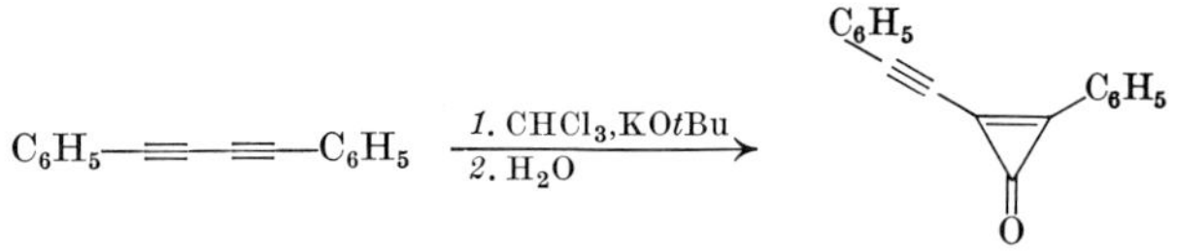

(23)

methide (33), a precursor of dichlorocarbene, at $-100°$ with terminal acetylenes gave, on acidification and work up, the corresponding cyclopropenone. Alternatively, the addition of hypobromous acid to a terminal acetylene, followed by a Favorski elimination on the resulting α,α-dibromoketone, also gave the cyclopropenone (37). The kinetic acidity of the cyclopropene hydrogen in these compounds is greater than that of acetylene (33).

(24a) R = CH_3
(24b) R = C_2H_5
(24c) R = nC_3H_7
(24d) R = nC_5H_{11}

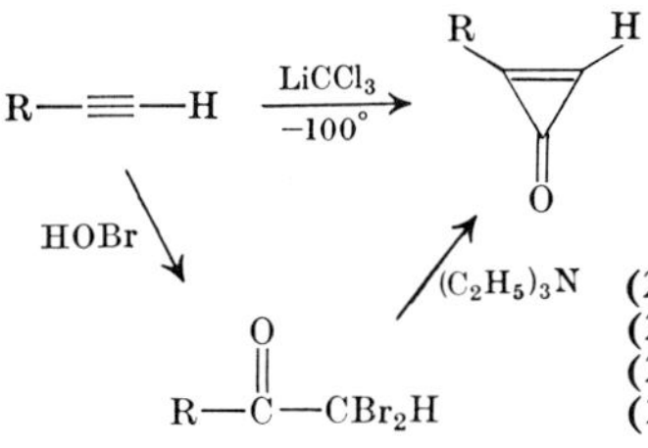

Diphenylquinocyclopropene **(27a)** and a substituted diphenylquinocyclopropene **27b** have been synthesized (38) by the addition of phenylchlorocarbene to the acetylenes **25a,** and **25b**, followed by treatment of the salts **26a** and **26b** with strong base. The dibromide **27b** is more basic than diphenylcyclopropenone **(19).**

(25a) X = H, R = $C_6H_5CH_2$
(25b) X = Br, R = $C_6H_5CH_2$

(26a) (26b)

(27a) (27b)

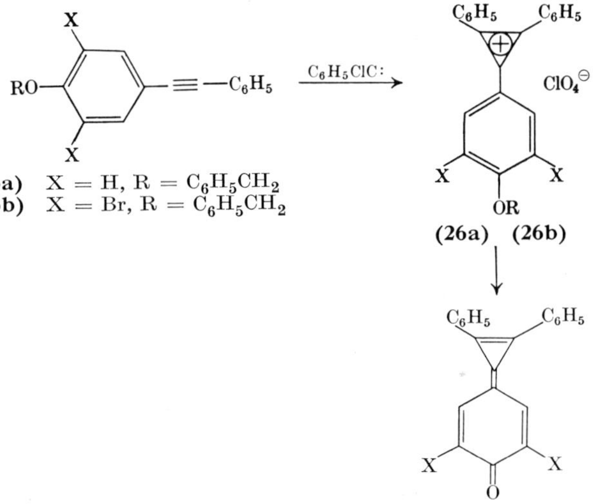

Farnum and his co-workers (39) have recently reported the synthesis of phenylhydroxycyclopropenone **(29)**, a derivative of the lower vinylog of tropolone. The compound **29** was prepared by treatment of 1,3,3-trichloro-2-phenylcyclopropene **(28)** with potassium *tert*-butoxide. Phenylhydroxycyclopropenone is an extremely strong acid, and the similarity of its UV spectrum to that of its sodium salt and methyl ether demonstrates that in aqueous solution **29** exists as the enol and not as the diketone **29a.**

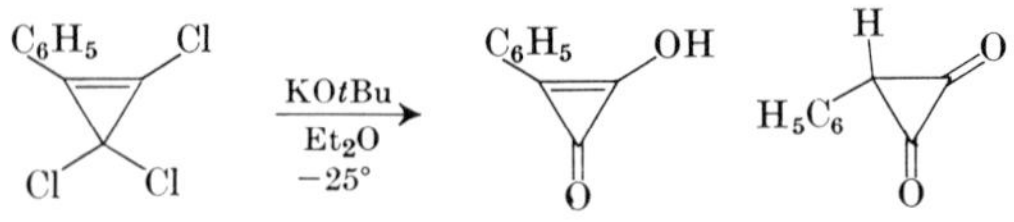

(28) → (29) (29a)

[KOtBu, Et₂O, −25°]

Methylene cyclopropene (30) is a lower homolog of fulvene. A number of substituted methylene cyclopropenes have been synthesized

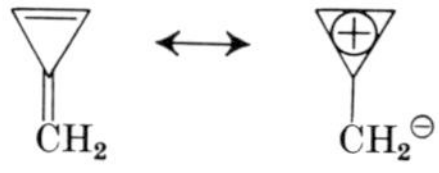

(30) ↔ (30a)

(33b, 40, 41). Diphenylcyclopropenone (19) reacts with the Wittig reagent 31 to give the methylene cyclopropene 32 (40). Treatment of the nitrosourea 33 with dimethylfumarate and potassium *tert* butoxide

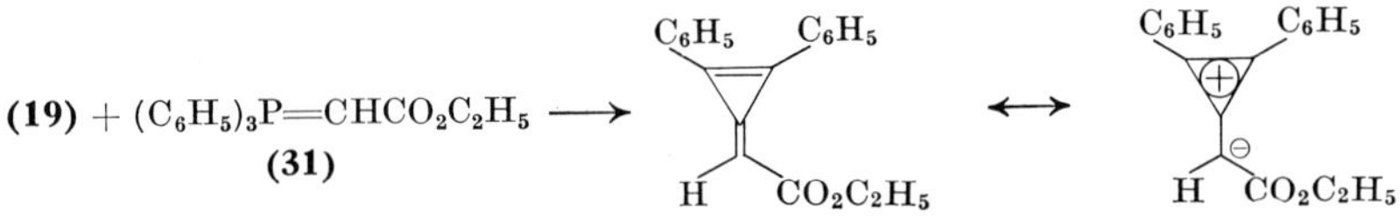

(19) + $(C_6H_5)_3P=CHCO_2C_2H_5$ ⟶ (32) ↔ (32a)
(31)

gave the methylenecyclopropene 34 (41). Both 32 and 34 have a complex electronic spectrum, which on addition of fluoroboric acid,

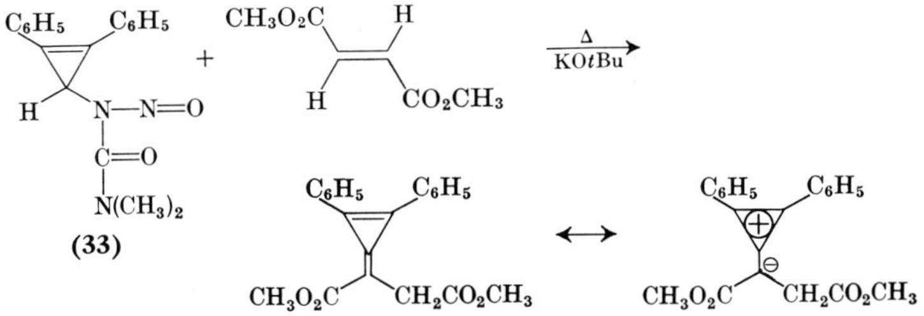

(33) + [dimethyl fumarate] $\xrightarrow[KOtBu]{\Delta}$ (34) ↔ (34a)

changed to that of the diphenylcyclopropenyl cation due to protonation of the exocyclic methylene group. The NMR spectrum of 32 showed a large upfield shift of the methylene proton, compared with the methylene protons of Feist's ester. This is in accordance with the resonance hybrid having a considerable contribution from the dipolar form 32a.

The aromatic 2 π system should also be attained by the removal of two electrons from cyclobutadiene, giving the cyclobutadienyl dication (35). The first attempted synthesis of a derivative of this system was

(35)

reported by Katz and his co-workers (42), who reacted 1,2,3,4-tetramethyl-3,4-dichlorocyclobutene (36) with silver hexafluoroantimonate in sulfur dioxide. Instead of the expected dication 38, the monocation 37a was obtained. The monocation 37b was more conveniently prepared by the reaction of aluminum trichloride in methylene chloride, and a number of analogous cyclobutenyl cations were prepared in this manner (43). The NMR spectrum of 37b shows three signals at τ 7.72(3H), 7.57(3H), and 7.09(6H), and the spectrum did not change over the temperature range investigated (43). It was suggested that the stability of the monocation is due to considerable 1,3-interaction, the species existing as the homocyclopropenyl cation (39, R = Cl). The UV spectra of a series of cyclobutenyl cations (37a–37e) gave considerable support to this view, and an estimate of 0.33β for the 1,3-interaction was made (43).

Treatment of the dichloride 36 with 97% sulfuric acid also gave 37, R = Cl (44). However, only a single methyl signal is observed in the NMR spectrum (τ 7.26), indicating that an equilibrium between the methyl groups occurs, presumably due to a rapid transfer of the chloride ion.

(37a) R = Cl, X = SbF$_6$
(37b) R = Cl, X = AlCl$_4$
(37c) R = CH$_3$, X = AlCl$_4$
(37d) R = H, X = AlCl$_4$
(37e) R = Br, X = AlCl$_4$

The report by Freedman and Frantz (45), in 1962, that the reaction of excess stannic chloride with 1,2,3,4-tetraphenyl-2,3-dibromocyclobutene (40), gave the dication 41a, appeared to indicate that in the cyclobutenyl system, unlike the cyclopropenyl system, phenyl substitution has a large stabilizing effect. However, an x-ray crystallographic study (46) of the salt revealed that in the solid state it existed as the monocation 42a. Whether the salt exists as 41a or 42a in solution is not known, but the present evidence suggests that the subsequently prepared fluoroborate exists as the dication 41b (47). On addition of silver fluoroborate to 40, two molar equivalents of silver bromide were precipitated. The ^{19}F NMR signal of the salt shows only

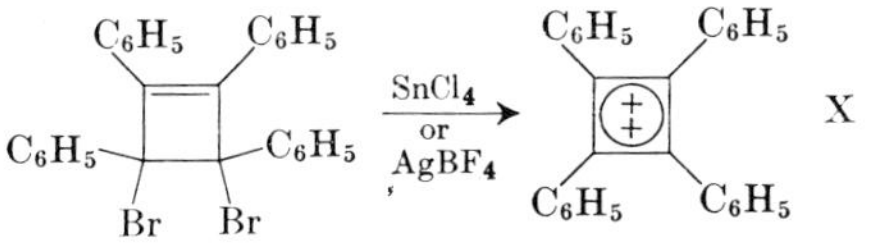

(40)

(41a) X = SnCl$_6^{\ominus}$
(41b) X = 2BF$_4^{\ominus}$

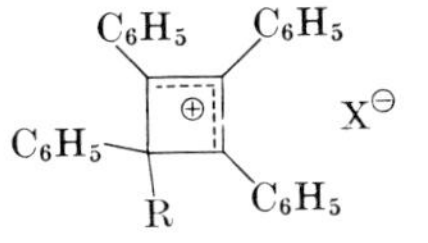

(42a) R = Cl, X = SnCl$_5$
(42b) R = F, X = BF$_4$

one type of fluorine, and the chemical shift value (+70.9 ppm from CF$_3$CO$_2$H) is in accordance with the known value for the fluoroborate anion. The equilibration of monocations of the type 42b has not, however, been rigorously excluded. Farnum and Webster (48) have reported that treatment of the cyclobutenone 43 with 96% sulfuric acid gave the dication 44. The NMR spectrum (a complex band from τ 1.5–2.0) at lower field than that of the protonated species 45 (signal at τ 2.1–2.7) supported this assignment.

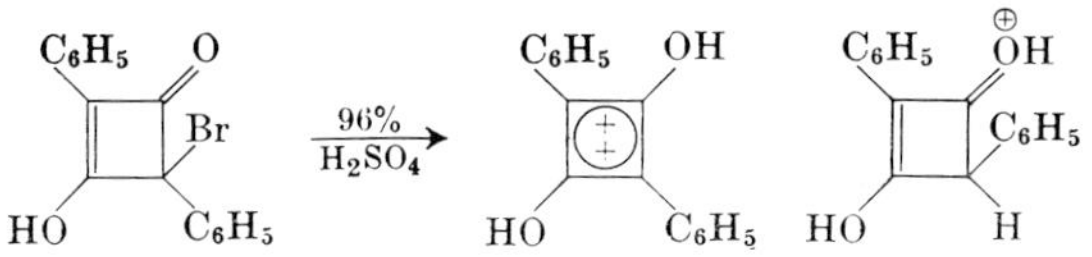

(43) (44) (45)

Cyclobutadienequinone (46) may have the polar structure 46a as a major resonance contributor. This contribution, which should find its expression in the physical properties of the cyclobutadienequinones, together with the possibility of the reduction of the quinones to cyclobutadienediols (47), has stimulated research in this area. Smutny

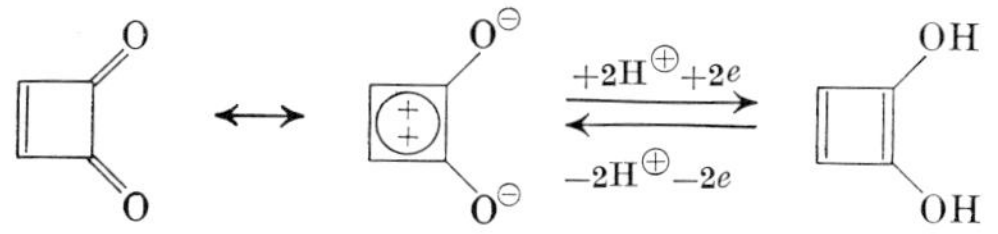

(46) ⟷ (46a) $\xrightarrow[-2H^{\oplus}-2e]{+2H^{\oplus}+2e}$ (47)

and Roberts (49) synthesized phenylcyclobutadienequinone (49) by treatment of the chlorocyclobutene 48, prepared from chlorotrifluoroethylene and phenylacetylene, with 92% sulfuric acid at 100°. The dipole moment of 49 was estimated to be 5.3 D, (50,51) but the

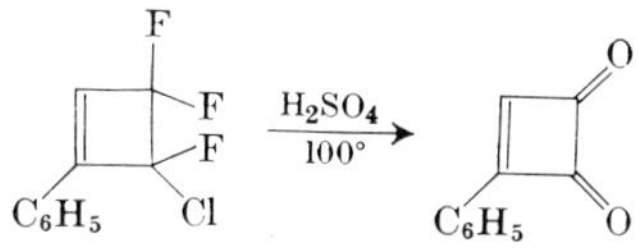

(48) $\xrightarrow[100°]{H_2SO_4}$ (49)

contribution of 46a could not be reliably estimated. Compound 49 could not be reduced to the hydroquinone, but it reacted readily with halogens to give the substituted cyclobutadienequinones 50. The halogen atom in 50 is extremely reactive, and it can be replaced by a variety of groups, e.g., 51a–51c. The alcohol 51a is an extremely strong acid (pK_a 0.37 ± 0.04).

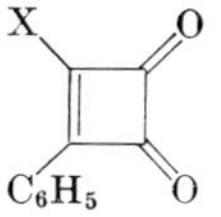

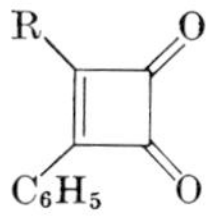

(50) X = Cl,Br   (51a) R = OH
                  (51b) R = NH_2
                  (51c) R = OCH_3

Blomquist and LaLancette (52) have prepared diphenylcyclobutadienequinone (54) by a similar route. Hexafluorocyclobutene (52) was treated with phenyllithium, and the resulting diphenyltetrafluorocyclobutene (53) gave 54 on reaction with concentrated sulfuric acid at 100°. The IR and NMR spectra were consistent with structure 54. Diethylcyclobutadienequinone (55) has also been prepared (53) and its structure confirmed by the IR and NMR spectra.

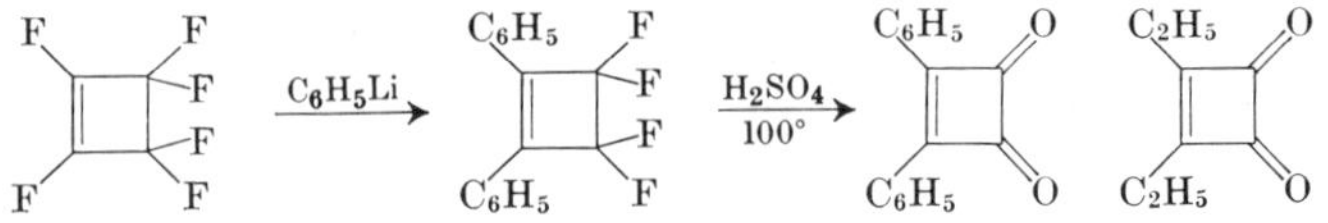

The synthesis of squaric acid (54) **(57)** has restored interest in the series of dianions of which its salt is a member. It has been suggested that this series forms a new aromatic group (55). Squaric acid was prepared by the hydrolysis of 1,2-diethoxy-3,3,4,4-tetrafluorocyclobutene **(56)** with 50% sulfuric acid at 100° (54). Squaric acid **(57)** (pK_2 2.2) is nearly as strong an acid as sulfuric acid (pK_2 1.5). The IR spectrum of the dipotassium salt shows no OH, C=O, or C=C stretching band, all of which are found in the acid, but a broad band from 1540 to 1490 cm^{-1} is present (54). The Raman spectrum is consistent with a symmetric structure for the dianion (55). A number of derivatives of squaric acid have recently been prepared (56). The croconate ($C_5O_5^{2-}$) and rhodizonate ($C_6O_6^{2-}$) dianions are other known members of the group **(57,58)**. MO calculations (59) predict the stability of these ions and also of the $C_3O_3^{2-}$ ion. The chemistry of these salts has been investigated (58). The ions may be considered as members of the 2 π series if structures such as **59** are considered.

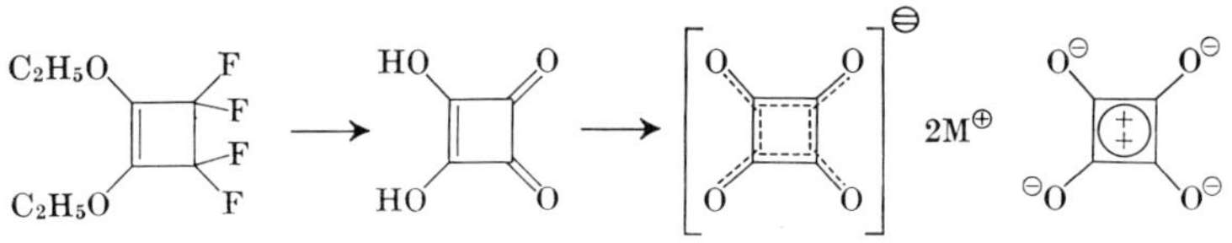

B. $n=1$

The $n = 1$ series contains both nonaromatic $4n$ and aromatic ($4n + 2$) members, the former with 4 π and the latter with 6 π electrons. Benzene, the cyclopentadienyl anion and the tropylium cation are all $n = 1$ species, possessing the "aromatic sextet."

The simplest member of the series is the cyclopropenyl anion **(60)** with 4 π electrons. Attempts to prepare this anion or a derivative have so far proved unsuccessful, but evidence for its transient formation has been presented (60). Treatment of the ester **61** with potassium tert-butoxide in deutero-tert-butanol for 31 hr gave 5% of the deuterium exchanged product **63**. By comparison, the cyclopropyl ester **64**, under the same conditions, exchanges 22% of its hydrogen for

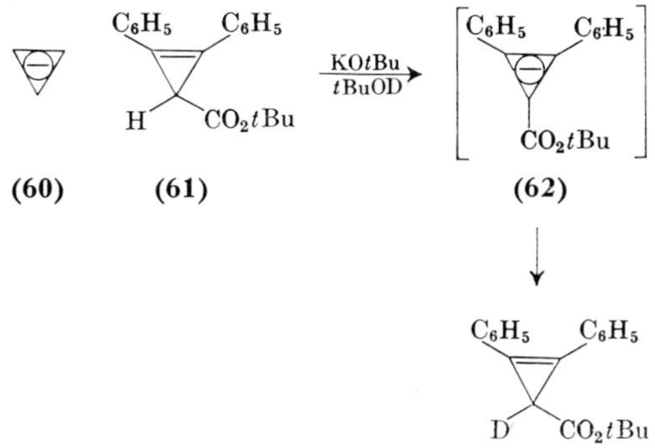

(60)   **(61)**   →(KOtBu/tBuOD)   **(62)**   ↓   **(63)**

deuterium in 30 min. The double bond thus destabilizes the anion **62** compared with the anion **65**.

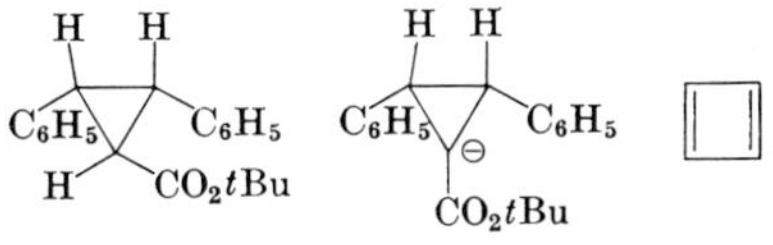

(64)   **(65)**   **(66)**

Cyclobutadiene **(66)** is the second member of the series with 4π electrons, and this molecule has been a synthetic goal for many years. Numerous theoretical calculations (61) have suggested that it will be unstable, due to the electronic configuration. It has been predicted that the molecule will distort from the square to a rectangular configuration with alternate single and double bonds, and even that it would dissociate into two molecules of acetylene. The simple MO theory predicts that cyclobutadiene will have zero DE, but more refined methods suggest that cyclobutadiene is an antiaromatic compound with a negative DE (61). A recent calculation (62) indicates that the singlet has virtually zero DE and is more stable than the triplet by about 14–21 kcal mole^{-1}. However, the heat of formation (830.1 kcal mole^{-1}) is greater than that of two moles of acetylene (778.9 kcal).

Longuet-Higgins and Orgel (63) predicted that cyclobutadiene would be stabilized by coordination with a suitable transition metal, and this concept was brilliantly exploited by Criegee and Schröder in 1959, by the synthesis of tetramethylcyclobutadiene nickel chloride (**68**) (64). 1,2,3,4-Tetramethyl-3,4-dichlorocyclobutene (**67a**) was reacted with nickel carbonyl in ether or benzene when **68** was precipitated. Treatment of **68** with sodium nitrite gave the diol, **67b**, while heating **68** to 200° yielded octamethylcyclooctatetraene. Heating **68** in solution gave

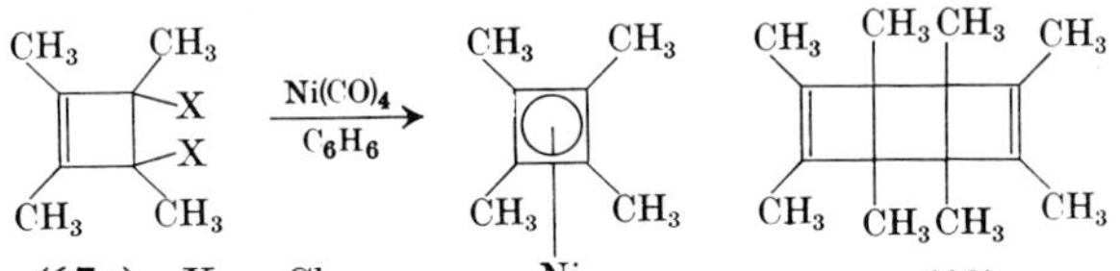

(**67a**) X = Cl
(**67b**) X = OH
(**67c**) X = I

(**68**)

(**69**)

the tricyclic dimer **69** (64). An interesting reaction was shown to take place (64) between **68** and sodium cyclopentadienide. Ring opening occurred, and the 4,5,6,7-tetramethyl-8,9-dihydroindene complex **70** was formed (65).

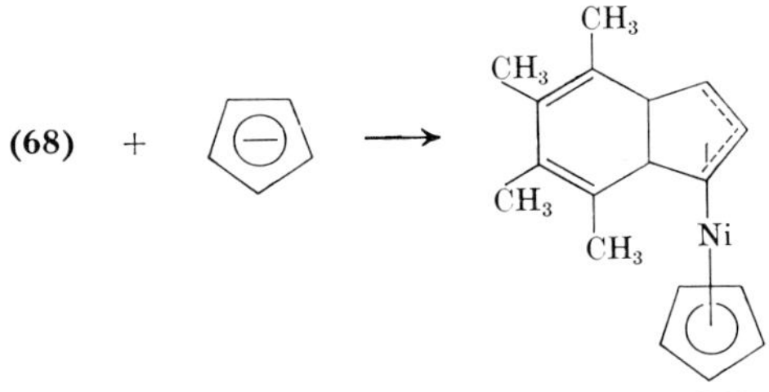

(**68**) + →

(**70**)

The successful application of the prediction of Longuet-Higgins and Orgel rapidly led to the synthesis of a number of complexed cyclobutadiene systems. Hübel and Braye (66) reported that the reaction of irondodecacarbonyl with diphenylacetylene gave a complex, which they suggested was either **71** or **72**. X-ray analysis (67) revealed that the compound had the structure **71** and indicated that the phenyl groups lie slightly out of the plane of the cyclobutadiene ring The structure of **68** was also confirmed by an x-ray study (68), the substituents again lying slightly out of the ring plane.

Malatesta et al. (69) reported a similar synthesis of the palladium complex **73a** by the reaction of diphenylacetylene with palladium chloride in ethanol. A dimer was formed initially, which gave **73a**

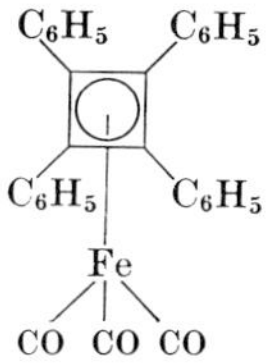

CONJUGATED CYCLIC HYDROCARBONS 15

(71) [Fe(CO)₃ tetraphenylcyclobutadiene complex]

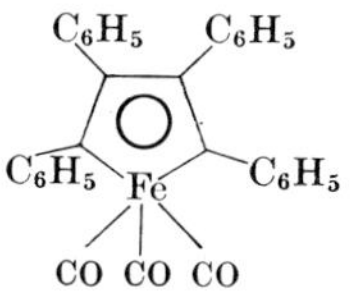

(72) [Fe(CO)₃ tetraphenylcyclopentadienone complex]

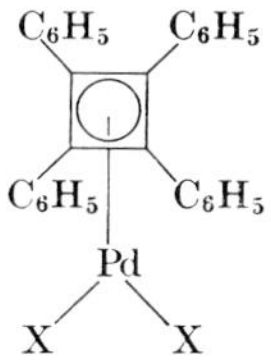

(73a) X = Cl
(73b) X = Br
(73c) X = I

on treatment with acid. The synthesis was subsequently modified (70) and an alternative formula for the dimer suggested. A cobalt complex **75** was prepared by the displacement of cyclooctatetraene (COT) or 1,5-cyclooctadiene from the complexes **74a** and **74b** with diphenylacetylene (71).

Freedman (72) prepared the tetraphenylcyclobutadiene nickel bromide complex **77** by treatment of 1,1-dimethyl-2,3,4,5-tetraphenylstannole (**76**) with bromine, and heating the product in the presence of nickel bromide at 125–140°.

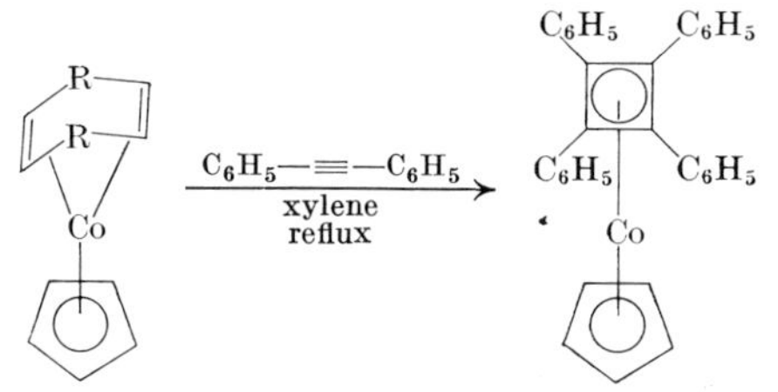

(74a) R = C₂H₂
(74b) R = C₂H₄

$\xrightarrow[\text{reflux}]{C_6H_5-\!\!\equiv\!\!-C_6H_5 \text{ xylene}}$

(75)

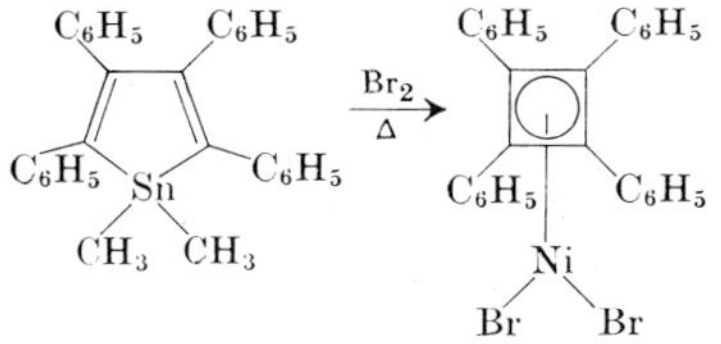

(76) → $\xrightarrow[\Delta]{Br_2}$ (77) 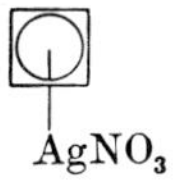 (78) AgNO₃

The palladium complexes **(73) (73)** can be synthesized by an alternative route and can be converted into the complexes of other metals by treatment with the appropriate metal carbonyl.

Subsequent work has shown that the reported (74) unsubstituted cyclobutadiene silver nitrate complex **78** is, in fact, the silver nitrate complex of a dimer, possibly COT (75). However, the synthesis of an unsubstituted cyclobutadiene complex has recently been reported by Pettit and his co-workers (76). *cis*-3,4-Dichlorocyclobutene **(79)** was treated with iron enneacarbonyl and the complex **80** isolated. Treatment of this complex with ferric chloride led to the previously unknown *trans*-3,4-dichlorocyclobutene **(81)**, which, as previously predicted (77), gave *trans,trans*-1,4-dichlorobutadiene **(82)** on warming (76). The complex **80** is aromatic in the sense that it undergoes electrophilic substitution and a number of substituted complexes have been prepared, e.g., **83a–83c** (78).

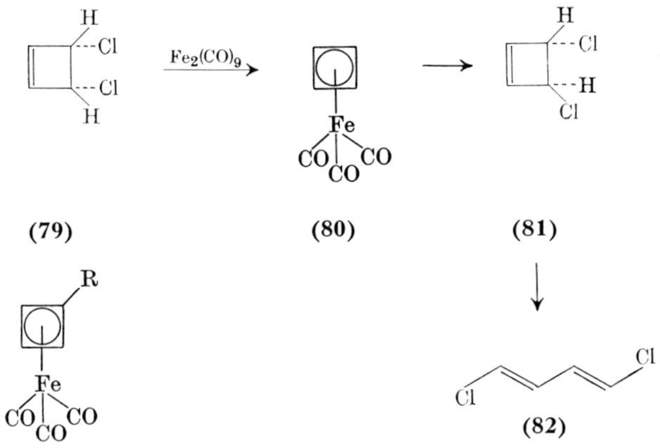

(79)   (80)   (81)

(82)

(83a) R = CHO
(83b) R = COCH$_3$
(83c) R = CH$_2$Cl

The chemistry of cyclobutadiene metal complexes has recently been reviewed (79a). The IR spectra of the cyclobutadiene complexes have received considerable attention, and the work in this area has also been reviewed (79b). Frequency assignments for $C_4(CH_3)_4NiCl_2$ have been made and correlated with the spectral expectations for a molecule M—C_4X_4 with C_{v4} symmetry.

Attempts to prepare noncomplexed derivatives of cyclobutadiene have continued. Blomquist and his co-workers (80,81) have investigated the addition of dienophiles to dimethylenecyclobutenes. Diphenyldimethylenecyclobutene **(84a)** (80) was found to require extremely reactive dienophiles, such as tetracyanoethylene (TCNE), for addition to occur, and the addition product **85** was that of 1,2 and not 1,4 addition. The unsubstituted dimethylenecyclobutene **84b** (81), synthesized by a fairly lengthy route, gave complex products with TCNE. A simple synthesis of **84b** by the thermal rearrangement of 1,5-hexadiyne has been described more recently (82).

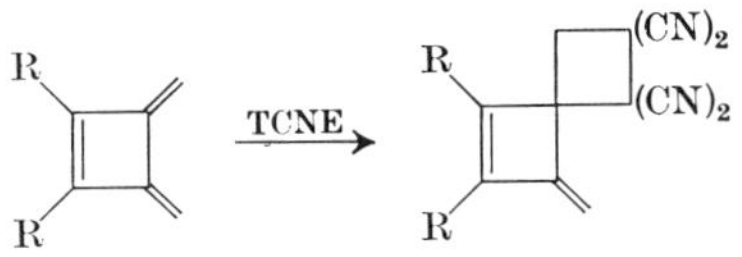

(84a) R = C₆H₅
(84b) R = H
(85)

Roberts et al. (83) treated 2,4-dichloro-3,3-difluoro-1-phenylcyclobutene **(86)** with phenyllithium and obtained the dimer **87**. They suggested that in general the destruction of cyclobutadienes occurs by dimerization at low temperatures and by ring opening at high tempera-

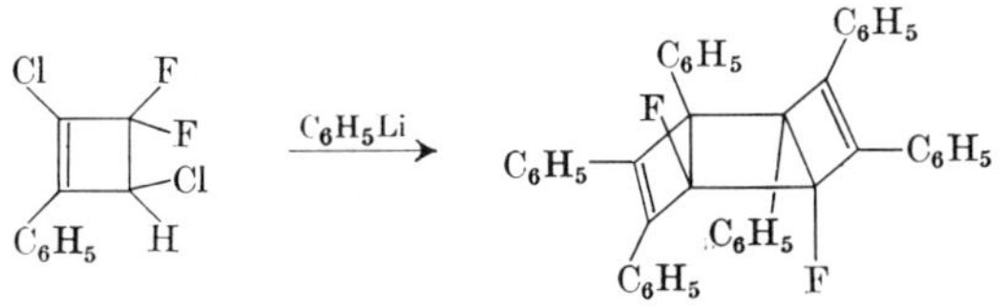

(86)   (87)

tures, and not by dissociation to acetylene (see above) (83). An analogy with the dimerization of cyclopentadiene, "homocyclobutadiene," was made.

White and Dunathan (84) have also obtained dimers **89–92** on treatment of the quaternary ammonium salt **88** with strong base. Under the Hofmann elimination conditions, only one of the quaternary ammonium groups was displaced, and the cyclobutene **93** was obtained. The tricyclic hydrocarbons **91** and **92** are converted, on warming, to **89** and **90**, respectively.

An elegant approach to cyclobutadiene has been made by Corey and Streith (27). 2-Pyrone **(94)** was photorearranged to the unstable 2-photopyrone **(95)**. 2-Photopyrone may be considered to be derived from cyclobutadiene and carbon dioxide. *N*-Methyl-2-pyridone **(96)** is similarly photorearranged to **97**, which can be conceived to be derived from cyclobutadiene and methyl isocyanate. The mass spectral decomposition shows a peak at m/e 52, which has been ascribed to the cyclobutadienyl cation **(98)**.

(88) (93) (91) (92) (89) (90)

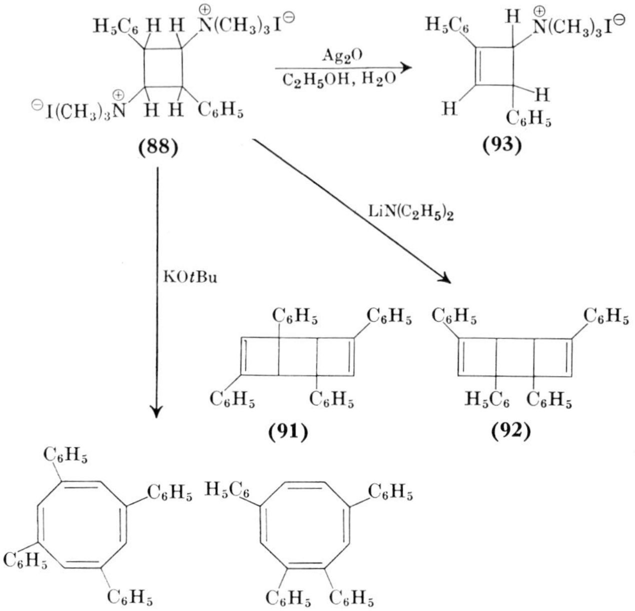

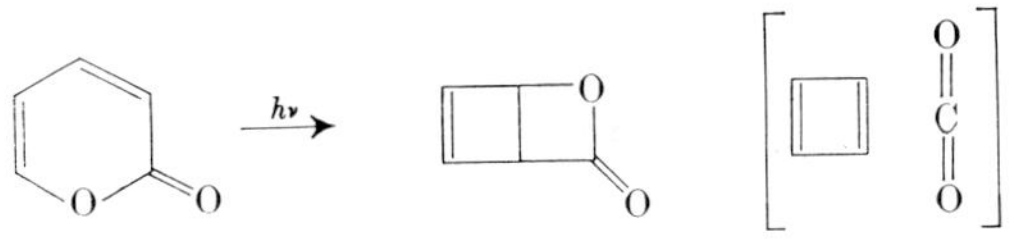

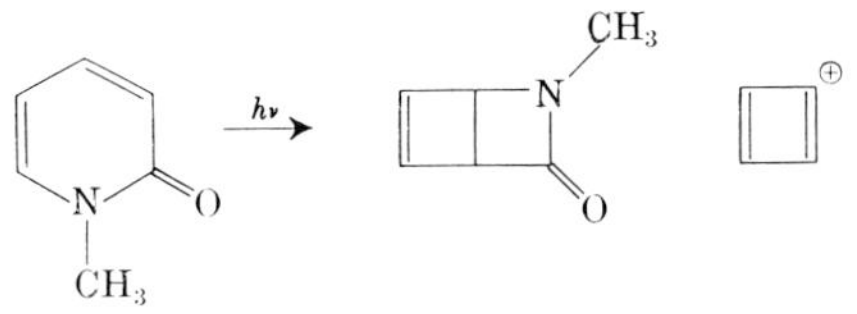

Evidence for the formation of cyclobutadiene has recently been reported by Pettit and his co-workers (85,86). When cyclobutadiene irontricarbonyl **(80)** is treated with ceric ammonium nitrate in the presence of methyl propiolate, the substituted bicyclo[2.2.0]hexadiene **99a** is formed, which, on warming to 90°, is rapidly converted to methyl benzoate **(100a)**. A similar reaction with phenyl acetylene

(94) (95)

(96) (97) (98)

gave the phenyl derivative **99b**, which gave biphenyl **(100b)** on warming. When the experiment was carried out by adding cold aqueous ceric salt to an ethereal solution of **80**, followed by distillation of the vapors into a liquid nitrogen trap, the subsequent addition of methyl propiolate to the condensed vapors gave small amounts of methyl benzoate. This suggests that cyclobutadiene has a finite existence, that it can be distilled, and that the formation of the bicyclohexadienes is not taking place through a metal complex. The cyclobutadiene produced in this manner reacts both as a diene and as a dienophile.

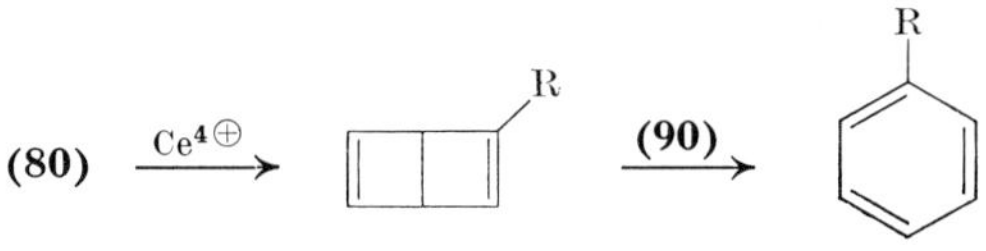

(80) $\xrightarrow{Ce^{4\oplus}}$ [cyclobutadiene-R] $\xrightarrow{(90)}$ [benzene-R]

(99a)	R = CO_2CH_3	**(100a)**	R = CO_2CH_3
(99b)	R = C_6H_5	**(100b)**	R = C_6H_5

Stereospecific addition occurs, and this supports the theory that cyclobutadiene has a singlet ground state (87).

A possible method of stabilizing cyclobutadiene is by substituting the opposite ends of the double bonds with an electron-donating and an electron-withdrawing group. This method has been extensively explored by Breslow and his co-workers (88). A number of cyclobutenes have been synthesized in which this "push–pull" effect can occur, e.g., **101** and **102**. The compound **102** should be further stabilized by the electron-withdrawing benzoyl group. However, all attempts to introduce the second double bond into either system have been unsuccessful.

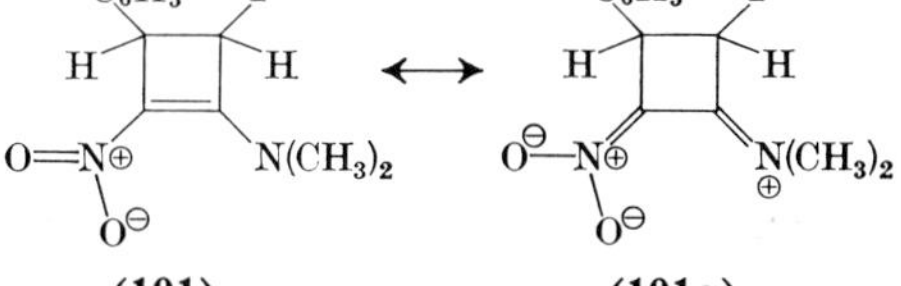

(101) ↔ (101a)

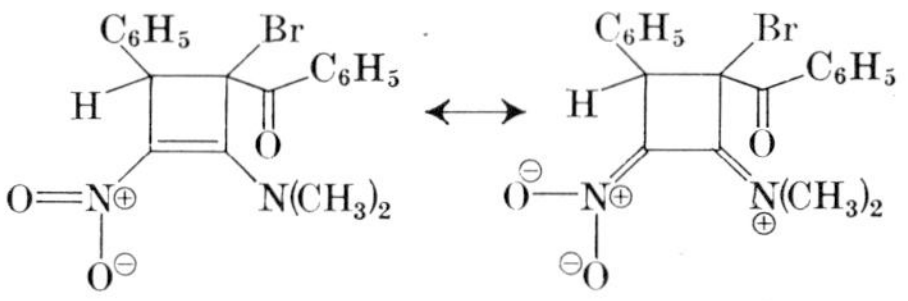

(102) ↔ (102a)

The cyclobutadiones and cyclobutenone can be considered to be the keto forms of cyclobutadienediols and cyclobutadienol. The cyclobuta-1,3-diones are readily available from the dimerization of ketenes. The parent compound cyclobuta-1,3-dione (103) has been prepared by the reaction of ketene with ethoxyacetylene, followed by hydrolysis (89). The IR spectrum shows virtually no hydroxyl absorption, and the NMR spectrum has a single peak at τ 6.14, which indicates the

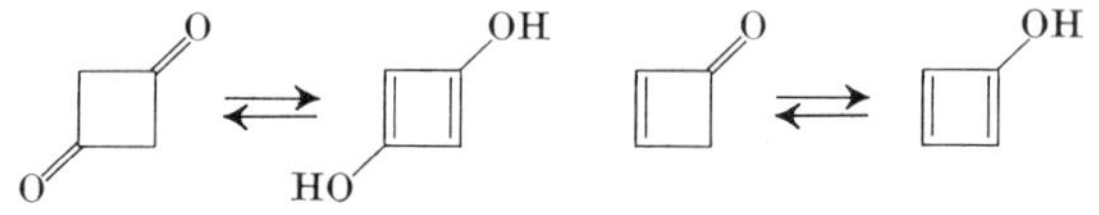

(103)   (103a)   (104)   (104a)

absence of any of the enol 103a. 2,4-Dichloro-3-phenylcyclobutenone (105), synthesized by Roberts and his co-workers (90), shows no indication (IR, OH stretch absent, no $FeCl_3$ color, no enol acetate) of existing in the enolic form 105a.

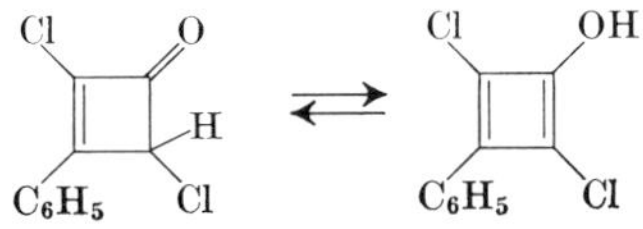

(105)   (105a)

Cyclobutadiene would give a $(4n + 2)$ system by either the removal or addition of two electrons. The cyclobutadienyl dication is a 2π electron system and has been discussed in the previous section. The cyclobutadienyl dianion (106) is a 6π electron system. Two electrons are in bonding orbitals, and four are in nonbonding orbitals, and the cyclobutadienyl dianion is thus the lower homolog of the cyclooctatetraenyl dianion (see below). Attempted syntheses of the dianion have been reported. Adam (91) reacted 3,4-di-iodo-1,2,3,4-tetramethylcyclobutene (67c) with n-butyllithium at −70°, and obtained the dimer 69 and the methylene compound 107. With lithium in liquid ammonia at −33°, 67a gave the dimer 69 as well as the hydrocarbon 108. Deuterium was not incorporated when the ammoniacal mixture was worked up with D_2O. Freedman et al. (92) have recently prepared the anion 110 by treatment of the tetraphenylcyclobutene 109 with butyllithium. The NMR spectrum is almost identical with that of the diphenylethyl anion. The dianion could not be prepared in this way, but more rewarding approaches were promised.

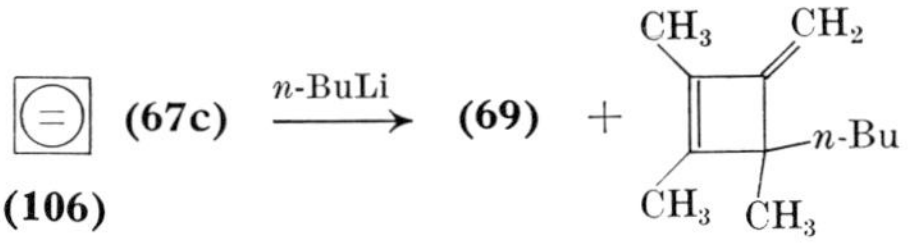

(106) (67c) —n-BuLi→ (69) + (107)

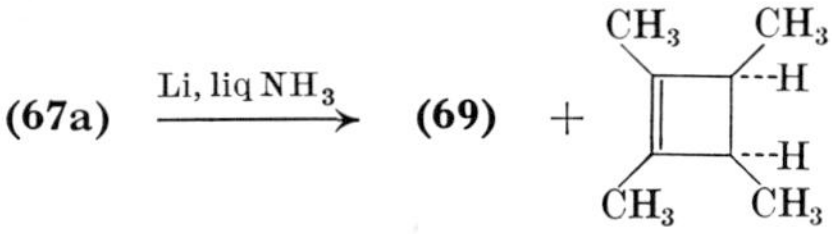

(67a) —Li, liq NH₃→ (69) + (108)

The cyclopentadienyl cation is a $4n$ system with 4 π electrons and, if planar, would, by simple Hückel theory, have a triplet ground state. The simple cation **111** has not been synthesized, but the pentaphenylcyclopentadienyl cation **113** was claimed by Ziegler and Schnell (93) in 1925 to be formed by treatment of pentaphenylcyclopentadienol (**112**) with concentrated sulfuric acid. This observation has recently

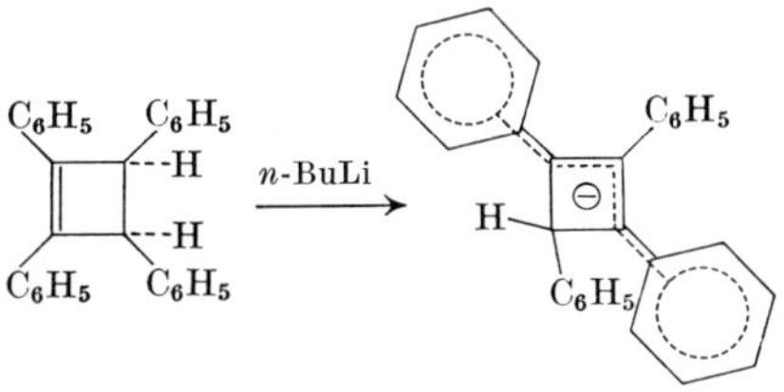

(109) —n-BuLi→ (110)

been shown to be incorrect (94), although the cation is probably a transient intermediate in the formation of the complex reaction products. However, if the alcohol is treated with boron trifluoride in methylene chloride at $-60°$, then the cation **113** is produced (95). The NMR spectrum of the solution shows only broad solvent lines, and no signals for the phenyl protons are observed. Addition of solutions of the cation to cold methanol gave the ether **114** in high yield. An ESR spectrum of the cation in methylene chloride at 77°K revealed that a triplet species was present, and from the absence of an NMR signal, a rapid equilibrium between **113** and **113a** must be involved. On raising the temperature, the amount of the triplet species increased, and the triplet must therefore lie above the singlet ground state (calc. 0.48 ± 0.05 kcal mole^{-1}). The zero E value was consistent with a C_5v symmetry. The cation is an antiaromatic species (95).

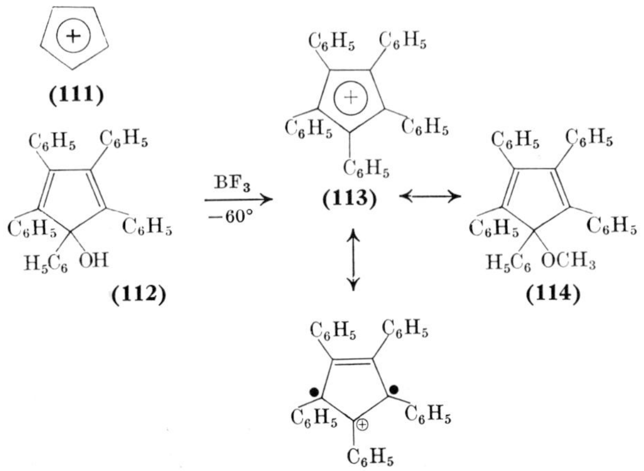

Hexachlorocyclopentadiene **(115)**, on treatment with antimony pentafluoride at room temperature, followed by rapid cooling, gave the pentachlorocyclopentadienyl cation **(116)** (96). The ESR spectrum at low temperature again showed the $\Delta m = 2$ line, indicative of a triplet species **116a**, and the low value of the E parameter (0.002 cm^{-1}) was again consistent with a C_{5v} symmetry. The intensity (I) of the signal obeyed the Curie law ($I = k/T$) over the temperature range 200–204°K. Since a triplet lying above the ground state would cause a deviation from the Curie law, it was concluded that the triplet is almost certainly the ground state of the molecule (96b). On reacting the cation with methanol, four dimeric chlorocyclopentenones were obtained, the structures of which have not yet been reported.

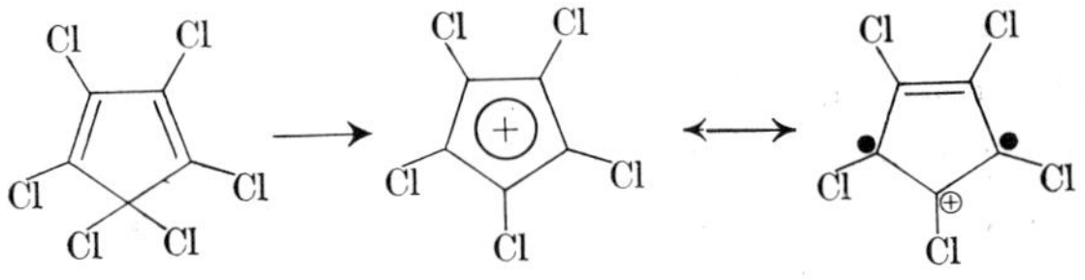

Snyder (97) has pointed out that the Hückel treatment greatly exaggerates the Jahn-Teller effect for neutral molecules with pseudodegenerate ground states. The cyclopentadienyl cations, although charged species, have pseudodegenerate ground states, and it appears that in these systems the energy gained by distortion is small.

Cyclopentadienone **(117)**, unlike cyclopropenone, is unstable and rapidly dimerizes to bicyclopentadienone **(118)**. The instability is a consequence of the unfavorable charge distribution in the dipolar form **117a**, which thus contributes little to the resonance structure.

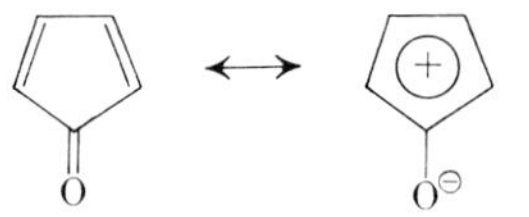

(117)   (117a) 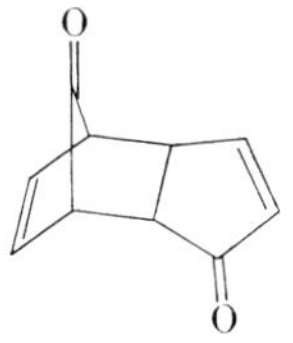   (118)

A number of investigations of the transient cyclopentadienyl radical **(119)** have been reported. Thrush (98) produced the radical by flash

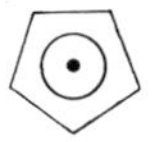

(119)

photolysis of cyclopentadiene or ferrocene in the gas phase. Pottie and Lossing (99) have detected the radical in the mass spectrum of the products arising from the pyrolysis of anisole at 1000°. The initially formed phenoxy radical dissociates to the cyclopentadienyl radical and carbon monoxide. The value of the ionization potential obtained (8.69 eV) was in good agreement with the theoretical value of 8.82 eV calculated by Streitwieser (100). The radical has also been prepared by the irradiation of cyclopentadiene with an electron beam (101), and by the pyrolysis of ferrocene above 800° (102). The ESR signal revealed 6 lines with a 5.98 G splitting, in the ratio of $1:5:10:10:5:1$, and gave a Q value of 29.9 G. The pentaphenyl cyclopentadienyl radical and its ESR spectrum have also been reported (103).

The first member of the 6 π electron aromatic series, the classical aromatic group, is the cyclopentadienyl anion **(120)**. The high acidity of cyclopentadiene was observed by Thiele, who showed this to be due to the stability of the conjugate base, the cyclopentadienyl anion **(120)**. The chemistry of this 6 π electron system is extensive and will not be reviewed here. Ferrocene **(121)**, the first of the sandwich molecules,

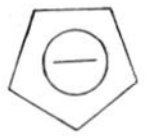

(120)

is stabilized by the interaction of the cyclopentadiene and the iron orbitals, forming a closed aromatic system.

Fulvene **(122)** has little aromatic character, but the dipole moment, though small, indicates that some contribution from the dipolar form **122a** occurs.

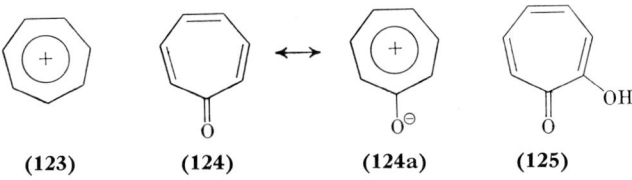

(121)   (122)   (122a)

The tropylium cation **(123)**, predicted to have aromatic stability by Hückel, was prepared by Doering and Knox (7) in 1954. A large number of subsequent preparations have been reported (104,105). Tropone **(124)** is stable, unlike cyclopentadienone, due to the favorable charge distribution in the dipolar form. Tropolone **(125)** is a third aromatic system of this type. These systems have been extensively reviewed (9,105), and will not be considered in detail here.

(123)   (124)   (124a)   (125)

Heptafulvene **(128)** may also be stabilized by the contribution from the dipolar form (106). The valence bond theory indicates that bond alternation will occur, which was also the conclusion of more refined MO calculations (107). Considerable divergence of opinion occurred in the prediction of the dipole moment; at one time even different directions were predicted. It now appears to be generally agreed that it will be small and directed towards the exocyclic methylene group (106,108). The MO calculations indicated a high reactivity towards radical reagents. The molecule was synthesized by Doering and Wiley in 1954 (104,109). Reaction of methyl diazoacetate with benzene yielded methyl 7-cycloheptatrienyl carboxylate **(126)**. Conversion to the amide, followed by reduction with lithium aluminium hydride at 0° gave the amine **127**. Finally, methylation and subsequent Hofmann elimination led to a solution of heptafulvene (**128**). Heptafulvene is very unstable and can only be obtained as deep red, dilute solutions. The heat of hydrogenation, 92.6 kcal mole^{-1}, gives an estimated DE of 13.2 kcal mole^{-1} (110). Heptafulvene has also been

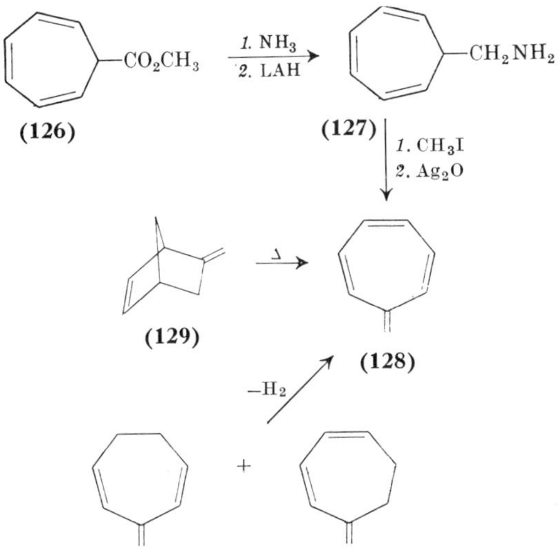

obtained in small yield from the pyrolysis of **129** (110), and by dehydrogenation of mixtures of **130a** and **130b** (111).

Derivatives of heptafulvene appear to be much more stable. A number of 8,8-disubstituted derivatives have been synthesized by Nozoe and his co-workers, and by Kitahara and Doi (105). The tropylium ion was reacted with malonitrile or diethyl malonate to give the cycloheptatrienes **131a** and **131b**, together with the dicycloheptatrienyl compounds **132a** and **132b**. Oxidation of **131a** and **131b**, or pyrolysis of **132a** and **132b**, gave the heptafulvenes **133a** and **133b**. The heptafulvene **133a** could be made directly by treatment of bromomalonitrile with tropylium bromide. The dipole moment of **133a** was 7.49 D, and that of **131a**, 4.12 D (112). An estimate of the dipole moment of the heptafulvene system of 3.07 D was made, with the ring positive. In the annelated heptafulvenes, **134** and **135**, synthesized by Bergmann and Ikan (113), the dipole moments are small but indicate a polarization such that the cycloheptatrienyl ring was again positive.

Hafner et al. (114) have synthesized the interesting heptafulvene **136** which appears to be considerably stabilized by resonance between structures **136a** and **136b**. Jutz (115) and Bertelli, Golino, and Dreyer (116) have synthesized a number of 8-vinyl derivatives, e.g., **137** and **138**.

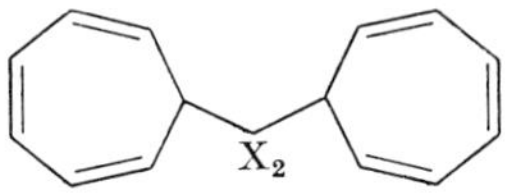

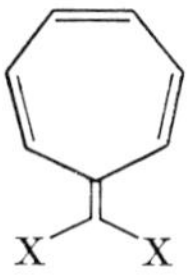

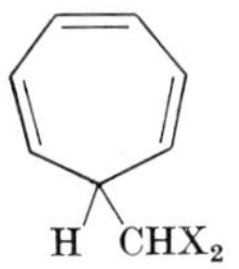

(131a) X = CN
(131b) X = $CO_2C_2H_5$

(132a) X = CN
(132b) X = $CO_2C_2H_5$

(133a) X = CN
(133b) X = $CO_2C_2H_5$

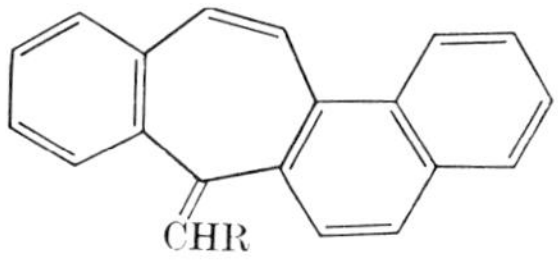

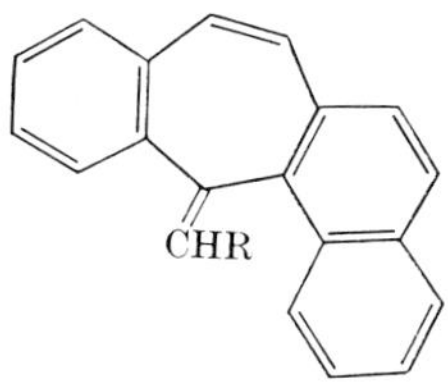

(134a) R = C_6H_5
(134b) R = p-ClC_6H_4

(135a) R = C_6H_5
(135b) R = p-ClC_6H_4

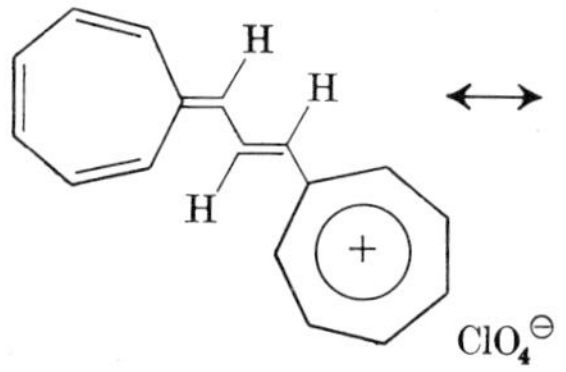

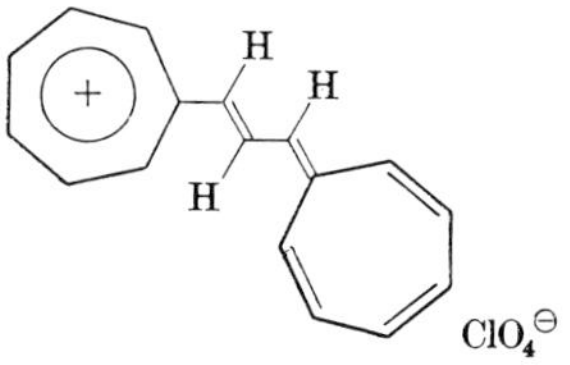

(136a) $ClO_4^{\ominus}$

(136b) $ClO_4^{\ominus}$

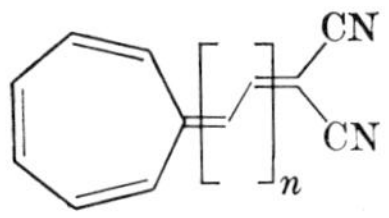

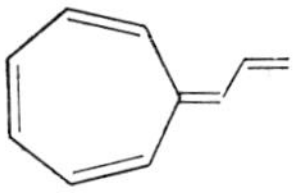

(137) $n = 1, 2$

(138)

The cyclooctatetraenyl dication **(139)** would, on simple MO grounds, be predicted to be a stable 6 π system. So far, this molecule has eluded synthesis. Bryce-Smith and Perkins (117) have reported the failure of a number of methods which were successful in the preparation of the tropylium ion. Pettit and his co-workers (118) treated COT with concentrated sulphuric acid and obtained a red solution which had an

NMR spectrum consistent with the bicyclo[5.1.0]octadienyl cation **(140)**. This appears to exist as the homoaromatic ion **140a** in which the σ electrons of the 1,7-bond form part of the 6 π system. Homotropone **(141)** has also been synthesized (119), and the cyclopropyl hydrogens H_A, H_B have different chemical shifts in the NMR. This difference is accentuated by treatment with acid. Protonation of tricarbonylcyclooctatetraenyl iron **(142)** also gives a carbonium ion, probably **143**, in which the σ electrons are not involved (120,121). However, tricarbonylcyclooctatetraenyl molybdenum **(144)** on acid treatment gives a cation, the NMR spectrum of which is consistent with the open homoaromatic structure **145** (122).

(139)

(140)

(140a)

(141)

(142) **(143)**

(144) **(145)**

(146) **(147)** **(148)**

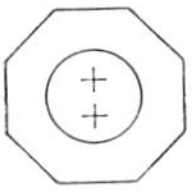

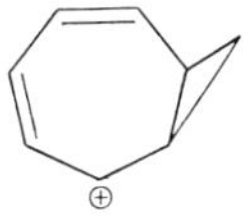

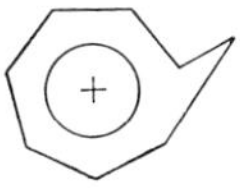

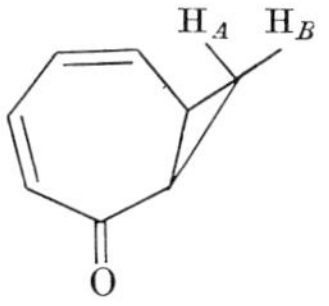

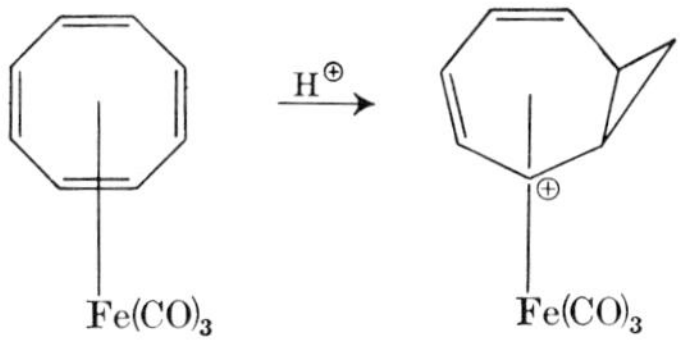

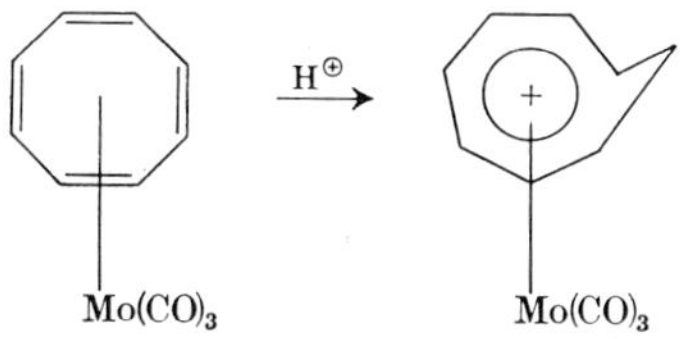

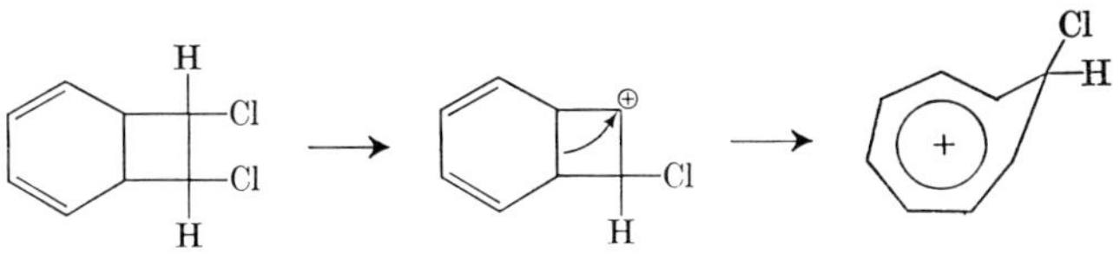

It has been suggested (123) that experiments designed to prepare **139** may, in some cases, be frustrated by the rearrangement of an initially formed monocation to the stable homotropylium ion, which does not proceed further. Thus, the dichloride **146** may lose one chloride ion to give the monocation **147** which rearranges to **148**.

C. $n = 2$

This series contains both molecules with $4n$ and $(4n + 2)$ π electrons. The tropenyl radical **(149)** has 7 π electrons, of which one, in simple MO theory, must occupy an antibonding orbital. However, Jahn-Teller distortion applies, and the nonplanar form has been calculated to be 0.859 kcal mole^{-1} more stable (124). The radical has been observed by both mass spectroscopic and ESR techniques in a number of reactions. It has been produced by photolysis (125) and by pyrolysis (126) of bitropenyl, the x-ray irradiation of cycloheptatriene (127), and by the oxidation of cycloheptatriene with titanous ion/hydrogen peroxide (128). The low value of the ionization potential (6.60 eV) (124), obtained by mass spectrometry, is in agreement with simple MO theory and indicates that the radical has a lower DE than the cation. The ESR spectrum shows eight equally spaced lines

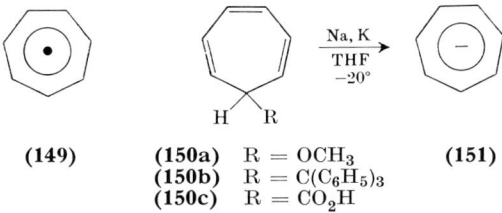

(149)   (150a) R = OCH$_3$ (151)
        (150b) R = C(C$_6$H$_5$)$_3$
        (150c) R = CO$_2$H

(3.9 gauss) (123,125–129) consistent with a molecule of D_{7h} symmetry. The temperature dependence of the spectrum indicates population of low-lying excited vibration states (130).

The tropenyl anion **(151)** has 8 π electrons, two of which would be in degenerate antibonding orbitals. This orbital degeneracy would be lost by symmetry perturbations, and Snyder (131) has estimated that Jahn-Teller bond-length distortion in the lowest singlet state would stabilize the two configurations of C_{2v} symmetry by approximately 6 kcal mole^{-1}. The calculated DE for the anion is low (C$_7$H$_7^+$ 2.99β > C$_7$H$_7^{\cdot}$ 2.54β > C$_7$H$_7^-$ 2.10β) (132).

The anion has recently been synthesized by Dauben and Rifi (132). Addition of either 7-methoxy-1,3,5-cycloheptatriene **(150a)** or 7-triphenylmethyl-1,3,5-cycloheptatriene **(150b)** in THF at $-20°$, to a suspension of sodium–potassium alloy in THF, gave a deep blue diamagnetic solution of the anion (λ_{max} 750 mμ). Carbonation of the solution yielded 7-carboxy-1,3,5-cycloheptatriene **(150c)**. From the pK_a of **151**, a value for the DE about 0.8–1.1β greater than that of cycloheptatriene has been calculated. Doering and Gaspar (133) have obtained evidence for the existence of the tropenyl anion in the base-catalyzed deuterium exchange of cycloheptatriene.

Treatment of triphenyltropylphosphonium tetrafluoroborate **(152)** with aqueous methanolic sodium hydroxide gave cycloheptatriene and triphenyl phosphine oxide, presumably through the existence of the tropenyl anion (134).

Breslow and Chang (135) have prepared the heptaphenyltropenyl anion **(154)** by the addition of potassium to a solution of heptaphenyl-cycloheptatrienyl bromide **(153)** in dimethoxyethane. The deep purple solution shows no solvent line broading, has no ESR signal, and is not paramagnetic. It thus appears to have a nonplanar singlet ground state.

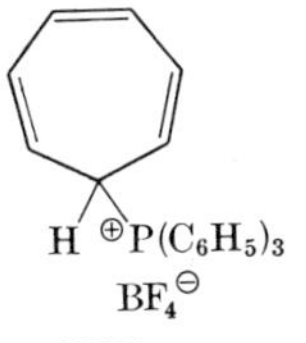

(152) 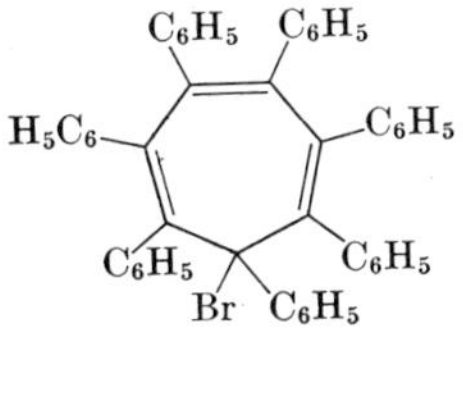 (153) 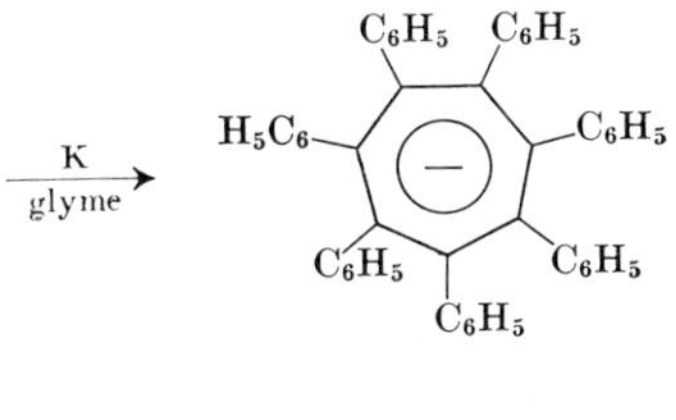 (154)

The addition of a further electron to the tropenyl anion has recently been reported. Tropyl methyl ether **(150a)** reacted in THF with a sodium mirror to give a deep green solution of the tropenide dianion radical **(155)** (136). The ESR spectrum at $-100°$ was an octet of equally spaced lines (3.48 G), which are further split into a septet (1.74 G), due to interaction with the two sodium ions.

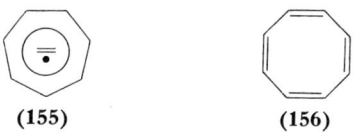

(155) (156)

The synthesis of COT **(156)** by Willstätter et al. (4) demonstrated that this hydrocarbon did not have the properties of a "super" benzene but resembled a polyolefin. The difference between the eight- and six-membered rings found a satisfying explanation in the MO theory. Reppe's commercial synthesis (137) of COT allowed a full study of its properties, and it was demonstrated to have the "tub" conformation **156a** (138). An extensive chemistry has developed (139).

The remarkable affinity of COT for electrons was attributed by Katz (140) to the formation of the planar 10 π aromatic dianion **157**. The dipotassium salt is a crystalline solid which is stable in solution. The NMR spectrum shows a sharp singlet which is almost coincident with the signal of COT, presumably due to the balance between the effects of ring current and electronic charge. The equilibrium between COT, the dianion and the radical anion **158** lies towards the right, in contradistinction to the polynuclear aromatic hydrocarbons (141). However, in the absence of alkali metal ions, the equilibrium lies towards the left (142). The ESR spectrum (141,142) of the radical anion **158** is

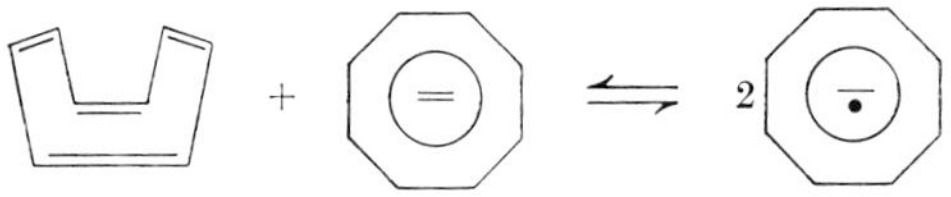

(156a)   (157)   (158)

consistent with a planar structure, and this is supported by the carbon-13 hyperfine splitting (143). Similar conclusions have been drawn from the ESR spectra of the radical anions of the monoalkyl COT's (144). Oscillopolaragraphic reduction of COT also supports this view (142,145).

It was predicted that the annelation of COT would decrease its affinity for electrons (146). However, *sym*-dibenzocyclooctatetraene **(159)** is easily reduced (147,148), either polarographically or with alkali metals, and the NMR spectrum of the dianion (148) and the ESR spectrum of the radical anion (147,148) are in accord with the planar structure. The COT dianion is carboxylated (137) to the cycloocta-2,5,7-triene-1,4-dicarboxylic acid **(160)** and alkylated (149) to give

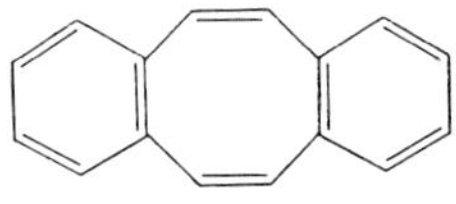

(159)

unspecified isomers of dialkyl cyclooctatrienes. The dianion reacts with *gem*-dihalides by 1,2-addition to give derivatives of bicyclo[6.1.0]-nonatriene (150,151) and provides a useful synthetic entry to these systems. Thus **157** with 1,1-dichloroethane gave *syn*-9-methylbicyclo[6.1.0]nonatriene **(161b)** (151), and analogous products **161a, 161c, 161e,** and **161f** with methylene chloride, chloroform, carbon tetrachloride, and dichloromethyl methyl ether (150). With dichlorophenylphosphine again, only 1,2-addition occurs (152), and 9-phenyl-9-phosphabicyclo[6.1.0]nonatriene **(162)** is formed, which is, however, easily thermally rearranged to 9-phenyl-9-phosphabicyclo[4.2.1]-nonatriene **(163)**. A large degree of stereoselectivity seems to be involved, and the reaction probably occurs by reduction of the dihalide to a species which adds to the concomitantly formed COT. Addition of the dianion to an excess of acetyl chloride gave a number of products (153), corresponding to both 1,2- and 1,4-addition **164** and **165**. Similarly 1,2- and 1,4-addition occur with aldehydes and ketones, for example, benzaldehyde gives both **166** and **167** (154).

The homocyclooctatetraenyl radical anion **(168)** and the homocyclooctatetraenyl dianion **(169)** have recently been reported (155). The radical anion was prepared from bicyclo[6.1.0]nonatriene **(161a)** by either reduction with potassium in 1,2-dimethoxyethane (155a) or by electrolytic reduction in liquid ammonia saturated with tetramethylammonium iodide (155b). The ESR spectrum is consistent with the monocyclic rather than the bicyclic species, but the C-9 protons are not equivalent, indicating that the anion is not planar (155). Further reduction of the anion with potassium in 1,2-dimethoxyethane gave the dianion **169** (155a), whereas further electrolytic reduction leads to the methylcyclooctatetraenyl anion radical, possibly through the existence of the dianion **169** (155b).

The next highest vinylog of the cyclopentadienyl anion, the cyclononatetraenyl anion **(170)**, was prepared in 1963 (150,156). Treatment of the ether **161e** with potassium in THF (150), or the chlorides **161c** and **161d** with lithium in THF (150,156), gave a solution of the anion **170**. Metathesis of the lithium salt with tetraethylammonium chloride gave the tetraethylammonium salt **171** as a crystalline solid, stable in an inert atmosphere (156). The NMR spectrum of **170** showed only a sharp singlet at ca. τ 3 when the reaction was carried out in perdeuterotetrahydrofuran, in excellent agreement with that predicted for the symmetrical anion (τ 2.9) (150). The symmetrical structure

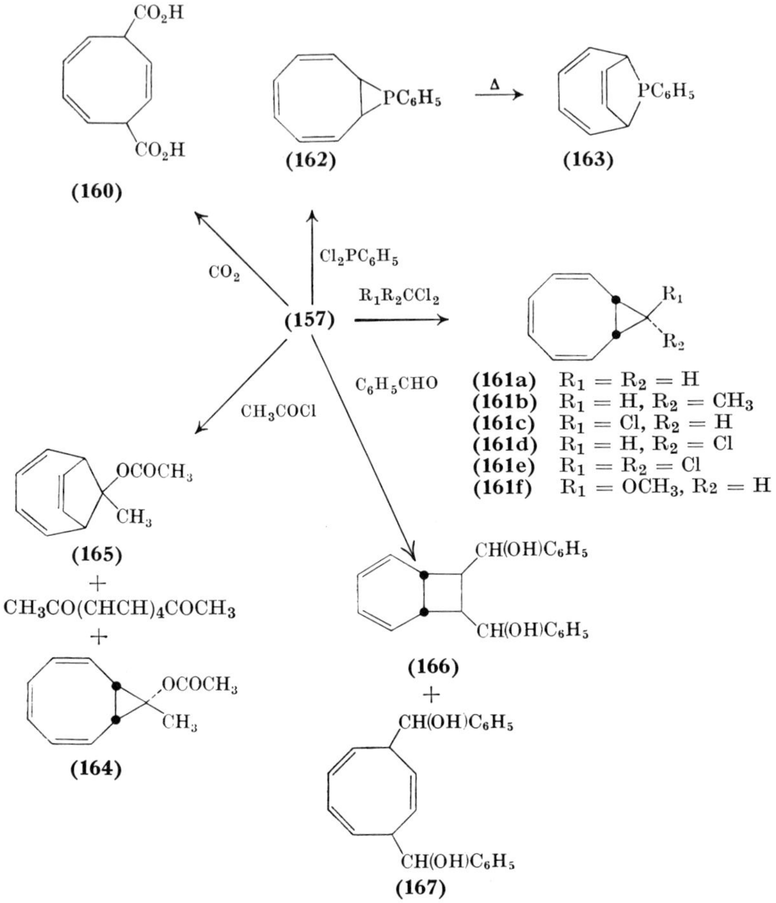

was further supported by the ^{13}C NMR spectrum (156), and by the IR and UV spectra. The UV spectrum was in good agreement with that calculated by the Pariser-Parr method for a molecule with D_9h symmetry (157). Quenching the anion with water gave 8,9-dihydroindene (**172a**) (150), and possibly cyclononatetraene (156), and with

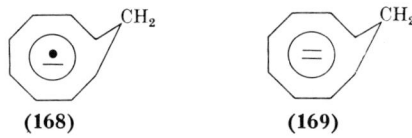

deuterium oxide 1-deutero-8,9-dihydroindene **(172b)** was obtained (150). Carbonation gave **172c** and methylation, **172d** (150). Hydrogenation of the anion gave a mixture containing some cyclononane (156). Proton exchange occurs with cyclopentadiene, but not with indene, which places the pK of cyclononatetraene between 16 and 21 on the Streitwieser scale (156). The synthesis of diazocyclononatetraene has been claimed, but the present evidence is slight (158).

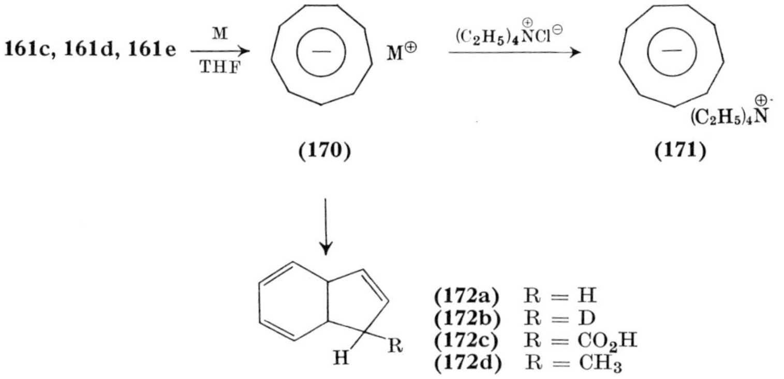

161c, 161d, 161e $\xrightarrow[\text{THF}]{\text{M}}$ (170) M$^\oplus$ $\xrightarrow{(C_2H_5)_4\overset{\oplus}{N}Cl^\ominus}$ (171) (C$_2$H$_5$)$_4$$\overset{\oplus}{N}$

(172a) R = H
(172b) R = D
(172c) R = CO$_2$H
(172d) R = CH$_3$

The bridged anion **174**, has recently been synthesized by two groups of workers (159). The tricyclic hydrocarbon **173**, obtained by a method analogous to the synthesis of 1,6-methano[10]annulene (*vide infra*), on proton abstraction with sodium methylsulfinylmethylide gave **174**. The NMR spectrum shows an upfield shift of the methano-protons, consistent with the presence of a ring current.

Cyclodecapentaene, [10]annulene, a monocyclic hydrocarbon with 10 π electrons, is the next higher homolog of benzene, and might be expected to have aromatic properties. However, such expectations are dimmed on closer examination of the molecule. In the configuration **175**, with 3 *cis*- and 2 *trans*-double bonds, which minimizes bond

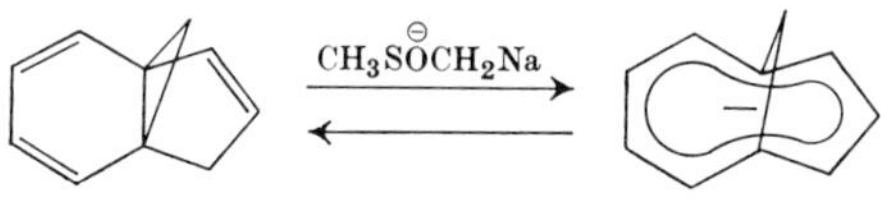

(173) $\xrightleftharpoons{CH_3\overset{\ominus}{S}OCH_2Na}$ (174)

angle strain, the van der Waals radii of the hydrogen atoms inside the ring seriously overlap, and little resonance stabilization can accrue

(160). If this internal interaction is removed by making the bonds all *cis* **(176)** considerable bond angle strain results. Other possible configurations (e.g., **177**) may minimize these difficulties.

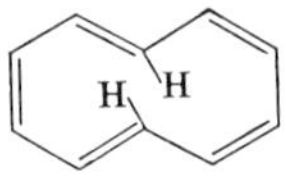

(175) 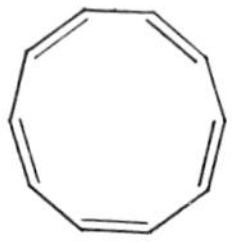   **(176)** 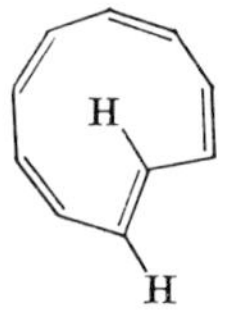   **(177)**

A large number of attempted syntheses have been reported (9,10a). Van Tamelen and Pappas (161) have synthesized the valence tautomer, *cis*-9,10-dihydronaphthalene **(181)** by the following sequence. The butadiene–benzoquinone adduct **(178)** was reduced with aluminum isopropoxide to a stereoisomeric mixture of diene diols **(179)**. One of these (mp 165°) was separated, which on treatment with hydrogen bromide and then NBS gave the tetrabromide **(180)**. Dehydrobromination of **180** led to **181**, but all attempts to valence tautomerize this to [10]annulene failed.

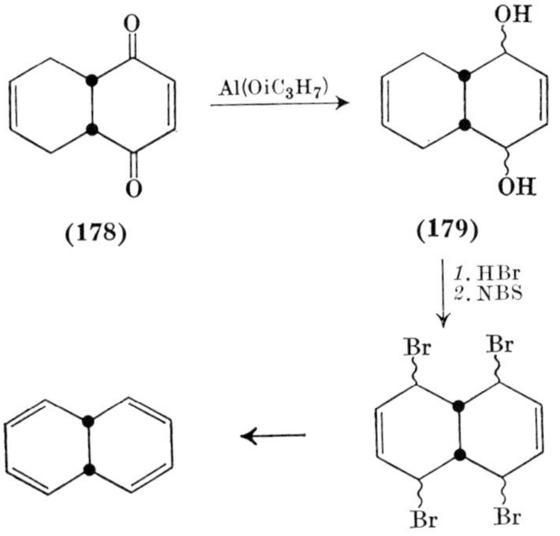

Johnson and his co-workers (162) synthesized the diene dione **182**, but could obtain no evidence for enolization to **183**.

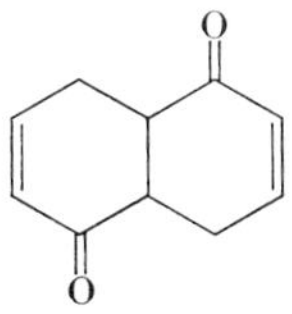

(182) 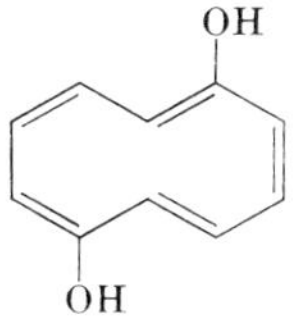   (183)

1,6-Steric interaction between the internal hydrogens on the *trans* double bonds of **175** might be removed by replacing them by a bridge. This view has been elegantly exploited by Vogel and his co-workers (163,164), who have synthesized a number of compounds of the type **184** and have shown that these spontaneously valence tautomerize to **185**. Addition of dichlorocarbene to isotetralin (**186**) gave the adduct

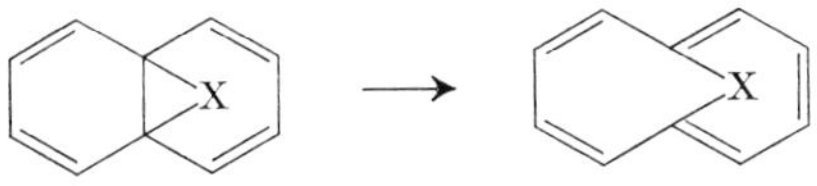

(184) → (185)

187, which on dechlorination with sodium in liquid ammonia led to **188**. Bromination gave the tetrabromide **189**, and subsequent dehydrobromination gave 1,6-methano[10]annulene (**190**) (163). The NMR spectrum, an A_2B_2 multiplet at τ 2.8 (8H) and a sharp singlet at τ 10.5 (165), and the UV spectrum [λ_{max} 256 mμ (ε 68,000), 259

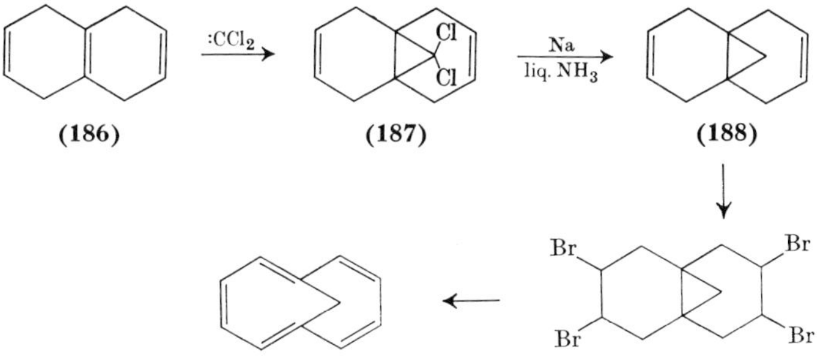

(186) → :CCl$_2$ → (187) → Na, liq. NH$_3$ → (188)

(190) ← (189)

(63,000), and 298 (6200)] support the aromatic, all conjugated structure **190** rather than the tetraene structure **184** (X = CH$_2$). An x-ray analysis (167) of 1,6-methano[10]annulene-2-carboxylic acid (**191a**) indicated that the perimeter is not quite planar, but that the bond lengths fall in the range 1.38–1.42 Å. 1,6-Methano[10]annulene exhibits some classical aromatic properties. It gives the monobromide **191b** and the dibromide **191c** with NBS. The monobromide **191b** can be dehydrobrominated to a transient monodehydro-1,6-methano-[10]annulene **192** (166). However, **190** does give a Diels-Alder

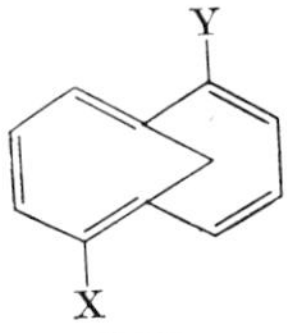

(191a) X = CO₂H, Y = H
(191b) X = Br, Y = H
(191c) X = Y = Br
(191d) X = COCH₃, Y = H
(191e) X = NO₂, Y = H
(191f) X = Y = NO₂
(191g) X = H, Y = NH₂
(191h) X = H, Y = OH

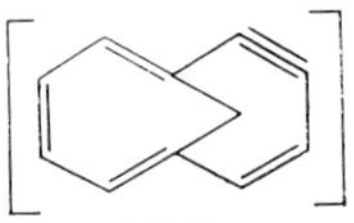

(191)   (192)

adduct with maleic anhydride in refluxing chlorobenzene, but not in refluxing benzene (168). With dimethyl acetylenedicarboxylate the adduct **193** is obtained, which decomposes at 400°/mm to give benzocyclopropene (**194**) (168). The amine **191g** and the enol **191h** have

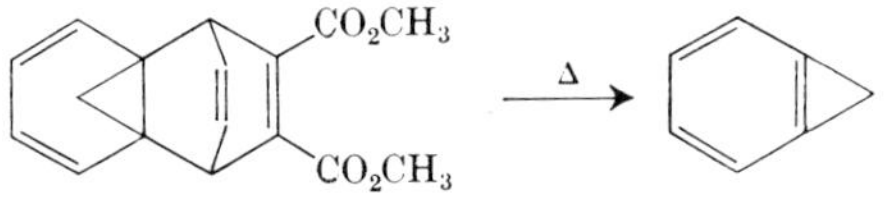

(193)   (194) 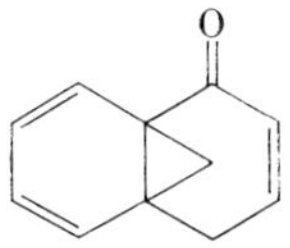   (195)

recently been prepared (169). The enol **191h** is in tautomeric equilibrium with the ketone **195**, the former being favored in polar, and the latter in nonpolar media.

A number of [10]annulenes with 1,6-heterobridges have been prepared. The NMR spectrum of 1,6-oxido[10]annulene (**196**) (170,171) supports the aromatic extended conjugated system. Nitration with cupric nitrate-acetic anhydride gave two isomeric mononitro compounds (169). In the NMR spectrum of 1,6-imino[10]annulene (**197**), the ring protons appear as a low field multiplet centered at τ 2.8, and the imino proton at τ 11.1 (172). The imine **197** forms a hydrochloride and can be N-methylated.

The ESR spectra of the radical anions of **190** and **196** and some of their deuterio derivatives have been reported (173). The observed spin

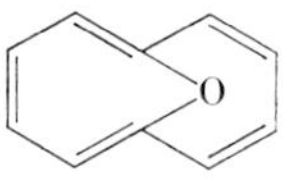

(196) 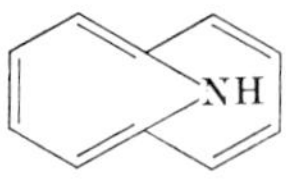   (197)

densities are in good agreement with those predicted by simple MO theory, provided that the electron repulsion of the bridging groups is taken into account.

The nature of the 1,6-bridge appears to have a profound effect on the valence tautomerism of these systems. It seems, at present, that the aromatic system is favored in those cases in which there is a one atom bridge, whereas a larger bridge favors the nonaromatic tetraene. Thus Bloomfield and Quinlin (174) have synthesized the ether **198**, which exists as thetetraene, and 9,10-dihydro-9,10-ethanonaphthalene **(199)** also shows no tendency to valence tautomerize to 1,6-ethano-[10]annulene (175,176).

A bridged isomer of the undecacyclopentadienyl cation **200** has been reported (177). Addition of methylene to **190** gave the bicyclo[5.4.1]-dodecapentaene **201** as a bright yellow oil. Treatment of this oil with

(198) **(199)**

triphenylmethylfluoroborate gave bicyclo[5.4.1]dodecapentaenylium fluoroborate **(202)** as a stable aromatic 10 π electron system. In the NMR spectrum the ring protons appear at low field (τ 0.4–1.7), and the methano-bridge protons, which are shielded by the ring current, appear at high field (τ 10.3–11.8). Comparison of the position of the resonance of the bridge protons in the cation **202** and the anion **174** (τ 10.7–11.2) suggests that little charge delocalization onto the bridge occurs.

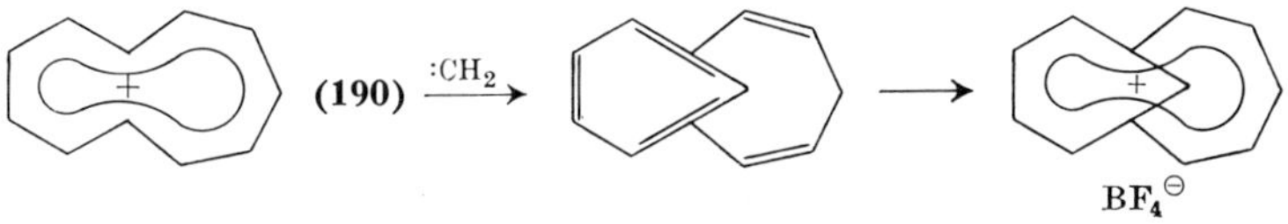

(200) (190) $\xrightarrow{:CH_2}$ **(201)** $\longrightarrow$ **(202)** $BF_4^{\ominus}$

The cation, uncharged species, and anion in the bridged 10 π electron series have thus all been synthesized and show the properties expected for aromatic systems. The synthesis of the unbridged [10]annulene and of the undecacyclopentadienyl cation remain to be accomplished, and is under investigation in many laboratories.

D. $n > 2$

The problem of the interaction of internal hydrogens is still present in the larger cyclic polyenes, considering structures in which bond angle distortion has been minimized. A number of predictions have been made regarding the ring size required for planarity to be attained. Mislow (160) suggested that [30]annulene would be the first cyclic polyene after benzene which could be planar, whereas Baker and McOmie (9) and Soldheimer et al. (178) proposed that the interactions in [18]annulene should not be extreme. The larger cyclic polyenes should also provide evidence for or against Longuet-Higgins and Salem's prediction (179) that bond alternation should occur in the larger cyclic $(4n + 2)$ π electron annulenes. A recent estimate by Dewar and Gleicher (180) suggests that bond alternation should commence between [22]- and [26]annulene.

The synthesis of these larger systems has mainly been carried out by Sondheimer and his co-workers (181–183). The basis of their method is the oxidative coupling of α,ω-diacetylenes. Under Glaser conditions (184) (oxygen with cuprous chloride and ammonium chloride in aqueous ethanol) terminal diacetylenes of the type **203** yield cyclic dimers **204**, as well as linear products. Under Eglinton conditions (185) (cupric acetate in pyridine), the terminal diacetylenes give a variety of cyclic products including monomers (if n is sufficiently large), dimers, trimers, tetramers, etc. With suitably chosen values of n, the cyclic products can be prototropically rearranged with base to give dehydroannulenes directly. The dehydroannulenes so formed are then partially reduced by catalytic hydrogenation to the respective annulenes.

$$\text{H}-\text{C}\equiv\text{C}-(\text{CH}_2)_n-\text{C}\equiv\text{C}-\text{H} \qquad \left(\text{C}\equiv\text{C}-(\text{CH}_2)_n-\text{C}\equiv\text{C}\right)_m$$

(203) (204)

Annelated annulenes have been synthesized by various groups of workers, and recently less general methods have been described for the synthesis of a number of specific annulenes. Systems in which the internal hydrogens have been removed by bridging have also been obtained.

1. $n = 3$

[14]Annulene, a $(4n + 2)$ system, and possibly [12]annulene have been synthesized. Both suffer from overcrowding of the internal hydrogens as typified by [10]annulene.

Sondheimer and Wolovsky (187) found that oxidative coupling of 1,5-hexadiyne **(205)** under Glaser conditions, with a large volume of benzene, gave the unstable cyclic dimer **206**, which on prototropic rearrangement gave a mixture of biphenylene **(207)**, and two dehydro-[12]annulenes. The latter were originally thought to be isomeric bisdehydro[12]annulenes, but they have recently been shown to be 1,5-bisdehydro[12]annulene **(208)** [1.5%] and the interesting 1,5,9-tri-dehydro[12]annulene **(209)** [0.65%] (187,188). Tridehydro[12]annulene **(209)** has been elegantly synthesized by Untch and Wysocki (188), starting from the readily available cyclododecatriene **(210)**. Bromination of **210** and dehydrobromination gave the tribromide **211** (189), which on treatment with NBS, followed by dehydrobromination, gave **209** directly (188).

Bisdehydro[12]annulene **(208)** is a highly unstable solid which is completely destroyed after 1 hr at room temperature. Its IR spectrum shows an acetylene band at 2170 cm^{-1} and a strong band at 980 cm^{-1} attributed to a conjugated *trans* double bond. The NMR spectrum

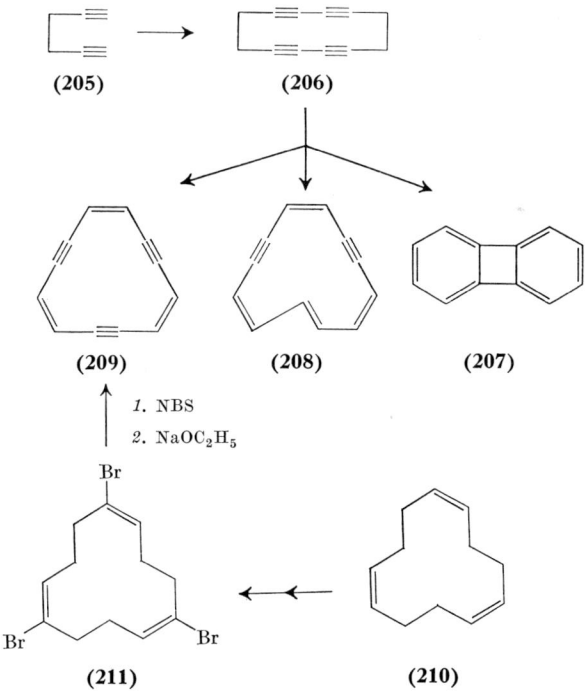

at room temperature is complex but is consistent with the 1,5-diyne structure with three *cis* and one *trans* double bonds. The equivalence and low field resonance of the *trans*-vinylic protons suggests that this is a time-averaged spectrum and that bond rotation occurs such that both protons spend part of their time inside the ring. The appearance of the internal protons in the $4n$ π electron series at *lower* field than the outer protons has recently been recognized (see below). Broadening and a downfield shift of the *trans*-vinylic resonance signal occurs on cooling to $-80°$ in hexadeuteroacetone (183).

1,5,9-Tridehydro[12]annulene **(209)** is more stable than the bisdehydro isomer. The UV spectrum is similar to that of bisdehydro[12]annulene **(208)**. The IR spectrum shows an acetylene band (2170 cm^{-1}), but no *trans* double bond absorption, and the NMR spectrum shows only one sharp singlet (τ 5.58) (187,188). The proton resonance signal is unaffected by change of solvent or temperature ($-80°$ to $+80°$) (187). The high field value of the vinylic proton may be due to the interaction with the acetylene, or it may be due to a paramagnetic ring current effect (see below). However, Sworski's view (190) that **209** may have the properties of a perturbed benzene is not correct.

Wittig and his co-workers (191) obtained both the *cis,cis*- and the *trans,trans*-1,2:3,4:7,8:9,10-tetrabenzo[12]annulenes **(212)** by a lengthy route. Both isomers gave diphenic acid on oxidation, and on hydrogenation the same tetrahydro product was obtained. On heating the *trans,trans* compound to 170–180°, the tetrahydrobiphenylene derivative **213** was formed.

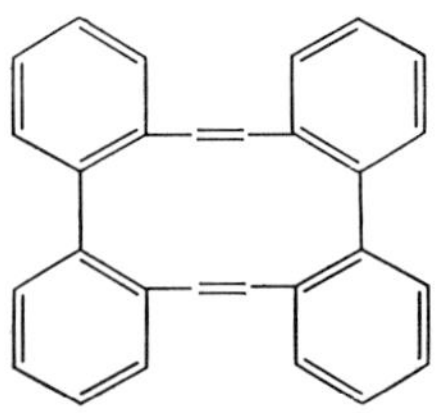

(212) 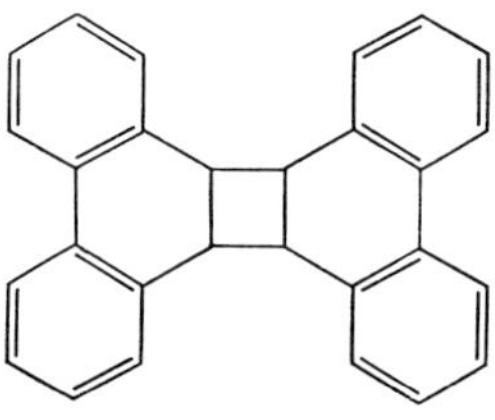   (213)

Eglinton, Raphael and their co-workers (192a) synthesized 1,2:7,8-dibenzo-3,5,9,11-tetradehydro[12]annulene **(215)** by oxidative coupling of *o*-diethynylbenzene **(214)**. The NMR spectrum had a single band, and the electronic spectrum was complex. Compound **215** was also obtained by oxidative cyclization of **216** (192b).

The tribenzo analogs of both the bis- and the tridehydro[12]annulenes have recently been reported (193,194). 1,2:5,6:9,10-Tribenzo-3,7,11-tridehydro[12]annulene **(217)** has a simple UV spectrum (λ_{max} 290 mμ, ε 370,000) and the IR spectrum is also simple, with bands at 2208 and 750 cm^{-1}. The Raman spectrum shows a totally symmetric acetylene stretching mode at 2221 cm^{-1}, and the NMR spectrum shows only aromatic protons. The radical anion can be prepared by addition of potassium in dimethoxyethane to the compound, and the ESR spectrum shows the expected seven-line splitting (195). In the NMR spectrum

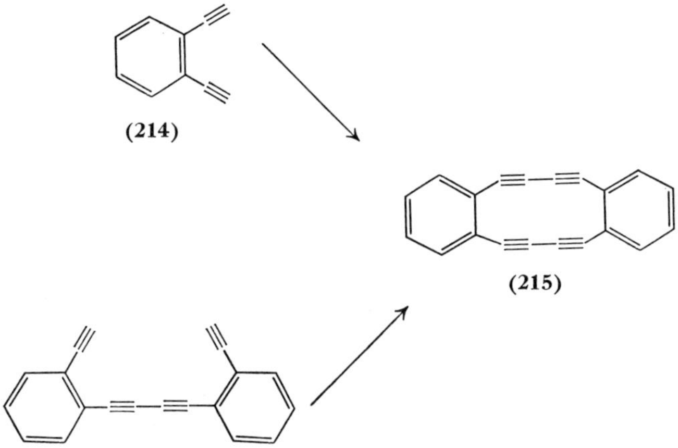

(214)

(215)

(216)

of **218**, which has also been prepared, the *trans*-vinylic proton appears as a single band at τ 1.34 (193). The low field position of this band may be attributed to a time averaging of the internal and external proton, and it would be of interest to investigate the effect of cooling on the spectrum of **218**.

Morimoto et al. (196) have coupled 9,10-diethynylphenanthrene to give the 9,10-phenanthro analog of **215**.

Attempts to convert **208** and **209** into [12]annulene by partial hydrogenation led to yellow oils, which showed the expected bathochromic shift in the UV. However, it was not unequivocally shown that [12]annulene had been obtained (186).

Tribenzo[12]annulene **(219)** has recently been prepared by Staab and his co-workers (197) by a Wittig reaction between o-phthalaldehyde and the bis-ylid prepared from 2,2'-bis(bromomethyl)-*trans*-stilbene.

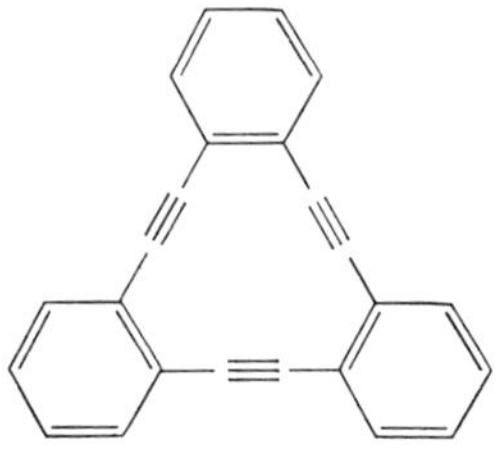

(217) 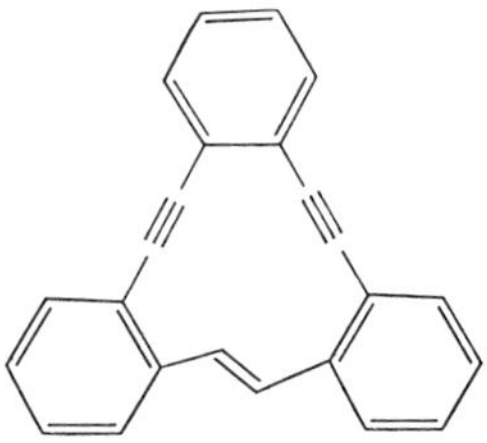 (218)

In the NMR spectrum the all *trans* isomer **219** showed the aromatic protons at τ 2.68, and the olefinic protons as a sharp singlet at τ 2.87. The UV spectrum indicated that the molecule is not planar.

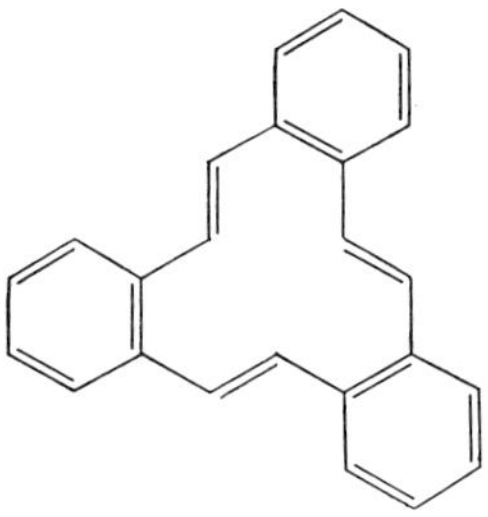

(219)

Entry into the [14]annulene series was achieved by the oxidative coupling of *trans,trans*-4,10-tetradecadiene-1,7,13-triyne **(220)** under Eglinton conditions, followed by prototropic rearrangement (181,182,198). Monodehydro[14]annulene **(221)** [2%], and 1,8-bis-dehydro[14]annulene **(222)** [0.4%] were formed. The NMR spectrum of **221** showed a complex signal between τ 1.2–2.7 (10H) and a double doublet at τ 10.70 (2H) (199). The large difference in proton shift is attributed to the induced diamagnetic ring current, which shields the inner protons and deshields the outer protons. Compound **222** is more stable, and its structure has been confirmed by x-ray crystallographic analysis (200). The NMR spectrum showed a high field multiplet at τ 15.54 (2H) for the inner protons, and low field multiplets at τ 1.57 (4H) and τ 0.45 (4H). The x-ray data indicated that the molecule is planar and centrosymmetric (200). The ring current contribution to the diamagnetic anisotropy is in good agreement with that predicted (201).

The preparation of 1,5,9-tridehydro[14]annulene **(224)** by base treatment of the cyclic dimethanesulfonate **223** has recently been reported (202). The NMR spectrum showed two multiplets at τ 0.5–0.86 (2H) and τ 1.46–1.92 (5H) and a triplet at τ 14.96 (1H), which is in accord with a structure containing one *trans* and three *cis* double bonds.

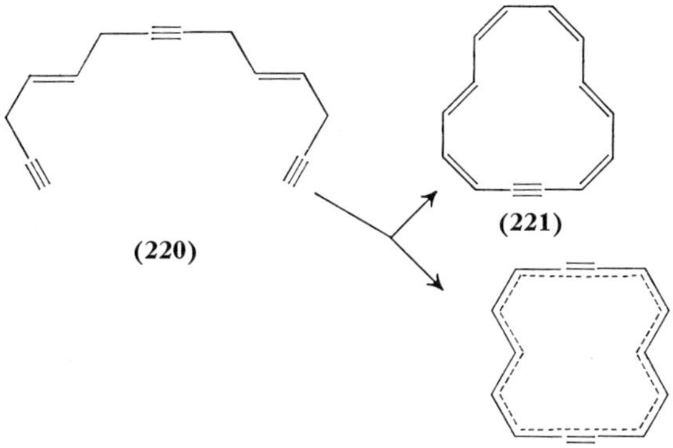

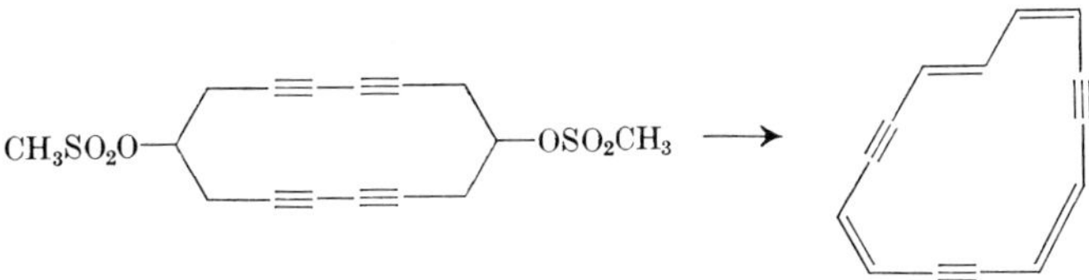

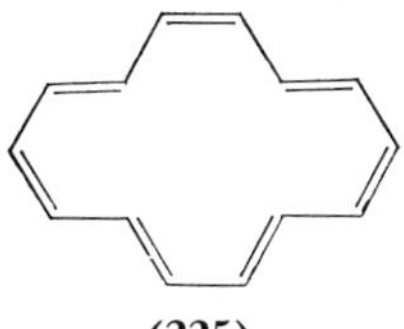

Partial hydrogenation of monodehydro[14]annulene **(221)** over Lindlar catalyst gave [14]annulene [15%] **(225)** (198). The NMR spectrum (203) at room temperature showed two sharp singlets at τ 4.42 and τ 3.93, which have been shown to be due to the two interconvertible conformational isomers. The equilibrium is in favor of the isomer with the higher field resonance (6:1); although both can be separated, in solution reequilibration occurs after about 30 min at room temperature (204). Since the x-ray crystallographic analysis of the isomer present in larger amount has indicated that it is centrosymmetric (205), it probably has the structure **226**, and the minor component is therefore **227**. The NMR spectrum of [14]annulene at

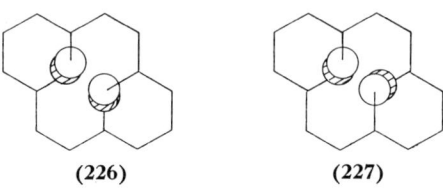

(226)   (227)

room temperature suggested that it did not have a ring current, presumably due to internal hydrogen interactions (181,199). However, a dramatic change occurs when the solution is cooled (183,206). The τ 4.42 band broadens at −20° and disappears at −30°. At −40° two new bands at τ 2.5 (10H) and τ 9.9 (4H) appear, and at −60° the spectrum shows bands at τ 2.4 and τ 10 due to **226**, with a broadened band at τ 3.9 due to **227**. At room temperature therefore, a time-averaged spectrum is being observed, but the rate of interchange of the internal and external protons on cooling slows sufficiently, in the case of isomer **226**, for the individual resonances to be observed. Thus [14]annulene does sustain a ring current, despite the large van der Waals interactions, and is an aromatic compound. It is of interest that the proton interchange does not destroy the cyclic delocalization of the π electrons, but the reason for this is not well understood. The NMR spectrum of [18]annulene shows a similar temperature dependence (see below).

Both **221** and **222** undergo electrophilic substitution (207). Nitration of **221** gave a mononitro compound, sulfonation gave two isomeric sulfonic acids, and acetylation gave an acetyl compound in low yield. The substituent in this case was shown to be in a position adjacent to the triple bond. Similar results were obtained for **222**, except that in this case one monosulfonic acid and two acetyl derivatives were obtained. [14]Annulene did not give isolable products under similar reaction conditions.

A number of interesting systems with a 14 π periphery have been synthesized by Boekelheide and Phillips (208,209) Cyclization of the diiodo compound **228** led to the metacyclophane **229**, which on oxidation gave the bis-dienone **230**. Dehydrogenation with NBS afforded the stable extended quinone **231**, which on reductive acetylation gave the diacetate **232**. The latter had an NMR spectrum consisting of signals at τ 1.42 and τ 1.63, with the internal methyl protons absorbing as a singlet at τ 14.03. Its electronic spectrum was similar to that of [14]annulene **(225)**. Reduction of the quinone **231** with lithium aluminum hydride gave the hexahydropyrene **233** which was dehydrogenated to *trans*-15,16-dimethyldihydropyrene **(234)**. In both physical (NMR) and chemical properties (electrophilic substitution) this molecule is aromatic. Substitution occurs at the 2 and 7 positions on nitration, bromination, and acylation. On irradiation with visible light (210), a fascinating valence tautomerization to the metacyclophane **(235)** occurs, which reverts to the more stable **234** in the dark. The ESR spectra (211) of the radical cation and anion of **234** are in good agreement with MO calculations based on a complete electron delocalization around the periphery.

The attempted preparation of *anti*-1,6:8,13-bismethano[14]annulene **(237a)**, and the successful preparation of 1,6:8,13-diepoxy[14]annulene **(237b)** have recently been reported (212). The diepoxide **236**, prepared by the peracid oxidation of hexahydroanthracene, on treatment with NBS followed by dehydrobromination with potassium *tert*-butoxide gave a 5% yield of **237b**. This is a red, crystalline compound, thermally stable and with a complex NMR and electronic spectrum.

2. $n = 4$

Representatives of both the $4n$ (16 π electrons) and ($4n + 2$) (18 π electrons) series have been synthesized.

Oxidative coupling of *trans*-4-octene-1,7-diyne **(238)** under the Glaser conditions gave 25% of the linear dimer *trans,trans*-4,12-hexadecadiene-1,7,9,15-tetrayne **(239)** and 10% of the cyclic dimer *trans,trans*-1,9-cyclohexadecadiene-4,6,12,14-tetrayne **(240)**(213). Prototropic rearrangement of the cyclic dimer resulted in a mixture of dehydro[16]annulenes and dibenzdihydropentalene **(241)**. The monocyclic compounds were at first thought to be isomeric bisdehydro[16]-annulenes, but these have more recently been shown to be in different oxidation states (214). 1,9-Bisdehydro[16]annulene **(242)** has been

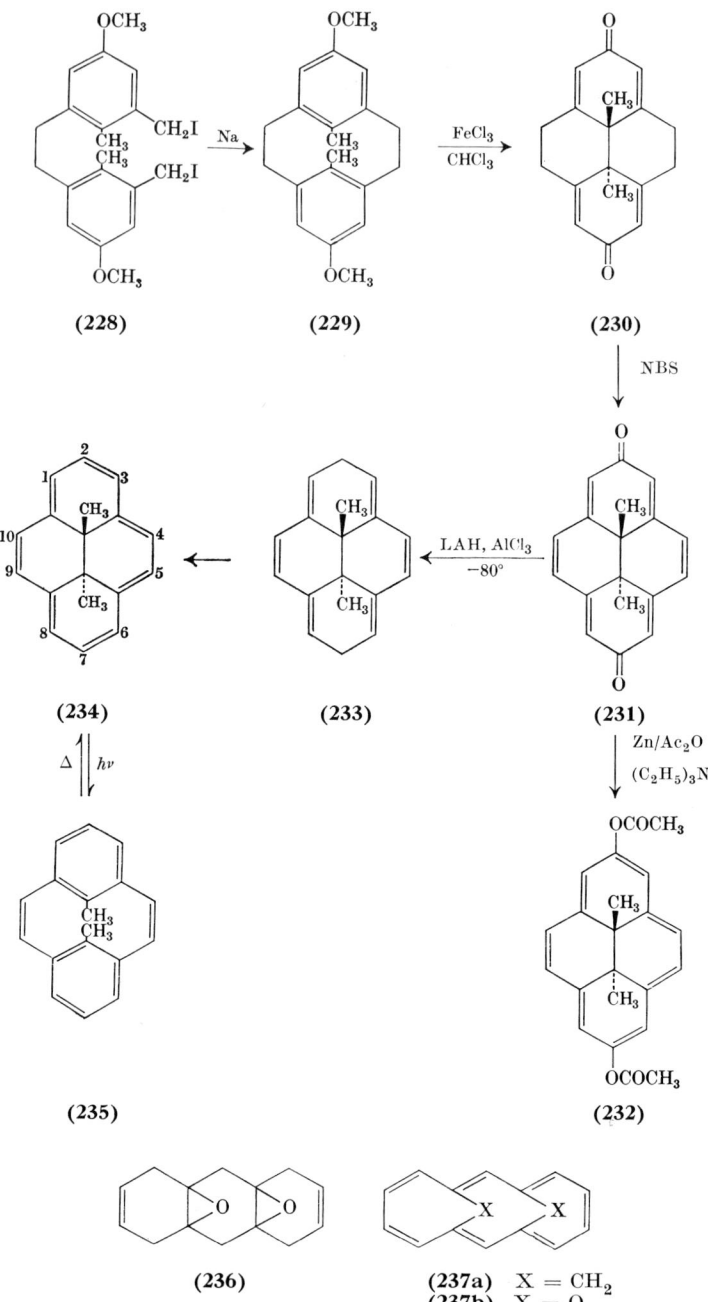

(228) (229) (230)

(234) (233) (231)

(235) (232)

(236) (237a) X = CH$_2$
(237b) X = O

characterized. Its NMR spectrum at room temperature shows a quartet at τ 2.25 (4H), attributed to the protons of the *trans* double bonds, an octet at τ 4.35 (4H), and a doublet at τ 4.93 (4H). The coupling constants, but not the chemical shifts, are almost identical to those of bisdehydro[12]annulene **(208)** [see above]. At $-80°$, the τ 2.25 peak has disappeared, a new peak at τ 0.2 (2H) has appeared, and the band at τ 4.35 now corresponds to six protons. This suggests that the *trans* protons are not equivalent, and that at low temperature the individual, rather than the time averaged, resonance is being observed (183). Thus **242** is a nonaromatic system.

A second bis- **(243)** and a tridehydro[16]annulene have also been isolated, and their structures characterized (214).

Partial hydrogenation of bisdehydro[16]annulene **242** yields about 20% of the crystalline [16]annulene **(244)** (181).

A recent elegant synthesis of [16]annulene has been described by Schröder and Oth (215). The thermal dimer of COT, **245**, on irradiation with UV light, valence tautomerizes to give [16]annulene, identical in all respects to that synthesized by Sondheimer and Gaoni.

The NMR spectrum of [16]annulene at room temperature shows only one peak at τ 3.27, and structure **244** was suggested on stereochemical grounds (181,182). On cooling the solution (215), the resonance signal broadens, and at $-120°$ two new signals replace the original singlet, one resonance at τ -0.32 (4H) and the other at τ 4.8 (12H). Again the internal protons of this $4n$ system are at very low field, as in bisdehydro[16]annulene **(242)**. The position of the internal protons is at complete variance to the position of the internal protons in the $(4n + 2)$ series. It has been suggested (216,217) that this is due to a paramagnetic ring current effect in the $4n$ series, due to the magnetically allowed transition between the highest occupied MO and the lowest unoccupied MO, the energy difference between these levels being small. The members of the $4n$ series are thus not only nonaromatic, but their behavior in a magnetic field is precisely the *opposite* to that found in aromatic systems.

The synthesis of 1,2:5,6:9,10:13,14-tetrabenzo-3,7,11,15-tetradehydro[16]annulene **(246)** has recently been reported (194). It was assigned the strainless D_2d symmetry on the basis of its spectroscopic properties. The *sym*-tetrabenzo[16]annulene **(247)** had previously been synthesized (218,219).

[18]Annulene is in the $(4n + 2)$ π electron series and should be aromatic. However, the possibility that internal hydrogen interactions may prevent the attainment of planarity still exists. The synthesis of [18]annulene and a number of dehydro[18]annulenes has been described (181,182). Oxidative coupling of 1,5-hexadiyne (205) under the Glaser

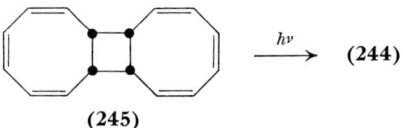

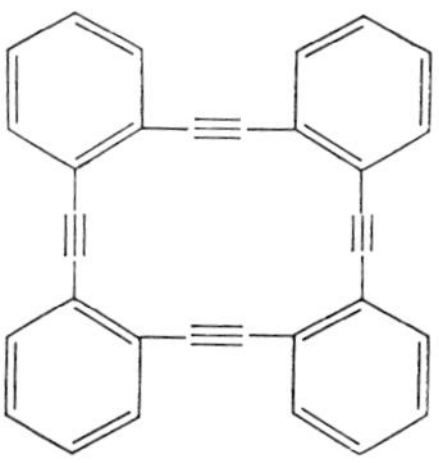

CONJUGATED CYCLIC HYDROCARBONS 49

(246) 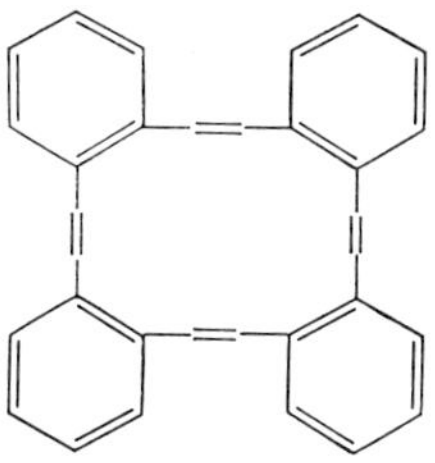   (247)

conditions gave a mixture of the linear dimer and the cyclic trimer, tetramer, pentamer, and hexamer. Prototropic rearrangement of the cyclic trimer **248** gave 50% of a mixture of dehydro[18]annulenes and triphenylene **(249)**. From the mixture of dehydro[18]annulenes two tri- and one tetradehydro[18]annulene were obtained (220). The

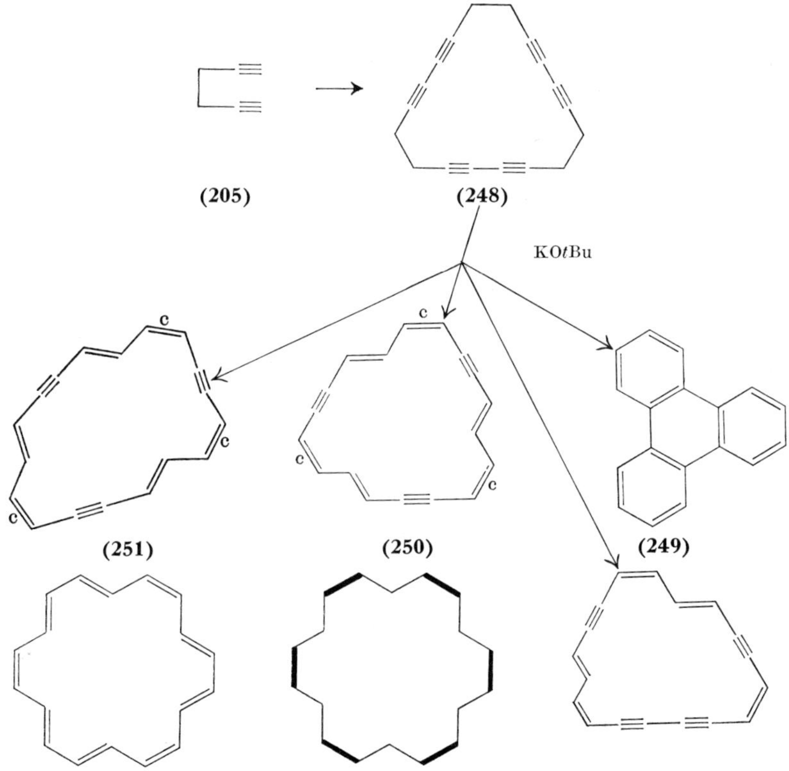

(205) → (248)

KO*t*Bu

(251)   (250)   (249)

(253)   (253a)   (252)

major component, a tridehydro[18]annulene, was assigned the structure **250** (220). The NMR spectrum shows a complex band at low field (τ 1.7–3.1), and a double doublet at high field (τ 8.26), assigned to the outer and inner protons, respectively. Tridehydro[18]annulene **(250)** is thus an aromatic compound. The minor components, a second tridehydro[18]annulene **(251)**, and a tetradehydro[18]annulene **(252)** were assigned the structures shown. The tridehydro[18]annulene **(250)** has also been synthesized by coupling of 1,5-hexadiyne-3-ol under Eglinton conditions, followed by LAH reduction and dehydration (221).

The dehydro[18]annulenes **(250–252)** could be converted to [18]-annulene by partial hydrogenation over 10% Pd/C (220,222). The electronic spectrum supports the structure **253**. The x-ray analysis (223) indicated that the molecule has a center of symmetry and is planar (deviation 0.1 Å). There are two types of bonds with different bond lengths ["cisoid" (1.419 $\pm$ 0.004 Å) and "transoid" (1.382 $\pm$ 0.003 Å)], but these are not alternate (see **253a**, dark lines "cisoid" bonds). The NMR spectrum (183) at room temperature shows two bands at τ 1.06 (12H) and τ 12.0 (6H) corresponding to the outer and inner protons, respectively. On cooling to $-60°$ the bands shift, the low-field band to τ 0.72 and the high-field band to τ 12.99. On heating, the bands broaden, and at 40° they can no longer be distinguished. At 70° a very broad band at τ 4.6 appears, the line width of which decreases with increasing temperature. This behavior is identical to that found with [14]annulene, except that the transition from the "individual" to the averaged spectrum occurs at higher temperature. This emphasizes that the presence of a "single" band cannot be taken as evidence for the absence of a diamagnetic ring current. By the NMR criterion, both [14]- and [18]annulene are aromatic compounds.

The chemical reactivity of [18]annulene is ambiguous. It undergoes nitration with cupric acetate in acetic anhydride, acetylation with acetic anhydride-boron trifluoride etherate (224), but it also forms a Diels-Alder adduct with maleic anhydride (222).

Hexamethyltridehydro[18]annulene has been synthesized and converted by partial hydrogenation to hexamethyl[18]annulene, although this was probably not homogeneous (225).

A number of systems with a peripheral 18 π electron system have been reported by Badger and his co-workers (226–228). In these systems the internal hydrogens have been replaced by heteroatom bridges. Perkin condensation of thiophen-2,5-diacetic acid (254) with the *cis*-dithienyl acrylate 255, followed by esterification, hydrolysis, and decarboxylation, gave the [18]annulene trisulfide (256a). The NMR spectrum indicated that it should be considered to be three thiophens joined by ethylene groups (227). A subsequent calculation (229) also concluded that delocalization should not occur. However when the [18]annulene trioxide (256b) was synthesized by a similar route it was found to have two signals in the NMR spectrum, at τ 1.32 (6H) and τ 1.34 (6H), indicating considerable delocalization (228). Its electronic spectrum was similar to that of tridehydro[18]annulene (251). The monooxide disulfide 256c is not aromatic (230) whereas the dioxide monosulfide 256b is aromatic. This difference in behavior may arise partially from the greater aromaticity of thiophen, and partially from the greater size of the sulfur atom. The x-ray analyses of these compounds should be of considerable interest in providing an estimate of the degree of planarity necessary for cyclic delocalization of the π electrons to occur.

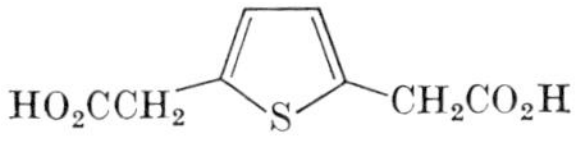

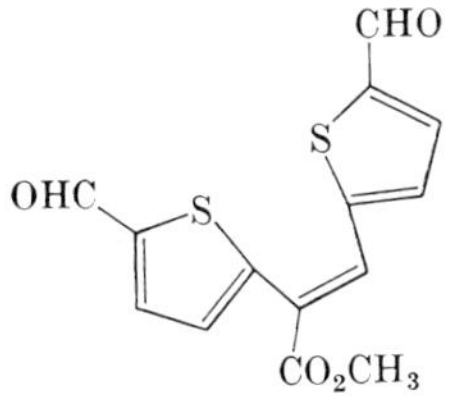

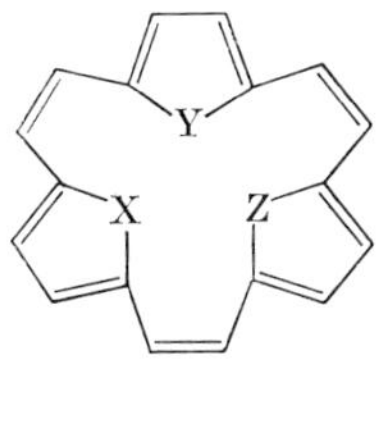

(256a) X = Y = Z = S
(256b) X = Y = Z = O
(256c) X = O, Y = Z = S
(256d) X = Y = O, Z = S

3. $n > 4$

It is in these larger monocyclic polyenes that the bond alternation effect predicted by Longuet-Higgins and Salem (179) should occur. Dewar and Gleicher (180) have suggested that this effect will occur between [22]annulene, which should have equivalent bonds, and [26]-annulene, which should have alternate double and single bonds. Neither of these systems has yet been synthesized.

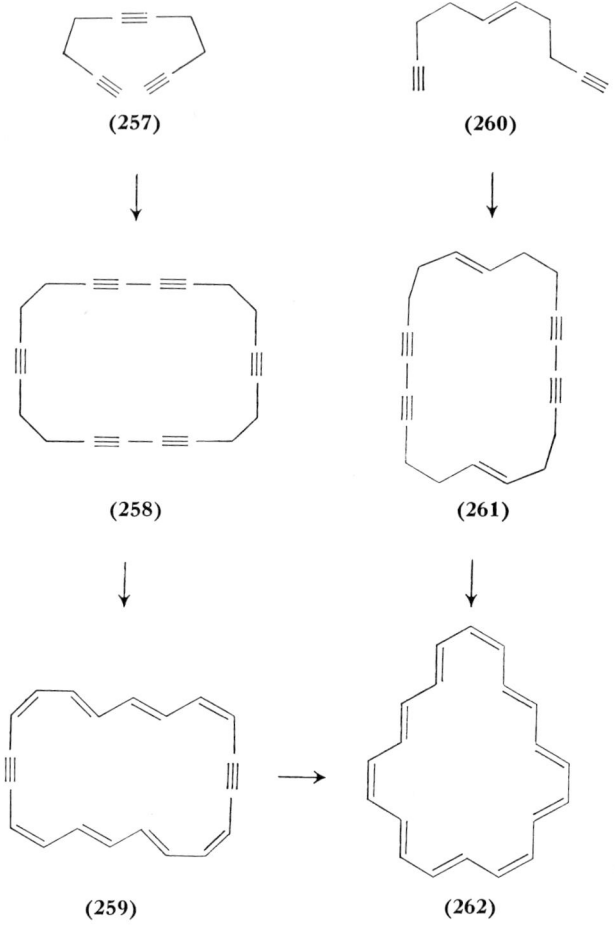

A number of attempts to prepare [20]annulene have been reported (231–233). Coupling of 1,5,9-decatriyne (257) under the Eglinton conditions (231,233) gave the cyclic dimer 258 which, on prototropic rearrangement, yielded 1,11-bisdehydro[20]annulene (259) as a crystalline solid. The NMR spectrum (183) at room temperature showed multiplets at τ 1.6 (4H) and τ 2.6 (4H), due to the protons on the *trans* double bonds, a triplet at τ 4.3 (4H) and a double doublet at τ 4.9 (4H), due to the *cis* vinylic protons. On cooling the solution, the resonance signals at τ 1.6 and τ 2.6 broaden, and eventually disappear at −60°. At −80°, two new signals at τ −1.6 (2H) and τ −0.4 (2H)

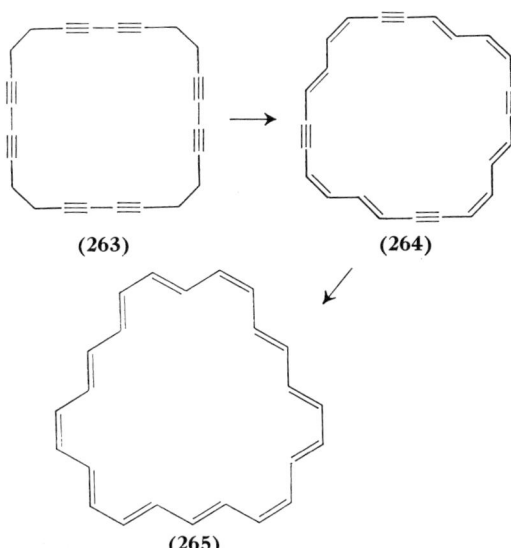

(263) (264)

(265)

have appeared, which are due to the inner protons, and the τ 4.3 band now corresponds to eight protons. This behavior is identical to that of bisdehydro[16]annulene, and, as the disappearance temperature is the same, it suggests that the increase in ring size has been balanced by the increase in the number of internal protons.

Coupling of *trans*-5-decene-1,9-diyne (260) under Eglinton conditions gave the cyclic dimer, trimer, tetramer, and pentamer (232). Protobropic rearrangement of the dimer 261, and partial hydrogenation of the bisdehydro[20]annulene (259), gave inhomogeneous yellow oils, which had the expected characteristics for [20]annulene (262) (232,233).

[24]Annulene, a member of the $4n$ series, has been synthesized (220,222). The cyclic tetramer 263, obtained from the Eglinton coupling of 1,5-hexadiyne, was rearranged with base to tetradehydro-[24]annulene (264). The NMR spectrum at room temperature showed a double doublet at τ 1.60 (4H), and a complex multiplet τ 4.40–5.02 (12H), indicating that the molecule is nonaromatic (183). Partial hydrogenation over Lindlar catalyst gave [24]annulene (15%), assigned the probable structure 265 (222). [24]Annulene is much less stable than [18]annulene. The NMR spectrum at room temperature shows only a broad singlet at τ 2.75 (183).

On cooling, the NMR signal broadens, disappears at −20°, and two new absorptions appear at τ −2.9 to −1.2 and at τ 5.27, corresponding to the internal and external protons, respectively. [24]Annulene thus exhibits the same properties as [16]annulene and the [16] and [20]-dehydroannulenes, and appears to be antiaromatic and possesses a paramagnetic ring current (234).

[30]Annulene is a member of the $(4n + 2)$ series ($n = 7$), but it may show bond alternation. It has been prepared from the cyclic pentamer obtained from 1,5-hexadiyne (220). Prototropic rearrangement of the total product from the oxidative coupling of 1,5-hexadiyne gave 1% of a crystalline pentadehydro[30]annulene as a mixture of isomers (220). Partial hydrogenation over Lindlar catalyst gave [30]annulene as a highly unstable, crystalline powder (222). The same compound was obtained from the prototropic rearrangement of the cyclic trimer of 1,5,9-decatriyne followed by partial hydrogenation (233). Its instability suggests that [30]annulene is not aromatic in the classical sense, but no information is available regarding bond alternation or ring current.

III. Polycyclic Systems

The simple Hückel MO theory does not apply to polycyclic hydrocarbons (10a). The $(4n + 2)$ rule can be applied to these systems, but numerous exceptions occur. Alternatively, the number of π electrons in the periphery of the molecule can be determined, considering the crosslinks as small perturbations. Again the simplification is extreme, and exceptions occur (10a). Valence bond (VB) calculations tend to be more satisfactory than simple MO methods. Craig has proposed a set of rules based on the VB treatment (10a,235).

Early MO calculations (236) on a number of then unknown hydrocarbons, e.g., pentalene, heptalene, and fulvalene, suggested that these might have considerable DE and exhibit aromatic properties. The free valence index (F), however, indicated a much greater reactivity to free-radical reagents compared with conventional aromatic systems. VB methods, in contrast, predicted that bond alternation would occur, and the systems would not exhibit aromatic stability (235,237). Later MO calculations (97,238), in which asymmetric structures were considered, agree with the predictions of the VB treatment. The nonequivalence of a theoretically large DE and aromatic stability has been emphasized (104).

A critique of MO calculations of alternant hydrocarbons has appeared (239).

A. SYSTEMS WITH 3-MEMBERED RINGS

Bicyclo[2.1.0]pent-2-ene **(266)**, "homocyclobutadiene," has recently been synthesized by the UV irradiation of cyclopentadiene (240). It has a half-life of 2 hr at room temperature, and the NMR spectrum suggests that there is little interaction between the cyclopropyl ring and the double bond. Bicyclo[3.1.0]hexatriene **(267)**, a lower homolog

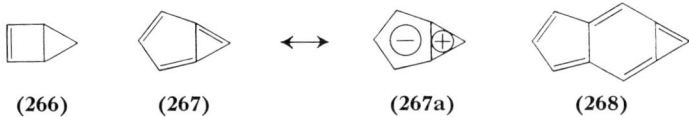

(266)   (267)   (267a)   (268)

of azulene, has not yet been synthesized. A considerable DE was predicted (12) (2.39 β), but bond angle strain and the high maximum electron density may render synthesis difficult (239). The 10 π electron system **268** has also not yet been synthesized and no calculations of its DE have been reported.

Triafulvalene **269** has not yet been synthesized. However, derivatives of triapentafulvalene* **(270)**, in which the dipolar form **270a** might be expected to contribute to the stability of the molecule, have recently been reported (241–247). Three synthetic methods have been described. The reaction (241a,241c) of a cyclopropyl cation **271a** with the indenyl **(272a)** or fluorenyl **(272b)** anion gave the dihydrocalicenes **273a–273d**; hydride abstraction, followed by

(269)   (270)   (270a)

deprotonation, then gave the triapentafulvalenes **274a–274d**. The reaction of di-n-propylcyclopropenone **(20)** with 1-carbomethoxy indene **(275)** in acetic anhydride gave the triapentafulvalene **(276)** directly (241b). The third method (242) involves the reaction of the tetraphenylcyclopentadienyl anion **(277)** with 3,3-dichloro-1,2-diphenylcyclopropene **(278)**. All the triapentafulvalenes react with strong acids to give the cyclopropenylium salts. The UV spectra show a

* The name calicene has been given to these compounds, but we prefer the name triapentafulvalene, which indicates their relationship to the fulvalenes.

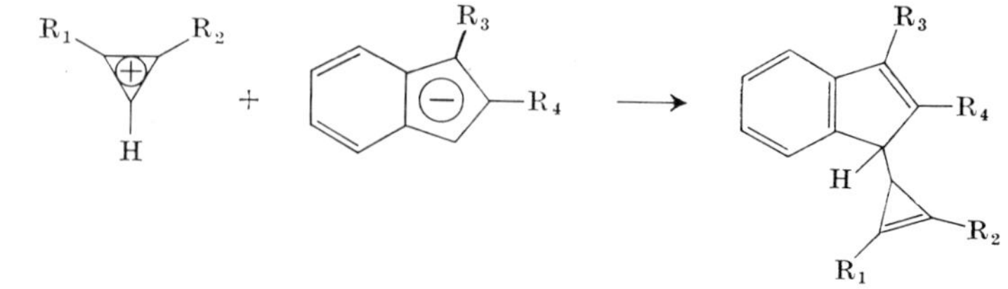

(271a) R$_1$ = R$_2$ = C$_6$H$_5$
(271b) R$_1$ = R$_2$ = CH$_3$

(272a) R$_3$ = R$_4$ = H
(272b) R$_3$, R$_4$ = —C$_4$H$_4$—

(273a)
(273b)
(273c)
(273d)

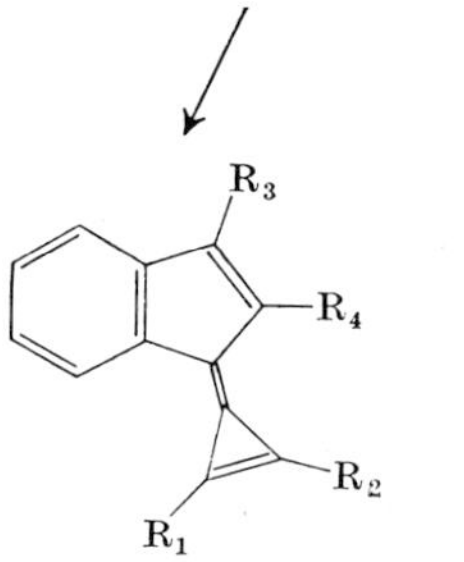

(274a) R$_1$ = R$_2$ = CH$_3$; R$_3$ = R$_4$ = H
(274b) R$_1$ = R$_2$ = C$_6$H$_5$; R$_3$ = R$_4$ = H
(274c) R$_1$ = R$_2$ = CH$_3$; R$_3$, R$_4$ = —C$_4$H$_4$—
(274d) R$_1$ = R$_2$ = C$_6$H$_5$; R$_3$, R$_4$ = —C$_4$H$_4$—

bathochromic shift on passing from a more to a less polar solvent, an effect which would be expected if the dipolar form contributes to the ground state. The size of the shift varies. Compound **279** has an extremely large dipole moment (6.3 D) for a hydrocarbon, which again suggests a large contribution from the dipolar form (242). The

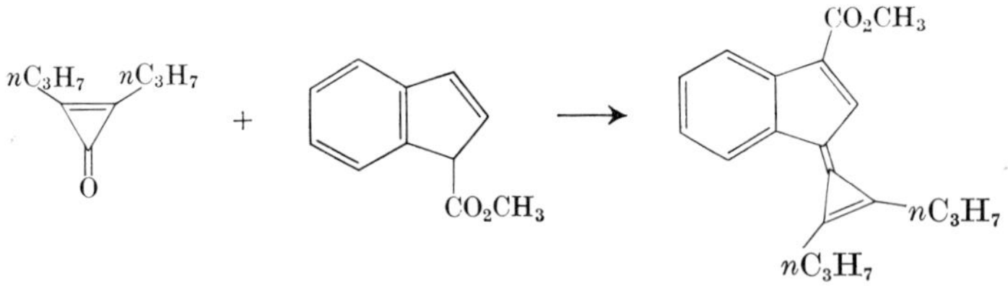

(20) (275) (276)

[Structures (278), (277), (279), (280), (281)]

acyltriapentafulvalenes, e.g., **281** (246,247) show a reduced double-bond character of the intercyclic bond, and from the coalescence temperature of the α-methylene proton signals in the NMR spectrum, an estimate of 19 kcal mole^{-1} for the *cis-trans* isomerization has been made. The acyltriapentafulvalenes undergo a wide range of electrophilic substitution reactions (247).

B. SYSTEMS WITH 4-MEMBERED RINGS

Calculations have been made for a number of systems with fused cyclobutadiene rings (12). Bicyclo[2.2.0]hexatriene **(282)** has been calculated to have a fairly large DE, but is unknown. Although it has a 6 π electron periphery, all of the canonical structures contain at least one cyclobutadiene ring. The tricyclooctatetraene **283** has a larger calculated DE, but it has an 8 π electron periphery. Bicyclo[2.2.0]-hexa-1,3-diene **(284)** and a number of its derivatives have recently

(282)   (283)

been synthesized (248). These, together with the prismanes **(285)** and benzvalenes **(286)**, are of interest as valence tautomers of benzene (249).

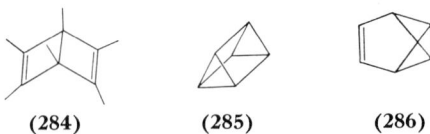

(284) (285) (286)

A possible method of stabilizing the cyclobutadiene ring is by annelation. Benzocyclobutadiene (288) has been prepared as a transient intermediate which rapidly dimerizes (250,251). Debromination of 1,2-dibromobenzocyclobutene (287) with zinc powder gave

6a,10a-dihydrobenzo[a]biphenylene (290), presumably by dimerization of 288 to 289 followed by subsequent rearrangement. Benzocyclobutadiene reacted as a dienophile with 2,3-dihydronaphthalene (291)

and formed the adduct **292** (250). A metal complex of benzocyclobutadiene has been prepared by Pettit et al. (76). When *trans*-1,2-dibromobenzocyclobutene **(287)** is treated with iron enneacarbonyl, a benzocyclobutadienyl iron carbonyl complex **293** is formed. This gave the dimer **294** on treatment with silver nitrate, and the complex **295** with triphenyl phosphine.

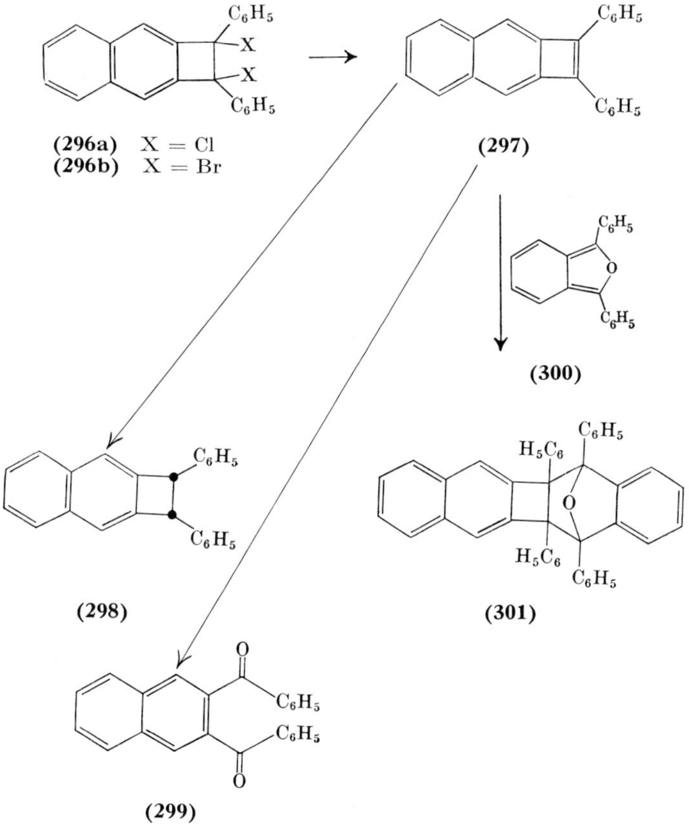

Cava and Nenitzescu and their respective co-workers have investigated, in detail, the chemistry of a number of naphthocyclobutadienes. 1,2-Diphenyl-1,2-dihalonaphthocyclobutene **(296a, 296b)** when reacted with zinc in boiling benzene for 3 min gave 1,2-diphenylnaphthocyclobutadiene **(297)** (252). The NMR spectrum of **297**, a low-field multiplet due to the aromatic protons (14H) and a singlet at τ 3.50 (2H), was in agreement with the assigned structure and resembled that of *cis*-stilbene. Hydrogenation over palladium gave *cis*-1,2-diphenylnaphthocyclobutene (298), oxidation with potassium permanganate gave the diketone 299 and treatment with 1,3-diphenylisobenzofuran (300) gave the adduct 301. Nenitzescu and his co-workers (253) have attempted to prepare 3,8-diphenylnaphthocyclobutadiene (304) by addition of 1,3-diphenylisobenzofuran (300) to 302, followed by dehydration and subsequent pyrolysis. It was not possible to isolate 304, but it could be trapped with 1,3-diphenylisobenzofuran to give an adduct, which on subsequent dehydration gave 1,4,1′,4′-tetraphenylbinaphthylene (305). Treatment of the dihalides 306 with lithium amalgam (253) also generated 304. Cava and Hwang (254) have succeeded in preparing the stable 1,2-dibromo-3,8-diphenylnaphthocyclobutadiene (308) by debromination of the tetrabromide 307 with zinc in boiling benzene for 10–15 sec.

The stabilization of the cyclobutadiene ring system must arise from the increasing contribution to the ground state of canonical structures

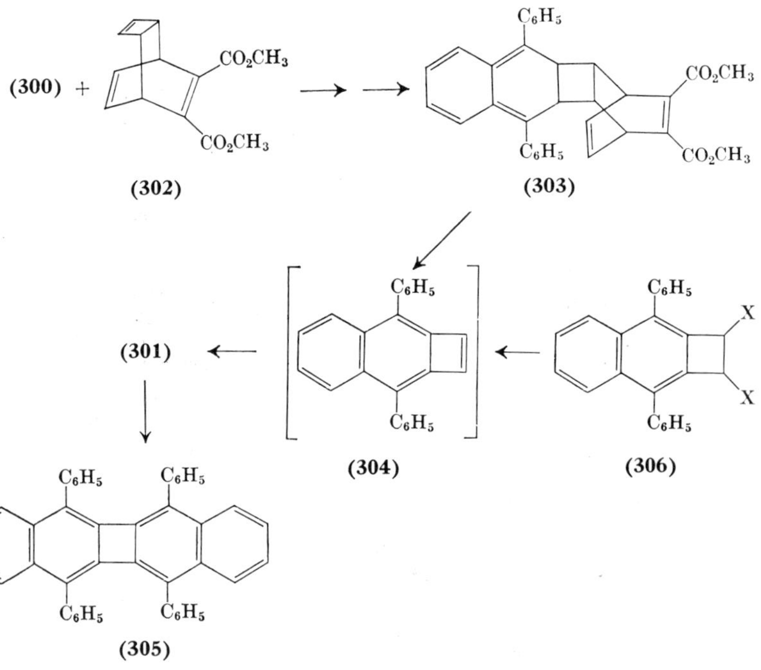

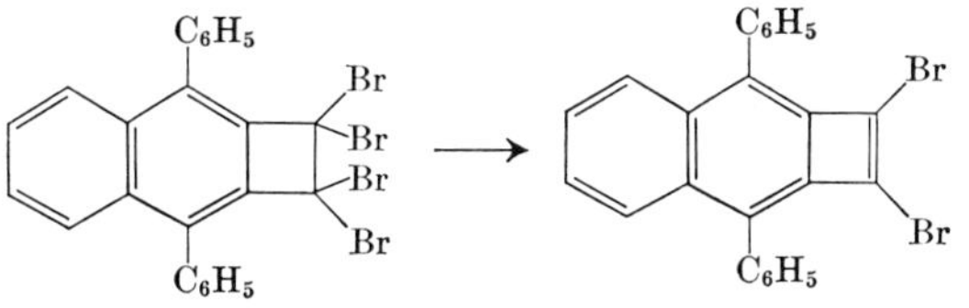

(307) (308)

in which there is no formal cyclobutadiene ring. This has been substantiated by an x-ray crystallographic study of biphenylene (309) (255). The bonds joining the two benzene rings are long (1.52 Å), in excellent agreement with the MO prediction. Structure 309a, with a 12 π electron periphery and a formal cyclobutadiene ring, thus contributes little to the ground state of the molecule.

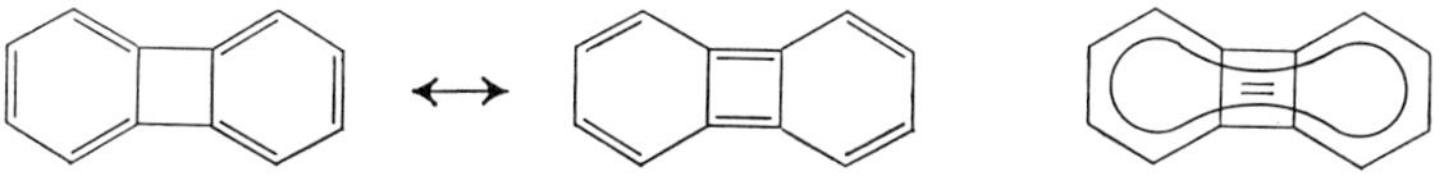

(309) (309a) (310)

The monoanion, dianion, and monocation of biphenylene have been prepared (256). The nature of the long wavelength electronic spectra of the monoanion and monocation was adduced to confirm the essentially aromatic character of the benzene rings in biphenylene, and the relative intensities of some of the bands supported the conclusion that biphenylene (309) is not fully characteristic of a benzenoid alternant hydrocarbon. Bauld and Banks (257) have prepared the dianion 310 in the same manner and have considered that the ease of reduction of 309 was due to the attainment of the 14 π electron aromatic system, but this has been disputed (258) on the grounds that the highest occupied orbital in biphenylene is bonding and not degenerate, unlike that of COT or cyclobutadiene.

Benzocyclobutadienequinone (313) was synthesized by Cava and Napier (259). Treatment of the diiodide 311 with silver nitrate yielded the dinitrates 312, which on refluxing with triethylamine in dichloromethane gave 313. In the IR spectrum of 313 the carbonyl stretching frequencies were high (1815, 1783 cm^{-1}), indicating a considerable ring strain, but the molecule was quite thermally stable.

An interesting MO comparison (12) has been made between the tricyclic 10 π systems 314 and 315, formally derived from the fusion of

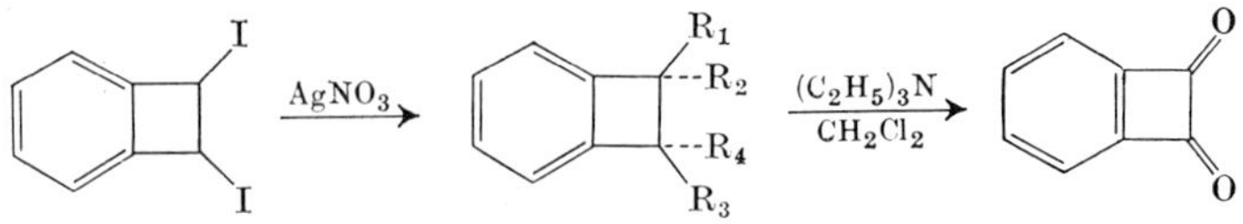

(311) →AgNO₃→ (312) →(C₂H₅)₃N / CH₂Cl₂→ (313)

$R_1 = R_3 = ONO_2$; $R_2 = R_4 = H$
$R_1 = R_4 = ONO_2$; $R_2 = R_3 = H$

one ($4n + 2$) and two $4n$ π electron systems. Both have a considerable calculated DE (2.68 and 3.07β, respectively), but the ground state of **314** is a triplet, whereas that of **315** is a singlet. A canonical form for **314** in which there is no cyclobutadiene ring cannot be written. Neither molecule has been synthesized.

(314) (315)

The fusion of COT with cyclobutadiene gives the 10 π system **316**. This can be written as **316a**, which does not have a formal cyclobutadiene ring. This suggests that the 9,10-bond should have single-bond character, as in azulene, rather than double-bond character, as in

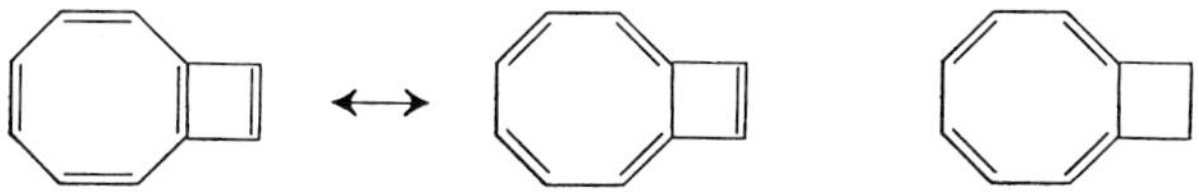

(316) ↔ (316a)   (317)

naphthalene. The dihydro compound **317** has recently been synthesized (260), but attempts to introduce a further double bond have so far been unsuccessful.

C. SYSTEMS WITH 5-MEMBERED RINGS

Armit and Robinson suggested that pentalene (**318**) might be an aromatic system, though they later withdrew this suggestion (3). Early MO treatments (236) predicted considerable DE, but the localization energies towards nucleophilic attack suggested that it might be easily polymerized by strong base (261). The VB treatment (235,237) predicted that bond alternation would occur, a view subsequently supported by more refined MO studies (238).

A number of annelated pentalenes have been known for many years (e.g., **319**) (262). These all have at least two sites of annelation, and all attempts to synthesize benzopentalene **(320)** have failed. However,

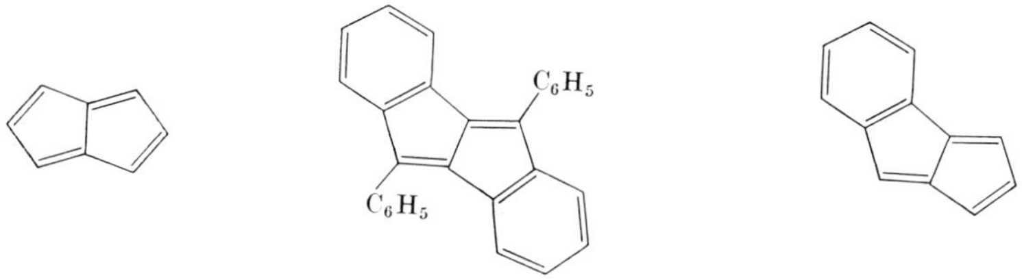

(318)   (319)   (320)

a derivative of benzopentalene has recently been reported by Le Goff (263). The triol **321** was dehydrated with phosphorus oxychloride in pyridine to give the triphenylbenzopentalene **322**. This is a green, crystalline hydrocarbon, stable to heat, oxygen, and moderately strong

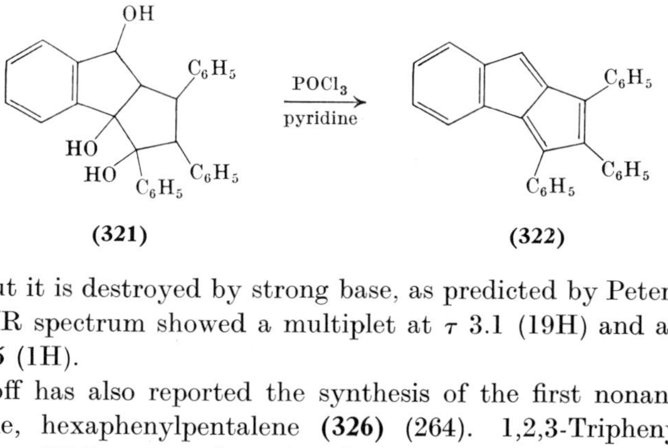

(321)   (322)

acids, but it is destroyed by strong base, as predicted by Peters (261). The NMR spectrum showed a multiplet at τ 3.1 (19H) and a singlet at τ 3.75 (1H).

Le Goff has also reported the synthesis of the first nonannelated pentalene, hexaphenylpentalene **(326)** (264). 1,2,3-Triphenylcyclopentadiene **(323)** was condensed with 1,2,3-triphenylpropenone **(324)**, using a potassium fluoride catalyst, and the resulting dihydrohexaphenylpentalene **(325)** was dehydrogenated with NBS to yield **326**. Hexaphenylpentalene is a stable, crystalline solid, which slowly oxidizes in solution, and has an extensive electronic spectrum. It adds methyl acetylenedicarboxylate to give the azulene **327a** or **327b**.

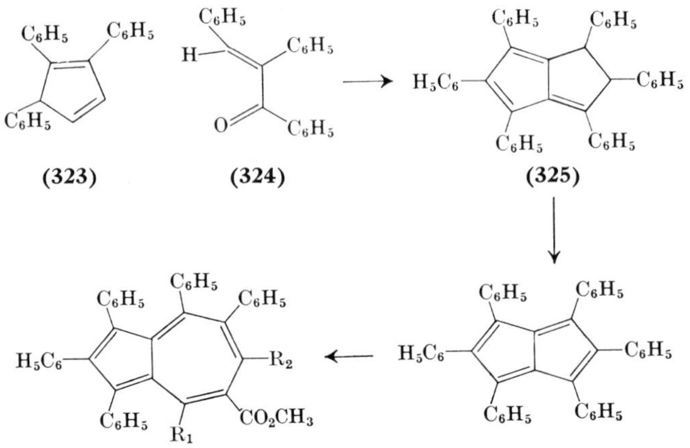

(323) (324) → (325)

(327a) $R_1 = C_6H_5$, $R_2 = CO_2CH_3$
(327b) $R_1 = CO_2CH_3$, $R_2 = C_6H_5$

(326)

Hafner and his co-workers (10d) have synthesized a large number of polycyclic systems which may be considered as pentalene derivatives. 4,6,8-Trimethylazulene (328) reacts with dimethylformamide and phosphorus oxychloride to give the immonium salt 329. Ring closure with sodium methoxide gave 330, which on Hofmann elimination gave 3′,5′-dimethylcycloheptatrieno-1′,7′,6′:1,7,6-pentalene (331) (10d). In the NMR spectrum (266) the protons on the seven-membered ring are at lower field than those of 4,6,8-trimethylazulene, and the protons on the five-membered ring are at slightly higher field. This suggests a greater contribution from the dipolar structure. The hydrocarbon does not show azulene like properties; it reacts readily with dienes or dienophiles across one of the double bonds of the five-membered rings to give an azulene. Thus with TCNE it gives the adduct 332. A theoretical study of 331 suggests it should be an olefin (267).

Utilizing a similar route, Hafner and co-workers (268) have also synthesized the hydrocarbon 333, which may be considered to be a derivative of pentalene, azulene, or heptalene. It is a thermostable solid which gives wine-red solutions. The NMR spectrum (268) shows a multiplet at τ 1.5–3.3 (9H), and a singlet at τ 7.25 (3H). Its stability and lack of reactivity towards electrophilic reagents suggests that it might best be considered as the combination of a peripheral 14 π and a central 2π electron system (cf. pyrene). Hydrogenation converts 333 to the azulene 334.

(328) (329)

(332) (331) (330)

(333) (334)

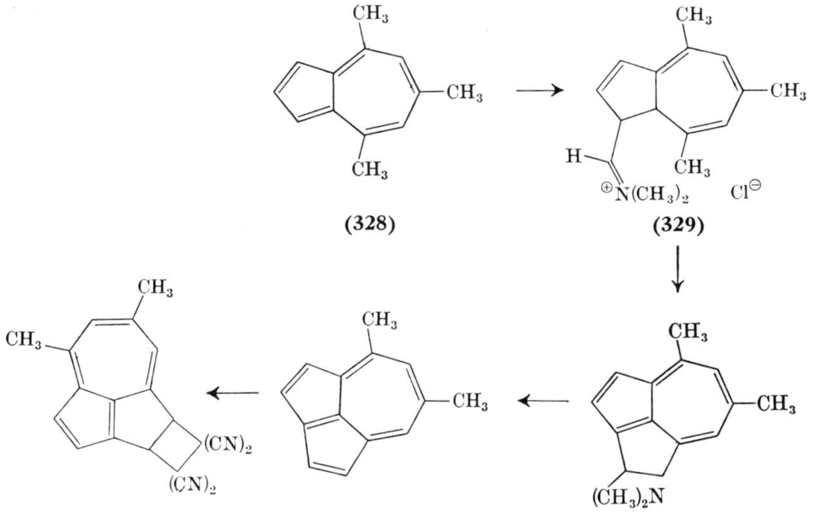

Considerable theoretical interest has been shown in the hydrocarbons **335** and **336**. VB and MO calculations are in disagreement about the possible DE (239). However, since these systems can be treated as central and peripheral $(4n + 2)$ π electron combinations, the stability of **333** should encourage renewed attempts at their synthesis.

(335)

(336)

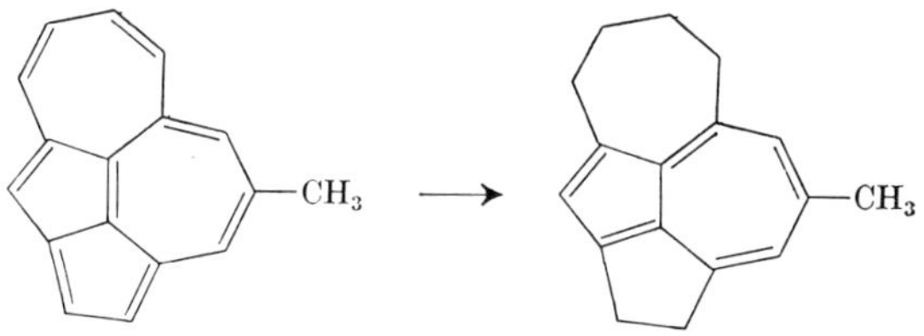

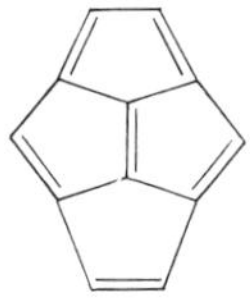

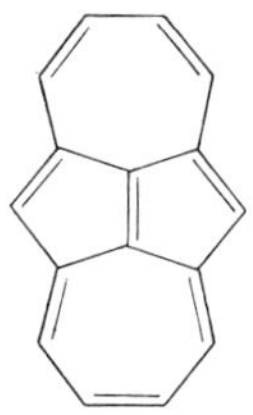

Pentalene is an 8 π electron system. If the crosslink is considered to be a small perturbation, then the system resembles cyclooctatetraene, and the 10 π electron dianion might be expected to be a stable aromatic system. An alternative view is to consider the dianion to be made up of two fused cyclopentadienyl anions. An elegant synthesis of this dianion has been described by Katz and co-workers (269). Isobicyclopentadiene (337) was pyrolyzed in a quartz tube at 575° under nitrogen, when dihydropentalene (338) was obtained. Deprotonation of 338 with n-butyl lithium gave pale yellow solutions of the pentalene dianion (339). The NMR spectrum shows a triplet resonance at τ 4.27 (2H) and a doublet at τ 5.02 (4H). Hydrogenation of the quenched dianion gave *cis*-bicyclo[3.3.0]octane (340). Treatment of

the dianion with methylene chloride gave indene (270). A number of metal complexes of the pentalene dianion have been synthesized (271,272) in which one of the cyclopentadienyl rings is coordinated to the metal atom e.g., 341 and 342. The dibenzopentalene dianion has been synthesized (273).

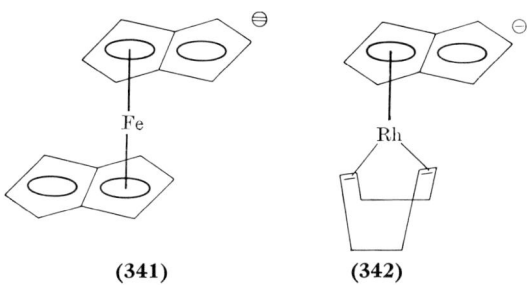

The interposition of a benzene ring between the two cyclopentadiene rings of pentalene was predicted to lead to an increase in the stability of the system. This prediction has been substantiated by the synthesis of s-indacene (**345**) by Hafner and co-workers (10d,274). The aldimino perchlorate **343** reacted with sodium cyclopentadienide in THF at −40° to give the fulvene **344**, which spontaneously lost dimethylamine and ring closed below 0° to give **345**. The structure was confirmed by full hydrogenation to s-hydrindacene (**346**), and bromination to hexabromo-s-hydrindacene (**347**). s-Indacene does not show aromatic properties, and forms a silver nitrate complex.

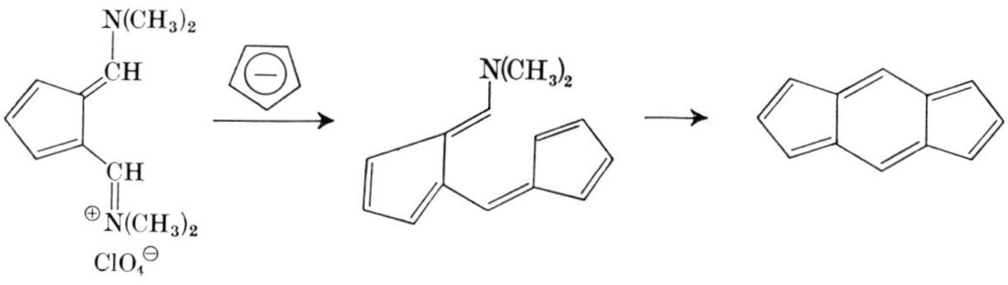

A substituted s-indacene has been prepared by Le Goff and La Count (275). Pentacarbomethoxycyclopentadiene (**348**) self-condensed at 150–160° to give the deep-red hexacarbomethoxy-s-indacene diol (**349**). Reaction with NBS gave a bromoquinone, assigned the structure **350a** or **350b**.

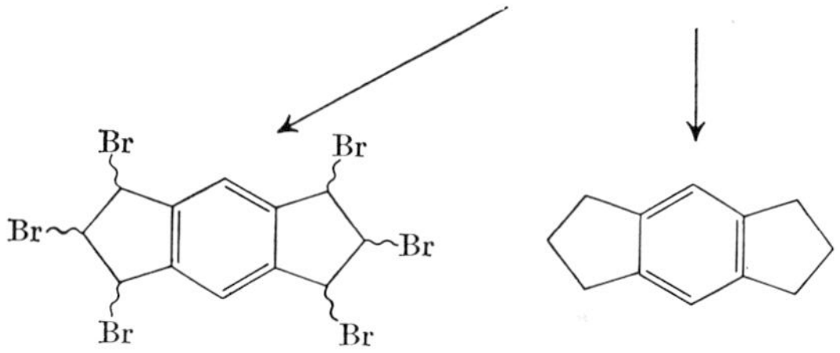

as-Indacene was predicted to be less stable than *s*-indacene, and it has so far not been synthesized.

The *s*- and *as*-indacenes might be expected to be easily reduced to the 14π electron dianions. Dianions from both systems have been synthesized. *s*-Indacene on treatment with lithium in liquid ammonia gave the *s*-indacenyl dianion (**351**) as a colorless, air-sensitive compound,

(348)

(349)

(350b)

(350a)

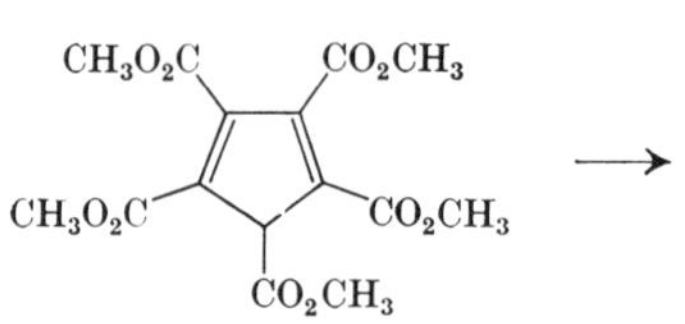

which on hydrolysis gave 1,5-dihydro-*s*-indacene (10d). The diol **349** on treatment with potassium fluoride in methanol gave the dianion **352**, which reacts with tropylium fluoroborate to give the salt **353** (275). The *as*-indacenyl dianion has been prepared by Katz and Schulman (276). The diasterioisomeric acetates **354** were pyrolyzed in a nitrogen stream at 630°, forming an isomeric mixture of

(351)

(352)

(353)

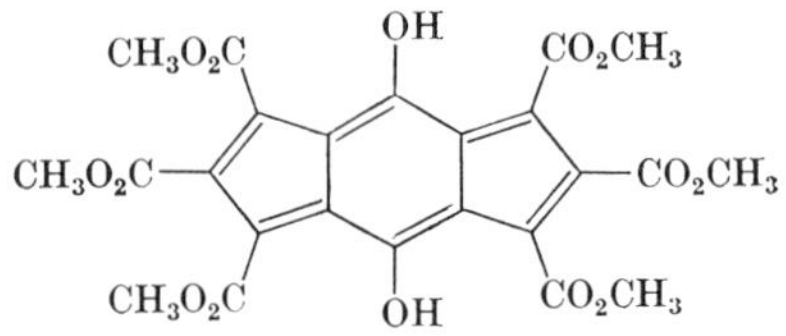

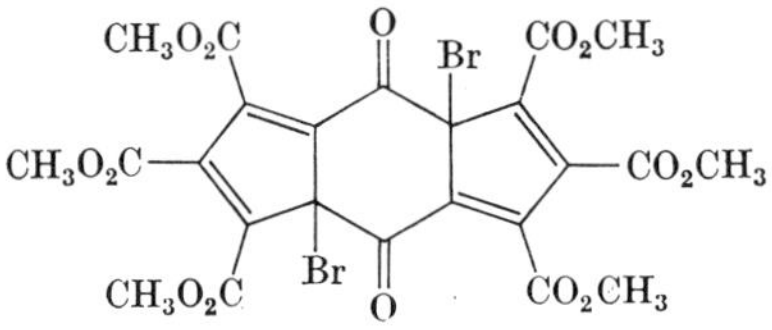

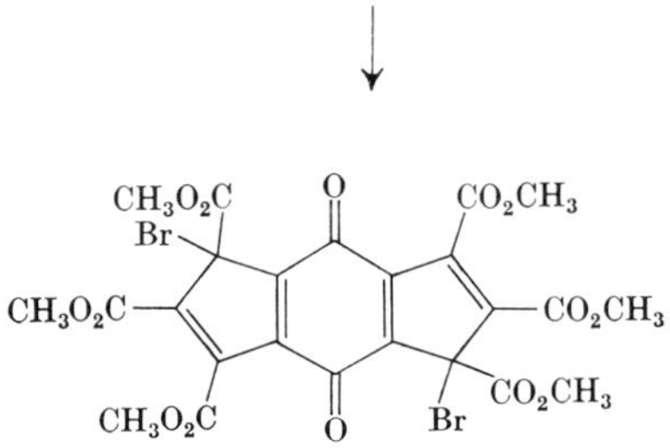

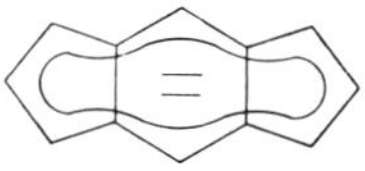

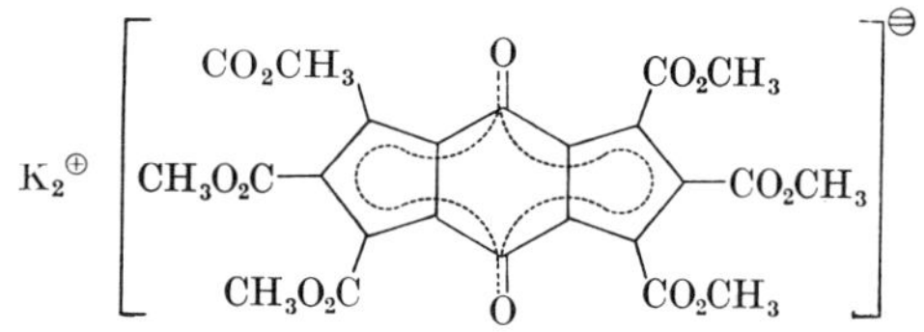

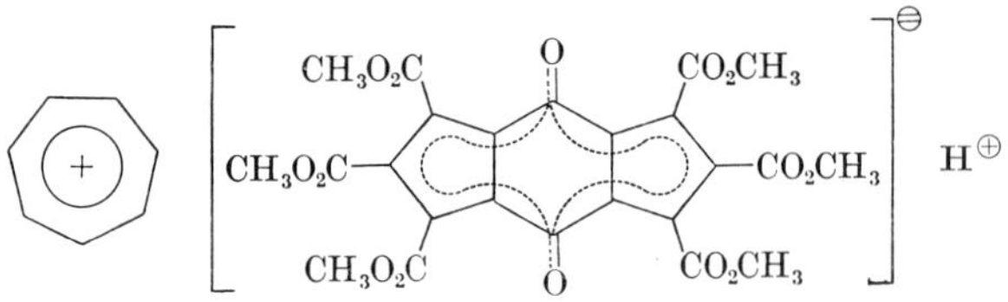

dihydro-*as*-indacenes (355). Deprotonation of the mixture with *n*-butyllithium in dimethoxyethane gave a white solid, soluble in THF. The NMR spectrum supported the dianion structure 356, and quenching the dianion with deuterium oxide gave dideuterated-dihydro-*as*-indacene.

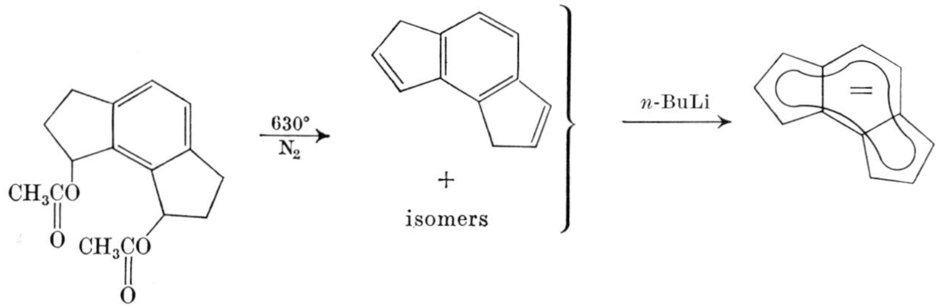

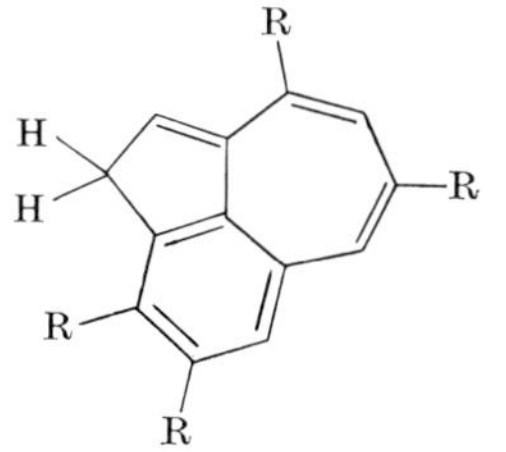

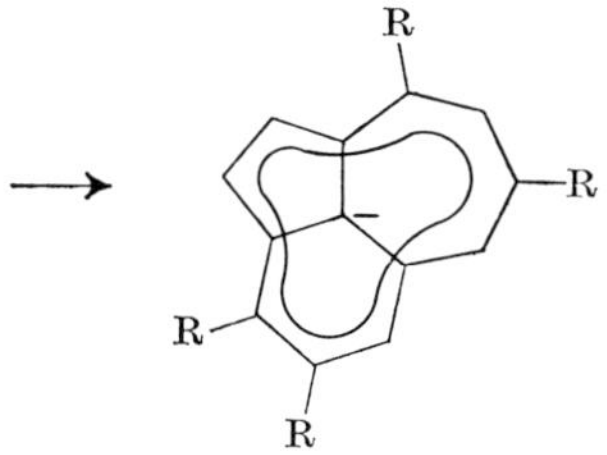

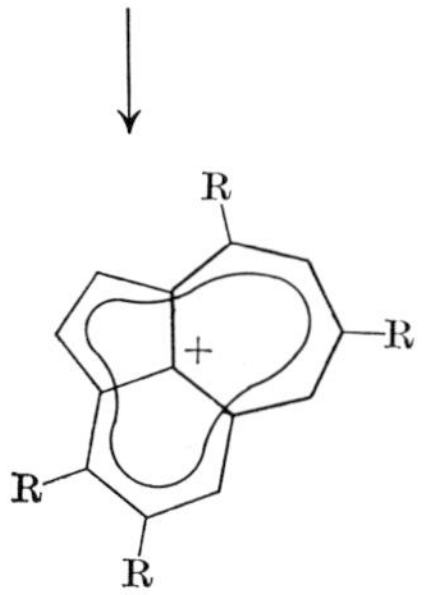

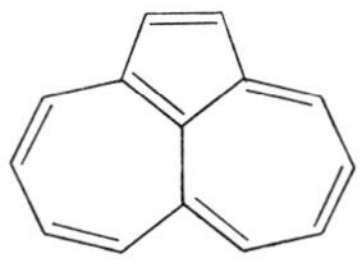

Hafner and Schaum (265) have prepared the hydrocarbon 357a with fused 5-, 6- and 7-membered rings. Deprotonation with methyllithium gave the 14 π electron anion 358a, and hydride abstraction with trityl perchlorate gave the 12 π electron cation **359a**. Both of these systems may be considered as having a 12 π electron periphery, with a centrally charged atom, in analogy with the phenalene system (see below). The unmethylated hydrocarbon **357b**, recently prepared by Boekelheide and Smith (277), has analogous properties, and the benz[c,d]azulenyl ions **358b** and **359b** have been prepared.

The tricyclic hydrocarbon **360**, synthesized by Hafner and Schneider (278), may be considered as an azulene or heptalene. Its spectroscopic and chemical properties resemble an azulene with a diene bridge, rather than a heptalene with an ethylene bridge, which is in accord with the MO calculations (267). The hydrocarbon **360** forms a Diels-Alder adduct with TCNE, and undergoes electrophilic substitution in the 5-membered ring.

Salts of the dibenz[c,d,h]azulenium cation (**361**) have recently been prepared (279) and these are stable in the absence of moisture. The system presumably exists with a periphery of 16 π electrons, by analogy with the phenalenyl and benz[c,d]azulenyl systems.

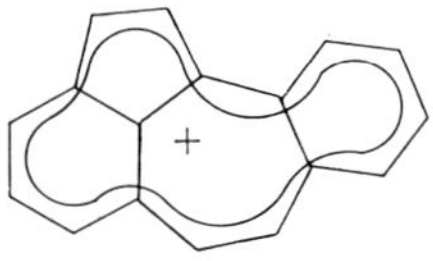

(**361**)

The three isomeric dicyclopentadienocyclooctatetranes **362–364** are 14 π electron systems. They are isoelectronic with the s- and as-indacenyl dianions, and the syntheses of the latter systems may stimulate interest in these fused cyclooctatetraenes.

A cyclooctatetraenocyclopentadienone has been synthesized by Breslow, Vitale and Wendel (280). The diketone **365** was cyclized with sodium methoxide to give **366a**, which was converted with thionyl chloride to the unstable chloride **366b**. Chromatography on alumina gave **367**. In the dipolar form, **367a**, this is a 10 π electron system and

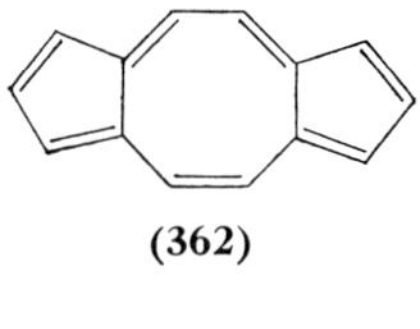

(**362**) 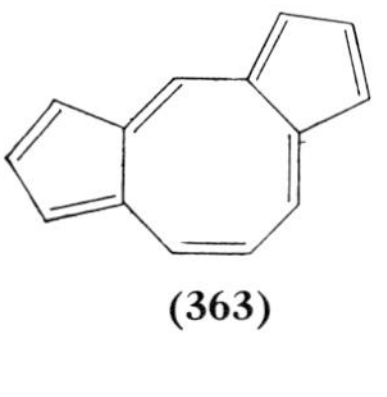   (**363**) 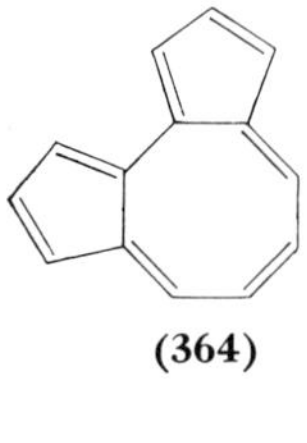   (**364**)

might show aromatic properties. However, the NMR spectrum has the vinylic proton band in the τ 3.5–4.5 region, indicating that the molecule is not aromatic. It is only stable in solution, thus resembling a cyclopentadienone rather than an aromatic system.

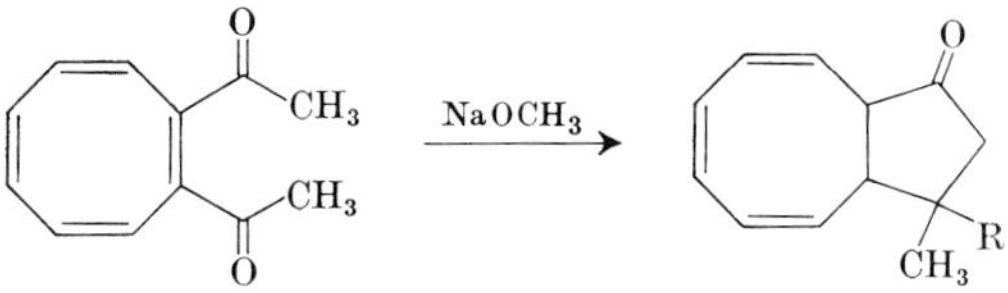

(365) (366a) R = OH
(366b) R = Cl

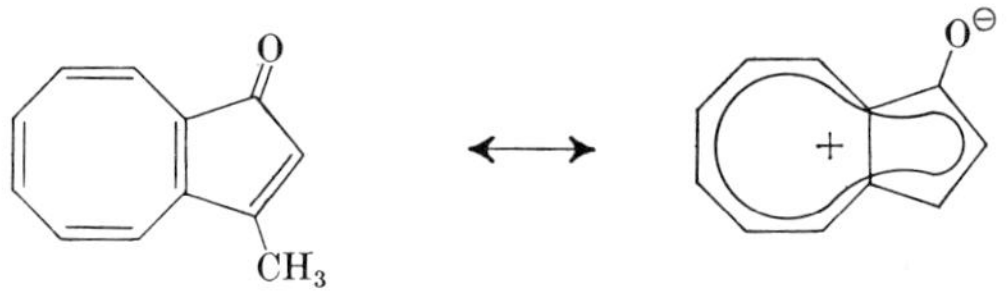

(367) (367a)

A higher homolog of azulene has recently been synthesized by Mayer and Sondheimer (202). Base treatment of the cyclic dimethane-sulphonate **223** yielded the bicyclic hydrocarbon **368**, besides the tridehydro[14]annulene **(224)** (see above). The hydrocarbon **368** is a dark green solid which decomposes rapidly. The NMR spectrum shows only aromatic protons (τ 2.1–3.2), and the IR spectrum has a strong acetylene band. The compound is basic, like azulene, and the low stability probably arises from the ease with which transannular reactions may occur.

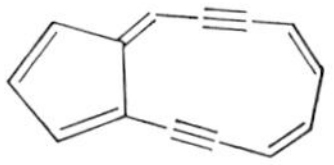

(368)

MO calculations (236) on fulvalene **(371)** suggested that this molecule might have a large DE. The parent compound was synthesized by Doering and Matzner (104). Treatment of a solution of sodium cyclopentadienide in THF with iodine gave a solution of dihydrofulvalene **(369)**, which gave the dianion **370** on deprotonation with n-butyllithium.

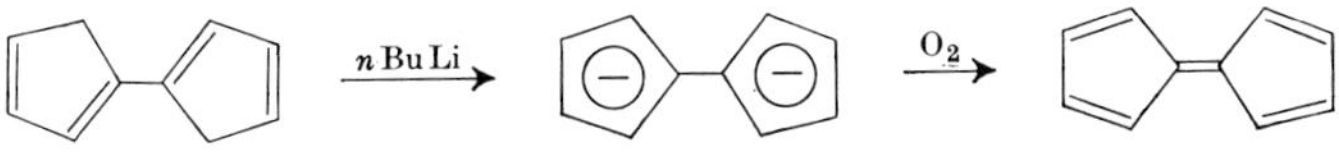

(369) (370) (371)

The dianion on shaking with oxygen gave an orange solution of fulvalene. Hydrogenation of the solution gave bicyclopentyl, and addition of TCNE gave the bis-adduct, from which fulvalene could be regenerated. Fulvalene is not destroyed by air or acids, but it polymerizes at concentrations greater than $0.001M$. Photolysis of diazocyclopentadiene at low temperature gave a product with an UV spectrum identical to that of fulvalene (281). *A posteriori* calculations conclude that fulvalene should exhibit bond alternation (282).

A number of annelated fulvalenes have been known for many years, and 1,2,3,4-tetraphenylfulvalene has also been known for some time (238). Perchlorofulvalene **(372)** has been prepared (283), and it is much more stable than fulvalene. An x-ray analysis (284) has shown that the central bond is long (1.49 Å), the rings are not in the same plane, being twisted through 41°, and the chlorine atoms lie out of the plane of the five-membered ring.

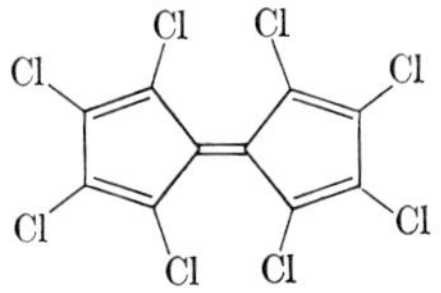

(372)

Sesquifulvalene **(373)** might be expected to be more stable than fulvalene, as the dipolar structure **373a** should contribute to the ground state. Prinzbach and his collaborators have synthesized a large number of substituted sesquifulvalenes, and the parent compound has been obtained in solution (285–288). Sodium tetraphenylcyclopentadienide was condensed with tropylium bromide to give the

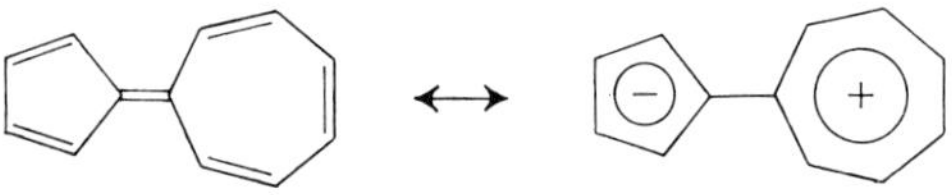

(373)   **(373a)**

dihydrotetraphenylsesquifulvalene **374** in high yield. Dehydrogenation with haloquinones led to 7,8,9,10-tetraphenylsesquifulvalene **(375)** as a green, crystalline solid, which gave red solutions in benzene (285). LAH and butyllithium reacted instantly with **375**, which also gave a Diels-Alder adduct with TCNE and was easily hydrogenated. It thus appears to have little aromatic character.

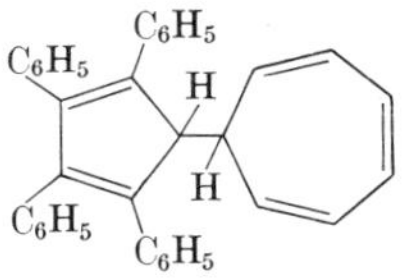

(374) 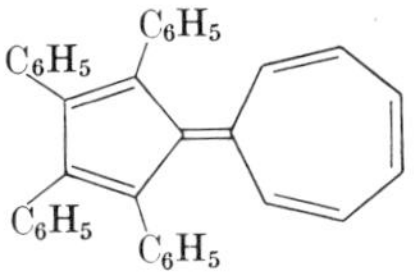 (375)

A number of benzosesquifulvalenes have been synthesized (286). Addition of sodium indenide to tropylium bromide gave the dihydrobenzosesquifulvalene **376**, which gave 8-benzylidene-9,10-benzosesquifulvalene **(377)** on base condensation with benzaldehyde. At higher temperatures in the presence of base, **377** was transformed into the benzosesquifulvalene **378**. This was sensitive to oxygen and gave a 1,3-bis adduct with TCNE.

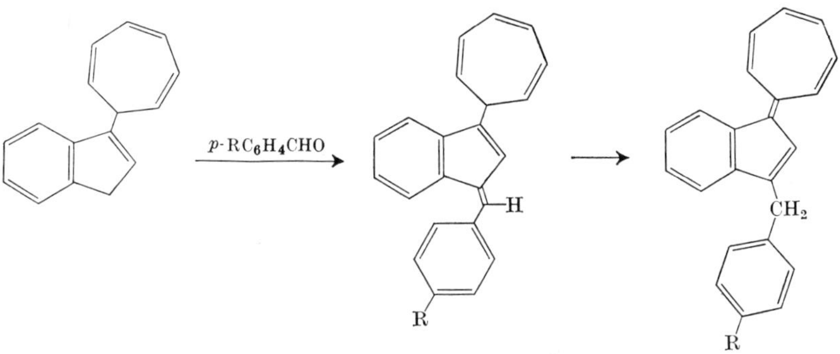

(376) $\xrightarrow{p\text{-}RC_6H_4CHO}$ (377) $\longrightarrow$ (378)

A large number of sesquifulvalenes have now been synthesized using this method (287). In the synthesis of nonannelated systems **379** ($R_1 = R_2 = H$) a competitive side reaction occurs and the vinylogous products **380** are also obtained. The side reaction increases with the

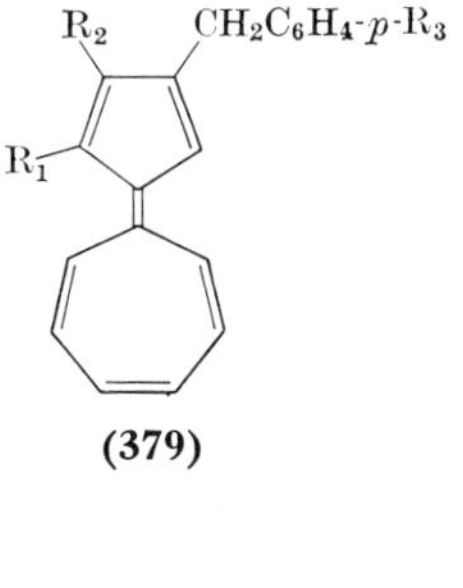

(379) 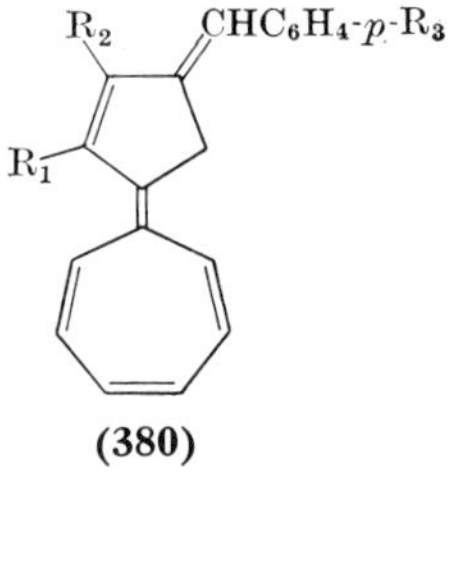 (380)

increasing electron-accepting power of R_3. The sesquifulvalenes are generally sensitive to oxygen, add bromine, form Diels-Alder adducts, and are thermally labile. The structure of the adducts with TCNE vary in a manner which is not easily rationalized. The NMR spectra of the nonannelated compounds suggest a considerable degree of bond localization.

The energy difference between the cycloheptatriene and the norcaradiene structures has recently been shown to be small (288). Molecular models suggested that in dimethyl dibenzosesquifulvalene (381), the 1,6-methyl interactions should prevent the coplanarity of the two rings and perhaps favor the norcaradiene structure 382. This concept was confirmed by synthesis of 382 by the addition of N,N-diethylbutadienylamine to the triafulvalene 274c, followed by acidification and pyrolytic elimination of diethylamine. The NMR, UV, and IR spectra were consistent with the norcaradiene formulation, and 382 showed no

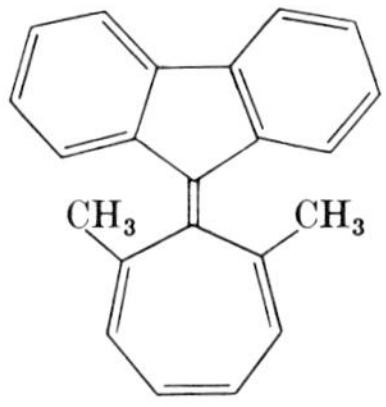

(381) 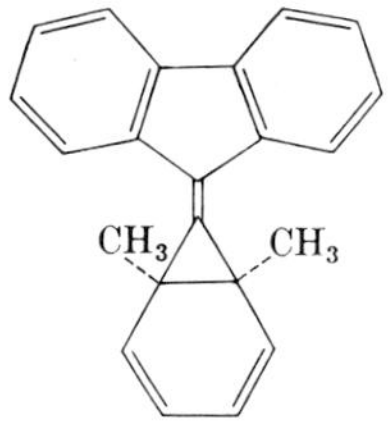   (382)

tendency to valence tautomerize to 381. It was thermally stable to 275°, and did not form Diels-Alder adducts with acetylenedicarboxylate or maleic anhydride (288).

The synthesis of a number of sesquifulvalene quinones has recently been reported (289). Indane-1,3-dione (383) reacted with two moles of tropylium bromide to give the 2,2-ditropylindan-1,3-dione (384), which on thermal decomposition gave 2,3-benzosesquifulvalene-1,4-quinone (385) as a red, crystalline solid. The parent compound, sesquifulvalene-1,4-quinone (386) was synthesized by the reaction of

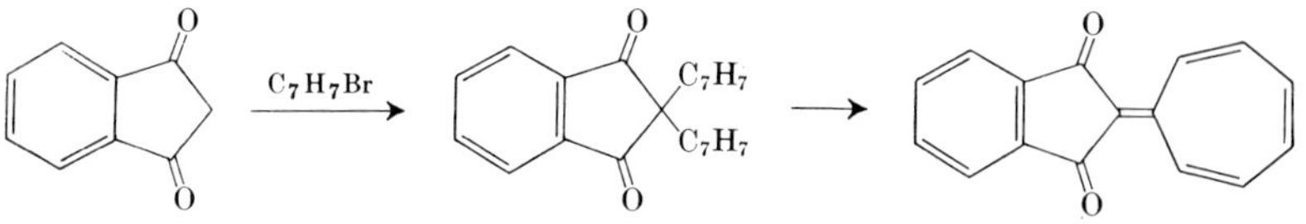

(383)   (384)   (385)

tropylium bromide with cyclopentene-3,5-dione, followed by dehydrogenation with chloranil. The quinones are high-melting, thermally stable, crystalline compounds, unaffected by light or oxygen. The double bond in the five-membered ring in **386** is reactive, and adds

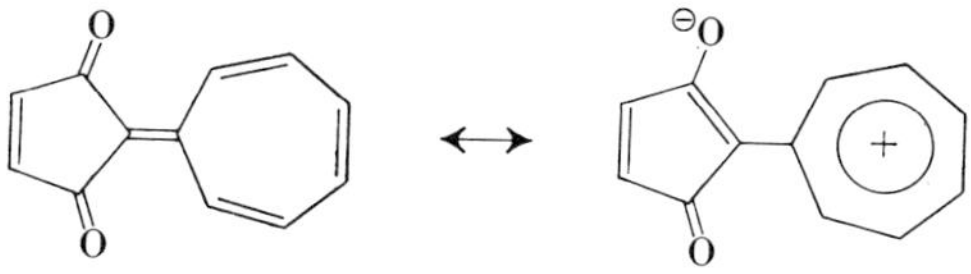

(386)   (386a)

bromine, cyclopentadiene, and diazomethane. The dipolar structure **386a** presumably contributes to the ground state stability of the system.

D. SYSTEMS WITH 6-MEMBERED RINGS

The phenalene system **(387)** is well known, and its chemistry has recently been reviewed (290). The cation **388a**, anion **388b**, and free radical **388c** are all known. There are a number of large

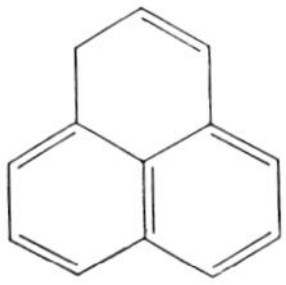

(387)

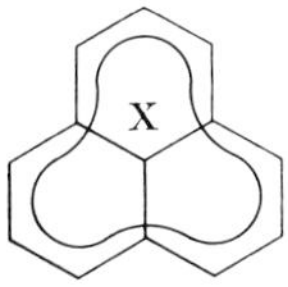

(388a) X = +
(388b) X = −
(388c) X = ·

polycyclic systems which, like phenalene, cannot be written with Kekulé structures. Triangulene **(389)** is such a system (291), and MO calculations predict that this hydrocarbon should exist as a triplet diradical (292). Clar and his co-workers have described an attempted synthesis (291).

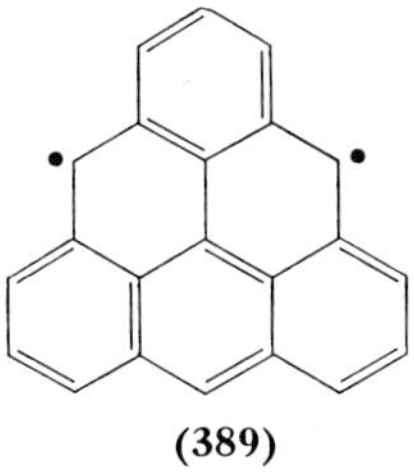

(389)

The synthesis of dicyclooctatetraeno[1,2:4,5]benzene **(393)** has recently been reported (293). 7,8-Dimethylenecyclo-1,3,5-triene **(390)** was reacted with cyclooctatrienyne **(391)** to give the Diels-Alder adduct **392**. Dehydrogenation with 2,3-dichloro-5,6-dicyano-p-benzoquinone in boiling benzene gave **393**. The NMR spectrum has the vinylic proton band at τ 3.47–4.12, indicating that **393** does not behave as an 18 π peripheral electron system. This suggests that structure **393a**, which does not contain a formal benzene ring, is not a significant contributor to the ground state of the molecule.

Staab and his co-workers (294) have synthesized a number of systems, such as **394**, in which the possibility exists of cyclic delocalization over the complete system. Such delocalization would take place at the expense of the discrete benzene structures, but no evidence for this has been detected.

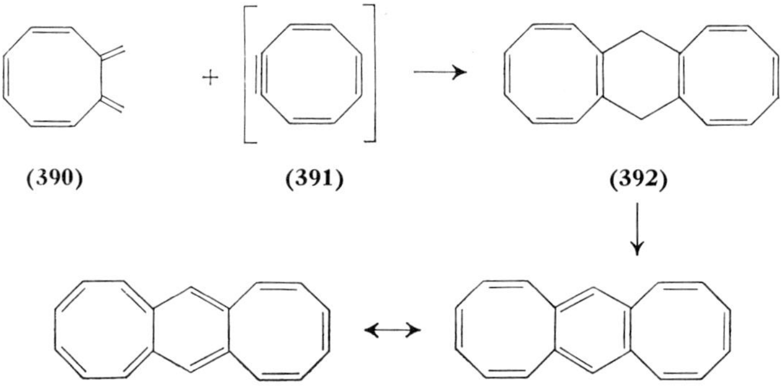

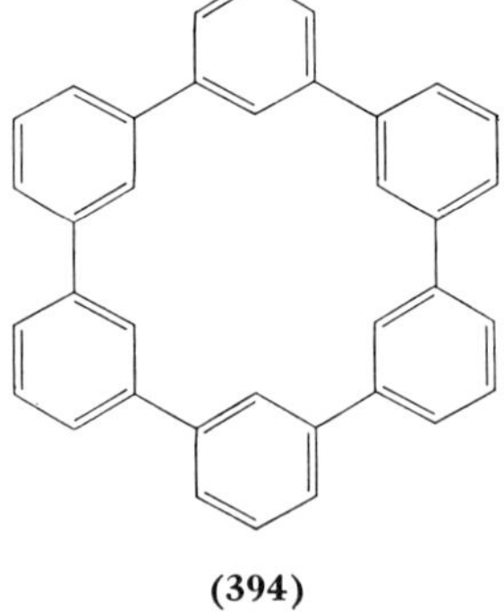

E. SYSTEMS WITH RINGS GREATER THAN 6-MEMBERED

Heptalene (**398**) has been the subject of a large number of theoretical calculations (97,235–9,282), and it is now generally agreed that the molecule will have alternant bonds and be of C_{2h} rather than D_{2h} symmetry. Heptalene has been prepared by Dauben and Bertelli (295). The ditosylate **395**, prepared in a three-step sequence from naphthalene-1,5-dicarboxylic acid, was solvolyzed with acetic acid, sodium dihydrogen phosphate to the dihydroheptalene **396**. Hydride abstraction gave the heptalinium ion (**397**) and subsequent deprotonation gave heptalene (**398**). Heptalene is more basic than azulene and reacts rapidly with oxygen, acids, and bromine. The NMR spectrum

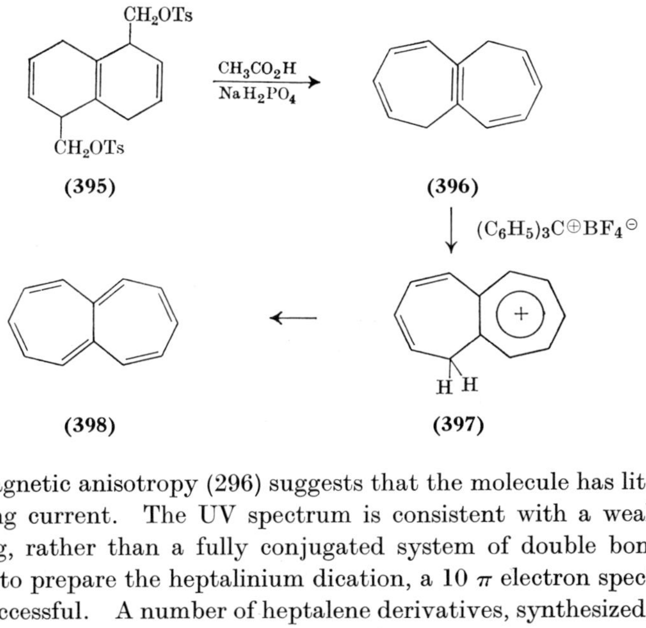

and diamagnetic anisotropy (296) suggests that the molecule has little, if any, ring current. The UV spectrum is consistent with a weakly interacting, rather than a fully conjugated system of double bonds. Attempts to prepare the heptalinium dication, a 10 π electron species, were unsuccessful. A number of heptalene derivatives, synthesized by Hafner et al., have been described previously.

Cyclooctatetraeno-cycloheptatriene (**401**) has been prepared by the reaction of 1,8-diformylcyclooctatetraene (**399**) with the bisphosphorane **400** (297). Removal of a proton from **401** would give the 14 π system **402**, consisting of fused $4n$ and $(4n + 2)\pi$ systems. However **401**, with potassium *tert*-butoxide in deuterated DMSO-*tert*-butyl alcohol, exchanges 20–30 times slower than cycloheptatriene.

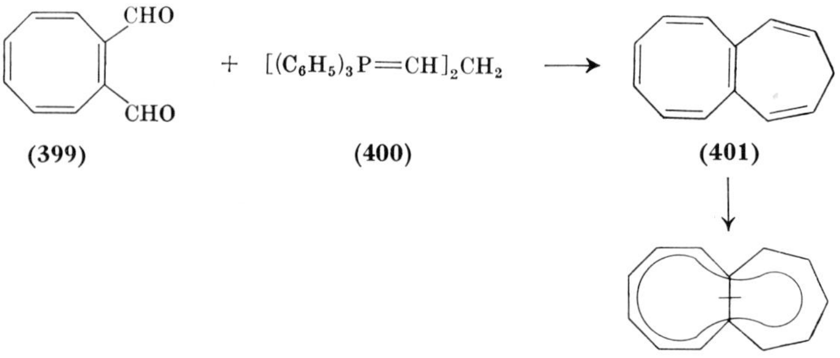

(399) + (400) [(C₆H₅)₃P=CH]₂CH₂ → (401)

↓

(402)

Heptafulvalene (404) was synthesized by Doering and Mayer (104), by reduction of the tropylium ion to give ditropyl (403), which on bromination and dehydromination gave 404

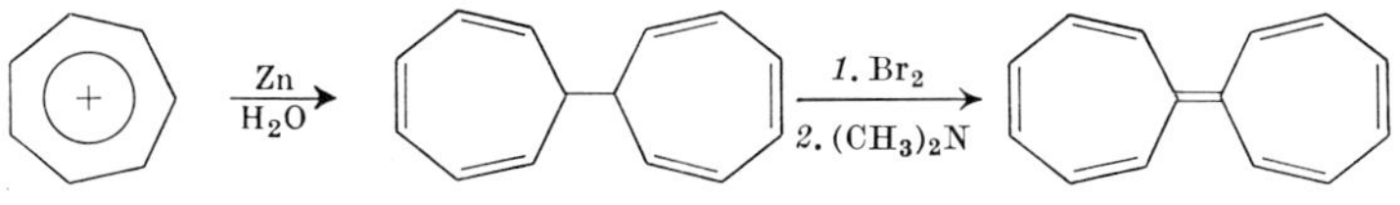

$$\underset{(403)}{\text{ditropyl}} \xrightarrow{\text{Zn/H}_2\text{O}} \underset{}{} \xrightarrow[2.\,(CH_3)_2N]{1.\,Br_2} \underset{(404)}{}$$

Heptafulvalene was obtained as almost black crystals, and was more stable than heptafulvene (128) towards acids and oxidizing agents. It had an extensive electronic spectrum, with maxima at 234 and 362 mμ, and did not give Diels-Alder adducts. The DE obtained from heat of hydrogenation measurements (110) was ca. 28 kcal mole^{-1}, considerably less than that predicted by simple MO calculations.

It was suggested (10a) that octalene (405) should have a large DE and might be considered to have a 14 π electron periphery. A more recent calculation (180), however, gives a low value for the DE, and this suggests that octalene will be a nonplanar polyolefin. The parent compound has not yet been synthesized, but hexabenzo-octalene (411)

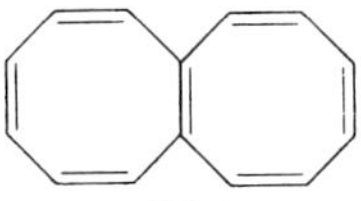

(405)

and benzo-octalene (407) have been reported. Benzo-octalene was prepared in low yield by the reaction of the diformyl compound 399 and the bisphosphorane 406. The NMR and UV spectra of 407 are

(399) + (406) [structure with =P(C₆H₅)₃ groups] → (407) [structure]

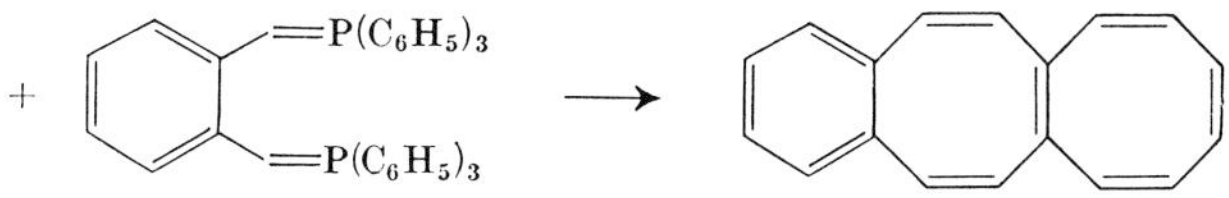

similar to benzocyclooctatetraene and indicate that **407** has the eight-membered rings in the tub conformations and is not an aromatic compound. Dihydrooctalene has been synthesized by a similar route, but the final double bond could not be introduced (297). Tochtermann (298) has prepared hexabenzo-octalene **(411)**, utilizing the ketone **408**, which was subjected to pinacolic reduction to give **409**. Rearrangement of **409** under strongly acidic conditions gave **410**, which on LAH reduction and acid rearrangement led to **411**. Hexabenzo-octalene is a colorless hydrocarbon with a UV spectrum similar to that of benzocyclooctatetraene.

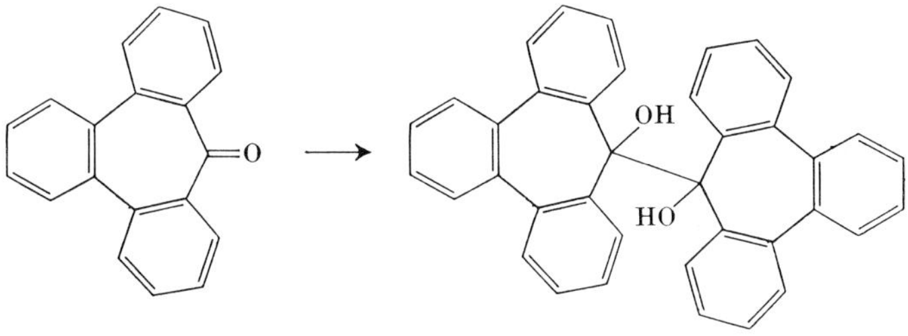

(408)   (409)

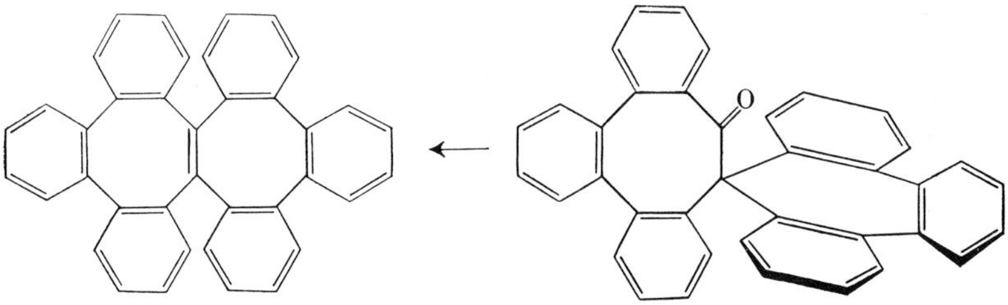

(411)   (410)

IV. Conclusion

The simple Hückel theory has been outstandingly successful in stimulating the experimental chemist to prepare new types of systems. In general, the predictions of the simple theory have been verified. The main areas of current interest are the preparation of medium ring annulenes; the synthesis of $4n\,\pi$ electron systems; the question whether there is a class of aromatic compounds formed by the fusion of $4n\,\pi$ electron systems; the preparation of aromatic systems with strained rings; and homoaromatic compounds. The preeminence of the $6\,\pi$ electron system for aromatic stability has been confirmed, and the properties of benzene and its derivatives appear to be unique. No satisfactory definition of aromaticity has yet been formulated, and it may well be that the range of properties exhibited by "aromatic" compounds is too great for them to be encompassed in any such comprehensive system.

V. Addendum

The addendum mainly covers work published between September 1966 and September 1967, as well as some earlier publications and privately communicated results.

The lectures presented at the International Symposium on Aromaticity, held at Sheffield in 1966, have now appeared (299).

A text on cyclobutadiene and related compounds has been published (300a). Dewar (300b) has outlined a perturbational MO method (PMO), based on HMO parameters, but which gives results in accord with SCF MO calculations. The same author has redefined aromaticity in terms of DE using a "real" classical molecule as the reference compound (300b).

Musher (301) has attacked the theoretical basis of the "ring current" concept, which has been defended (302).

The bond lengths, obtained by x-ray studies, of a series of compounds which differ only in bond hybridization, give some support to the view of Dewar and Schmeising that hybridization, rather than conjugation, is responsible for bond shortening 303).

II. MONOCYCLIC SYSTEMS

$A.\ n = 0$

Both the parent cyclopropenyl cation (1) (305) and cyclopropenone (17) (306) have been synthesized.

Reduction of tetrachlorocyclopropene (13) with tri-n-butyl tin hydride gave a mixture of mono-, di-, and trichlorocyclopropenes (411). 3-Chlorocyclopropene (411a) was isolated by preparative GLC. The NMR spectrum in SO_2 shows a single proton resonance at $3.28\,\tau$, presumably due to the rapid transfer of the chlorine between the three carbon atoms. Treatment of 411a with antimony pentachloride in

CH$_2$Cl$_2$ gave a quantitative yield of cyclopropenyl hexachloroantimonate (1a). The IR and NMR (singlet $-1.1\,\tau$, $J_{^{13}C-H}$ 265 cps) spectra are in accord with the assigned structure.

Hydrolysis of the mixture of chlorocyclopropenes (411) with cold water gave cyclopropenone (17), presumably arising from 411b, identified by its NMR (singlet $1.0\,\tau$, $J_{^{13}C-H}$ 230 cps) and IR (1870, 1835 cm^{-1}) spectra. Attempts to isolate 17 have so far been unsuccessful.

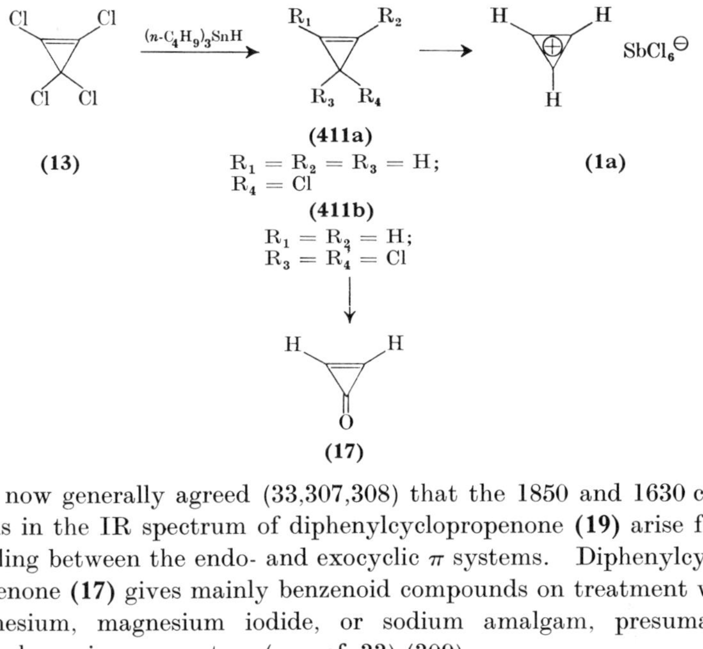

It is now generally agreed (33,307,308) that the 1850 and 1630 cm^{-1} bands in the IR spectrum of diphenylcyclopropenone (19) arise from coupling between the endo- and exocyclic π systems. Diphenylcyclopropenone (17) gives mainly benzenoid compounds on treatment with magnesium, magnesium iodide, or sodium amalgam, presumably through a prismane system (see ref. 33) (309).

A number of methylene cyclopropene derivatives, of the type 412, have been reported (310). The IR and NMR spectra suggest a large contribution from the dipolar form 412a.

The dipole moment of 413 (5.9 D in C$_6$H$_6$ at 25°) is also consistent with a considerable charge separation (310).

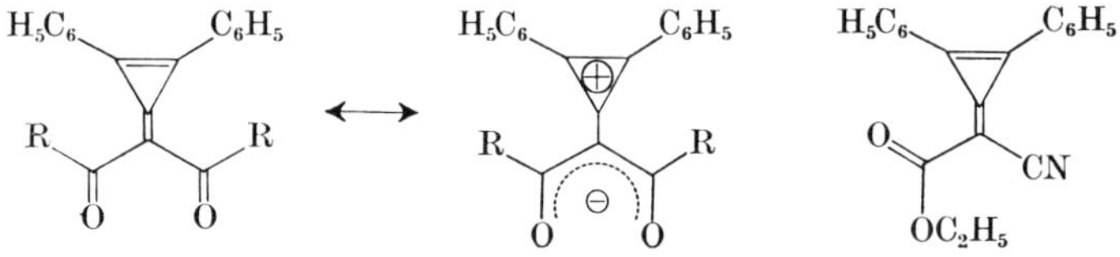

1-Dicyanomethylene-2,3-diphenylcyclopropene **(414)** reacts with enamines (e.g., **415**) to give ring-opened products (e.g., **417**), presumably through the intermediacy of the bicyclic system **416** (311).

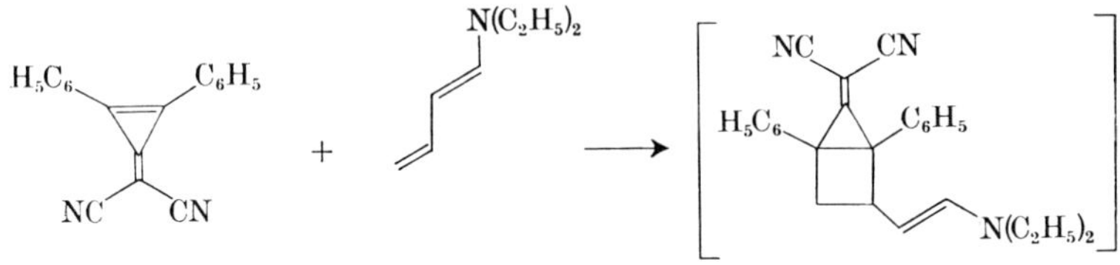

A short review on squaric acid **(57)** has appeared (312). A variety of compounds with active hydrogens condense with squaric acid to give highly colored compounds, for which structures such as **418** and **419** have been suggested (see ref. 59, p. 96) (313).

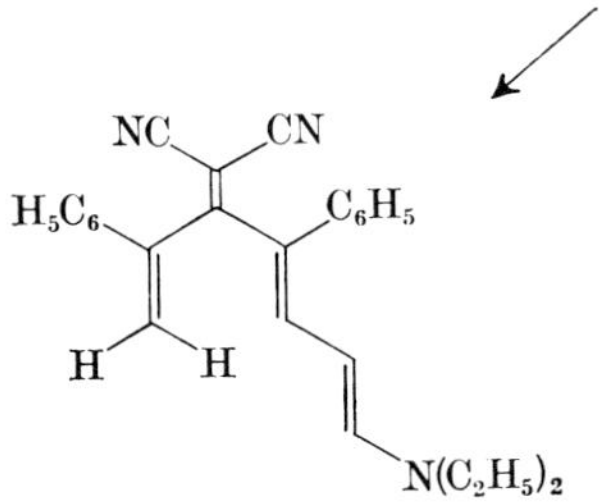

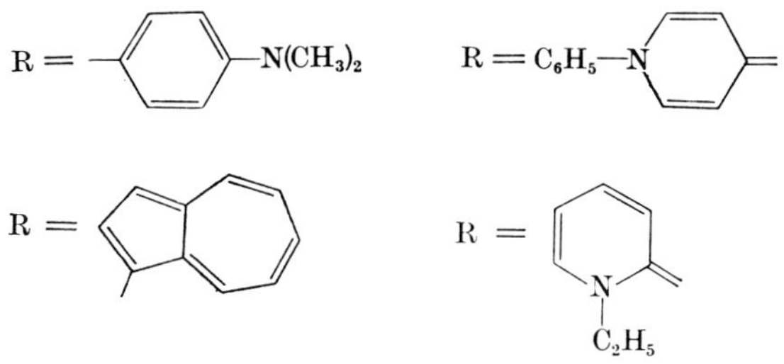

B. $n = 1$

The NMR spectrum of orientated cyclobutadiene iron tricarbonyl (71) in a nematic solvent has an eight-line spectrum, which is consistent with a square, rather than rectangular, cyclobutadienyl ring (314). A full paper on the interconversion of cyclobutadienyl complexes has appeared (see ref. 73) (315).

Some evidence for free cyclobutadiene has been inferred in the flash photolysis of cyclobutadiene iron tricarbonyl (71) by examining the change of the mass spectrum of the products with time (316). The m/e 52 signal decayed rapidly, and the peaks attributed to benzene and acetylene increased.

The possible intermediacy of chlorotrimethylcyclobutadiene (421) in the rearrangement of 3-dichloromethyl-1,2,3-trimethyl-cyclopropene (420) has been reported (317).

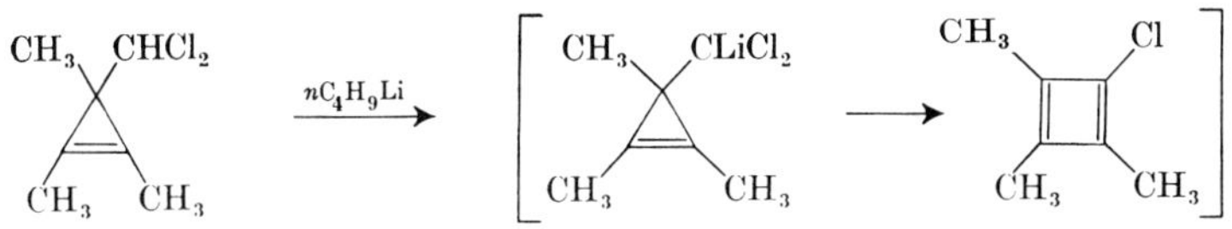

[Scheme: (420) → [intermediate] → (421) → Dimers]

The possible intermediacy of the bishomocyclopentadienide anion (424) was postulated by Brown and Occolowitz in the solvolysis of the bicyclic diene 422a (318). They found that the rate of exchange was 3×10^4 times as fast as that of the monoene 423. The anion 424 has now been observed directly by treatment of the methyl ether 422b with sodium potassium alloy, and its NMR and UV spectra have been reported (319,320).

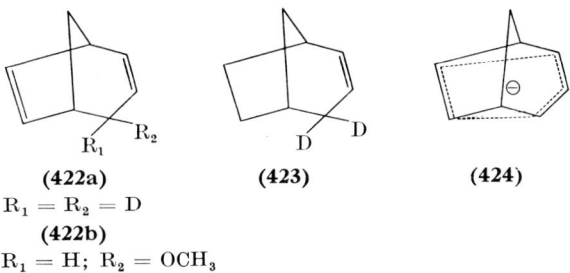

(422a) $R_1 = R_2 = D$
(422b) $R_1 = H; R_2 = OCH_3$
(423)
(424)

An x-ray structural analysis of 8,8-dicyanoheptafulvalene **(133a)** confirms that bond alternation occurs, and the length of the exocyclic double bond, 1.42 Å, supports the contention that the dipolar form makes a large contribution to the structure (321).

Cyclooctatrienone **(425)** was protonated with fluorosulfonic acid (FSO_3H) in sulfur dioxide to give the hydroxyhomotropylium cation **(426)** (322). The NMR spectrum shows a large chemical shift difference between H_b (8.68 τ) and H_a (5.6 τ).

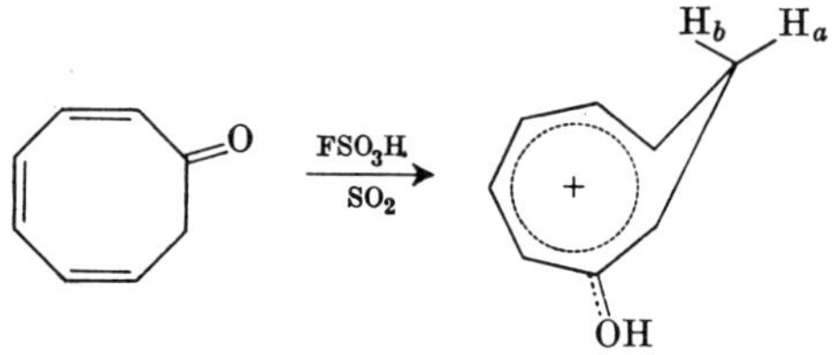

Treatment of *cis*-7,8-dichlorocyclooctatriene **(427)** with FSO_3H gave the *exo*-8-chlorohomotropylium cation **(428)** (323). The *endo* isomer **(429)** was obtained by the reaction of **427** with antimony pentafluoride (323). Evidence has been presented to indicate that **428** is an intermediate in the chlorination of cyclooctatetraene (324).

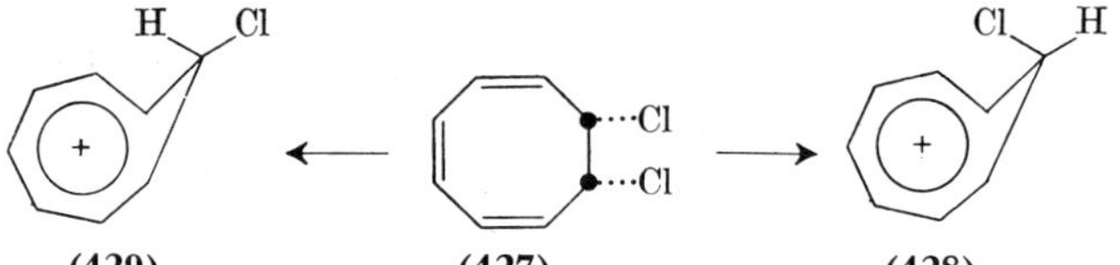

The electrochemical oxidation of COT in acetic acid gives products which can be accounted for by the intermediacy of either the cation radical or dication **139** (325).

C. $n = 2$

The ESR spectrum of the phenylcyclooctatetraene anion radical has been reported (326). Theoretical treatments of the ESR spectra of the alkyl cyclooctatetraene (327) and of the dibenzocyclooctatetraene (328) anion radicals have appeared.

[10] Annulene (175,176) has been prepared in solution at −190° by the photolysis of *trans*-9,10-dihydronaphthalene **(430)** (329a). On

warming the solution of [10]annulene to room temperature, *cis*-9,10-dihydronaphthalene **(181)** was obtained, and on treatment of the solution at −75° with diimide, a 40% yield of cyclodecane **(431)** was isolated.

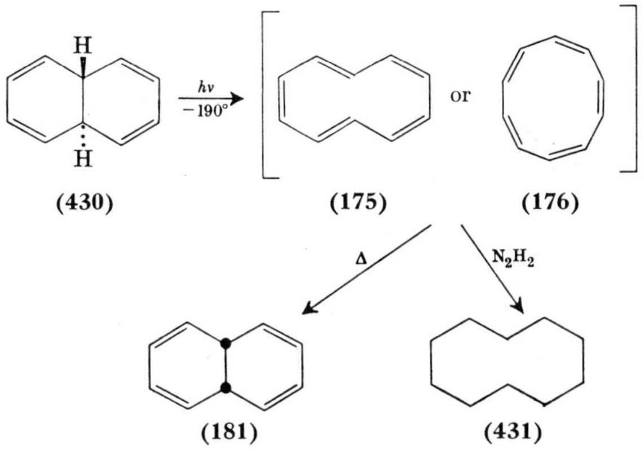

Masamune and his co-workers (329b) have recently prepared bicyclo[6.2.0]deca-2,4,6,9-tetraene **(433)** by low temperature photolysis of **432** in the presence of sodium methoxide. Thermal isomerization of **433** gave *trans*-9,10-dihydronaphthalene **(430)** quantitatively, possibly by a conrotatory opening of the cyclobutene ring to give **177** as an intermediate.

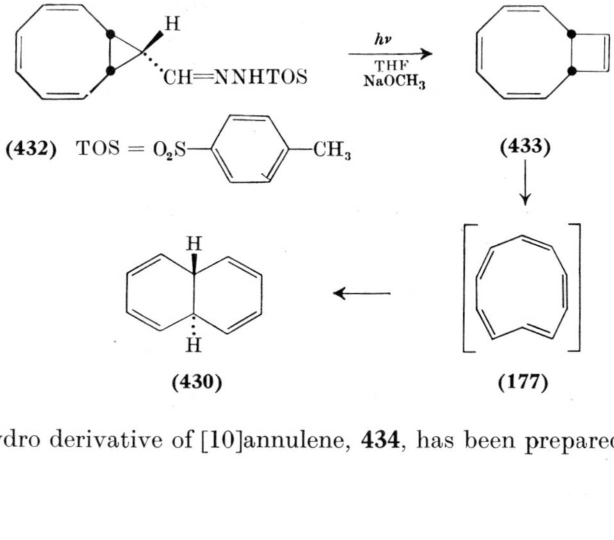

A dihydro derivative of [10]annulene, **434**, has been prepared (330)·

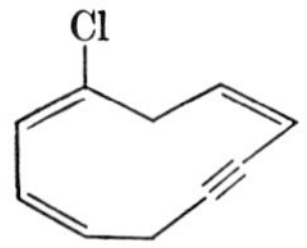

(434)

The thermal rearrangement of dimethyl 9,10-dicarboxy-9,10-dihydronaphthalene **(435)** gave a mixture of esters from which the disubstituted naphthalenes **436, 437**, and **438** were isolated (331). The presence of **438** indicates that a simple valence tautomerism to a substituted [10]annulene is not responsible for the products. The mechanism suggested for the pyrolysis of the Diels-Alder adducts of COT (332,333) may also be oversimplified.

The substituted [10]annulene **439** has been prepared by a Wittig reaction between naphthalene-1,8-dialdehyde and the ylid obtained from 1,8-bis(bromomethyl)naphthalene (334).

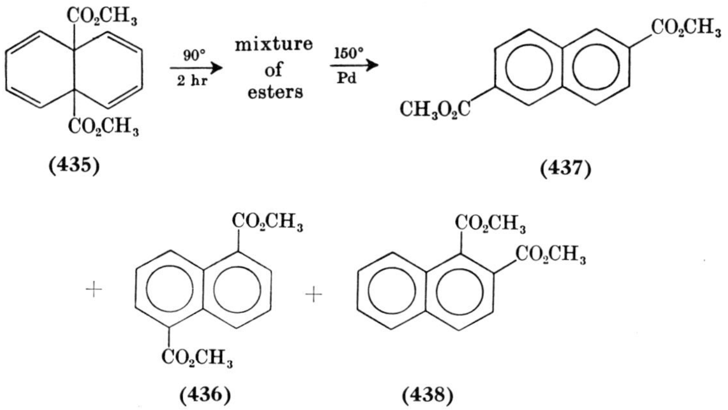

(435) → (90°, 2 hr) mixture of esters → (150°, Pd) **(437)**

(436) + **(438)**

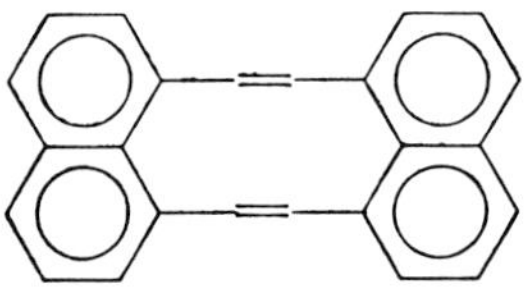

(439) 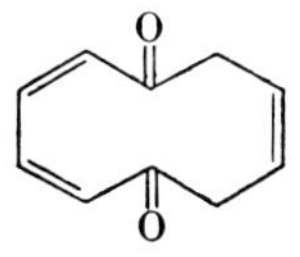 **(440)**

The diketone **440** does not enolize to [10]annulene hydroquinone (335).

Mono-*trans*-1,2:3,4:7,8-Tribenzo[10]annulene **(441)** has been prepared by a Wittig reaction between phthaldehyde and the ylid derived from 2,2'-bis-(bromomethyl)biphenyl **(336)**.

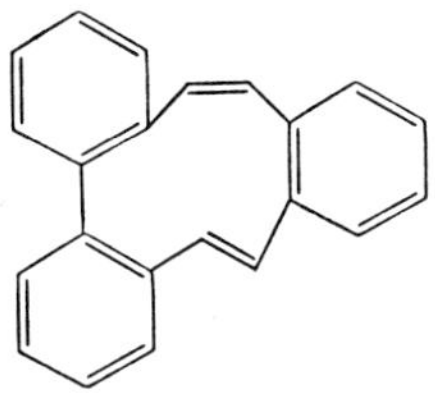

(441)

The dipole moments of a number of bridged [10]annulenes **(190, 191b, 191c, 196, 197)** are in agreement with the previously established structures if a partial moment of ca. 0.8 D is assigned to the nonplanar π-electron system **(337)**. An NMR **(338)** and x-ray **(339)** study of 1,6-methano[10]annulene chromium tricarbonyl shows that the extended aromatic structure is maintained and that the ring is asymmetrically bonded to the metal. The substituted 1,6-oxide[10]annulene **442** has been prepared **(340)**, and the NMR spectrum is similar to that of 1,6-oxido[10]-annulene **(196)**, but the UV spectrum shows much less intense bands. The change in the electronic spectrum on protonation suggests that the 10 π system is converted into the 14 π *cis*-15,16-epoxy-15,16-dehydropyrene **(443)**.

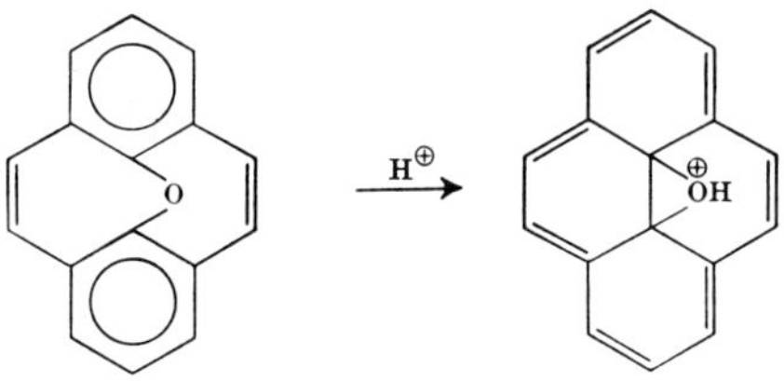

(442)   **(443)**

D.

The energy barriers to interconversion of external and internal protons for a number of annulenes and dehydroannulenes have been determined by NMR methods, and have low values (9–14 kcal/mole) **(341)**. The energy barrier of the $4n + 2$ π compounds is only slightly higher than that of the equivalent $4n$ compound.

1. $n = 3$

The ESR spectrum of the radical anion obtained by treatment of 1,8-bisdehydro[14]annulene **(222)** with sodium in dimethoxyethane or THF has been reported, and the spin densities agree with the HMO, but not the SCF calculations (342).

Full accounts of the preparation (343) and properties (344) of *trans*-15,16-dimethyldihydropyrene **(234)** have appeared. The preparation and properties of *trans*-15,16-diethyldihydropyrene **(444)** have also been reported (345). From the NMR spectrum the methylene protons on the ethyl group are more "inside" the ring than the methyl protons. The electronic spectrum of 2-acetamino-*trans*-15,16-dimethyldihydropyrene **(445)** resembles that of **234** and **444**, and is in agreement with theoretical predictions deduced from a configuration interaction model with a D_2h π-perimeter (346).

Vogel and Günther (347) have reported that the *cis*-diepoxide **446**, but not the *trans*-diepoxide **447**, will dehydrogenate to 1,6:8,13-diepoxy[14]annulene **(237b)**.

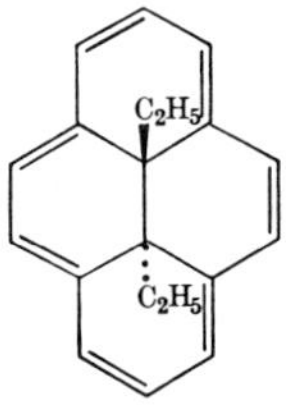

(444) 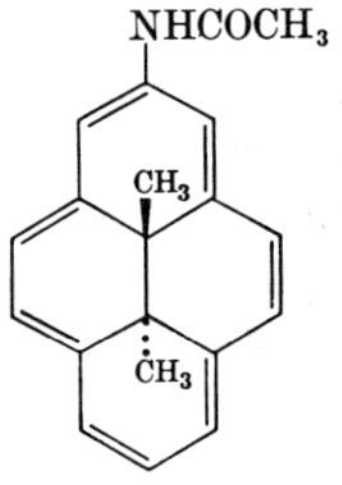   **(445)**

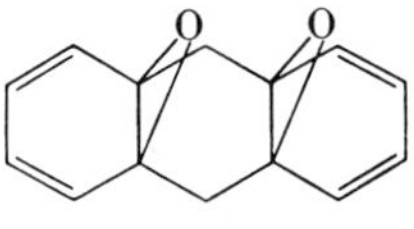

(446) 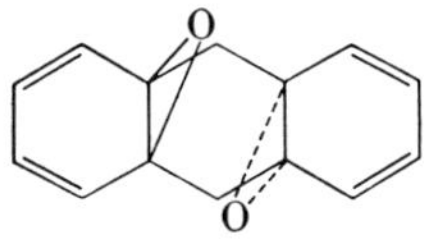   **(447)**

2. $n = 4$

A Pople-Santry calculation suggests that the difference in the bond lengths of [18]annulene **(253a)** is due to differences in σ bond strength arising from a distortion of the bond angle from 120° (348). Novel conformational effects have been observed in substituted [18]annulenes

(448), which can be accounted for by supposing that the substituent and its five associated protons cannot be transferred to a position inside the ring (449) (349).

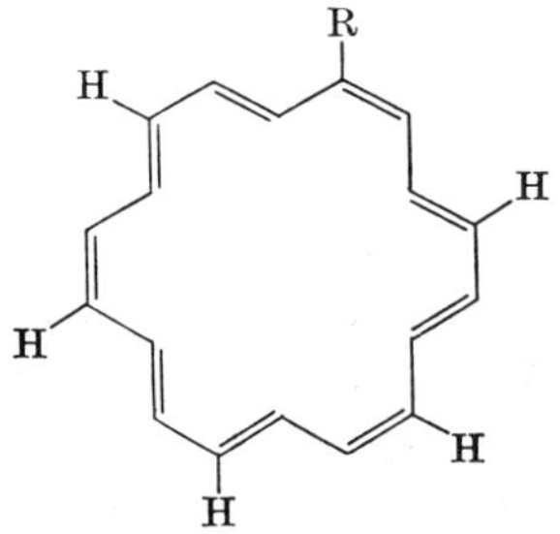

(448a) R = NO$_2$
(448b) R = COCH$_3$ (449)

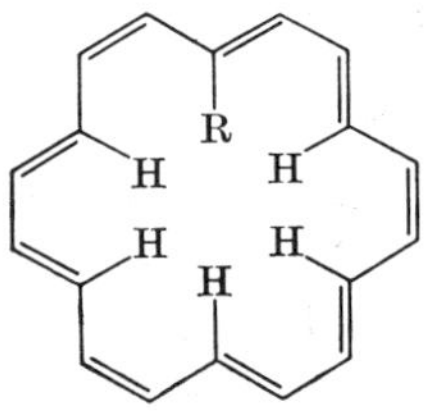

Hexadehydro[18]annulene (450) has been synthesized (350), and the NMR spectrum, a singlet at 3.0 τ, shows a remarkable chemical shift difference from that of 1,5,9-tridehydro[12]annulene (209), 5.58 τ, as predicted by the paramagnetic ring current theory (216,217,351).

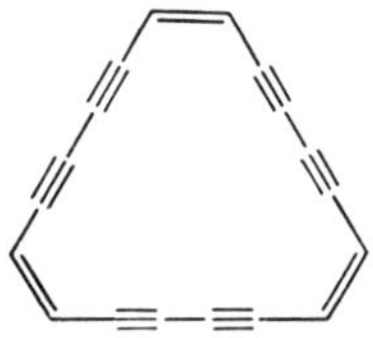

(450)

A tridehydro[26]annulene has been prepared (352). Its NMR spectrum, resembles that of a linear polyolefin rather than one of the smaller annulenes.

III. POLYCYCLIC SYSTEMS

The PMO method (300b) can be applied to polycyclic, as well as monocyclic, systems; it predicts that pentalene and heptalene will be antiaromatic.

HMO calculations (353), with the addition of σ-bond compression effects, indicate that methylenecyclopropene (30), triafulvalene (269), and triapentafulvalene (270) will show considerable bond fixation, and that the DE and diamagnetic anisotropy will be much lower than that predicted by the simple HMO theory.

Zahradnik and his co-workers have continued their theoretical studies on nonalternant hydrocarbons (354). Boyd (355) considers that pentalene and heptalene are representatives of two classes of hydrocarbons, and reports calculations for other members of the series, all of which are derived from perturbed $4n$ systems.

B. Systems with 4-Membered Rings

The products obtained from oxidizing (benzocyclobutadiene)iron tricarbonyl **(293)** are derived from benzocyclobutadiene **(288)**, but depend on the nature of the oxidizing agent (356a). Lead tetraacetate in pyridine gave the dimer **290**, whereas using silver ions as the oxidant gave **294**. The silver ion was shown to catalyze the conversion of the Diels-Alder intermediate **289** into **451**, which, on subsequent rearrangement to **452** followed by intramolecular Diels-Alder addition, gave **294**.

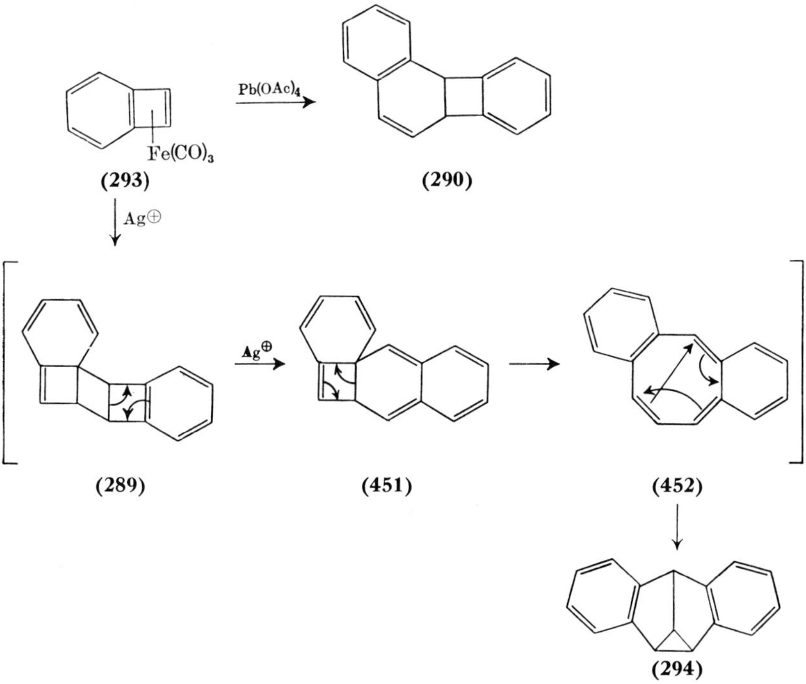

Blomquist and Hruby (356b) prepared 1,2-bis(triphenylphosphoranyl)-benzocyclobutene **(453)**, in which the dipolar form **(454)**, a 10π system, is an important resonance contributor. This system is a benzannelated derivative of the cyclobutadienyl dianion **(106)**.

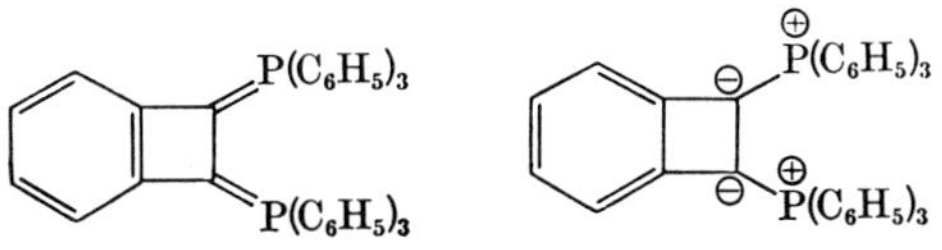

(453) **(454)**

C. Systems with 5-Membered Rings

1,3-Bis(dimethylamino)pentalene **(460)** has been prepared by Hafner and his co-workers (357). Sodium cyclopentadienide **(455)** reacts with the complex **456**, prepared from tetra-*N*-methyl-malondiamide and triethyloxonium tetrafluoroborate, to give the fulvene **457**. This, when boiled in xylene, loses dimethylamine and gives 3-(dimethylamino)-1(2*H*)pentalenone **(458)**, which forms the immonium perchlorate **(459)** on treatment with dimethyl ammonium perchlorate. Deprotonation gave **460** as a dark blue crystalline solid with the expected

(455) **(456)** **(457)** **(459)** **(458)** **(460)** **(461)**

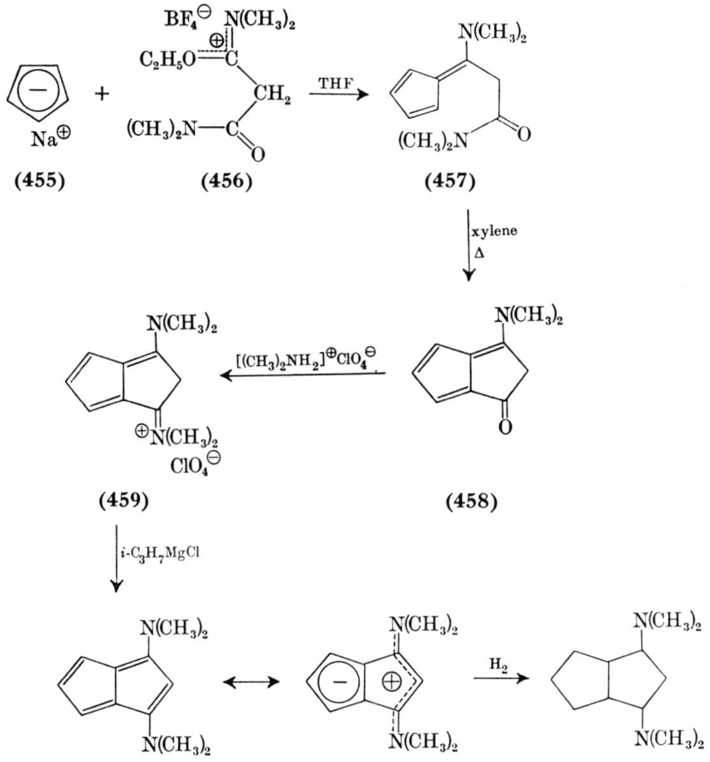

UV and NMR spectral properties. The compound **460** is stable in oxygen, gives deep blue solutions in aprotic solvents, and on full hydrogenation gives **461**. The pentalenone **458** is easily enolized to **462**, in contrast to 1,4-pentalenedione **(463)** (358).

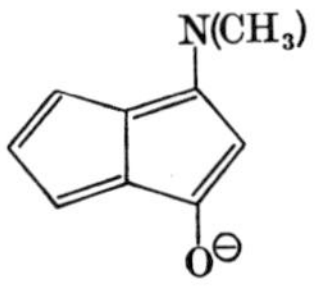

(462) 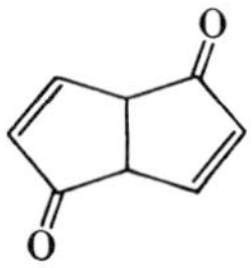   **(463)**

Pyracylene **(466a)** (359) and 1,2-dibromopyracylene **(466b)** (360) have been prepared. Bromination of pyracene **(464)** with NBS gave the tetrabromide **(465)**, which on treatment with potassium iodide gave a red solution of **466a**. The NMR spectrum showed two singlets of equal intensity at 3.48 and 3.99 τ, and hydrogenation gave a quantitative yield of pyracene. The upfield shift of the NMR spectrum is consistent with the system possessing a 12 π periphery. Attempts to isolate solid pyracylene were unsuccessful. The dibromide **466b** was prepared in a similar manner.

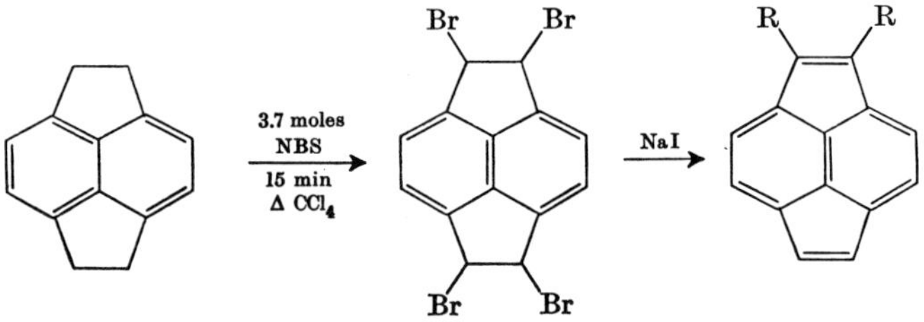

(464)   **(465)**   **(466a)** R = H
                            (466b) R = Br

Corannulene **(467)** (361) and the corannulene anion radical **(468)** (362) have been prepared. The ESR spectrum of the dark green

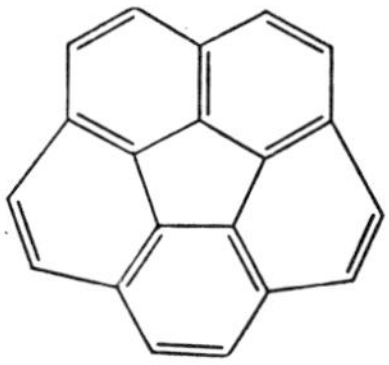

(467) 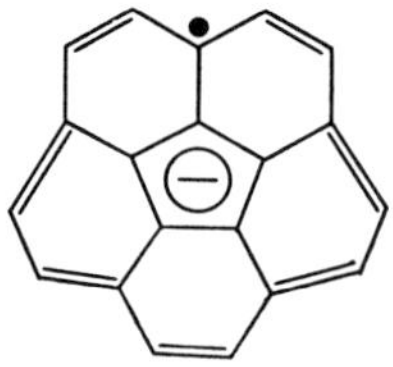   **(468)**

solutions of the anion radical show 11 equally spaced lines, and the bowl shaped anion may be considered to have a 15π electron peripheral system.

The ESR spectra of the dianions of fluorene and a number of fluorene derivatives have been obtained (363,364).

Octabromofulvalene **(469)** has been prepared, and it has properties similar to those of octachlorofulvalene **(372)** (365).

The preparation of *sym*-dibenzfulvalene **(470)** (366) has been reported.

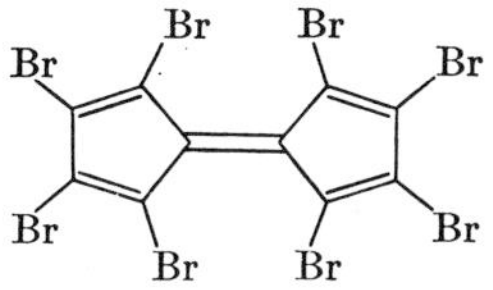

(469) 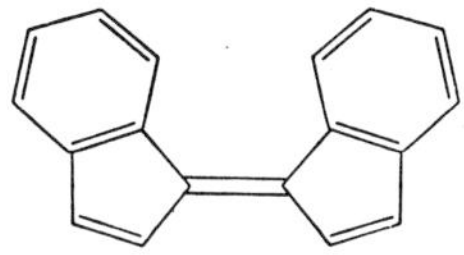   **(470)**

Prinzbach and his co-workers have given full details of their preparation of sesquifulvalenes (367). The NMR spectra of a number of substituted sesquifulvalenes have been correlated with the π-electron distribution (368).

The interesting pentaundecafulvalene **(471)**, together with the isomers **472** and **473**, was synthesized by treatment of lithium fluorenide with bicyclo[5.4.1]dodecapentaenylium fluoroborate **(202)**, followed by oxidation (369). The NMR spectrum is in accord with the proposed structure **(471)**. The compound **(471)** has a low basicity and does not react with dimethyl acetylenedicarboxylate.

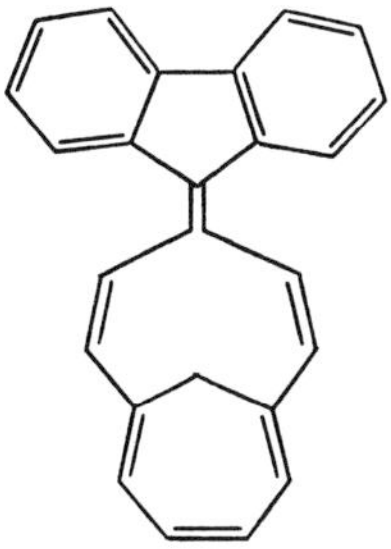

(471) 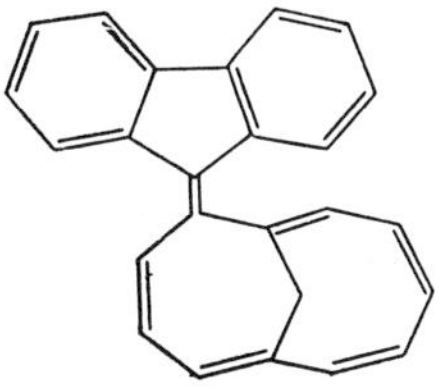   **(472)** 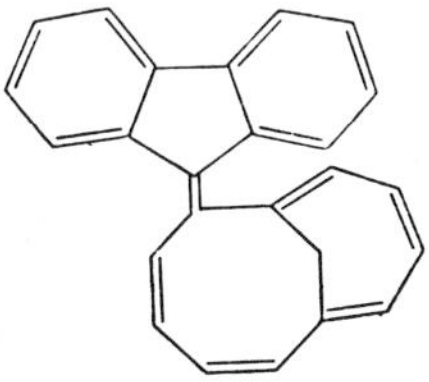   **(473)**

D. Systems with 6-Membered Rings

Staab and his co-workers have described the preparation and properties of a number of cyclic phenylenes, none of which exhibit delocalization over the complete system (370). The electronic spectra of a number of phenalenyl ions have been analyzed theoretically (371).

The bicyclic ketone **474a** (372) and the methoxy ketone **474b** (373) have recently been prepared, and the dipolar structure **475** appears to make a considerable contribution to the ground state.

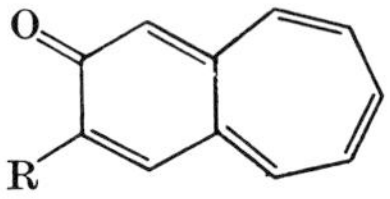

(**474a**) R = H
(**474b**) R = OCH$_3$

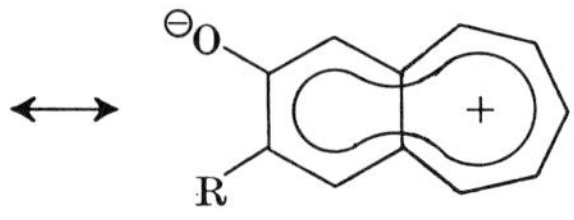

(**475**)

E. Systems with Rings Greater than 6-Membered

A new synthesis of heptafulvalene (**404**) has been reported (374). The octalene derivative **476** has been prepared (375).

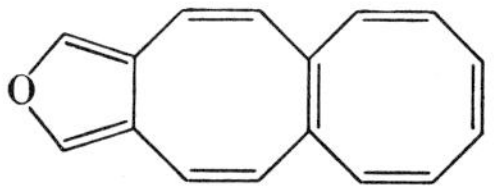

(**476**)

ACKNOWLEDGMENTS

The authors wish to thank Professors R. Breslow, T. J. Katz, and F. Sondheimer for kindly reading the manuscript and for making many helpful suggestions.

REFERENCES

1. J. R. Partington, *A History of Chemistry*, Vol. 4, Macmillan, London, 1964, p. 553.
2. J. R. Partington, *A History of Chemistry*, Vol. 4, Macmillan, London 1964, p. 841.
3. J. W. Armit and R. Robinson, *J. Chem. Soc.*, **1922**, 827; **1925**, 1604.
4. R. Willstätter and E. Waser, *Ber.*, **44**, 3423 (1911); R. Willstätter and M. Heidelberger, *Ber.*, **46**, 517 (1913).
5. E. Hückel, *International Conference on Physics, London*, **1934**, Vol. 2, The Physical Society, London, 1935.
6. M. J. S. Dewar, *Nature*, **155**, 50,141,479 (1945).
7. W. von E. Doering and L. J. Knox, *J. Am. Chem. Soc.*, **76**, 3203 (1954).
8. R. Breslow, *Chem. Eng. News*, **43**, xxvi, 90 (1965).
9. D. Ginsburg, *Non-Benzenoid Aromatic Compounds*, Interscience, New York, 1959.

10(a) A. Streitwieser, *Molecular Orbital Theory for Organic Chemists*, Wiley, New York, 1961, Chap. 10; (b) M. E. Vol'pin, *Russ. Chem. Rev.*, **29**, 129 (1960); (c) W. Baker, *Chem. Brit.*, **1965**, 191,250; (d) K. Hafner, *Angew. Chem.*, **75**, 1041 (1963); *Angew. Chem. Intern. Ed. Engl.*, **3**, 165 (1964).

11. D. M. G. Lloyd, *Carbocyclic Non-Benzenoid Aromatic Compounds*, Elsevier, London, 1966.
12. J. D. Roberts, A. Streitwieser, and C. M. Regan, *J. Am. Chem. Soc.*, **74**, 4579 (1952).
13. R. Breslow and C. Yuan, *J. Am. Chem. Soc.*, **80**, 5991 (1958).
14. M. Sundaralingam and L. H. Jensen, *J. Am. Chem. Soc.*, **88**, 198 (1966).
15. (a) R. Breslow and H. Höver, *J. Am. Chem. Soc.*, **82**, 2644 (1960); (b) R. Breslow, H. Höver, and H. W. Chang, *J. Am. Chem. Soc.*, **84**, 3168 (1962).
16. These values have been converted to the τ scale from the shifts given in ref. 15b in ppm from benzene (taken as 2.73 τ).
17. D. G. Farnum and M. Burr, *J. Am. Chem. Soc.*, **82**, 2651 (1960).
18. R. Breslow, J. Lockhart, and H. W. Chang, *J. Am. Chem. Soc.*, **83**, 2375 (1961).
19. R. Breslow and H. W. Chang, *J. Am. Chem. Soc.*, **83**, 2367 (1961).
20. S. L. Manatt and J. D. Roberts, *J. Org. Chem.*, **24**, 1336 (1959).
21. R. Breslow, W. Bahary, and W. Reinmuth, *J. Am. Chem. Soc.*, **83**, 1763 (1961).
22. R. Breslow and P. Dowd, *J. Am. Chem. Soc.*, **85**, 2729 (1963); R. Breslow, P. Gal, H. W. Chang, and L. J. Altman, *J. Am. Chem. Soc.*, **87**, 5139 (1965).
23. S. W. Tobey and R. West, *J. Am. Chem. Soc.*, **88**, 2481 (1966); R. West, A. Sado, and S. W. Tobey, *J. Am. Chem. Soc.*, **88**, 2488 (1966).
24. G. L. Closs and V. N. M. Rao, *J. Am. Chem. Soc.*, **88**, 4116 (1966).
25. (a) G. B. Kistiakowsky and J. V. Michael, *J. Chem. Phys.*, **40**, 1447 (1964), and refs. therein; (b) G. P. Glass and G. B. Kistiakowsky, *J. Chem. Phys.*, **40**, 1448 (1964).
26. *Catalogue of Mass Spectral Data*, Vol. 2, Ann. Pet. Inst., Project 44, p. 508; R. Grigg, M. V. Sargent, D. H. Williams, and J. A. Knight, *Tetrahedron*, **21**, 3441 (1965); however see W. H. Pirkle, *J. Am. Chem. Soc.*, **87**, 3022 (1965).
27. E. J. Corey and J. Streith, *J. Am. Chem. Soc.*, **86**, 950 (1964).
28. Cyclopropanones have recently been reported in solution. See W. B. Hammond and N. J. Turro, *J. Am. Chem. Soc.*, **88**, 2880 (1966).
29. D. N. Kursanov, M. E. Vol'pin, and Yu. D. Kovenshkov, *J. Gen. Chem. USSR (Eng. Transl.)*, **30**, 2855 (1960).
30. R. Breslow, R. Haynie, and J. Mirra, *J. Am. Chem. Soc.*, **81**, 247 (1959).
31. A. Krebs, *Angew. Chem.*, **77**, 10 (1965); *Angew. Chem. Intern. Ed. Engl.*, **4**, 10 (1965).
32. R. Breslow, T. Eicher, A. Krebs, R. A. Peterson, and J. Posner, *J. Am. Chem. Soc.*, **87**, 1320 (1965).

33. (a) R. Breslow and L. J. Altman, *J. Am. Chem. Soc.*, **88**, 504 (1966); (b) S. Andreas, *J. Am. Chem. Soc.*, **87**, 3941 (1965).
34. G. Quinkert, K. Opitz, W. W. Wiersdorff, and J. Weinlich, *Tetrahedron Letters*, **1963**, 1863.
35. R. Breslow, L. J. Altman, A. Krebs, E. Mohacsi, I. Murata, R. A. Peterson, and J. Posner, *J. Am. Chem. Soc.*, **87**, 1326 (1965).
36. E. V. Dehmlow, *Tetrahedron Letters*, **1965**, 2317; **1966**, 3763.
37. N. J. McCorkindale, R. A. Raphael, W. T. Scott, and B. Zwanenburg, *Chem. Commun.*, **1966**, 133.
38. A. S. Kende, *J. Am. Chem. Soc.*, **85**, 1882 (1963).
39. D. G. Farnum, J. Chickos, and P. E. Thurston, *J. Am. Chem. Soc.*, **88**, 3075 (1966).
40. M. Battiste, *J. Am. Chem. Soc.*, **86**, 942 (1964).
41. W. M. Jones and J. M. Denham, *J. Am. Chem. Soc.*, **86**, 944 (1964).
42. T. J. Katz, J. R. Hall, and W. C. Neikam, *J. Am. Chem. Soc.*, **84**, 3199 (1962).
43. T. J. Katz and E. H. Gold, *J. Am. Chem. Soc.*, **86**, 1600 (1964); *J. Org. Chem.*, **31**, 372 (1966).
44. C. F. Wilcox and D. L. Nealy, *J. Org. Chem.*, **28**, 3446 (1963).
45. H. H. Freedman and A. M. Frantz, *J. Am. Chem. Soc.*, **84**, 4165 (1962).
46. R. F. Bryan, *J. Am. Chem. Soc.*, **86**, 733 (1964).
47. H. H. Freedman and A. E. Young, *J. Am. Chem. Soc.*, **86**, 734 (1964).
48. D. G. Farnum and B. Webster, *J. Am. Chem. Soc.*, **85**, 3504 (1963).
49. E. J. Smutny and J. D. Roberts, *J. Am. Chem. Soc.*, **77**, 3420 (1955).
50. E. J. Smutny, M. C. Caserio, and J. D. Roberts, *J. Am. Chem. Soc.*, **82**, 1793 (1960).
51. C. M. Sharts and J. D. Roberts, *J. Am. Chem. Soc.*, **83**, 871 (1961).
52. A. T. Blomquist and E. A. LaLancette, *J. Am. Chem. Soc.*, **83**, 1387 (1961).
53. A. T. Blomquist and R. A. Vierling, *Tetrahedron Letters*, **1961**, 655.
54. J. D. Park, S. Cohen, and J. R. Lacher, *J. Am. Chem. Soc.*, **84**, 2919 (1962).
55. R. West, H. Y. Niu, D. L. Powell, and M. V. Evans, *J. Am. Chem. Soc.*, **82**, 6204 (1960).
56. S. Cohen and S. G. Cohen, *J. Am. Chem. Soc.*, **88**, 1533 (1966).
57. K. Yamada, N. Mizuno, and Y. Hirata, *Bull. Chem. Soc. Japan*, **31**, 543 (1958); M. Washino, K. Yamada, and K. Kurita, *Bull. Chem. Soc. Japan*, **31**, 552 (1958).
58. R. West, H. Y. Niu, and M. Ito, *J. Am. Chem. Soc.*, **85**, 2584 (1963); M. Ito and R. West, *J. Am. Chem. Soc.*, **85**, 2580 (1963).
59. R. West and D. L. Powell, *J. Am. Chem. Soc.*, **85**, 2577 (1963).
60. R. Breslow and M. Battiste, *Chem. Ind. (London)*, **1958**, 1143.

61. For example J. E. Lennard Jones and J. Turkevich, *Proc. Roy. Soc. (London)*, *Ser. A.*, **158**, 297 (1937); G. W. Wheland, *Proc. Roy. Soc. (London), Ser. A.*, **164**, 397 (1938); C. A. Coulson and W. E. Moffitt, *Phil. Mag.*, **40**, 1 (1949); A. D. Liehr, *Z. Naturforsch.*, **16a**, 641 (1961); L. C. Snyder, *J. Chem. Phys.*, **33**, 619 (1960).
62. M. J. S. Dewar and G. J. Gleicher, *J. Am. Chem. Soc.*, **87**, 3255 (1965).
63. H. C. Longuet-Higgins and L. E. Orgel, *J. Chem. Soc.*, **1956**, 1969.
64. R. Criegee and G. Schröder, *Ann. Chem.*, **623**, 1 (1959); R. Criegee, *Angew. Chem.*, **74**, 703 (1962); *Angew. Chem. Intern. Ed. Eng.*, **1**, 521 (1962).
65. R. Criegee and P. Ludwig, *Chem. Ber.*, **94**, 2038 (1961).
66. W. Hübel and E. H. Braye, *J. Inorg. Nucl. Chem.*, **10**, 250 (1959).
67. R. P. Dodge and V. Schomaker, *Nature*, **186**, 798 (1960).
68. J. D. Dunitz, H. C. Mez, O. S. Mills, and H. M. M. Shearer, *Helv. Chim. Acta*, **45**, 647 (1962).
69. L. Malatesta, G. Santarella, L. Vallarino, and F. Zingales, *Angew. Chem.*, **72**, 34 (1960).
70. A. T. Blomquist and P. M. Maitlis, *J. Am. Chem. Soc.*, **84**, 2329 (1962).
71. A. Nakamura and N. Hagihara, *Bull. Chem. Soc. Japan*, **34**, 452 (1961).
72. H. H. Freedman, *J. Am. Chem. Soc.*, **83**, 2194, 2195 (1961).
73. P. M. Maitlis and M. L. Games, *Can. J. Chem.*, **42**, 183 (1964).
74. M. Avram, H. P. Fritz, H. Keller, G. Mateescu, J. F. W. McOmie, N. Sheppard, and C. D. Nenitzescu, *Tetrahedron*, **19**, 187 (1963).
75. M. Avram, H. P. Fritz, H. Keller, C. G. Kreiter, G. Mateescu, J. F. W. McOmie, N. Sheppard, and C. D. Nenitzescu, *Tetrahedron Letters*, **1963**, 1611.
76. G. F. Emerson, L. Watts, and R. Pettit, *J. Am. Chem. Soc.*, **87**, 131 (1965).
77. M. Avram, I. Dinulescu, M. Elian, M. Farcasiu, E. Marica, G. Mateescu, and C. D. Nenitzescu, *Chem. Ber.*, **97**, 372 (1964).
78. J. D. Fitzpatrick, L. Watts, G. F. Emerson, and R. Pettit, *J. Am. Chem. Soc.*, **87**, 3254 (1965).
79. (a) P. M. Maitlis, *Advan. Organometal. Chem.*, **4**, 95 (1966); (b) H. P. Fritz *Advan. Organometal. Chem.*, **1**, 239 (1964).
80. A. T. Blomquist and Y. C. Meinwald, *J. Am. Chem. Soc.*, **81**, 667 (1959).
81. A. T. Blomquist and P. M. Maitlis, *Proc. Chem. Soc.*, **1961**, 332.
82. W. D. Huntsman and H. J. Wristers, *J. Am. Chem. Soc.*, **85**, 3308 (1963).
83. K. Nagarajan, M. C. Caserio, and J. D. Roberts, *J. Am. Chem. Soc.*, **86**, 449 (1964).
84. E. H. White and H. C. Dunathan, *J. Am. Chem. Soc.*, **86**, 453 (1964).
85. L. Watts, J. D. Fitzpatrick, and R. Pettit, *J. Am. Chem. Soc.*, **87**, 3253 (1965).
86. G. D. Burt and R. Pettit, *Chem. Commun.*, **1965**, 517.
87. L. Watts, J. D. Fitzpatrick, and R. Pettit, *J. Am. Chem. Soc.*, **88**, 623 (1966).

88. R. Breslow, D. Kivelevich, M. J. Mitchell, W. Fabian, and K. Wendel, *J. Am. Chem. Soc.*, **87**, 5132 (1965).
89. H. H. Wasserman and E. V. Dehmlow, *J. Am. Chem. Soc.*, **84**, 3786 (1962).
90. J. D. Roberts, G. B. Kline, and H. E. Simmons, *J. Am. Chem. Soc.*, **75**, 4765 (1953).
91. W. Adam, *Tetrahedron Letters*, **1963**, 1387.
92. H. H. Freedman, G. A. Dvorakian, and V. R. Sandel, *J. Am. Chem. Soc.*, **87**, 3019 (1965).
93. K. Ziegler and B. Schnell, *Ann. Chem.*, **445**, 266 (1925).
94. R. Breslow and H. W. Chang, *J. Am. Chem. Soc.*, **83**, 3727 (1961).
95. R. Breslow, H. W. Chang, and W. A. Yager, *J. Am. Chem. Soc.*, **85**, 2033 (1963).
96. (a) R. Breslow, R. Hill, and E. Wasserman, *J. Am. Chem. Soc.*, **86**, 5349 (1964); (b) R. Breslow, H. W. Chang, R. Hill, and E. Wasserman, *J. Am. Chem. Soc.*, **89**, 1112 (1967).
97. L. C. Snyder, *J. Phys. Chem.*, **66**, 2299 (1963).
98. B. A. Thrush, *Nature*, **178**, 155 (1956).
99. R. F. Pottie and F. P. Lossing, *J. Am. Chem. Soc.*, **85**, 269 (1963).
100. A. Streitwieser, *J. Am. Chem. Soc.*, **82**, 4123 (1960).
101. S. Ohnishi and I. Nitta, *J. Chem. Phys.*, **39**, 2848 (1963).
102. P. J. Zandstra, *J. Chem. Phys.*, **40**, 612 (1964).
103. D. C. Reitz, *J. Chem. Phys.*, **34**, 701 (1961).
104. W. von E. Doering, in *Theoretical Organic Chemistry, Kekulé Symposium*, Butterworth, London, 1959, p. 35.
105. T. Nozoe, *Prog. Org. Chem.*, **5**, 132 (1961).
106. G. Berthier and B. Pullman, *Trans. Faraday. Soc.*, **45**, 484 (1949).
107. T. Nakajima and S. Katagiri, *Mol. Phys.*, **7**, 149 (1963–1964).
108. A. Julg, *J. Chim. Phys.*, **52**, 50 (1955); **59**, 759 (1962).
109. W. von E. Doering and D. W. Wiley, *Tetrahedron*, **11**, 183 (1960).
110. R. B. Turner, W. R. Meador, W. von E. Doering, L. H. Knox, J. R. Mayer, and D. W. Wiley, *J. Am. Chem. Soc.*, **79**, 4127 (1957).
111. D. S. Matteson, J. J. Drysdale, and W. H. Sharkey, *J. Am. Chem. Soc.*, **82**, 2853 (1960).
112. M. Yamakawa, H. Watanabe, T. Mukai, T. Nozoe, and M. Kubo, *J. Am. Chem. Soc.*, **82**, 5665 (1960).
113. E. D. Bergmann and R. Ikan, *J. Org. Chem.*, **28**, 3341 (1963).
114. K. Hafner, H. W. Riedel, and M. Danielisz, *Angew. Chem.*, **75**, 344 (1963); *Angew. Chem. Intern. Ed. Eng.*, **2**, 215 (1963).
115. C. Jutz, *Chem. Ber.*, **97**, 2050 (1964).
116. D. J. Bertelli, C. Golino, and D. L. Dreyer, *J. Am. Chem. Soc.*, **86**, 3329 (1964).
117. D. Bryce-Smith and N. A. Perkins, *J. Chem. Soc.*, **1962**, 1339.

118. J. L. von Rosenberg, J. E. Mahler, and R. Pettit, *J. Am. Chem. Soc.*, **84**, 2842 (1962); C. E. Keller and R. Pettit, *J. Am. Chem. Soc.*, **88**, 604, 606 (1966). See also S. Winstein, C. G. Kreiter, and J. I. Brauman, *J. Am. Chem. Soc.*, **88**, 2047 (1966).
119. J. D. Holmes and R. Pettit, *J. Am. Chem. Soc.*, **85**, 2531 (1963).
120. A. Davison, W. McFarlane, L. Pratt, and G. Wilkinson, *J. Chem. Soc.*, **1962**, 4821.
121. G. N. Schrauzer, *J. Am. Chem. Soc.*, **83**, 2966 (1961).
122. S. Winstein, H. D. Kaesz, C. G. Kreiter, and E. C. Freidrich, *J. Am. Chem. Soc.*, **87**, 3267 (1965).
123. J. Schulman, private communication, see also ref. 43.
124. W. Hobey and A. D. McLachlan, *J. Chem. Phys.*, **33**, 1695 (1960).
125. G. Vincow, M. L. Morrell, W. V. Volland, H. J. Dauben, and F. R. Hunter, *J. Am. Chem. Soc.*, **87**, 3527 (1965).
126. A. G. Harrison, L. R. Honnen, H. J. Dauben, and F. P. Lossing, *J. Am. Chem. Soc.*, **82**, 5593 (1960).
127. D. E. Wood and H. M. McConnell, *J. Chem. Phys.*, **37**, 1150 (1962).
128. A. Carrington and I. C. P. Smith, *Mol. Phys.*, **7**, 99 (1963–1964).
129. S. Arai, J. Shida, K. Yamaguchi, and Z. Kuri, *J. Chem. Phys.*, **36**, 1885 (1962).
130. R. W. Fessenden and S. Ogawa, *J. Am. Chem. Soc.*, **86**, 3591 (1964).
131. L. C. Snyder, footnote 6, ref. 132.
132. H. J. Dauben and M. R. Rifi, *J. Am. Chem. Soc.*, **85**, 3041 (1963).
133. W. von E. Doering and P. P. Gaspar, *J. Am. Chem. Soc.*, **85**, 3043 (1963).
134. A. W. Johnson, *Chem. Ind. (London)*, **1964**, 504.
135. R. Breslow and H. W. Chang, *J. Am. Chem. Soc.*, **87**, 2200 (1965).
136. N. L. Bauld and M. S. Brown, *J. Am. Chem. Soc.*, **87**, 4390 (1965).
137. W. Reppe, O. Schlichting, K. Klager, and T. Toepel, *Ann. Chem.*, **560**, 1 (1948).
138. O. Bastiansen, L. Hedberg, and K. Hedberg, *J. Chem. Phys.*, **27**, 1311 (1957).
139. G. Schröder, *Cyclooctatetraen*, Verlag Chemie, Würzburg, 1965.
140. T. J. Katz, *J. Am. Chem. Soc.*, **82**, 3784, 3785 (1960).
141. H. L. Strauss, T. J. Katz, and G. K. Fraenkel, *J. Am. Chem. Soc.*, **85**, 2360 (1963).
142. R. D. Allendoerfer and P. H. Rieger, *J. Am. Chem. Soc.*, **87**, 2336 (1965).
143. H. L. Strauss and G. K. Fraenkel, *J. Chem. Phys.*, **35**, 1738 (1961).
144. A. Carrington and P. F. Todd, *Mol. Phys.*, **7**, 533 (1963–1964); **8**, 299 (1964).
145. T. J. Katz, W. H. Reinmuth, and D. E. Smith, *J. Am. Chem. Soc.*, **84**, 802 (1962).
146. K. Mislow and H. D. Perlmutter, *J. Am. Chem. Soc.*, **84**, 3591 (1962).
147. A. Carrington, H. C. Longuet-Higgins, and P. F. Todd, *Mol. Phys.*, **8**, 45 (1964).

148. T. J. Katz, M. Yoshida, and L. C. Siew, *J. Am. Chem. Soc.*, **87**, 4516 (1965).
149. V. D. Azatyan, *Dokl. Akad. Nauk SSSR*, **98**, 1403 (1954); *Chem. Abstr.*, **49**, 12318 (1955).
150. T. J. Katz and P. J. Garratt, *J. Am. Chem. Soc.*, **85**, 2852 (1963); **86**, 5194 (1964).
151. T. J. Katz and P. J. Garratt, *J. Am. Chem. Soc.*, **86**, 4876 (1964).
152. T. J. Katz, C. Nicholson, and C. A. Reilly, *J. Am. Chem. Soc.*, **88**, 3832 (1966).
153. T. S. Cantrell and H. Shechter, *J. Am. Chem. Soc.*, **85**, 3300 (1963).
154. T. S. Cantrell and H. Schechter, *J. Am. Chem. Soc.*, **87**, 136 (1965).
155. (a) R. Rieke, M. Oligaruso, R. McClung, and S. Winstein, *J. Am. Chem. Soc.*, **88**, 4729 (1966); M. Oligaruso, R. Rieke, and S. Winstein, *ibid.*, **88**, 4731 (1966); (b) T. J. Katz and C. Talcott, *ibid.*, **88**, 4732 (1966).
156. E. A. LaLancette and R. E. Benson, *J. Am. Chem. Soc.*, **85**, 2853 (1963); **87**, 1941 (1965).
157. H. E. Simmons, D. B. Chesnut, and E. A. LaLancette, *J. Am. Chem. Soc.*, **87**, 982 (1965).
158. D. Lloyd and N. W. Preston, *Chem. Ind. (London)*, **1966**, 1039.
159. (a) W. Grimme, M. Kaufhold, U. Dettmeier, and E. Vogel, *Angew. Chem.*, **78**, 643 (1966); *Angew. Chem., Intern. Ed Engl.*, **5**, 604 (1966). (b) P. Radlick and W. Rosen, *J. Am. Chem. Soc.*, **88**, 3461 (1966).
160. K. Mislow, *J. Chem. Phys.*, **20**, 1489 (1952).
161. E. E. van Tamelen and B. Pappas, *J. Am. Chem. Soc.*, **85**, 3296 (1963).
162. W. S. Johnson, J. Dolf Bass, and K. L. Williamson, *Tetrahedron*, **19**, 861 (1963).
163. E. Vogel and H. D. Roth, *Angew. Chem.*, **76**, 145 (1964); *Angew. Chem. Intern. Ed. Engl.*, **3**, 228 (1964).
164. E. Vogel and W. A. Böll, *Angew. Chem.*, **76**, 784 (1964); *Angew. Chem. Intern. Ed. Engl.*, **3**, 642 (1964).
165. G. Günther, *Z. Naturforsch.*, **20b**, 948 (1965).
166. W. A. Böll, *Angew. Chem.*, **78**, 755 (1966); *Angew. Chem. Intern. Ed. Engl.*, **5**, 733 (1966).
167. M. Dobler and J. D. Dunitz, *Helv. Chim. Acta*, **48**, 1429 (1965).
168. E. Vogel, W. Grimme, and S. Korte, *Tetrahedron Letters*, **1965**, 3625.
169. E. Vogel, W. Schröch, and W. A. Böll, *Angew. Chem.*, **78**, 753 (1966); *Angew. Chem. Intern. Ed. Engl.*, **5**, 732 (1966).
170. F. Sondheimer and A. Shani, *J.Am. Chem. Soc.*, **86**, 3168 (1964).
171. E. Vogel, M. Kiskup, W. Pretzer, and W. A. Böll, *Angew. Chem.*, **76**, 785 (1964); *Angew. Chem. Intern. Ed. Engl.*, **3**, 642 (1964).
172. E. Vogel, W. P. Pretzer, and W. A. Böll, *Tetrahedron Letters*, **1965**, 3613.
173. F. Gerson, E. Heilbronner, W. A. Böll, and E. Vogel, *Helv. Chim. Acta*, **48**, 1494 (1965).

174. J. J. Bloomfield and W. J. Quinlin, *J. Am. Chem. Soc.*, **86**, 2738 (1964).
175. E. Vogel, W. Maier, and J. Eimer, *Tetrahedron Letters*, **1966**, 655.
176. J. J. Bloomfield and J. R. Smiley Irelan, *Tetrahedron Letters*, **1966**, 2971.
177. W. Grimme, H. Hoffman, and E. Vogel, *Angew. Chem.*, **77**, 348 (1965); *Angew. Chem. Intern. Ed. Engl.*, **4**, 354 (1965).
178. F. Sondheimer, R. Wolovsky, and Y. Amiel, *J. Am. Chem. Soc.*, **84**, 274 (1962).
179. H. C. Longuet-Higgins and L. Salem, *Proc. Roy. Soc. (London), Ser. A*, **251**, 172 (1959).
180. M. J. S. Dewar and G. J. Gleicher, *J. Am. Chem. Soc.*, **87**, 685 (1965).
181. F. Sondheimer, *Pure Appl. Chem.*, **7**, 363 (1963).
182. F. Sondheimer, *Proc. Roy. Soc. (London), Ser. A*, **297**, 173 (1967).
183. F. Sondheimer, I. C. Calder, J. A. Elix, Y. Gaoni, P. J. Garratt, K. Grohmann, G. Di Maio, J. Mayer, M. V. Sargent, and R. Wolovsky, *Chem. Soc. Spec. Publ.*, **21**, 75 (1967).
184. C. Glaser, *Ber.*, **2**, 422 (1869); *Ann. Chem.*, **154**, 137 (1870).
185. G. Eglinton and A. R. Galbraith, *J. Chem. Soc.*, **1959**, 889.
186. R. Wolovsky and F. Sondheimer, *J. Am. Chem. Soc.*, **87**, 5720 (1965).
187. F. Sondheimer, R. Wolovsky, P. J. Garratt, and I. C. Calder, *J. Am. Chem. Soc.*, **88**, 2610 (1966).
188. K. G. Untch and D. C. Wysocki, *J. Am. Chem. Soc.*, **88**, 2608 (1966).
189. K. G. Untch and D. J. Martin, *J. Am. Chem. Soc.*, **87**, 3518 (1965).
190. T. J. Sworski, *J. Chem. Phys.*, **16**, 550 (1948).
191. G. Wittig, G. Koenig, and K. Clauss, *Ann. Chem.*, **593**, 127 (1955).
192. (a) O. M. Behr, G. Eglinton, A. R. Galbraith, and R. A. Raphael, *J. Chem. Soc.*, **1960**, 3614; (b) O. M. Behr, G. Eglinton, I. A. Lardy, and R. A. Raphael, *J. Chem. Soc.*, **1964**, 1151.
193. H. A. Staab and F. Graf, *Tetrahedron Letters*, **1966**, 751.
194. I. D. Campbell, G. Eglinton, W. Henderson, and R. A. Raphael, *Chem. Commun.*, **1966**, 87.
195. H. Brunner, K. H. Hausser, M. Rawitscher, and H. A. Staab, *Tetrahedron Letters*, **1966**, 2775.
196. M. Morimoto, S. Akiyama, S. Misumi, and M. Nakagawa, *Bull. Chem. Soc. Japan*, **35**, 857 (1962).
197. H. A. Staab, F. Graf, and B. Junge, *Tetrahedron Letters*, **1966**, 743.
198. F. Sondheimer and Y. Gaoni, *J. Am. Chem. Soc.*, **82**, 5765 (1960).
199. F. Sondheimer, Y. Gaoni, L. M. Jackman, N. A. Bailey, and R. Mason, *J. Am. Chem. Soc.*, **84**, 4595 (1962).
200. N. A. Bailey and R. Mason, *Proc. Roy. Soc. (London), Ser. A*, **290**, 94 (1966).
201. N. A. Bailey, M. Gerloch, and R. Mason, *Mol. Phys.*, **10**, 327 (1966).
202. J. Mayer and F. Sondheimer, *J. Am. Chem. Soc.*, **88**, 602, 603 (1966).

203. L. M. Jackman, F. Sondheimer, Y. Amiel, D. A. Ben-Efraim, Y. Gaoni, R. Wolovsky, and A. A. Bothner-By, *J. Am. Chem. Soc.*, **84**, 4307 (1962).
204. Y. Gaoni and F. Sondheimer, *Proc. Chem. Soc.*, **1964**, 299.
205. J. Bregman, *Nature*, **194**, 679 (1962).
206. Y. Gaoni, A. Malera, F. Sondheimer, and R. Wolovsky, *Proc. Chem. Soc.*, **1964**, 397.
207. Y. Gaoni and F. Sondheimer, *J. Am. Chem. Soc.*, **86**, 521 (1964).
208. V. Boekelheide and J. B. Phillips, *J. Am. Chem. Soc.*, **85**, 1545 (1963).
209. V. Boekelheide and J. B. Phillips, *Proc. Natl. Acad. Sci., U.S.*, **51**, 550 (1964).
210. H. R. Blattman, D. Meuche, E. Heilbronner, R. J. Molyneux, and V. Boekelheide, *J. Am. Chem. Soc.*, **87**, 130 (1965).
211. F. Gerson, E. Heilbronner, and V. Boekelheide, *Helv. Chim. Acta*, **47**, 1123 (1964).
212. E. Vogel, M. Biskup, A. Vogel, and H. Günther, *Angew. Chem.*, **78**, 755 (1966); *Angew. Chem. Intern. Engl. Ed.*, **5**, 734 (1966).
213. F. Sondheimer and Y. Gaoni, *J. Am. Chem. Soc.*, **83**, 4863 (1961).
214. I. C. Calder, Y. Gaoni, P. J. Garratt, and F. Sondheimer, unpublished observations.
215. G. Schröder and J. F. M. Oth, *Tetrahedron Letters*, **1966**, 4083.
216. J. A. Pople and K. G. Untch, *J. Am. Chem. Soc.*, **88**, 4811 (1966).
217. H. C. Longuet-Higgins, *Chem. Soc., Spec. Publ.* **21**, 109 (1967).
218. E. D. Bergmann and Z. Pelchowicz, *J. Am. Chem. Soc.*, **75**, 4281 (1953).
219. C. E. Griffin, K. R. Martin, and B. E. Douglas, *J. Org. Chem.*, **27**, 1627 (1962).
220. F. Sondheimer and R. Wolovsky, *J. Am. Chem. Soc.*, **84**, 260 (1962); R. Wolovsky, *J. Am. Chem. Soc.*, **87**, 3638 (1965).
221. F. Sondheimer, Y. Amiel, and Y. Gaoni, *J. Am. Chem. Soc.*, **84**, 270 (1962).
222. F. Sondheimer, R. Wolovsky, and Y. Amiel, *J. Am. Chem. Soc.*, **84**, 274 (1962).
223. J. Bregman, F. L. Hirschfeld, D. Rabinovich, and G. M. J. Schmidt, *Acta Cryst.*, **19**, 227 (1965); F. L. Hirschfeld and D. Rabinovich, *Acta Cryst.*, **19**, 235 (1965).
224. I. C. Calder, P. J. Garratt, F. Sondheimer, and R. Wolovsky, unpublished observations.
225. F. Sondheimer and D. A. Ben-Efraim, *J. Am. Chem. Soc.*, **85**, 52 (1963).
226. G. M. Badger, J. A. Elix, and G. E. Lewis, *Proc. Chem. Soc.*, **1964**, 82.
227. G. M. Badger, J. A. Elix, and G. E. Lewis, *Australian J. Chem.*, **18**, 71 (1965); *Australian J. Chem.*, **19**, 1221 (1966).
228. G. M. Badger, J. A. Elix, G. E. Lewis, U. P. Singh, and T. M. Spotswood, *Chem. Commun.*, **1965**, 269.
229. C. A. Coulson and M. D. Poole, *Proc. Chem. Soc.*, **1964**, 220.

230. G. M. Badger, G. E. Lewis, and U. P. Singh, *Australian. J. Chem.*, **19**, 257, 1461 (1966).
231. F. Sondheimer, R. Wolovsky, and D. A. Ben-Efraim, *J. Am. Chem. Soc.*, **83**, 1686 (1961).
232. F. Sondheimer and Y. Gaoni, *J. Am. Chem. Soc.*, **83**, 1259 (1961).
233. F. Sondheimer and Y. Gaoni, *J. Am. Chem. Soc.*, **84**, 3520 (1962).
234. I. C. Calder and F. Sondheimer, *Chem. Commun.*, **1966**, 904.
235. D. P. Craig, in *Theoretical Organic Chemistry, Kekulé Symposium*, Butterworths, London, 1959, p. 10.
236. R. D. Brown, *Trans. Faraday Soc.*, **45**, 296 (1949); **46**, 146 (1950); *Nature*, **165**, 566 (1950); G. Berthier and B. Pullman, *Trans. Faraday Soc.*, **45**, 484 (1949); *Compt. Rend.*, **229**, 717 (1949).
237. P. C. den Boer, D. H. W. den Boer, C. A. Coulson, and T. H. Godwin, *Tetrahedron*, **19**, 2163 (1963).
238. (a) T. Nakajima, Y. Yaguchi, R. Kaeriyama, and Y. Nemoto, *Bull. Chem. Soc. Japan*, **37**, 272 (1964); and previous papers. (b) P. C. den Boer-Veenendaal, J. A. Vliegenthart, and D. H. W. den Boer, *Tetrahedron*, **18**, 1325 (1962) and previous papers.
239. R. Zahradnik, *Angew. Chem.*, **77**, 1097 (1965); *Angew. Chem. Intern. Ed. Engl.*, **4**, 1039 (1965).
240. J. I. Brauman, L. E. Ellis, and E. E. van Tamelen, *J. Am. Chem. Soc.*, **88**, 846 (1966).
241. (a) W. M. Jones and R. S. Pyron, *J. Am. Chem. Soc.*, **87**, 1608 (1965). (b), A. S. Kende and P. T. Izzo, *J. Am. Chem. Soc.*, **87**, 1609 (1965). (c) H. Prinzbach, D. Siep, and U. Fischer, *Angew. Chem.*, **77**, 219, 621 (1965); *Angew. Chem. Intern. Ed. Engl.*, **4**, 242, 598 (1965).
242. E. D. Bergmann and I. Agranat, *Chem. Commun*, **1965**, 512.
243. M. Ueno, I. Murata, and Y. Kitahara, *Tetrahedron Letters*, **1965**, 2967.
244. E. D. Bergmann and I. Agranat, *Tetrahedron*, **22**, 1275 (1966).
245. H. Prinzbach and U. Fischer, *Angew. Chem.*, **78**, 642 (1966); *Angew. Chem. Intern. Ed. Engl.*, **5**, 602 (1966).
246. A. S. Kende, P. T. Izzo, and P. T. MacGregor, *J. Am. Chem. Soc.*, **88**, 3359 (1966).
247. A. S. Kende, P. T. Izzo, and W. Falmar, *Tetrahedron Letters*, **1966**, 3697.
248. E. E. van Tamelen, *Angew. Chem.*, **77**, 759 (1965); *Angew. Chem. Intern. Ed. Engl.*, **4**, 738 (1965).
249. H. G. Viehe, *Angew. Chem.*, **77**, 768 (1965); *Angew. Chem. Intern. Ed. Engl.*, **4**, 746 (1965).
250. M. Avram, I. G. Dinulescu, D. Dinu, G. Mateescu, and C. D. Nenitzescu, *Tetrahedron*, **19**, 309 (1963).
251. M. P. Cava and D. R. Napier, *J. Am. Chem. Soc.*, **79**, 1701 (1957).

252. M. P. Cava, B. Hwang, and J. P. van Meter, *J. Am. Chem. Soc.*, **85**, 4032 (1963).
253. C. D. Nenitzescu, M. Avram, I. G. Dinulescu, and G. Mateescu, *Ann. Chem.*, **653**, 79 (1962).
254. M. P. Cava and B. Hwang, *Tetrahedron Letters*, **1965**, 2297.
255. T. C. W. Mak and J. Trotter, *Proc. Chem. Soc.*, **1965**, 163; J. Waser and C.-S. Lu, *J. Am. Chem. Soc.*, **66**, 2035 (1944).
256. N. S. Hush and J. R. Rowland, *Mol. Phys.*, **6**, 317 (1963).
257. N. L. Bauld and D. Banks, *J. Am. Chem. Soc.*, **87**, 128 (1965).
258. R. Waack, M. A. Doran, and P. West, *J. Am. Chem. Soc.*, **87**, 5508 (1965).
259. M. P. Cava and D. R. Napier, *J. Am. Chem. Soc.*, **79**, 3606 (1957).
260. J. A. Elix, M. V. Sargent, and F. Sondheimer, *J. Am. Chem. Soc.*, **89**, 180 (1967).
261. D. Peters, *J. Chem. Soc.*, **1958**, 1028, 1039.
262. See E. D. Bergmann in ref. 9, p. 141.
263. E. Le Goff, *J. Am. Chem. Soc.*, **84**, 1505 (1962).
264. E. Le Goff, *J. Am. Chem. Soc.*, **84**, 3975 (1962).
265. K. Hafner and H. Schaum, *Angew. Chem.*, **75**, 90 (1963); *Angew. Chem. Intern. Ed. Engl.*, **2**, 95 (1963).
266. E. G. Hoffman, *Ann. Chem.*, **624**, 47 (1959).
267. M. A. Ali and C. A. Coulson, *Mol. Phys.*, **4**, 65 (1961).
268. K. Hafner, R. Fleischer, and K. Fritz, *Angew. Chem.*, **77**, 42 (1965); *Angew. Chem. Intern. Ed. Engl.*, **4**, 69 (1965).
269. T. J. Katz, M. Rosenberger, and R. K. O'Hara, *J. Am. Chem. Soc.*, **86**, 249 (1964).
270. T. J. Katz and W. H. Okamura, *Tetrahedron*, **23**, 2941 (1967).
271. T. J. Katz and M. Rosenberger, *J. Am. Chem. Soc.*, **85**, 2030 (1963).
272. T. J. Katz, and J. T. Mrowca, *J. Am. Chem. Soc.*, **89**, 1105 (1967).
273. A. J. Silvestri, *Tetrahedron*, **19**, 855 (1963).
274. K. Hafner, K. H. Häfner, C. Hönig, M. Kreuder, G. Ploss, G. Shulz, E. Sturm, and K. H. Vöpel, *Angew. Chem.*, **75**, 35 (1963); *Angew. Chem. Intern. Ed. Engl.*, **2**, 123 (1963).
275. E. Le Goff and R. B. La Count, *Tetrahedron Letters*, **1964**, 1161.
276. T. J. Katz and J. Schulman, *J. Am. Chem. Soc.*, **86**, 3169 (1964).
277. V. Boekelheide and C. D. Smith, *J. Am. Chem. Soc.*, **88**, 3950 (1966).
278. K. Hafner and G. Schneider, *Ann. Chem.*, **672**, 194 (1964).
279. E. Galantay, H. Agahigian, and N. Paolella, *J. Am. Chem. Soc.*, **88**, 3875 (1966).
280. R. Breslow, W. Vitale, and K. Wendel, *Tetrahedron Letters*, **1965**, 365.
281. W. B. deMore, H. O. Pritchard, and N. Davidson, *J. Am. Chem. Soc.*, **81**, 5874 (1959).

282. T. Nakajima and S. Katagiri, *Mol. Phys.*, **7**, 149 (1963–1964); O. Chalvet, R. Daudel, and J. J. Kaufman, *J. Phys. Chem.*, **68**, 490 (1964).
283. V. Mark, *Tetrahedron Letters*, **1961**, 333.
284. P. J. Wheatley, *J. Chem. Soc.*, **1961**, 4936.
285. H. Prinzbach, *Angew. Chem.*, **73**, 169 (1961).
286. H. Prinzbach and D. Seip, *Angew. Chem.*, **73**, 169 (1961).
287. H. Prinzbach, *Angew. Chem.*, **76**, 235 (1964); *Angew. Chem. Intern. Ed. Engl.*, **3**, 319 (1964).
288. H. Prinzbach, U. Fischer, and R. Cruse, *Angew. Chem.*, **78**, 268 (1966); *Angew. Chem. Intern. Ed. Engl.*, **5**, 251 (1966).
289. Y. Kitahara, I. Murata, and T. Asano, *Bull. Chem. Soc. Japan*, **37**, 924 (1964).
290. D. H. Reid, *Quart. Rev.*, **19**, 274 (1965).
291. E. Clar, W. Kemp, and D. G. Stewart, *Tetrahedron*, **3**, 325 (1958).
292. H. C. Longuet-Higgins, *J. Chem. Phys.*, **18**, 265 (1950).
293. J. A. Elix, M. V. Sargent, and F. Sondheimer, *Chem. Commun.*, **1966**, 509.
294. H. A. Staab and F. Binnig, *Tetrahedron Letters*, **1964**, 319.
295. H. J. Dauben and D. J. Bertelli, *J. Am. Chem. Soc.*, **83**, 4657, 4659 (1961).
296. H. J. Dauben, International Symposium on Aromaticity, Sheffield, 1966.
297. R. Breslow, W. Horspool, H. Sugiyama, and W. Vitale, *J. Am. Chem. Soc.*, **88**, 3677 (1966).
298. W. Tochtermann, *Angew. Chem.*, **75**, 418 (1963); *Angew. Chem. Intern. Ed. Engl.*, **2**, 265 (1963).
299. *Chem. Soc. Spec. Publ.*, **21** (1967).
300a. M. P. Cava and M. J. Mitchell, *Cyclobutadiene and Related Compounds*, Academic Press, New York, 1967.
300b. M. J. S. Dewar, *Tetrahedron, Suppl.* 8, **1**, 75 (1966).
301. J. I. Musher, *J. Chem. Phys.*, **43**, 4081 (1965); **46**, 1219 (1967); *Advances in Magnetic Resonance*, J. S. Waugh, Ed., Academic Press, New York, 1967.
302. J. M. Gaitlis and R. West, *J. Chem. Phys.*, **46**, 1218 (1967).
303. R. Alden, J. Kraut, and T. G. Traylor, *J. Phys. Chem.*, **71**, 2379 (1967).
304. S. Winstein, E. C. Friedrich, R. Baker, and Y. Lin, *Tetrahedron, Suppl.* 8, **2**, 621 (1966).
305. R. Breslow, J. T. Groves, and G. Ryan, *J. Am. Chem. Soc.*, **89**, 5048 (1967); D. G. Farnum, G. Mehta, and R. G. Silberman, *J. Am. Chem. Soc.*, **89**, 5049 (1967).
306. R. Breslow and G. Ryan, *J. Am. Chem. Soc.*, **89**, 3073 (1967).
307. A. Krebs and B. Schrader, *Z. Naturforsch.*, **21b**, 194 (1966); Ann. Chem., **709**, 46 (1967).
308. I. Agranat and E. D. Bergmann, *Tetrahedron Letters*, **1966**, 2373.

309. N. Toshima, I. Moritani, and S. Nishida, *Bull. Chem. Soc. Japan*, **40**, 1245 (1967).
310. T. Eicher and A. Loshner, *Z. Naturforsch.*, **21b**, 295, 899 (1966).
311. J. Ciabattoni and E. C. Nathan, *J. Am. Chem. Soc.*, **89**, 3081 (1967).
312. S. Maahs and P. Hegenberg, *Angew. Chem.*, **78**, 927 (1966); *Angew. Chem. Intern. Ed. Engl.*, **5**, 888 (1966).
313. H. E. Sprenger and W. Ziegenbein, *Angew. Chem.*, **79**, 581 (1967); *Angew. Chem. Intern. Ed. Engl.*, **6**, 553 (1967).
314. C. S. Yannoni, G. P. Ceasar, and B. P. Dailey, *J. Am. Chem. Soc.*, **89**, 2833 (1967).
315. A. Efraty and P. M. Maitlis, *J. Am. Chem. Soc.*, **89**, 3744 (1967).
316. W. J. R. Tyerman, M. Kato, P. Kebarle, S. Masamune, O. P. Strausz, and H. E. Gunning, *Chem. Commun.*, **1967**, 497.
317. G. L. Closs and V. N. M. Rao, *J. Am. Chem. Soc.*, **88**, 4116 (1966).
318. J. M. Brown and J. L. Occolowitz, *Chem. Commun.*, **1965**, 376.
319. J. M. Brown, *Chem. Commun.*, **1967**, 638.
320. S. Winstein, M. Ogliaruso, M. Sakai, and J. M. Nicholson, *J. Am. Chem. Soc.*, **89**, 3656 (1967).
321. H. Shimanouchi, T. Ashida, Y. Sasada, M. Kakudo, I. Murata, and Y. Kitahara, *Bull. Chem. Soc. Japan*, **39**, 2322 (1966).
322. M. Brookhart, M. Ogliaruso, and S. Winstein, *J. Am. Chem. Soc.*, **89**, 1965 (1967).
323. G. Boche, W. Hechte, H. Huber, and R. Huisgen, *J. Am. Chem. Soc.*, **89**, 3344 (1967).
324. R. Huisgen, G. Boche, and H. Huber, *J. Am. Chem. Soc.*, **89**, 3345 (1967).
325. L. Eberson, K. Nyberg, M. Finkelstein, R. C. Petersen, S. D. Ross, and J. J. Uebel, *J. Org. Chem.*, **32**, 16 (1967).
326. A. Carrington, R. E. Moss, and P. F. Todd, *Mol. Phys.*, **12**, 95 (1967).
327. R. E. Moss, *Mol. Phys.*, **10**, 501 (1966).
328. J. F. Garst, *Mol. Phys.*, **10**, 207 (1966).
329a. E. E. van Tamelen and T. L. Burkoth, *J. Am. Chem. Soc.*, **89**, 151 (1967).
329b. S. Masamune, C. G. Chin, K. Hojo, and R. T. Seidner, *J. Am. Chem. Soc.*, **89**, 4804 (1967).
330. K. Grohmann and F. Sondheimer, *Tetrahedron Letters*, **1967**, 3121.
331. E. Vogel, W. Meckel, and W. Grimme, *Angew. Chem.*, **76**, 786 (1964); *Angew. Chem. Intern. Ed. Engl.*, **3**, 643 (1964).
332. M. Avram, G. Mateescu, and C. D. Nenitzescu, *Ann. Chem.*, **636**, 174 (1960); M. Avram, C. D. Nenitzescu, and E. Marica, *Chem. Ber.*, **90**, 1857 (1957).
333. R. C. Cookson, J. Hudec, and J. Marsden, *Chem. Ind. (London)*, **1961**, 21.
334. R. H. Mitchell and F. Sondheimer, *J. Am. Chem. Soc.*, **90**, 530 (1968).
335. P. J. Mulligan and F. Sondheimer, *J. Am. Chem. Soc.*, **89**, 7118 (1967).

336. K. Grohmann and F. Sondheimer, *J. Am. Chem. Soc.*, **89,** 7119 (1967).
337. W. Bremser, H. T. Gründer, E. Heilbronner, and E. Vogel, *Helv. Chim. Acta,* **50,** 84 (1967).
338. H. Günther and W. Grimme, *Angew. Chem.*, **78,** 1063 (1966); *Angew. Chem. Intern. Ed. Engl.*, **5,** 1043 (1966).
339. P. E. Baikie and O. S. Mills, *Chem. Commun.*, **1966,** 683.
340. B. A. Hess, A. S. Bailey, and V. Boekelheide, *J. Am. Chem. Soc.*, **89,** 2746 (1967).
341. I. C. Calder and P. J. Garratt, *J. Chem. Soc., B,* **1967,** 660.
342. N. M. Atherton, R. Mason, and R. J. Wratten, *Mol. Phys.*, **11,** 525 (1966).
343. V. Boekelheide and J. B. Phillips, *J. Am. Chem. Soc.*, **89,** 1695 (1967).
344. J. B. Phillips, R. J. Molyneux, E. Strum, and V. Boekelheide, *J. Am. Chem. Soc.*, **89,** 1704 (1967).
345. V. Boekelheide and T. Miyasaka, *J. Am. Chem. Soc.*, **89,** 1709 (1967).
346. H. R. Blattman, V. Boekelheide, E. Heilbronner, and J. P. Weber, *Helv. Chim. Acta,* **50,** 68 (1967).
347. E. Vogel and H. Günther, *Angew. Chem.*, **79,** 429 (1967); *Angew. Chem. Intern. Ed. Engl.*, **6,** 385 (1967).
348. J. N. Murrell and A. Hinchcliffe, *Trans. Faraday Soc.*, **62,** 2011 (1966).
349. I. C. Calder, P. J. Garratt, H. C. Longuet-Higgins, F. Sondheimer, and R. Wolovsky, *J. Chem. Soc., C,* **1967,** 1041.
350. W. H. Okamura and F. Sondheimer, *J. Am. Chem. Soc.*, **89,** 5991 (1967).
351. F. Baer, H. Kuhn, and W. Regal, *Z. Naturforsch.*, **22a,** 103 (1967).
352. C. C. Leznoff and F. Sondheimer, *J. Am. Chem. Soc.*, **89,** 4247 (1967).
353. T. Nakujima, S. Kohda, A. Tajiri, and S. Karasawa, *Tetrahedron,* **23,** 2189 (1967).
354. J. Michl and R. Zahradnik, *Coll. Czech. Chem. Commun.*, **31,** 3478 (1966), and preceding papers.
355. G. V. Boyd, *Tetrahedron,* **22,** 3409 (1966).
356a. W. Merk and R. Pettit, *J. Am. Chem. Soc.*, **89,** 4787 (1967).
356b. A. T. Blomquist and V. J. Hruby, *J. Am. Chem. Soc.*, **86,** 5041 (1964), **89,** 4996 (1967).
357. K. Hafner, K. F. Bangert and V. Orfanos, *Angew. Chem.*, **79,** 414 (1967); *Angew. Chem. Intern. Ed. Engl.*, **6,** 451 (1967).
358. H. J. Dauben, S. H. K. Jiang, and V. R. Ben, *Hua Hsueh Hsueh Pao,* **23,** 411 (1957); *Chem. Abstr.*, **52,** 16309h (1958).
359. B. M. Trost and G. M. Bright, *J. Am. Chem. Soc.*, **89,** 4244 (1967).
360. B. M. Trost and D. R. Brittelli, *Tetrahedron Letters,* **1967,** 119.
361. W. E. Barth and R. G. Lawton, *J. Am. Chem. Soc.*, **88,** 380 (1966).
362. J. Janata, J. Gendell, C.-Y. Ling, W. Barth, L. Backes, H. B. Mark, and R. G. Lawton, *J. Am. Chem. Soc.*, **89,** 3056 (1967).

363. E. G. Janzen, J. G. Pacifici, and J. L. Gerlock, *J. Phys. Chem.*, **70**, 3021 (1966).
364. N. L. Bauld and J. H. Zoeller, *Tetrahedron Letters*, **1967**, 885.
365. P. T. Kwitowski and R. West, *J. Am. Chem. Soc.*, **88**, 4541 (1966).
366. A. G. Anastassiou, F. L. Setliff, and G. W. Griffin, *J. Org. Chem.*, **31**, 2705 (1966).
367. H. Prinzbach, D. Seip, L. Knothe, and W. Faisst, *Ann. Chem.*, **698**, 34 (1966); H. Prinzbach, D. Seip, and G. Englert, *Ann. Chem.*, **698**, 57 (1966).
368. H. Prinzbach, V. Freudenberger, and U. Scheidegger, *Helv. Chim. Acta*, **50**, 1087 (1967).
369. H. Prinzbach and L. Knothe, *Angew. Chem.*, **79**, 620 (1967); *Angew. Chem. Intern. Ed. Engl.*, **6**, 632 (1967).
370. H. A. Staab and F. Binnig, *Chem. Ber.*, **100**, 293, 889 (1967); H. Bräunling, F. Binnig, and H. A. Staab, *Chem. Ber.*, **100**, 880 (1967).
371. R. Zahradnik, M. Tichý, P. Hochmann, and D. H. Reid, *J. Phys. Chem.*, **71**, 3040 (1967).
372. A. M. Khan, G. R. Proctor, and L. Rees, *J. Chem. Soc., C*, **1966**, 990.
373. G. R. Proctor and A. H. Renfrew, *Chem. Commun.*, **1966**, 696.
374. W. M. Jones and C. L. Ennis, *J. Am. Chem. Soc.*, **89**, 3069 (1967).
375. J. A. Elix, M. V. Sargent, and F. Sondheimer, *J. Am. Chem. Soc.*, **89**, 5080 (1967).

ORGANIC SYNTHESES BY MEANS OF NOBLE METAL COMPOUNDS

By JIRO TSUJI, *Basic Research Laboratories, Toyo Rayon Company, Kamakura, Japan*

CONTENTS

I. Introduction	110
II. Complex Formation by Noble Metal Compounds	112
III. Reactions Involving the Reduction of Divalent Palladium	117
A. Chemical Properties of Palladium Compounds Useful for Organic Syntheses	117
B. Oxidation of Olefins to Carbonyl Compounds	119
1. Oxidation of Olefins to Saturated Carbonyl Compounds	119
2. Mechanism of the Olefin Oxidation Reaction	122
3. Oxidation of Olefins via π-Allylic Complexes	126
4. Oxidation of Alcohols	131
C. Vinylation Reactions	132
1. Vinyl Ester Formation	132
2. Vinyl Ether and Vinyl Amine Formations	141
3. Displacement Reactions of Vinyl Chloride Catalyzed by Palladium Chloride	142
4. Unsaturated Nitrile Formation	143
5. Reactions of Olefins with Aromatic Rings	144
D. Reactions of Aromatic Compounds	145
E. Reactions of Carbanions with Palladium Compounds	147
IV. Palladium-Catalyzed Carbonylations and Decarbonylations	150
A. Introduction	150
B. Carbonylations of Simple Olefins	151
1. Carbonylation of Olefin-Palladium Chloride Complexes	151
2. Catalytic Carbonylation of Olefins	153
C. Aldehyde Formation	159
D. Mechanism of the Palladium-Catalyzed Carbonylation Reactions	160
E. Decarbonylation Reactions	161
F. Carbonylations of Allylic Compounds	166
G. Carbonylations of Conjugated Dienes	171
H. Carbonylations of Allene Complexes	176
I. Carbonylations of Acetylenic Compounds	177
J. Carbonylation of the Azobenzene Complex	183
K. Carbonylations of Amines	184

110 J. TSUJI

 V. Carbonylation and Decarbonylation Reactions Catalyzed by Other Noble Metal Compounds 186
  A. Platinum-Catalyzed Carbonylations 186
  B. Carbonylation and Decarbonylation Reactions by Using Rhodium Complexes 187
   1. Carbonylation Reactions 187
   2. Decarbonylation Reactions 189
  C. Ruthenium-Catalyzed Carbonylations 198
 VI. Homogeneous Hydrogenations 199
 VII. Hydrosilation Reactions Catalyzed by Noble Metal Compounds . . 206
 VIII. Addition Reactions of Olefinic and Acetylenic Compounds . . . 213
 IX. Resolution of Diastereoisomers by Complex Formation with Platinum Compounds 220
 X. Miscellaneous Reactions 227
 XI. Experimental 232
  A. Preparation of Palladium Chloride Complexes 232
  B. Preparation of 2-Dodecanone from 1-Dodecene on a Laboratory Scale 233
  C. Preparation of *exo*-2-Chloro-*syn*-7-acetoxynorbornane . . . 233
  D. Carbonylation of Allyl Chloride 234
  E. Decarbonylation of Octanoyl Bromide with Chlorocarbonylbis-(Triphenylphosphine)Rhodium 234
  F. Reaction of Benzenesulfonyl Chloride with Chlorotris(Triphenylphosphine)Rhodium 234
  G. Dimerization of Methyl Acrylate by Using Ruthenium Chloride 235
 References 235
 Supplementary References 247

I. Introduction

In organic chemistry laboratories, palladium and other noble metals and their compounds are familiar reagents as hydrogenation catalysts, and sometimes they are used for the preparation of aromatic compounds by catalytic dehydrogenation of certain alicyclic compounds. They are rather expensive and are rarely used in synthesis other than as hydrogenation and dehydrogenation catalysts. Recently, however, noble metal compounds, especially palladium compounds, have attracted much attention from the standpoint of synthetic organic chemistry as well as that of industrial chemistry. For this sudden development of palladium chemistry as a synthetic tool, two main impetuses can be cited. The first epoch-making discovery responsible for the emergence of palladium chemistry is the invention of the so-called "Wacker process," in which palladium chloride is used as an essential catalyst to produce acetaldehyde from ethylene and other carbonyl compounds from olefinic materials. It is rather surprising to find that even palladium can be used in the industrial production of such a cheap material as acetaldehyde. The second impetus for the development has been provided by the recent renaissance of the chemistry of transition metal complexes (including noble metal complexes) especially those formed with olefinic compounds. Recently, numerous noble metal complexes having organic ligands have been prepared, and the theoretical understanding of the bonding and electronic structure of the coordination compounds has been elucidated, mainly by inorganic chemists. Now it has been established that the above-mentioned Wacker process proceeds through the formation of an olefin–palladium chloride complex as an intermediate. The accumulation of knowledge on the coordination chemistry of noble metal compounds certainly has contributed to the rapid development of organic syntheses by means of these compounds.

The present article deals with the application of noble metal compounds, mainly those of palladium, to organic syntheses. There is much interesting chemistry involved in noble metal complexes having organic ligands; however, it is discussed here only when quite useful in organic syntheses. In other words, only the synthetic and preparative usefulness of noble metal compounds will be dealt with. Some important reactions catalyzed by noble metal compounds are omitted or referred to only briefly. For example, olefin isomerization is one of the important reactions catalyzed by noble metal compounds and has been studied extensively. In general, a terminal olefin is isomerized to nonterminal olefins, or a single olefin to a mixture of isomers; however, this topic has only limited use in organic syntheses and is not included. A review on olefin isomerization has been published (1). Also, catalytic hydrogenation and dehydrogenation using noble metals, and oxidation using osmium tetroxide (2) or platinum (3) are not included, because they are well-known reactions. Addition reactions or polymerizations of olefins are also important, but they are discussed only briefly. Patent literature is mentioned in some cases but, in general, the numerous patents covering this field are not referred to.

This is a rapidly developing field of research, and in most cases the problem of reaction mechanism has not been settled. Nevertheless, many controversial mechanisms are discussed with the hope that a better understanding of the reactions might result, and further, that these discussions may serve as valuable hints for future development of new synthetic reactions. It should be added that there are many reactions which are not very useful for organic syntheses at present, but the reactions involved are quite unique in some instances. It is highly probable that these reactions will be the seeds of future developments in organic chemistry. Consideration of the change in chemical properties of olefins and some other unsaturated compounds by complex formation would lead to a fruitful field of future studies. It is the author's hope that more organic chemists will be interested in this fascinating area of noble metal complexes, in order that many new organic reactions may be discovered. An interesting article discussing the analogy between the species of organic and coordination chemistry has been given by Halpern (4).

II. Complex Formation by Noble Metal Compounds

In organic syntheses by means of noble metal compounds, the formation of complexes with various unsaturated compounds is essential. In other words, the mechanism of many noble metal-catalyzed reactions can be explained in terms of complex formation. Many reactions carried out in the presence of noble metal compounds are possible because of the change in chemical properties which results from complex formation with unsaturated compounds. To understand the known reactions and to devise a new reaction, some knowledge of noble metal complexes with organic ligands is indispensable. Therefore, the typical complexes formed by noble metal compounds are briefly summarized at first. The coordination chemistry of noble metal compounds is of course a vast topic and requires a book of its own (5-8); thus, the summary here is not a complete one. It is only intended to give organic chemists a minimum knowledge of the complexes in order to understand the reactions discussed in this article.

In most of the reactions catalyzed by noble metal compounds, π-complex formation with an olefin is assumed. It is known that palladium, platinum, rhodium, ruthenium, and iridium form various kinds of π-complexes with olefins (8). The most typical and well-known one is the so-called Zeise salt, $K[C_2H_4-PtCl_3]$ **(1)**, which was

[structure of Zeise salt (1)]

synthesized as early as 1827 from ethanol and platinum chloride (9). Its bonding nature was suggested by Chatt and Duncanson (10). In addition, the corresponding propylene and amylene complexes were prepared by Birnbaum (11). The π-complexes of simple olefins with different noble metals have varying stabilities. Platinum complexes are rather stable and can be recrystallized and the olefins can be recovered from them by treatment of the complexes with a potassium cyanide solution. By virtue of this property, a platinum–olefin complex, coordinated with an optically active amine (2), is useful for the resolution of asymmetric olefins.

```
        Cl                     R    H                         Cl    R    H
         |                      \  /                    Cl    \    /
amine—Pt—Cl                      C          Cl          \      C
         |                      ‖ ·······Pd      Pd·······    ‖
       olefin                    C        \    /         C
                                / \        Cl           / \
                               H   H                   H   H
        (2)                              (3)
```

Olefin–palladium chloride complexes have a dimeric structure (3). They are not as stable as those of platinum. Although the isolation of stable palladium–olefin complexes is not possible in some cases, π-complex formation is assumed in many reactions of olefins in the presence of palladium compounds. There are several synthetic methods for the preparation of these olefin complexes. The Kharasch method is the most widely used for the preparation of a palladium chloride complex (12). In this method, the palladium chloride–benzonitrile complex, dissolved in benzene, is treated with an olefin. Also, olefin complexes of palladium can be prepared by direct reaction of olefins with palladium chloride (13–15). Other preparative methods of various olefin complexes have been summarized (8).

Unconjugated dienes form π-complexes. In contrast to the monoolefins, the complexes derived from some dienes are very stable. This is especially true when the two olefinic bonds behave as a bidentate ligand. Examples are the complexes of 1,5-hexadiene, 1,5-cyclooctadiene, dicyclopentadiene, and norbornadiene (4).

(4)

In addition to the above-mentioned π-complexes, there is another class of stable complexes of noble metal compounds, mainly of palladium chloride. These are called π-allyl complexes (16). They can be considered for convenience to involve a hybridization and delocalization of the π-electron pair and the free electrons of the allyl anion; the carbon–carbon distance in the complex is equal to that in a benzene ring. The simplest one is formed from allyl chloride and palladium chloride (17,18), and has the sandwiched dimer structure (5). Allylic

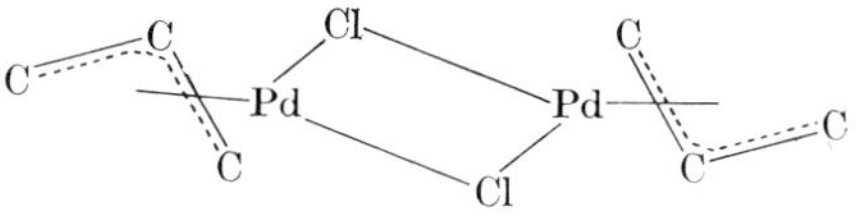

(5)

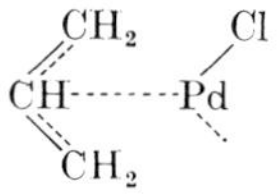

(5)
(abbreviated form)

compounds such as allylic halides, alcohols (19), and esters are commonly used in syntheses of π-allylic complexes of palladium. In addition, some other compounds such as conjugated dienes (20,21), allene (22,23), α,β- and β,γ- unsaturated carbonyl compounds (24,25), and some substituted olefins (26–31) form π-allylic complexes with various substituents.

In addition to the above-mentioned rather stable π- and π-allyl complexes, some noble metal compounds form σ-alkyl complexes. σ-Complexes are stable only when they are coordinated with phosphine or other appropriate ligands (32). However, they play a very important role in the transition metal-catalyzed reactions of olefins. In many cases, a σ-complex (7) is formed from an olefin π-complex (6) by an insertion reaction as shown in eq. (1) (33). In the insertion reaction, a group (A) on a metal migrates to a π-bonded olefin. In many

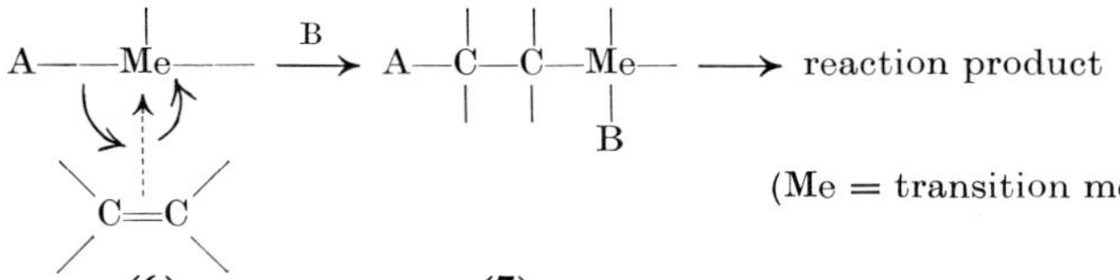

$$A\text{---}Me \xrightarrow{B} A\text{---}C\text{---}C\text{---}Me \longrightarrow \text{reaction product} \quad (1)$$

(Me = transition metal)

(6) (7)

cases, A is hydrogen. It can also be a chlorine, hydroxyl, alkyl, or other group. Many transition metal-catalyzed reactions of olefins proceed through the transformation of an olefin π-complex to a σ-complex. More generally, the *cis* ligand insertion is frequently found in many transition metal-catalyzed reactions, and the general scheme is shown in eq. (2). The ligand L is inserted between the metal and the

$$\begin{array}{c}A\\ |/\\ -Me-L\\ /|\end{array} \longrightarrow \begin{array}{c}|/\\ -Me-L-A\\ /|\end{array} \qquad (2)$$

ligand A, originally attached to the metal by a σ-bond (6,34). As will be discussed later, a large number of reactions catalyzed by noble metal compounds follow this pathway, and this transformation is an essential step in most of the noble metal-catalyzed reactions.

Like olefinic bonds, acetylenic bonds also form complexes with noble metal compounds. Different structures have been proposed for different metals and few studies have been carried out on their reactions.

Metal carbonyls form another important class of organometallic compounds. Carbonyl complex formation with rhodium, iridium, osmium, and ruthenium is definitely known (35,36). Typical examples are $Rh_2(CO)_8$, $Ir_2(CO)_8$, $Ru(CO)_5$, and $Os(CO)_5$. Palladium and platinum do not form simple carbonyls, but carbonyl derivatives of palladium and platinum are known.

It can be said that in the above-mentioned olefin complexes and metal carbonyls, olefins and carbon monoxide are activated by complex formation. In addition to olefins and carbon monoxide, some other molecules are activated by coordination with noble metal compounds. The most important example is the activation of hydrogen by coordination to form a hydride complex (37). The formation of hydride complexes is easily recognized by NMR, if the complexes have enough solubility in organic solvents. Hydride complexes are formed by the addition of molecular hydrogen, as shown by the general scheme in eq. (3).

$$\begin{array}{c}L_1L_4\\ \diagdown\diagup\\ Me\\ \diagup\diagdown\\ L_2L_3\end{array} + H_2 \rightleftarrows \begin{array}{c}L_1HH\\ \diagdown|\diagup\\ Me\\ \diagup|\diagdown\\ L_2L_3L_4\end{array} \qquad (3)$$

Hydride complexes are also formed by abstracting hydrogen from other compounds, such as alcohols, olefins, or silanes. For example, when cis-$PtCl_2(PEt_3)_2$ is heated in ethanol with potassium hydroxide, trans-$PtHCl(PEt_3)_2$ is produced in 90% yield, together with an equivalent amount of acetaldehyde (38) [eq. (4)]. As will be described later, hydrogen shifts, both intramolecular and intermolecular, are very

$$\underset{\underset{PEt_3}{|}}{\overset{\overset{Cl}{|}}{Cl-Pt-PEt_3}} + C_2H_5OH + KOH \longrightarrow \underset{\underset{PEt_3}{|}}{\overset{\overset{PEt_3}{|}}{Cl-Pt-H}} + CH_3CHO + KCl + H_2O \qquad (4)$$

important steps in noble metal compound-catalyzed reactions, and the hydrogen shift is possible during the formation of hydride complexes by abstraction of a hydrogen from a coordinated molecule, followed by the addition of the hydrogen to the other part of the molecule (intramolecular) or the other molecule (intermolecular).

Intermolecular hydrogen shift

$$H-A-\overset{|}{Me}-B \longrightarrow A'-\overset{\overset{H}{|}}{\underset{|}{Me}}-B \longrightarrow A'-\overset{|}{Me}-B-H \qquad (5)$$

Intramolecular hydrogen shift

$$\overset{H-X}{\underset{|}{Y-Me-}} \longrightarrow \overset{\overset{H}{|}}{\underset{\underset{|}{Y}}{\overset{X}{\|}-Me-}} \longrightarrow \underset{\underset{H-Y}{|}}{X-Me-} \qquad (6)$$

Furthermore, complex formations with nitrogen **(8)** (39,40), oxygen **(9)** (41-43), sulfur dioxide **(10)** (44-46), and carbene **(11)** (47) have

$$\underset{(8)}{\begin{array}{c} Ph_3P \diagdown \quad \diagup Cl \\ Ir \\ N \diagup \quad \diagdown PPh_3 \\ \| \\ N \end{array}} \qquad \underset{(9)}{\begin{array}{c} OC \quad PPh_3 \\ \diagdown | \quad O \\ Ir—\| \\ \diagup | \quad O \\ Cl \quad PPh_3 \end{array}}$$

$$\underset{(10)}{\begin{array}{c} OC \quad SO_2 \quad PPh_3 \\ \diagdown | \diagup \\ Ir \\ \diagup \quad \diagdown \\ Cl \quad \quad PPh_3 \end{array}} \qquad \underset{(11)}{\begin{array}{c} CH_2 \\ \| \\ Ph_3P—Ir—Cl \\ \diagup \quad \diagdown \\ OC \quad PPh_3 \end{array}}$$

been reported. Takahashi, Sonogashira, and Hagihara reported that tetrakis(triphenylphosphine)platinum and -palladium catalyze the oxygenation of phosphine to phosphine oxide and isocyanide to isocyanate with molecular oxygen, and that the oxygen is activated by complex formation: $Pt(PPh_3)_2O_2$ and $Pd(PPh_3)_2O_2$ (42). Until now, there have been few definite reports that these complexed molecules are "activated" and participate in useful synthetic reactions. However, the chemical properties of these complexes are very important topics of current studies, and it may be possible in the future that nitrogen or oxygen will be activated by complex formation towards participation in reactions such as nitrogen fixation or mild specific oxidation reactions.

III. Reactions Involving the Reduction of Divalent Palladium

A. CHEMICAL PROPERTIES OF PALLADIUM COMPOUNDS USEFUL FOR ORGANIC SYNTHESES

One of the essential properties of palladium compounds useful for organic syntheses is that palladium compounds, originally divalent, are reduced to the zerovalent state easily. This property of palladium compounds is important as the driving force of some reactions carried out in the presence of palladium chloride. An olefinic molecule π-complexed to divalent palladium is susceptible to a nucleophilic attack. In other words, by coordinating with palladium chloride, the olefinic bond, which is usually susceptible to electrophilic attack when not complexed, now reacts with nucleophiles. It is reasonably expected that the complex formation would greatly reduce the tendency to react with an electrophile due to lower electron density than in the free olefin. Such an olefin π-complex is comparable to the bridged bromonium ion postulated as an intermediate in electrophilic bromination of an olefin.

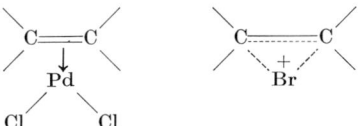

In another description, the olefin complex formation is somewhat similar to acid–base neutralization where the olefin (base) coordinates with palladium (acid).

Thus it becomes possible for various nucleophiles to attack the palladium–olefin complex. In this case, it should be considered that there are two possible sites for the nucleophilic attack, namely the metal and the ethylenic carbon. Nucleophiles which do not form a strong coordination bond with palladium, preferentially attack the ethylenic carbon. For such nucleophiles, we can cite OH^-, RCO_2^-,

RO⁻, amines, carbanions, and others. This type of nucleophilic reaction is not commonly encountered in usual organic chemistry. Although there have been several recent studies of nucleophilic attacks on π-bonded olefins, it is not certain whether the nucleophiles first coordinate with the metal and then migrate to the σ-bonded ligand (insertion reaction) or whether a direct intermolecular reaction is involved.

With the attack of the nucleophiles, palladium accepts two electrons and is converted into the zerovalent state. Thus, by the reaction of palladium–olefin complexes with a variety of nucleophiles in non-aqueous media, it is possible to prepare vinyl compounds by substitution at the double bond. Usually in organic chemistry, addition reactions are common with aliphatic double bonds, while substitution reactions are prevalent with aromatic compounds. On the other hand,

$$\underset{\substack{Cl \quad Cl}}{\overset{\overset{\displaystyle C=C}{\downarrow}}{Pd}} H + X^- \longrightarrow C=C\underset{X}{} + Pd + HCl + Cl^- \tag{7}$$

with the palladium-complexed reactions, it is possible to carry out nucleophilic substitution reactions on aliphatic double bonds by virtue of the facile reduction of divalent palladium to the zerovalent state. This type of vinylation reaction constitutes a new organic reaction and the synthetic usefulness of this reaction is quite significant. As will be described later, many interesting reactions are possible by virtue of this reactivity, and palladium complexes are very useful in organic syntheses.

However, palladium is still an expensive material for common use in organic chemistry laboratories. Divalent palladium is reduced to zerovalent palladium as described above by the reaction of an olefin with the nucleophiles. Fortunately, however, zerovalent palladium can be reoxidized easily to divalent palladium chloride by treatment with a mixture of hydrochloric acid and nitric acid. When *in situ* oxidation of the reduced palladium to divalent palladium (with some other metal ions such as Cu^{2+} or Fe^{3+} present in the reaction medium) is possible without precipitating metallic palladium, only a catalytic amount of palladium chloride is necessary. In turn, reduced Cu^{1+} or Fe^{2+} is reoxidized with molecular oxygen in the reaction medium as shown in eq. (8). In addition to cupric and ferric ions, the *in situ*

$$Pd^{2+} \rightarrow Pd^0 \qquad (8a)$$

$$Pd^0 + 2CuCl_2 \rightarrow PdCl_2 + 2CuCl \qquad (8b)$$

$$2CuCl + \tfrac{1}{2}O_2 + 2HCl \rightarrow 2CuCl_2 + H_2O \qquad (8c)$$

reoxidation of palladium can be carried out by using *p*-benzoquinone. Thus, when this recycling process is achieved by a proper choice of the reaction conditions, the unique oxidation reaction can be carried out with the consumption of molecular oxygen in the presence of a catalytic amount of palladium chloride. In this case, it can be said that palladium is not a very expensive reagent, and this is apparent from the examples described later.

B. OXIDATION OF OLEFINS TO CARBONYL COMPOUNDS

1. *Oxidation of Olefins to Saturated Carbonyl Compounds*

In 1934, Anderson, while investigating the structure of Zeise salt, observed that acetaldehyde was formed with the deposition of metallic platinum by heating an aqueous solution of Zeise salt at 100°, and gave eq. (9) for the observed reaction (48). Also, the formation of

$$\begin{bmatrix} Cl & & CH_2 \\ | & & \| \\ Cl-Pt & \leftarrow & \| \\ | & & CH_2 \\ Cl & & \end{bmatrix}^- K^+ + H_2O \longrightarrow KCl + 2HCl + Pt + CH_3CHO \qquad (9)$$

acetaldehyde with the precipitation of metallic palladium when ethylene was passed into an aqueous solution of palladium chloride has been known since 1894 (49). Actually, this reaction was used for the quantitative determination of palladium by means of ethylene (50).

These interesting oxidation reactions remained buried in the chemical literature for a long time without attracting the attention of organic chemists until the researchers of the Consortium für Elektrochemische Industrie (Research Institute of the Wacker Company) in München invented the process now called the Wacker process (51,52). The invention of the Wacker process is a good example of what sometimes happens in industrial research; the search for one thing failed, but led to something unexpected and possibly of greater value. In 1956, in the hope of preparing ethylene oxide, Smidt and co-workers were passing a gas mixture of ethylene, oxygen, and hydrogen over a palladium–charcoal catalyst. In this experiment, no ethylene oxide was formed, but a trace of acetaldehyde was observed. Smidt and coworkers were able to show that the palladium chloride–ethylene complex was an intermediate. They found that the reaction proceeded even more rapidly in an aqueous solution. In this reaction, a stoichiometric amount of palladium chloride was reduced and the rate of reoxidation of metallic palladium with molecular oxygen was too slow. Later they found ingeniously that metallic palladium can be readily reoxidized by cupric or ferric chloride in solution, thus opening up the possibility of using palladium in a catalytic amount. This oxidation reaction seems rather strange at first glance, because a noble metal is oxidized by a base metal ion. It should be said that this was a great invention introducing an entirely new process into the chemical industry and organic syntheses. Cuprous ion can be reoxidized by molecular oxygen and its rate of reoxidation is faster than that of other comparable metal ion systems. Within a relatively short period, this reaction was developed into a technical process. At present, the industrial production of acetaldehyde from acetylene is being replaced by this process all over the world. Also, acetone is produced from propylene. A review on these olefin oxidations will be given shortly (53).

The stoichiometry of the reaction is shown in eqs. (10). Instead of

$$CH_2=CH_2 + PdCl_2 + H_2O \rightarrow CH_3CHO + Pd + 2HCl \qquad (10a)$$

$$Pd + 2CuCl_2 \rightarrow PdCl_2 + 2CuCl \qquad (10b)$$

$$2CuCl + \tfrac{1}{2}O_2 + 2HCl \rightarrow 2CuCl_2 + H_2O \qquad (10c)$$

$$CH_2=CH_2 + \tfrac{1}{2}O_2 \rightarrow CH_3CHO \qquad (10)$$

cupric and ferric chloride, Moiseev, Vargaftik, and Syrkin utilized p-benzoquinone or hydrogen peroxide to reoxidize the palladium metal (54).

This oxidation reaction of olefins can be carried out with various unbranched olefins and olefins with various functional groups. Formally, the reaction proceeds by nucleophilic attack of hydroxide anion on an olefinic carbon (52), and the position of the hydroxide anion attack on an asymmetrically substituted olefin is predicted by Markownikoff's rule. Methyl ketones are the main products from terminal olefins (other than ethylene), indicating that the reaction involves a nucleophilic attack by hydroxide anion. However, by adjusting the reaction conditions, a considerable amount of aldehyde can be formed (55). It is known that a considerable amount of chloroacetaldehyde is formed as a by-product in the industrial production of acetaldehyde (56). The chlorination occurs under the influence of cupric chloride.

Compared with the great industrial success for the acetaldehyde and acetone productions, the application of this unique oxidation method to organic synthesis of methyl ketones from other terminal olefins on a laboratory scale has not been thoroughly studied. One reason is that with higher olefins (1-hexene and higher), the rate of the reaction decreases greatly. The higher terminal olefins do not react as readily in an aqueous solution of palladium chloride as do the lower olefins. This difficulty can be overcome by employing aqueous dimethylformamide (DMF) as solvent with a regulated feed of an olefin into the catalyst solution. In this way, Clement and Selwitz reported that it is possible to prepare methyl ketones in more than 80% yield (57).

$$CH_3-(CH_2)_9-CH=CH_2 \xrightarrow{PdCl_2,\ CuCl_2\ \text{in DMF}} CH_3(CH_2)_9COCH_3 \quad (11)$$
$$(87\%\ \text{yield})$$

The oxidation of various olefinic compounds has been studied by Smidt and co-workers (51,58). For example, when butadiene is oxidized, crotonaldehyde is the primary product by C-1 attack; then crotonaldehyde is reoxidized to form 3-ketobutyraldehyde which cyclizes in acidic solution by an aldol condensation to form 1,3,5-triacetylbenzene. In the same way, α,β-unsaturated acids are oxidized

$$CH_2=CH-CH=CH_2 \xrightarrow{OH^-} CH_3-CH=CH-CHO$$
$$\xrightarrow{OH^-} CH_3-CO-CH_2-CHO \longrightarrow \text{1,3,5-triacetylbenzene} \quad (12)$$

to keto acids. Since the reaction medium is acidic, the keto acids are easily decarboxylated to form ketones. With crotonic acid, attack on the β-carbon, followed by decarboxylation, gives acetone. The

$$CH_3-CH=CH-CO_2H \xrightarrow{OH^-} CH_3-CO-CH_2CO_2H \longrightarrow CH_3COCH_3 + CO_2 \quad (13)$$

isomeric methacrylic acid forms propionaldehyde. Some nitrogen-containing compounds are oxidized to give aldehydes or ketones free of nitrogen (58). For example, methacrylamide gives propionaldehyde. On the other hand, acrylonitrile is converted into 2-oxopropionitrile by α-carbon attack in 88% yield. The products obtained by the oxidation

$$CH_2=CH-CN \xrightarrow{OH^-} CH_3-CO-CN \qquad (14)$$

of various olefinic compounds are shown in Table I.

2. Mechanism of the Olefin Oxidation Reaction

The mechanism of the olefin oxidation reaction was studied at first by Smidt and Moiseev and their respective co-workers, and an olefin–palladium complex has been suggested as an intermediate. Smidt and co-workers proposed that the reaction proceeds through intramolecular reaction of the coordinated ethylene with an OH⁻ ligand. It was shown that the formation of acetaldehyde from the ethylene complex involves the intramolecular migration of a hydrogen atom from one carbon of the ethylene to the other. Another possibility is

$$\begin{array}{c}H\\ \diagdown\\ C\leftarrow OH^-\\ \|\rightarrow PdCl_3^-\\ C\\ \diagup \diagdown\\ H\quad H\end{array}\quad\longrightarrow\quad\left[\begin{array}{c}H\quad O-H\\ \diagdown |\diagup\\ C\\ \|\rightarrow PdCl_3^-\\ H-C\\ \diagup\diagdown\\ H\quad H\end{array}\right]^-\quad\longrightarrow\quad\begin{array}{c}H\\ |\\ +C-O-H\\ |\\ H-C-H\\ |\\ H\end{array}\quad\longrightarrow\quad\begin{array}{c}H\\ |\\ C=O\\ |\\ H-C-H\\ |\\ H\end{array}\qquad (15)$$

that vinyl alcohol is formed by OH⁻ attack on the ethylene with hydrogen abstraction from the ethylenic carbon with palladium chloride, and then vinyl alcohol rearranges to acetaldehyde (59). This possibility was ruled out by the fact that the reaction carried out in D_2O yielded acetaldehyde free of deuterium, indicating that all four hydrogens in the acetaldehyde must come from the ethylene (52). Therefore, the question to be answered is how hydrogen transfer from one carbon to the other takes place by the action of palladium chloride.

Kinetic studies of the ethylene oxidation reaction were carried out by several workers, and it was shown that the reaction is first order in ethylene and palladium ion (59,60), and that the reaction is inhibited by protons and chloride ion (59,61). In the ethylene oxidation, an isotope effect $k_H/k_D = 4.05$ was found by Moiseev, Vargaftik, and Syrkin (62) when the reaction was carried out in D_2O. Thus they

TABLE I
Oxidation of Various Unsaturated Compounds with $PdCl_2$ and Oxidation–Reduction Systems in Aqueous Solution (51,58)

Starting materials	Reaction Temp.	Reaction Time, min	Products	Conversion, %
Monoolefins				
Ethylene	20	5	Acetaldehyde	85
Propylene	20	5	Acetone	90
1-Butene	20	10	2-Butanone	80
1-Pentene	20	20	2-Pentanone	81
1-Hexene	30	30	2-Hexanone	75
1-Heptene	50	30	2-Heptanone	65
1-Octene	50	30	2-Octanone	42
1-Nonene	70	45	2-Nonanone	35
1-Decene	70	60	2-Decanone	34
Diolefins				
Butadiene	80	30	Crotonaldehyde	34
1,4-Pentadiene	20	15	2-Penten-1-al	91
Cyclo- and araliphatic olefins				
Cyclopentene	30	30	Cyclopentanone	61
Cyclohexene	30	30	Cyclohexanone	65
Indene	50	60	β-Indanone	66
Styrene	50	180	Acetophenone	57
Allylbenzene	40	30	Benzyl methyl ketone	76
Unsaturated carboxylic acids				
Acrylic acid	50	186	Acetaldehyde	50
Crotonic acid	50	60	Acetone	75
2-Pentenoic acid	35	45	2-Butanone	88
Methacrylic acid	40	60	Propionaldehyde	61
Cinnamic acid	50	10 hr	Acetophenone	35
Sorbic acid	65	15	Ethylideneacetone	35
Maleic acid	50	180	Pyruvic acid	
Itaconic acid	50	60	β-Formylpropionic acid	30
Unsaturated oxygenated compounds				
Allyl alcohol	25	5	Acrolein	75
Crotonaldehyde	25	180	Triacetylbenzene	35
Vinyl acetate	20	60	Acetaldehyde	73
Isopropenyl acetate	25	5	Acetone	94

(*continued*)

TABLE 1 (*Continued*)

Starting materials	Reaction Temp.	Time, min	Products	Conversion, %
Halogenated olefins				
Vinyl chloride	20	Short time	Acetaldehyde	100
Vinyl bromide	10	15	Acetaldehyde	98
1-Bromo-1-propene	30	15	Acetone	65
1-Bromo-1-butene	30	15	2-Butanone	67
1-Bromo-1-hexene	50	45	2-Hexanone	88
1-Chloro-2-methyl-1-propene	40	30	α-Methacrolein	45
α-Chlorostyrene	40	30	Acetophenone	55
Allyl chloride	50	30	Methylglyoxal	65
Allyl bromide	50	30	Methylglyoxal	80
Unsaturated halogenated acids				
α-Bromoacrylic acid	25	1 hr	Acetaldehyde	60
α-Chlorocrotonic acid	50	1 hr	Acetone	70
2-Bromo-2-pentenoic acid	80	1 hr	2-Butanone	62
α-Bromocinnamic acid	70	2 hr	Acetophenone	64
p-Chlorocinnamic acid	70	9 hr	*p*-Chloroacetophenone	25
Unsaturated amines				
Allylamine	25	60	Propionaldehyde	14.6[a]
(amine/PdCl$_2$ = 1:1)			Methylglyoxal	0.6[a]
(amine/PdCl$_2$ = 1:2)	25	60	Acetaldehyde	29.6[a]
			Methylglyoxal	7.3[a]
Allylurea	50	10	Propionaldehyde	24[a]
Unsaturated nitro compounds				
Nitroethylene	70	60	Nitroacetaldehyde	5.5[a]
1-Nitropropylene	70	60	Nitroacetone	37[a]
Unsaturated nitrile				
Acrylonitrile	30	30	2-Ketopropionitrile	88[a]
Unsaturated amides				
Methacrylamide	50	30	Propionaldehyde	82[a]
Crotonamide	50	30	Acetone	80[a]
Cinnamamide	50	80	Acetophenone	48[a]

[a] Yield (%).

proposed the mechanism in Scheme 1 to account for these experimental

$$C_2H_4 + PdCl_4{}^{2-} \rightleftharpoons C_2H_4PdCl_3{}^- + Cl^- \qquad (a)$$

$$C_2H_4PdCl_3{}^- + H_2O \rightleftharpoons C_2H_4PdCl_2H_2O + Cl^- \qquad (b)$$

$$C_2H_4PdCl_2H_2O + H_2O \rightleftharpoons C_2H_4PdCl_2OH^- + H_3O^+ \qquad (c)$$

$$C_2H_4PdCl_2OH^- \rightleftharpoons Cl_2Pd\text{---}CH_2CH_2OH^- \qquad (d)$$
$$(12)$$

$$\underset{Cl}{\overset{Cl}{\diagup}}Pd\text{---}CH_2\text{---}CH\text{---}O\text{---}H + H_2O \longrightarrow Cl^- + PdCl^- + CH_3CHO + H_3O^+ \qquad (e)$$

(12)   Scheme 1

results (63). The first step is the formation of the palladium chloride–ethylene π-complex (step a), which is then converted into a hydrated palladium dichloride π-complex (step b). Step c is the formation of a hydroxo species. The insertion of the π-complexed ethylene into the Pd—OH bond gives σ-complex (12), which has the structure of an oxypalladation adduct (step d). Acetaldehyde is formed by the irreversible breakdown of the oxypalladation product (step e).

In order to evaluate the formation and decomposition of the complex formed during the oxidation of ethylene in the presence of palladium chloride, Moiseev and Vargaftik carried out the reaction of β-hydroxyethylmercuric chloride with palladium chloride in ether. The reaction supposedly led to the formation of Cl—Pd—CH₂CH₂OH, which is postulated as an intermediate of the oxidation reaction. Then this complex decomposed to give acetaldehyde and metallic palladium (64). This result seems to support the intermediacy of the complex (12) in the ethylene oxidation.

$$Cl\text{---}Hg\text{---}CH_2\text{---}CH_2\text{---}OH + PdCl_2 \rightarrow (Cl\text{---}Pd\text{---}CH_2CH_2\text{---}OH) \rightarrow$$
$$CH_3CHO + Pd + HCl \qquad (16)$$

Henry carried out detailed kinetic studies and also comparative studies on the olefin oxidation reactions by palladium chloride and thallic ion. He observed that the isotope effect k_H/k_D is only 1.07 when deuterated ethylene was used for the oxidation reaction, showing that the hydride shift is not a slow step. In order to account for his experimental results, he proposed a somewhat different mechanism for the formation and decomposition of the oxypalladation product (65–67). In this mechanism, the oxypalladation step, or the conversion of the π-complex to the σ-complex, is the rate-determining step and it proceeds through a concerted nonpolar four-centered addition as shown in eq. (17). It is important in this mechanism that the decom-

$$\begin{array}{c}\text{Cl} \quad\quad \text{H}_2\text{C} \\ \diagdown\,\text{Pd}\,\diagup \quad\quad \diagdown\,\text{CH}_2 \\ \diagup \quad\quad \diagdown \\ \text{Cl} \quad\quad \text{HO}\end{array} \xrightarrow{\text{H}_2\text{O}} \begin{array}{c}\text{Cl} \quad\quad \text{CH}_2\text{CH}_2\text{OH} \\ \diagdown\,\text{Pd}\,\diagup \\ \diagup \quad\quad \diagdown \\ \text{Cl} \quad\quad \text{OH}_2 \\ \mathbf{(13)}\end{array} \quad (17)$$

position of the σ-complex **(13)** does not involve a carbonium ion; decomposition is possible through the activated complex **(14)**, in which palladium is assisting the transfer of the hydrogen from the hydroxy-bearing carbon as it leaves with its electrons.

$$\mathbf{13} \longrightarrow \left[\begin{array}{c} \text{H} \quad \text{H} \\ | \quad\quad | \\ \text{H—C—C=O—H} \\ | \quad\quad | \\ \text{Cl—Pd---H} \\ \mathbf{(14)} \end{array}\right] \longrightarrow \text{CH}_3\text{CHO} + \text{HCl} + \text{Pd}^0 \quad (18)$$

By further kinetic studies, Jira, Sedlmeier, and Smidt proposed the following mechanism to account for their experimental results (68). In their mechanism, the *trans*-monohydroxodichloro–olefin complex **(15)** is formed at first. The *trans* complex **(15)** is then converted into the *cis*-monohydroxodichloro–olefin complex **(17)** via the dihydroxo complex **(16)**. In the *cis* complex **(17)** the ethylene is activated by the *trans* chlorine and it is favorably situated for the insertion into the Pd—OH bond by the *cis*-ligand insertion to form σ-complex **(18)**. The hydrogen transfer from one carbon to the other is explained in the following elimination and readdition mechanism. The σ-complex **(18)** is converted into π-olefin–hydride complex **(19)** by abstraction of hydrogen from the hydroxy-bearing carbon. Then hydride is transferred to the other carbon with the simultaneous transformation of the π-complex **(19)** to a σ-complex **(20)**. Finally, acetaldehyde is formed by solvolytic decomposition of the σ-complex **(20)** through carbonium ion species **(21)** (Scheme 2).

3. *Oxidation of Olefins via π-Allylic Complexes*

Simple olefins form π-complexes easily. With some olefins, the initially formed π-complex is converted into a π-allylic complex with elimination of hydrogen chloride under certain conditions. Several

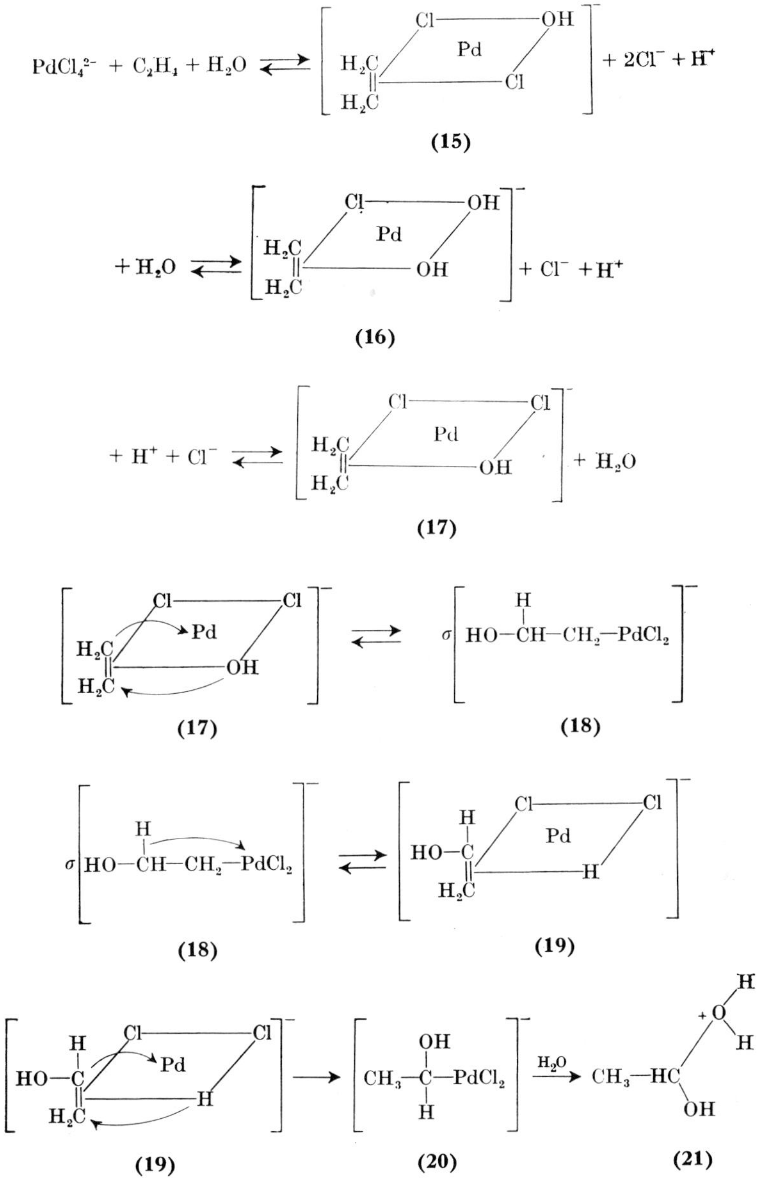

$PdCl_4^{2-} + C_2H_4 + H_2O \rightleftharpoons$ [structure **(15)**] $+ 2Cl^- + H^+$

$+ H_2O \rightleftharpoons$ [structure **(16)**] $+ Cl^- + H^+$

$+ H^+ + Cl^- \rightleftharpoons$ [structure **(17)**] $+ H_2O$

(17) $\rightleftharpoons$ **(18)** $\sigma[HO-CH(H)-CH_2-PdCl_2]^-$

(18) $\sigma[HO-CH(H)-CH_2-PdCl_2]^- \rightleftharpoons$ **(19)**

(19) $\rightarrow$ **(20)** $[CH_3-C(OH)(H)-PdCl_2]^- \xrightarrow{H_2O}$ **(21)** $CH_3-HC\begin{smallmatrix}+OH_2\\OH\end{smallmatrix}$

(21) $\longrightarrow CH_3CHO + H_3O^+$

Scheme 2

branched-chain olefins such as 2-methyl-1-butene or 2-methyl-1-pentene were tested for this π-allylic complex formation. It was found

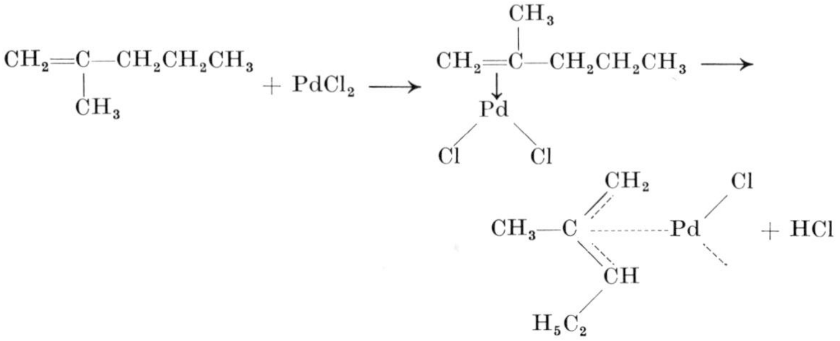

$$CH_2=C(CH_3)-CH_2CH_2CH_3 + PdCl_2 \longrightarrow$$

[π-olefin complex with Pd and two Cl ligands] $\longrightarrow$

[π-allyl complex: $CH_3-C(=CH_2)\cdots CH(C_2H_5)\cdots Pd(Cl)$] + HCl   (19)

that the larger the alkyl groups of the olefins and the higher the degree of branching, the larger the extent of π-allylic complex formation (26–31). For example, isobutene gave 2-methyl π-allyl complex in 27% yield by treatment with palladium chloride in 50% acetic acid at 90°. On the other hand, 3-ethyl-2-pentene gave 1,3-dimethyl-2-ethyl π-allyl complex in 98% yield under the same conditions.

In the oxidation of some substituted olefins, the reaction proceeds through the formation of a π-allylic complex, rather than a π-olefin complex, giving unsaturated carbonyl compounds. This is another type of oxidation by palladium chloride, which was studied mainly by Hüttel and co-workers (28). The oxidation of propylene in an aqueous or acetic acid medium affords a trace of acrolein, which is assumed to be formed via π-allyl complex formation. By a separate experiment, it was confirmed that hydrolysis of the π-allyl complex gave acrolein and propylene (69).

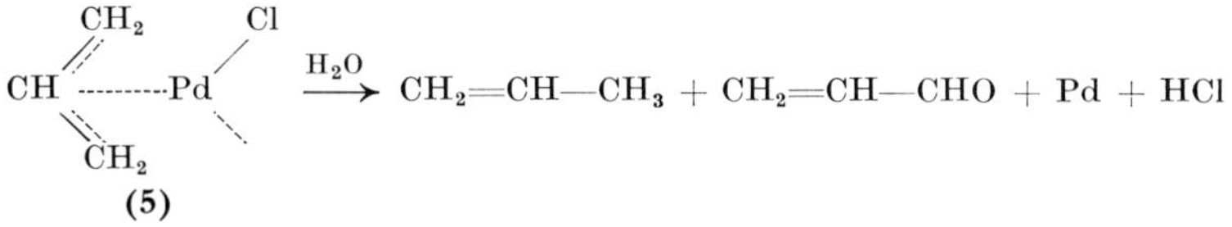

[π-allyl Pd Cl complex] (5) $\xrightarrow{H_2O}$ $CH_2=CH-CH_3 + CH_2=CH-CHO + Pd + HCl$ (20)

In the usual oxidation of olefins, hydrogen migration is essential for the formation of saturated carbonyl products. But when isobutene is oxidized, the products are α-methacrolein and a small amount of isobutyraldehyde. The latter is formed by non-Markownikoff addition followed by a hydride shift. The former is formed via a π-allylic complex as an intermediate in the oxidation, eq. (21). With isobutene, there is no hydrogen on the center carbon, and hence the normal (Markownikoff type) oxidation is impossible.

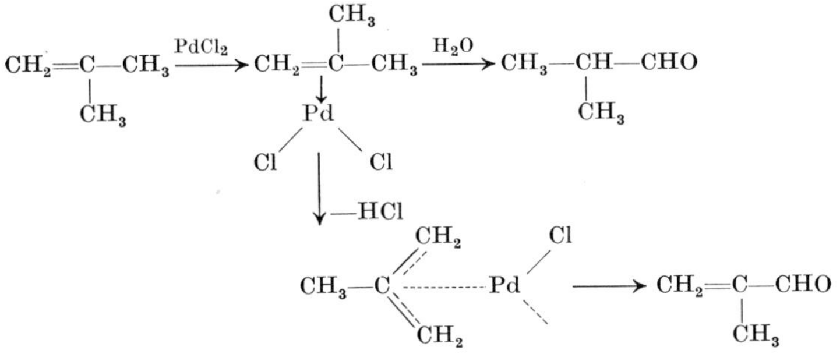

$$CH_2=C-CH_3 \xrightarrow{PdCl_2} CH_2=\underset{\underset{Pd}{|}}{\overset{\overset{CH_3}{|}}{C}}-CH_3 \xrightarrow{H_2O} CH_3-\underset{\underset{CH_3}{|}}{CH}-CHO$$

with Pd coordinated by Cl, Cl

$$\downarrow -HCl$$

$$CH_3-\underset{CH_2}{\overset{CH_2}{C}} \cdots Pd\overset{Cl}{\diagup} \longrightarrow CH_2=\underset{\underset{CH_3}{|}}{C}-CHO \quad (21)$$

Higher branched olefins undergo a somewhat different course of oxidation, giving unsaturated carbonyl compounds. 2-Methyl-1-pentene and 2-methyl-2-pentene produce mesityl oxide by oxidation in acetic acid. Mesityl oxide is formed by attack of OH⁻ at the position α to the allylic system of the complex as in eq. (22). The mechanism of this reaction seems complicated.

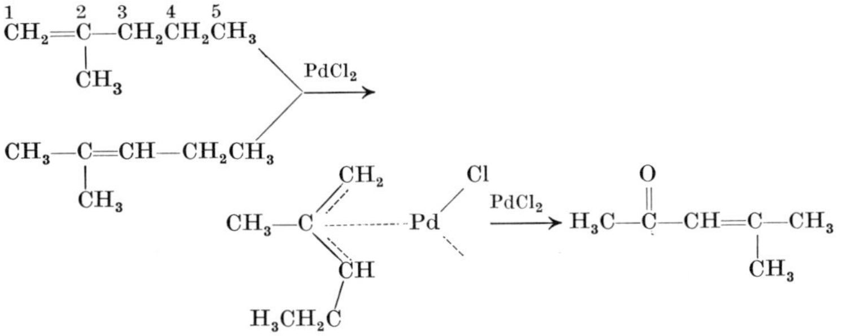

$$\overset{1}{C}H_2=\underset{\underset{CH_3}{|}}{\overset{2}{C}}-\overset{3}{C}H_2\overset{4}{C}H_2\overset{5}{C}H_3$$

$$CH_3-\underset{\underset{CH_3}{|}}{C}=CH-CH_2CH_3 \quad\xrightarrow{PdCl_2}$$

$$CH_3-\underset{\underset{H_3CH_2C}{}}{\overset{CH_2}{\underset{CH}{C}}} \cdots Pd\overset{Cl}{\diagup} \xrightarrow{PdCl_2} H_3C-\underset{}{\overset{\overset{O}{\|}}{C}}-CH=\underset{\underset{CH_3}{|}}{C}-CH_3 \quad (22)$$

Furthermore, Hüttel and Christ found that the branched π-allylic complex can be oxidized with palladium chloride to give two types of unsaturated carbonyl compounds depending on the reaction conditions. For example, the π-allylic complex derived from 2-methyl-1-butene [eq. (23)] afforded α-methylcrotonaldehyde in an unbuffered solution and β-methylcrotonaldehyde in a buffered solution.

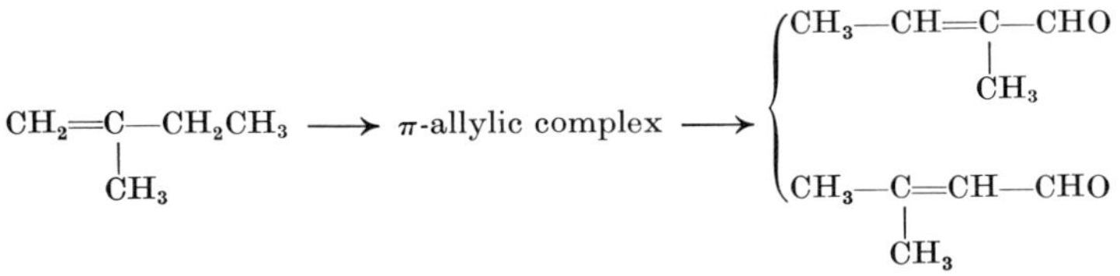

$$CH_2=\underset{\underset{CH_3}{|}}{C}-CH_2CH_3 \longrightarrow \pi\text{-allylic complex} \longrightarrow \begin{cases} CH_3-CH=\underset{\underset{CH_3}{|}}{C}-CHO \\ \\ CH_3-\underset{\underset{CH_3}{|}}{C}=CH-CHO \end{cases} \quad (23)$$

From these results, the olefin oxidation reaction can be summarized as in eq. 24 (28). At first, an olefin and palladium chloride form a

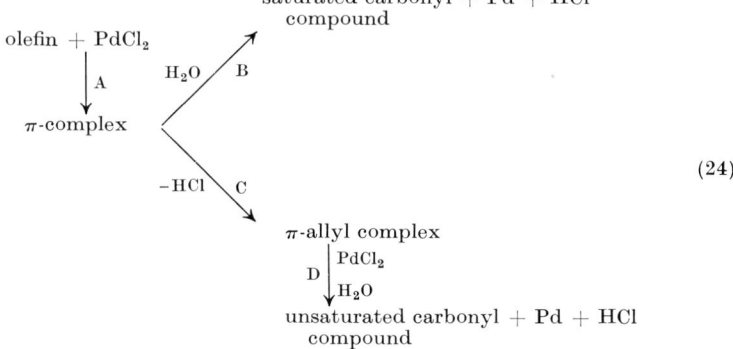

π-olefin complex (process A). The next step is normal OH⁻ attack, followed by hydrogen migration to give a saturated carbonyl compound (process B). When the olefin is branched, it does not follow process B; instead, the π complex is transformed into a π-allylic complex by elimination of hydrogen chloride (process C). When the olefin is highly branched, the π-allylic complex formed from it is very stable and the reaction stops at this stage. If the π-allylic complex is not very stable, it undergoes further oxidation with the help of another molecule of palladium chloride to form unsaturated carbonyl compounds (process D).

In addition, some interesting reactions were observed with branched olefins conjugated with a phenyl group (27,70). Thus, when 1,1-diphenylethylene was heated with one mole of palladium chloride in 50% acetic acid for 30 hr, benzophenone (16.4%) and 1,1,4,4-tetraphenylbutadiene (33.3%) were obtained. Analogously, α-methylstyrene was converted into acetophenone and 2,5-diphenyl-2,4-hexadiene. Thus, with these olefins, two new reactions were observed,

$$\begin{array}{c}C_6H_5\\ \diagdown\\ C=CH_2 + PdCl_2 \longrightarrow C_6H_5-CO-C_6H_5 + \begin{array}{c}C_6H_5\\ \diagdown\\ C=CH-CH=C\\ \diagup\\ C_6H_5\end{array}\begin{array}{c}C_6H_5\\ \diagup\\ \diagdown\\ C_6H_5\end{array}\\ \diagup\\ C_6H_5\end{array} \quad (25a)$$

$$C_6H_5-\underset{\underset{CH_3}{|}}{C}=CH_2 + PdCl_2 \longrightarrow C_6H_5-CO-CH_3$$

$$+ \; C_6H_5-\underset{\underset{CH_3}{|}}{C}=CH-CH=\underset{\underset{CH_3}{|}}{C}-C_6H_5 \quad (25b)$$

namely head-to-head dimerization with dehydrogenation to form the butadiene derivative and oxidation to form the ketone with the elimination of a methylene group, instead of giving an aldehyde. It seems that no reasonable mechanism of these reactions can be given on the basis of present knowledge.

4. *Oxidation of Alcohols*

In addition to the oxidation of olefins to aldehydes, Moiseev, Nikiforova, and Syrkin reported that alcohols can be oxidized with palladium chloride (71). When palladium chloride is heated in an alcohol, it is reduced rapidly to metallic palladium and the product is an aldehyde from a primary alcohol and a ketone from a secondary alcohol. It was proved that the oxidation is due to palladium chloride, and that dehydrogenation by metallic palladium is not responsible for the oxidation, at least with aliphatic alcohols. Furthermore, when the

$$R\text{—}CH(R')\text{—}OH + PdCl_2 \longrightarrow R\text{—}CO\text{—}R' + 2HCl + Pd \qquad (26)$$

temperature of the reaction is high, the aldehyde is oxidized further to an acid by the action of palladium chloride, eq. (27). Probably the

$$R\text{—}CHO + PdCl_2 + H_2O \rightarrow RCO_2H + Pd + 2HCl \qquad (27)$$

reaction proceeds through the mechanism in eq. (28). This oxidation

$$R\text{—}CH_2\text{—}OH + PdCl_2 \longrightarrow R\text{—}CH_2\text{—}O\text{—}PdCl + HCl$$

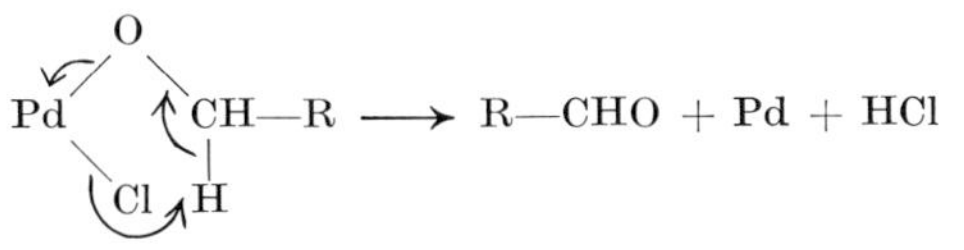

$$\begin{array}{c}\text{Pd}\diagup^{O}\diagdown\text{CH—R} \\ \diagdown_{Cl}\diagup_{H}\end{array} \longrightarrow R\text{—}CHO + Pd + HCl \qquad (28)$$

reaction can be made catalytic by using cupric chloride. However, the oxidation of an alcohol to an aldehyde is much slower than the oxidation of olefinic compounds to carbonyl compounds. Also, it is claimed in a patent that an ester is formed by the oxidation of an aldehyde with palladium chloride carried out in an alcohol and that this oxidation of an aldehyde can be made catalytic by using an excess of cupric chloride in the reaction medium (72).

$$R\text{—}CHO + R'OH + PdCl_2 \rightarrow R\text{—}CO_2\text{—}R' + Pd + 2HCl \qquad (29)$$

C. VINYLATION REACTION

1. *Vinyl Ester Formation*

The Wacker process described in the preceding section is the reaction which results in a formal sense from a nucleophilic attack by OH^-. Other anions might also be expected to attack the olefin complex. In 1960 Moiseev, Vargaftik, and Syrkin tried the reaction of ethylene with acetate anion in the presence of palladium chloride, and confirmed the formation of vinyl acetate with precipitation of metallic palladium (73). Later, Stern and Spector reported the same reaction under somewhat different conditions (74). In this reaction, the role of

$$CH_2=CH_2 + AcO^- + PdCl_2 \rightarrow CH_2=CH-OAc + Pd + HCl + Cl^- \quad (30)$$

sodium acetate is essential; without sodium acetate, the olefin–palladium chloride complex remains almost intact in acetic acid. But in the presence of sodium acetate, a very rapid reaction is observed with the separation of black metallic palladium. Different from the acetaldehyde formation, carbonyl formation by a hydride shift is not possible in this reaction; instead, vinyl acetate is formed by removal of a proton from the olefin. In addition to vinyl acetate, considerable amounts of acetaldehyde and ethylidene diacetate are formed. Also, acetic anhydride is formed in an amount equimolecular to acetaldehyde. In one experiment, ethylene at atmospheric pressure was bubbled into a solution of palladium chloride (9.0×10^{-2} moles) and sodium acetate (3.33×10^{-1} moles) in acetic acid at $105°$. After 3 hr, 8.96×10^{-2} moles of metallic palladium precipitated, and vinyl acetate (3.5×10^{-2} moles), acetaldehyde (3.86×10^{-2} moles), acetic anhydride (4×10^{-2} moles), and ethylidene diacetate (1.25×10^{-2} moles) were formed (75). Also, the formation of ethylene glycol monoacetate and diacetate in the presence of cupric salt has been reported [eq. (31)] (76).

$$CH_2=CH_2 + AcO^- + CH_3CO_2H \xrightarrow[CuCl_2]{PdCl_2} \begin{cases} CH_7=CH-OAc, CH_3CHO \\ CH_3-CH(OAc)_2, (CH_3CO)_2O \\ \underset{OH}{CH_2}-\underset{OAc,}{CH_2} \; \underset{OAc}{CH_2}-\underset{OAc}{CH_2} \end{cases} \quad (31)$$

Therefore, the yield of vinyl acetate in the stoichiometric method is not very high. According to Clement and Selwitz (77), palladium chloride catalyzes the acetylation of acetic acid by vinyl acetate to give acetaldehyde and acetic anhydride in an acetic acid–sodium acetate medium.

Encouraged by the great success of the Wacker process, several groups have successfully developed the industrial production of vinyl acetate by this method. In this reaction, as in the Wacker process, the reduced palladium is reoxidized to palladium chloride by the action of cupric chloride. At present, the industrial process of vinyl acetate production from ethylene catalyzed by palladium chloride is replacing the old process using acetylene.

The mechanism of this apparently simple reaction to form vinyl acetate seems to be quite complex. Moiseev and Vargaftik carried out the reaction of ethylene with palladium chloride in CH_3CO_2D and observed that vinyl acetate and ethylidene diacetate formed by the reaction were practically devoid of deuterium. To account for this result, the carbonium ion intermediate (23) was proposed (78); see eqs. (32). 23 then reacts with acetic acid to yield ethylidene diacetate.

$$CH_2=CH_2 + PdCl_2 + AcO^- \longrightarrow$$

$$\left(\begin{array}{c} Cl-Pd-CH_2-CH-OAc \\ | \\ H \end{array} \right) \longrightarrow CH_3-\overset{+}{C}H-OAc \quad (32a)$$

$$(22) (23)$$

$$23 \begin{array}{c} \nearrow CH_2=CH-OAc \\ {}^{-H^+} \\ \\ {}_{+OAc^-} \\ \searrow CH_3-CH(OAc)_2 \end{array} \quad (32b)$$

Vinyl acetate is formed by deprotonation. In order to prove the intermediacy of complex 22, they carried out the reaction of β-acetoxyethylmercuric chloride with palladium chloride, and the formation of vinyl acetate was confirmed (64). Palladium-assisted hydride

$$AcO-CH_2CH_2-Hg-Cl + PdCl_2 \rightarrow (AcO-CH_2CH_2-PdCl) \rightarrow$$
$$CH_2=CH-OAc + Pd + HCl \quad (33)$$

transfer is another possible route for vinyl acetate formation from complex 22, as proposed by Henry (66).

Propylene, deuterated at the center carbon, was mixed with non-deuterated propylene and the mixture was allowed to react with acetic acid in the presence of palladium chloride and sodium phosphate (79).

By this reaction, Stern and Spector found that the rate of the reaction decreased 2.8 fold by the deuteration. Therefore, it seems probable that the rate-determining step is the rupture of the C—H bond at the center carbon of propylene. In addition, it was found that deuterium was retained 75% in the propenyl acetate and isopropenyl acetate formed in the reaction, supporting a mechanism involving a 1,2 shift of the hydride from the attacked carbon, followed by proton loss from the adjacent carbon atom. In examining the results of the deuterium experiment, however, it has to be considered that deuterium can migrate to the other carbon by the catalytic action of palladium chloride (80,81), and that retention of the deuterium may not always be due to hydride migration.

The reaction of various olefins with acetate anion was studied by using palladium chloride and sodium acetate. In addition, the reaction of olefins with palladium acetate was studied in order to compare its reactivity with that of lead tetraacetate, mercuric acetate, and thallic acetate. With higher olefins, a complex mixture of acetates was obtained. Different authors gave different results from the reaction of acetate ion with higher olefins, and different mechanisms have been proposed. It seems likely that the course of the reaction is very dependent on the reaction conditions. It is probable that the reaction systems: (1) palladium chloride + sodium acetate, (2) palladium acetate, and (3) palladium chloride + sodium acetate + cupric salt, give different products, respectively. Also it is probable that changes in temperature, solvent, and time have some effect on the reaction products.

For example, Bryant and McKeon reported that when propylene was allowed to react with palladium acetate in acetic acid, allyl acetate constituted 90% of the products, and isopropenyl acetate (9%) and propenyl acetate (1%) were minor products (82). In marked contrast, the reaction of propylene with palladium chloride, disodium hydrogen phosphate, and acetic acid in isooctane gave 64% of isopropenyl acetate and 36% propenyl acetate (79). The results of the oxidation reaction of propylene under different conditions reported by several workers are summarized in Table II.

The mechanism of the reaction of olefins with palladium acetate was studied by Winstein and co-workers for comparison with the mechanism of the reaction of mercuric acetate, thallic acetate, and lead tetraacetate (83). Oxidations of propylene, 1-butene, *cis*- and *trans*-2-butenes,

TABLE II

Reaction of Acetate with Propylene

Pd compd.	Base	Solvent	Products, %				Ref.
			$CH_2=CH-CH_2OAc$	$CH_2=C-CH_3$ $\underset{OAc}{\|}$	$CH_3CH=CH-OAc$		
					cis	trans	
$Pd(OAc)_2$		CH_3CO_2H	90	9		1	82
$Pd(OAc)_2$		CH_3CO_2H	0.9	98.6		0.5	83
$PdCl_2$	Na_2HPO_4	CH_3CO_2H isooctane		64	36	36	79
$PdCl_2$	CH_3CO_2Na	CH_3CO_2H	3	44	36	17	84,85

1-pentene, and *cis*-2-pentene by palladium acetate proceeded smoothly at 25° to give high yields of monoacetates. By the analysis of the reaction products, Winstein found that from 1-olefins, the predominant product was an enol acetate and the minor product was an allylic acetate. Thus from propylene, isopropenyl acetate (98.6%), *cis*- and *trans*-propenyl acetate (0.5%), and allyl acetate (0.9%) were obtained. On the other hand, *cis*- and *trans*-2-butenes were oxidized nearly exclusively to a secondary allylic acetate (97%). From these experimental results, the following mechanism was proposed. At first, the oxypalladation of an olefin gives the adducts from which the element of H—Pd—OAc is eliminated to yield the enol acetates or allyl acetates. In the oxypalladation step, Markownikoff addition is preferred over non-Markownikoff addition, and elimination to give the allylic acetates is preferred somewhat over the alternative one leading to the enol acetates. This mechanism does not involve a hydride transfer step; see Scheme 3.

However, Bryant and McKeon gave different results (82). They obtained *trans*-crotyl acetate (58%) and 3-buten-2-ol acetate (40%) and some enol acetate by the reaction of palladium acetate in acetic acid with *cis*- and *trans*-2-butenes, eq. (34). To account for their

$$CH_3-CH=CH-CH_3 \longrightarrow \begin{array}{l} CH_3-CH=CH-CH_2OAc \quad (58\%) \\ CH_2=CH-\underset{\underset{OAc}{|}}{CH}-CH_3 \quad (40\%) \end{array} \quad (34)$$

results, they proposed the formation of an unsymmetrically bonded three-carbon intermediate. Moiseev, Vargaftik, and Syrkin obtained allylic acetates and the acetate of 2-hexen-1-ol in 68% yield by the reaction of 1-hexene. Analogously, 1-heptene gave the acetate of 2-hepten-1-ol (66%), and they proposed the intermediate formation of a π-allylic complex (86). Later, it was definitely shown that the reaction does not proceed through the formation of a π-allylic complex.

In these cases, the reaction conditions were probably different. Experimental results obtained under different reaction conditions can not be compared. Sometimes the separation and identification of the products are not easy, since they all have isomeric structures. Also, in the presence of palladium chloride, the primary product isomerizes easily. The possibilities of olefin isomerization and allylic isomerization of the ester must be considered when explaining the results.

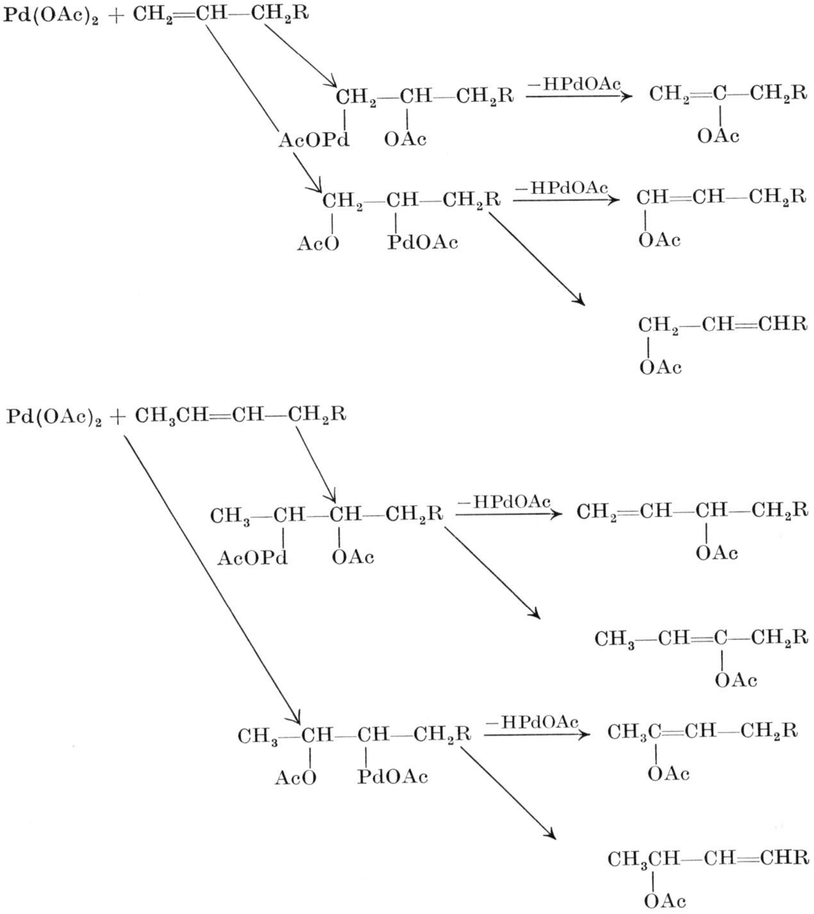

$Pd(OAc)_2 + CH_2=CH-CH_2R$

$$\begin{array}{c} CH_2-CH-CH_2R \\ | \quad\quad | \\ AcOPd \quad OAc \end{array} \xrightarrow{-HPdOAc} \begin{array}{c} CH_2=C-CH_2R \\ | \\ OAc \end{array}$$

$$\begin{array}{c} CH_2-CH-CH_2R \\ | \quad\quad | \\ AcO \quad PdOAc \end{array} \xrightarrow{-HPdOAc} \begin{array}{c} CH=CH-CH_2R \\ | \\ OAc \end{array}$$

$$\begin{array}{c} CH_2-CH=CHR \\ | \\ OAc \end{array}$$

$Pd(OAc)_2 + CH_3CH=CH-CH_2R$

$$\begin{array}{c} CH_3-CH-CH-CH_2R \\ | \quad\quad | \\ AcOPd \quad OAc \end{array} \xrightarrow{-HPdOAc} \begin{array}{c} CH_2=CH-CH-CH_2R \\ | \\ OAc \end{array}$$

$$\begin{array}{c} CH_3-CH=C-CH_2R \\ | \\ OAc \end{array}$$

$$\begin{array}{c} CH_3-CH-CH-CH_2R \\ | \quad\quad | \\ AcO \quad PdOAc \end{array} \xrightarrow{-HPdOAc} \begin{array}{c} CH_3C=CH-CH_2R \\ | \\ OAc \end{array}$$

$$\begin{array}{c} CH_3CH-CH=CHR \\ | \\ OAc \end{array}$$

(Scheme 3)

Schultz and Gross studied the reaction of acetate anion with 1-hexene and investigated the effect of the reaction conditions on the products (87). Actually, they found 24 peaks in the hexenyl acetate fraction by gas chromatographic analysis of the reaction products. It was shown clearly that reaction temperature, reaction time, acetate–chloride ratio, solvents, and other conditions have profound effects on the products. They especially emphasized the formation of hexan-1,2-diol-1-acetate, hexan-1,2-diol-2-acetate, and hexan-1,2-diol-diacetate. The formation of these products was explained by the mechanism of neighboring-group participation of acetate [eq. (35)]. It should be noticed that these bifunctional products are formed only when both palladium chloride and cupric chloride are used. It was observed that low acetate–chloride ratio and short reaction time favor neighboring-group displacement of palladium by acetate, instead of hydride transfer, to give the cyclic intermediate [eq. (35)].

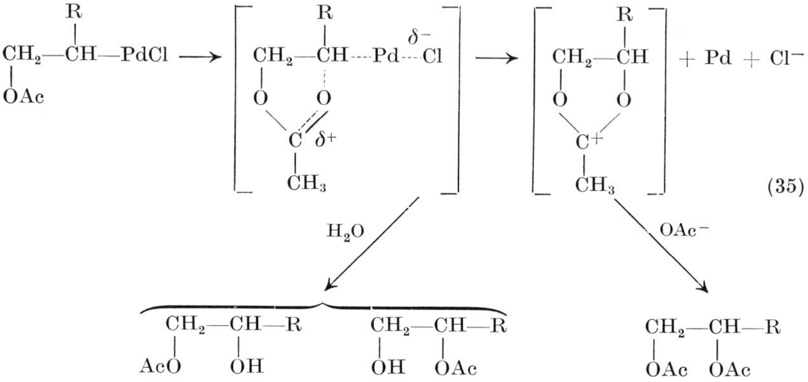

$$
\begin{array}{c}
\text{CH}_2\text{—CH—PdCl} \\
\phantom{CH_2\text{—}}| \\
\phantom{CH_2\text{—}}\text{R} \\
\phantom{CH_2\text{—}}| \\
\text{OAc}
\end{array}
\longrightarrow
\left[\text{cyclic Pd···Cl intermediate}\right]
\longrightarrow
\left[\text{cyclic cation} + \text{CH}_3\right] + \text{Pd} + \text{Cl}^-
$$

Products:

- $\text{CH}_2\text{—CH—R}$ with AcO, OH (from H_2O)
- $\text{CH}_2\text{—CH—R}$ with OH, OAc (from H_2O)
- $\text{CH}_2\text{—CH—R}$ with OAc, OAc (from OAc^-)

(35)

In order to explain gross changes in the product distribution as the reaction conditions were changed, Schultz and Gross proposed a one-carbon insertion mechanism. In this mechanism, the one-carbon insertion product **(24)** is formed by a neighboring-group five-centered

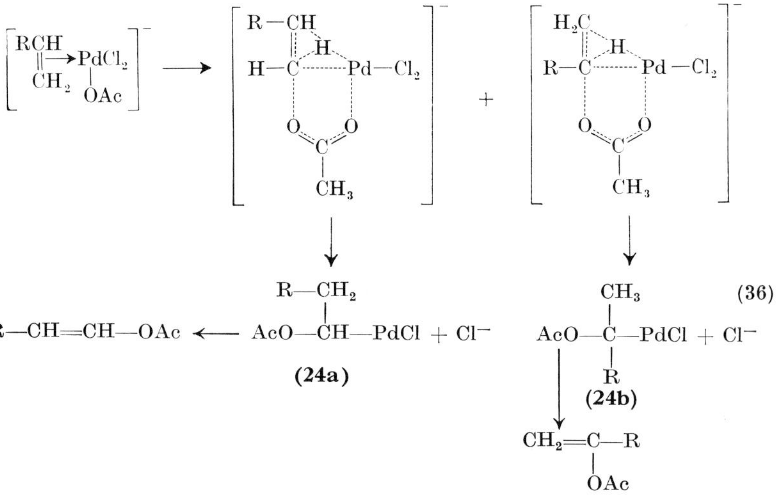

$$
\left[\begin{array}{c}\text{RCH}\\ \| \rightarrow \text{PdCl}_2 \\ \text{CH}_2 \ \text{OAc}\end{array}\right]^{-}
\longrightarrow
\left[\text{5-centered intermediate A}\right]
+
\left[\text{5-centered intermediate B}\right]
$$

(36)

$\text{R—CH=CH—OAc} \longleftarrow \text{AcO—CH—PdCl} + \text{Cl}^-$ with R—CH_2 substituent
(24a)

$\text{AcO—C—PdCl} + \text{Cl}^-$ with CH_3 and R substituents
(24b)
$\downarrow$
$\text{CH}_2\text{=C—R}$ with OAc

reaction, combined with concurrent palladium-assisted hydride transfers. This intermediate (24) then loses a proton and displaces palladium to form the vinylation products [eq. (36)].

The reaction of cyclohexene was also studied. Anderson and Winstein found the exclusive formation of 2-cyclohexenyl acetate by using palladium acetate in acetic acid (88). Green, Haszeldine, and Lindley obtained 2-cyclohexenyl acetate (76%) and 3-cyclohexenyl acetate (24%), rather than the expected 1-cyclohexenyl acetate (89). The proposed intermediate is (25), and in this intermediate, palladium interacts with the hydrogens at positions 3 and 4, leading to the products [eq. (37)].

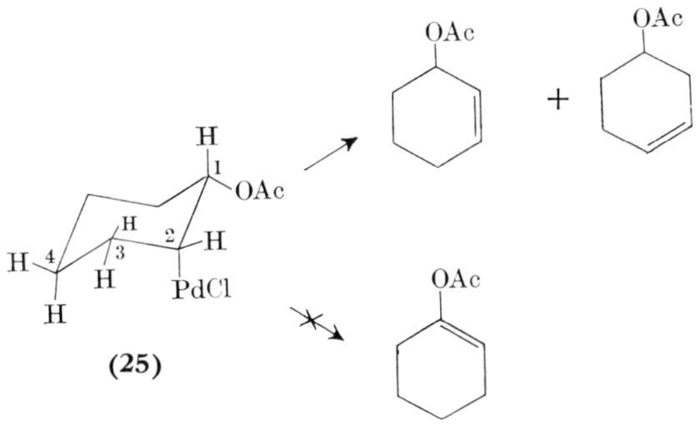

$$(37)$$

Baird found that the vinylation reaction of olefins higher than ethylene is sensitive to olefin structure and reaction medium. In addition to the unsaturated acetate formation, Baird, like Schultz and Gross, observed the formation of saturated bifunctional compounds such as diacetate and haloacetate by the reaction of palladium chloride and cupric chloride (90). Applying this reaction to norbornene, difficultly accessible *syn*-norbornenol was synthesized by a two-step reaction. When norbornene was heated with sodium acetate and cupric chloride in acetic acid containing a catalytic amount of palladium chloride, *exo*-2-chloro-*syn*-7-acetoxynorbornane was formed in 84% yield [eq. (38)]. This compound was converted into *syn*-7-norbornenol in 70% yield by treatment with potassium-*t*-butoxide. The mechanism in

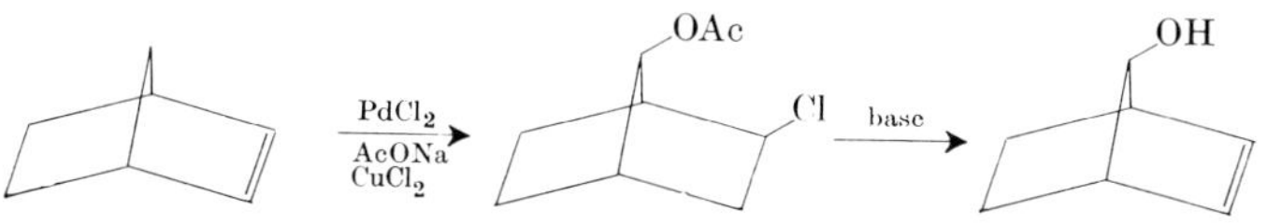

$$(38)$$

eq. (39) was proposed for the formation of chloroacetoxynorbornane, and Baird emphasized that the reaction provides important evidence in support of the carbonium-ion mechanism in the reaction of an olefin

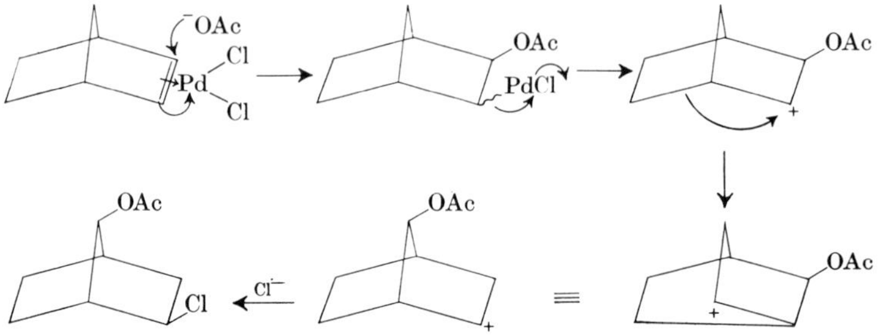

(39)

with acetate anion. Certainly, *exo*-2-chloro-*syn*-7-acetoxynorbornane was obtained by the rearrangement of norbornyl cation. It should be noticed that in many cases, norbornene undergoes reactions which are not observed with other olefins and it seems likely that this result does not necessarily mean that the carbonium-ion mechanism can be applied to all cases.

This rather lengthy description of confusing experimental results shows that it is premature to give a definite mechanism for the vinyl acetate formation from olefins and acetate ion.

In the course of these investigations of vinyl acetate formation, it was found that palladium chloride also catalyzes the transesterification

TABLE III

Preparation of Vinyl Esters by Transesterification (52)

Acid	Mole ratio vinylacetate/acid	Moles of catalyst $\times 10^2$/mole of acid	Temp., °C	Time, hr	Conversion, %	Yield, %
Propionic acid	3	Pd 0.5	76–80	3	45	96
Propionic acid	3	Pt 0.5	76–80	5	38	97
Lauric acid	3	Pd 1.4	76–80	5	77	98
Lauric acid	6	Pd 1.4	25	8	55	96
Lauric acid	3	Rh 1.3	76–80	5	28	99
α-Chloropropionic acid	3	Pd 0.5	76–80	2	65	95
Crotonic acid	3	Pd 0.8	76–80	5	55	90
Sorbic acid	3	Pd 1.0	76–80	4	39	92
Stearic acid	6	Pd 1.4	76–80	3.5	70	90
Oleic acid	3	Pd 1.6	76–80	5.5	70	—
Benzoic acid	3	Pd 1.2	76–80	3	53	98

of vinyl esters. When a vinyl ester was allowed to react with a carboxylic acid in the presence of palladium chloride, a new vinyl ester was formed in good yield at room temperature according to eq. (40)

$$R-CO_2CH=CH_2 + R'-CO_2H \xrightleftharpoons{PdCl_2} R-CO_2H + R'CO_2CH=CH_2 \quad (40)$$

(52). Smidt and co-workers carried out an experiment by treating vinyl propionate with acetic acid labeled with ^{18}O and it was found that ^{18}O was equally distributed over the propionic acid and vinyl acetate formed, showing that there was no attack of acetate ion on the vinyl carbon atom. Examples of the transesterification reaction are shown in Table III. In this reaction, palladium chloride is not reduced and the reaction is catalytic.

2. Vinyl Ether and Vinyl Amine Formations

Nucleophilic attack by an alkoxide anion has also been studied, and vinyl ethers can be prepared in the same way as vinyl acetate (73,74). In this reaction, however, the main product is an acetal, rather than a vinyl ether. When the reaction of ethylene with palladium chloride

$$CH_2=CH_2 + ROH \xrightarrow{PdCl_2} CH_2=CH-OR + CH_3CH(OR)_2 + (Pd + 2HCl) \quad (41)$$

was carried out in CH_3OD, Moiseev and Vargaftik found that the acetaldehyde dimethyl acetal formed by the reaction was devoid of deuterium (78). From this result, they proposed that the reaction proceeds through the intermediate formation of carbonium ion (26) from a palladium σ-complex. The addition of alcohol to 26 gives the acetal and deprotonation of the carbonium ion (26) produces vinyl ether. The acetal is not formed by the addition of alcohol to the

$$Cl-Pd-CH_2CH_2OCH_3 \longrightarrow CH_3\overset{+}{C}H-OCH_3 \xrightarrow{CH_3OD} CH_3-CH(OCH_3)_2$$
$$(26) \quad \underset{-H^+}{\searrow}$$
$$CH_2=CH(OCH_3) \quad (42)$$

vinyl ether [eq. (42)]. Also, the formation of a vinyl ether by the reaction of β-ethoxyethylmercuric chloride with palladium chloride in ether was confirmed as supporting evidence for the intermediate formation of the β-ethoxyethyl–palladium complex (64).

The reaction of other nucleophiles, butylamine and acetamide, with propylene in tetrahydrofuran in the presence of palladium chloride and sodium phosphate was reported by Stern and Spector (74). Isolation and analysis of the products were complicated by the fact that both the nucleophiles and the products apparently form complexes with palladium chloride. Hydrogenation of the complexes yielded butylisopropylamine and N-isopropylacetamide. Hirai, Sawai, and Makishima reported the formation of N-ethylidenebutylamine by the reaction of palladium chloride ethylene complex with n-butylamine in tetrahydrofuran (yield, ca. 20%, based on palladium chloride) (91).

$$\underset{Cl\quad Cl}{\overset{CH_2=CH_2}{\underset{\downarrow}{Pd}}} + Bu-NH_2 \longrightarrow CH_3CH=N-Bu + Pd + 2HCl \qquad (43)$$

3. Displacement Reactions of Vinyl Chloride Catalyzed by Palladium Chloride

Although the reactions to be described now, like the transesterification of vinyl esters, do not involve the reduction of divalent palladium, they are closely related with the other reactions and hence are discussed in this chapter.

It is well known that the chlorine atom of vinyl chloride is inert to nucleophilic attack. However, interesting displacement reactions of the chlorine of vinyl chloride with nucleophiles were reported by Stern, Spector, and Leftin (92). In the presence of disodium hydrogen phosphate and palladium chloride in isooctane and acetic acid, vinyl chloride was converted into vinyl acetate at room temperature [eq. (44)]. Under similar reaction conditions, vinyl chloride was converted

$$CH_2=CH-Cl + CH_3CO_2H \xrightarrow{PdCl_2} CH_2=CH-OCOCH_3 + HCl \qquad (44)$$

into isopropyl acetal by reaction with isopropyl alcohol. These displacement reactions do not involve the reduction of palladium chloride.

$$CH_2=CH-Cl + 2(CH_3)_2CHOH \xrightarrow{PdCl_2} CH_3CH[OCH(CH_3)_2]_2 + HCl \qquad (45)$$

The exact mechanism of the reactions is not known, but it is probable that the reaction proceeds via the formation of a π-complex of vinyl chloride with palladium chloride. The complex formation facilitates the replacement of the chlorine by changing the electron density on the carbon holding the chlorine. This reaction is apparently related to the palladium chloride-catalyzed transesterification of vinyl esters described before.

4. Unsaturated Nitrile Formation

Odaira and co-workers found that, in another vinylation reaction, olefinic cyanide can be prepared by the reaction of an olefin with palladium cyanide with the evolution of hydrogen cyanide (93). The

TABLE IV

Cyanation of Ethylene with $Pd(CN)_2$ (93)

Solvent	Yield, %[a]	
	Acrylonitrile	Propionitrile
C_6H_5CN	50.8	6.9
CH_3CN	17.2	2.7
DMF	7.7	15.6
DMSO	12.6	2.4

[a] Based on $Pd(CN)_2$ used.

reaction proceeds only in polar solvents such as dimethylformamide, dimethyl sulfoxide, and benzonitrile. Polymerization of olefins was observed in the reaction carried out in nonpolar solvents such as benzene and cyclohexane. Thus, acrylonitrile and propionitrile were obtained from ethylene [eq. (46)]. Table IV shows the results of the

$$CH_2=CH_2 + Pd(CN)_2 \longrightarrow \begin{cases} CH_2=CH-CN, Pd \\ CH_3-CH_2-CN, HCN \end{cases} \quad (46)$$

cyanation reaction of ethylene carried out in various solvents at 150° for 5 hr under 55 kg/cm² of ethylene pressure.

The reaction of propylene with palladium cyanide gave methacrylonitrile(I), 3-butenenitrile(II), crotononitrile(III), isobutyronitrile(IV), and butyronitrile(V). The yields of these products varied with the solvents used as shown in Table V. The formation of acrylonitrile from ethylene and hydrogen cyanide catalyzed by palladium was claimed in a patent (94). Similarly, the formation of vinyl chloride from ethylene and hydrogen chloride was claimed in a patent (95,96).

TABLE V

Cyanation of Propylene with $Pd(CN)_2$ (93)

Solvent	Temp., °C	Yield, %[a]				
		I	II	III	IV	V
C_6H_5CN	150	3.6	0.1	2.5	0.7	0.5
C_6H_5CN	210	20.5	4.5	Trace	6.4	None
DMF	210	20.0	12.0	None	2.5	None
C_2H_5CN	210	22.2	4.5	7.7	None	2.3

[a] Based on $Pd(CN)_2$ used.

5. *Reactions of Olefins with Aromatic Rings*

In addition to the above-mentioned vinylation reactions using various nucleophiles, it was found that olefin–palladium chloride complexes react with benzene derivatives to give styrene derivatives. The reaction should be carried out in acetic acid; in the absence of acetic acid, no reaction takes place (97). Thus, when the styrene–palladium chloride complex was refluxed in a mixture of benzene and acetic acid until metallic palladium precipitated, *trans*-stilbene was obtained in 28% yield. When ethylene was allowed to react with benzene in

$$\underset{PdCl_2}{C_6H_5CH{=}CH_2} + C_6H_6 \longrightarrow C_6H_5{-}CH{=}CH{-}C_6H_5 + Pd + 2HCl \quad (47)$$

acetic acid in the presence of palladium chloride in an autoclave, styrene and *sec*-butylbenzene were obtained. Some of the experimental results are shown in Table VI.

TABLE VI

Reactions of Olefins with Aromatic Compounds (97)

Olefin	Comp. aromatic	Reaction temp.	Product	Yield, %
Styrene	Benzene	Reflux	Stilbene	28
Styrene	Toluene	Reflux	*p*-Methylstilbene	25
Styrene	*p*-Xylene	Reflux	2.5-Dimethylstilbene	25
Styrene	Mesitylene	110°	No reaction	
Cyclohexene	Benzene	Reflux	1-Phenylcyclohexene	Trace
Ethylene	Benzene	250°	Styrene	Trace
			sec-Butylbenzene	32

In these reactions, two hydrogens are abstracted from benzene and the olefin by palladium chloride; it is probable that the benzene ring forms some sort of complex with palladium chloride. This is a new type of aromatic reaction and further studies are necessary before the mechanism of the reaction will be clear.

The last two reactions involve formation of a new carbon–carbon bond. In addition to these reactions, it might be possible to form carbon–carbon bonds by the reaction of carbanions with π-complexes of simple olefins, but so far, no reaction of carbanions with π-olefin–palladium chloride complexes has been reported, probably due to the difficulty of finding proper reaction conditions; a π-complex is too reactive to be selective for the reaction of carbanions.

D. REACTIONS OF AROMATIC COMPOUNDS

In the preceding section, the reaction of olefin complexes with benzene rings was described. The reaction indicates that a benzene ring and palladium chloride interact in some way before coupling takes place. By investigating the possibility of nucleophilic attack on palladium salt-complexed aromatic compounds, van Helden and Verberg found that aromatic compounds react in acetic acid–sodium acetate system to yield biphenyl derivatives (98). When benzene was allowed to react in acetic acid solution containing sodium acetate and palladium chloride at 90°, metallic palladium and biphenyl were formed according to (48). In the absence of sodium acetate, no coupling reaction took place.

$$2C_6H_6 + PdCl_2 + 2CH_3CO_2Na \rightarrow C_6H_5\text{—}C_6H_5 + Pd + 2NaCl + 2CH_3CO_2H \tag{48}$$

The following mechanism was suggested by van Helden and Verberg. In the first slow step, a complex is formed between the aromatic ring and palladium chloride. The bonding in this complex may be described as a donation of two π electrons of the aromatic ring to the empty σ orbital of the metal, e.g., in a similar way as between ethylene and palladium chloride. In a fast step, the intermediate reacts with acetate anion to yield a π-cyclohexadienyl–palladium chloride complex. The monomeric species is rapidly converted to the dimeric complex **(27)** with a structure similar to that of a π-allyl–palladium complex. This complex is not stable and decomposes to yield palladium, palladium chloride, acetic acid, and biphenyl. The biphenyl is formed via coupling of the allylic end. However, it is rather difficult to assume that allylic coupling gives biphenyl, since no allylic coupling has been observed in the decomposition of chlorine-bridged π-allylic complexes (99).

Davidson and Trigg proposed that this type of reaction proceeds via the formation of a very unstable σ-phenyl–palladium complex (100).

$$C_6H_5\text{-PdCl}_2 \xrightarrow{-OAc} C_6H_5(\text{H})\text{-PdCl(OAc)} \rightarrow (27) \rightarrow (49)$$

A phenyl radical is not generated in the reaction mixture since the dimerization is insensitive to scavengers such as oxygen. At 100°, palladium acetate reacts with an excess of benzene yielding biphenyl and palladium metal. On the other hand, benzene reacts with palladium acetate in acetic acid at 100° to give biphenyl and phenyl acetate.

$$C_6H_6 + Pd(OAc)_2 \longrightarrow \begin{cases} C_6H_5\text{—}C_6H_5,\ Pd \\ C_6H_5OAc,\ CH_3CO_2H \end{cases} \qquad (50)$$

The addition of perchloric acid accelerates the reaction and increases the yield of biphenyl. From these experimental results, it is apparent that palladium acetate behaves much like mercuric acetate. These results suggest the interesting possibility of new reactions of aromatic compounds by using palladium salts. In other words, a hydrogen on an aromatic ring can be abstracted by palladium salts quite easily. The nature of the interaction or complex formation between palladium salts and benzene rings seems to be a very interesting topic for further studies.

In this connection, it should be mentioned that the protons of benzene rings can be replaced with tritium easily in the presence of metallic palladium (101). Also, it is known that bromobenzene is converted into biphenyl by the catalytic action of palladium in methanol in the presence of potassium hydroxide (102). The exact mechanism of these palladium-catalyzed reactions is not known, but the hydrogen exchange and hydrogenation reactions of aromatic rings in the presence of noble metal catalysts have been explained in terms of π-complex adsorption (103). It is apparent that noble metal compounds interact with aromatic rings before the reaction takes place. Thus, it is probable that new aromatic reactions will be found in which palladium chloride or metallic palladium may complex with aromatic rings and abstract hydrogens from the ring very easily.

E. THE REACTIONS OF CARBANIONS WITH PALLADIUM COMPOUNDS

It is known that π-allylic complexes react with various nucleophiles, but the reactions are slower than those of olefin π-complexes; this is because π-allyl palladium complexes are more stable and less reactive than the π-complexes. For example, the π-allyl–palladium chloride complex does not react with water at room temperature.

The reaction of π-allylic complexes with carbanions was studied by Tsuji, Morikawa, and Takahashi. In the reactions of the complex with carbanions, attack at the allylic position was observed with the precipitation of metallic palladium. For example, π-allyl–palladium chloride and ethyl malonate in dimethyl sulfoxide gave allyl- and diallylmalonate as shown in eq. (51) (104,105). It is probable that

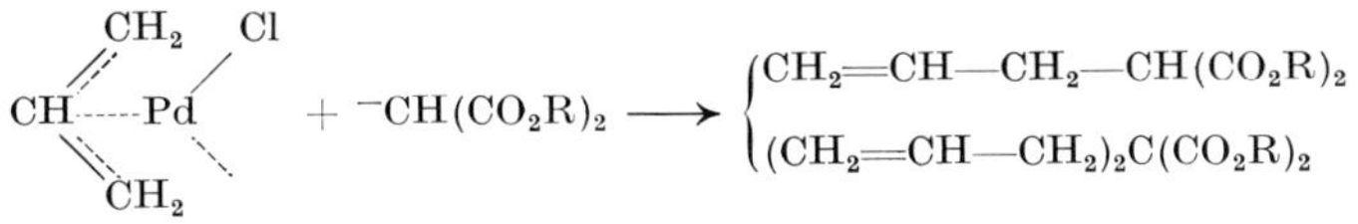

$$\text{CH}_2\text{=CH-CH}_2\text{-Pd-Cl} + {}^-\text{CH}(\text{CO}_2\text{R})_2 \longrightarrow \begin{cases} \text{CH}_2\text{=CH-CH}_2\text{-CH}(\text{CO}_2\text{R})_2 \\ (\text{CH}_2\text{=CH-CH}_2)_2\text{C}(\text{CO}_2\text{R})_2 \end{cases} \quad (51)$$

malonate anion at first coordinates to palladium and then the coupling between malonate and the allyl group takes place, but no conclusive evidence was given.

An example of another carbanion, an enamine, was found to react with the complex. The morpholine enamine of cyclohexanone reacts with the π-allyl complex and the allyl group is introduced into the α position of cyclohexanone. In this reaction it is rather unusual that

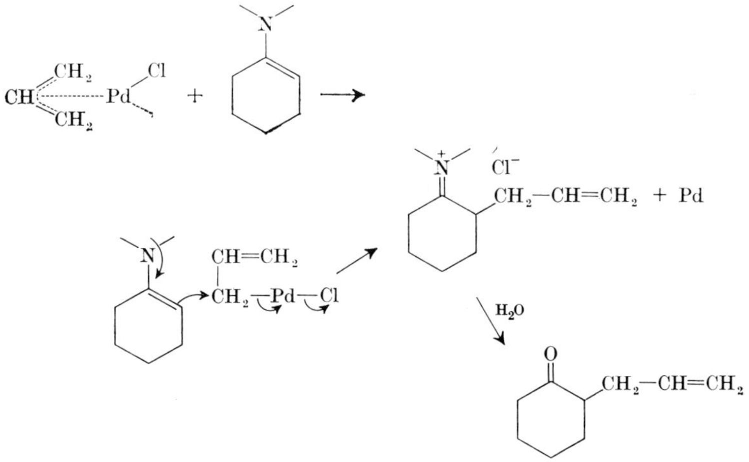

(52)

the enamine, which is an amine and is expected to react with the palladium to expel the allyl group, attacks carbon instead, eq. (52). Alkoxide anion reacts with the complex, but in this case, the oxidation of the alkoxide to a carbonyl compound is the main reaction and the expected allyl ether is a minor product [eq. (53)].

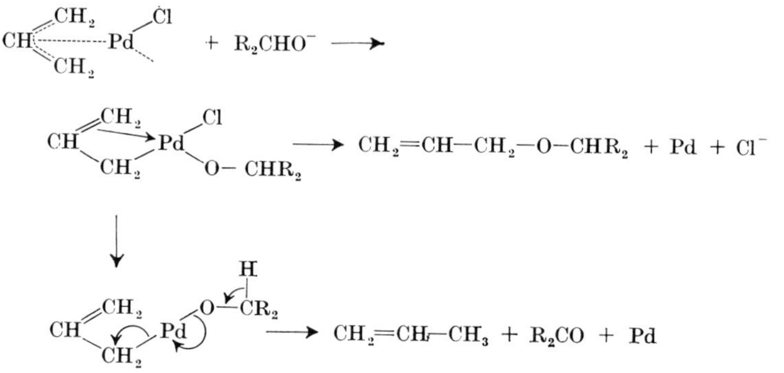

$$CH_2=CH-CH_2-Pd(Cl)(CH_2) + R_2CHO^- \longrightarrow$$

$$\longrightarrow CH_2=CH-CH_2-O-CHR_2 + Pd + Cl^- \quad (53)$$

$$\downarrow$$

$$\longrightarrow CH_2=CH-CH_3 + R_2CO + Pd$$

These reactions of the π-allyl complex with nucleophiles show that the palladium complexes differ from the usual organometallic compounds. For example, the allyl group of allyl Grignard reacts with electrophiles. On the other hand, when the allyl group is coordinated with palladium, it reacts with nucleophiles. Thus, the carbon–metal bonds in the Grignard and palladium complexes have opposite properties. This is due to the fact that divalent magnesium tends to make the carbon quite anionic, whereas palladium is easily reduced from divalent to zerovalent by abstracting two electrons from the carbanion.

$$CH_2=CH-CH_2-Mg-X \qquad CH_2=CH-CH_2-Pd-Cl$$
$$\qquad\qquad A^+ \qquad\qquad\qquad\qquad\qquad B^-$$

Of course, as long as the π-allylic complexes are derived from various allyl halides, the reactions mentioned here are not useful, because the allyl halides themselves react with nucleophiles without complexing with palladium. However, the π-allylic type complexes can be prepared from various types of compounds which do not react with nucleophiles by themselves. In these cases, the reactions of π-allylic complexes with nucleophiles are useful.

The reactions of carbanions with palladium complexes can also be applied to other stable palladium complexes. 1,5-Cyclooctadiene

forms a very stable complex with palladium chloride through two
π-olefin bonds. Chatt, Vallarino, and Venanzi found that the complex
reacts with alcohol in the presence of a weak base to form a new dimeric

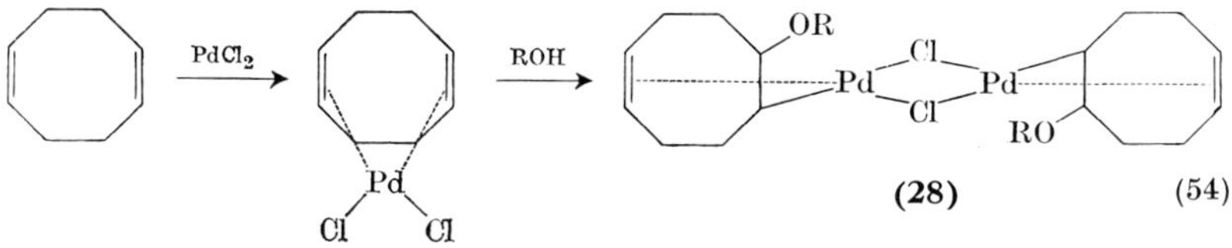

(28)   (54)

complex (28) (106,107). Tsuji and Takahashi found that active methylene compounds react easily with this complex to form new carbon–carbon bonds (108). Malonate or acetoacetate reacts smoothly with the complex in the presence of sodium carbonate in ether under heterogeneous conditions at room temperature. By this reaction, a new complex (29) which has a new carbon–carbon bond was isolated in almost quantitative yield. The ease of the nucleophilic attack at the double bond to form the new carbon–carbon bond is quite remarkable, showing that the palladium–olefin bond is very reactive to carbanions [eq. (55)].

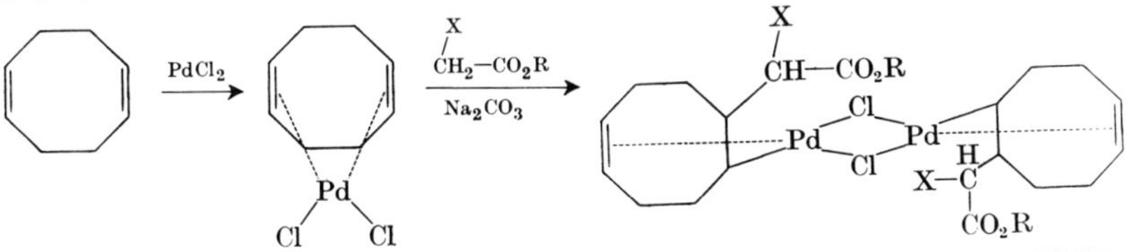

(29a) $X = CO_2R$,   (29b) $X = COCH_3$
(55)

The new complex (29) still has a palladium–carbon σ- and π-bond from the remaining double bond with palladium and undergoes further transformations by treatment with various bases. By an attack of a weak base such as sodium carbonate, or an amine which seems to coordinate with palladium, the palladium–carbon bond is cleaved and

(29) 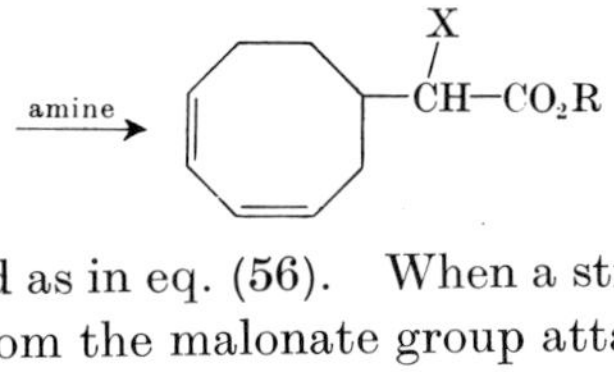 $\xrightarrow{\text{amine}}$ —CH—CO$_2$R   (56)

the compound is obtained as in eq. (56). When a stronger base (which can abstract hydrogen from the malonate group attached to the eight-membered ring) is used, a cyclopropane ring is formed by nucleophilic attack of the anion on the carbon σ-bonded to palladium with precipitation of metallic palladium to form a bicyclo(6,1,0)-nonene derivative.

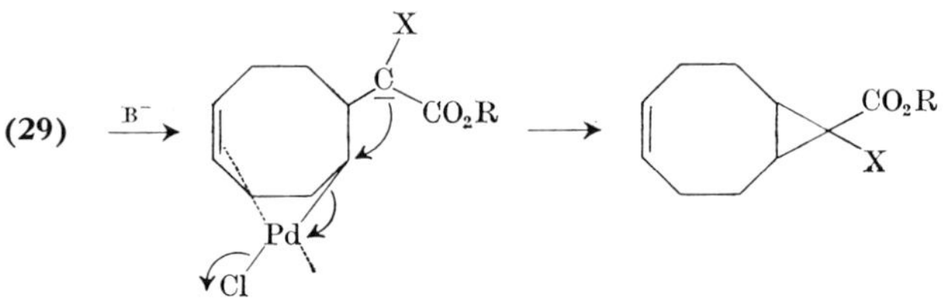

$$(29) \xrightarrow{B^-} \quad \longrightarrow \quad \tag{57}$$

When another molecule of malonate anion is allowed to react in dimethyl sulfoxide solution with the complex **29**, attack occurs at the π-complexed olefinic bond, followed by a transannular reaction of the eight-membered ring to form a bicyclo(3,3,0)octane having two malonate groups introduced. Also, malonate reacts with **29** to form an asymmetrically substituted bicyclo(3,3,0)octane. The reaction gives a single product, but the stereochemistry of the products is not known. This will be very interesting to study, for it will indicate whether the attack of the carbanion takes place directly or after coordination to the palladium.

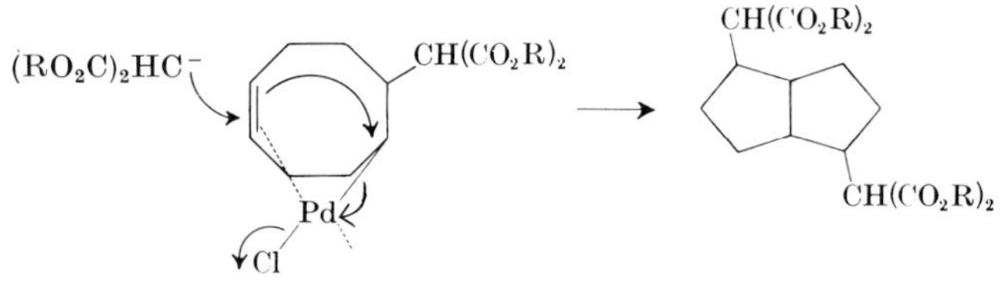

$$\tag{58}$$

IV. Palladium-Catalyzed Carbonylations and Decarbonylations

A. INTRODUCTION

Carbonylation, or the addition of carbon monoxide to various unsaturated bonds, has been studied extensively using several metal carbonyls; nickel, cobalt, and iron carbonyls have been most extensively studied (109). Some noble metals form carbonyls and they catalyze carbonylation in a few cases. On the other hand, palladium forms no simple carbonyls, but carbonyl derivatives such as $Pd_2(CO)_2Cl$ (110), or PdClCO (111) are known.

Recently, it has been found that palladium chloride or metallic palladium can be used for the carbonylation reaction and extensive studies have been carried out. Palladium complexes such as π-complexes of simple olefins and π-allyl complexes can be carbonylated with the concomitant reduction of divalent palladium. These reactions can be regarded as oxidation reactions in certain respects. Also, metallic palladium combined with hydrogen halides is an active catalyst for carbonylation.

B. CARBONYLATIONS OF SIMPLE OLEFINS

1. Carbonylation of Olefin–Palladium Chloride Complexes

The reaction of the ethylene–palladium chloride complex with carbon monoxide in benzene proceeds smoothly at room temperature to give β-chloropropionyl chloride (112,113). The reaction was applied

$$\begin{array}{c} CH_2\!=\!\!=\!\!CH_2 \\ \downarrow \\ PdCl_2 \end{array} + CO \longrightarrow Cl\!-\!CH_2\!-\!CH_2COCl + Pd \qquad (59)$$

to other olefins, especially α-olefins. In this reaction, carbon monoxide is always introduced at the terminal carbon giving a straight-chain acid

TABLE VII
Carbonylation of Olefins and Subsequent Esterification Reactions (113)

Olefin, excess	$PdCl_2$, g	CO pressure, kg/cm^2	Products	Yields, %[a]
Ethylene	5	55	$CH_2(Cl)CH_2COOC_2H_5$	41
Propylene	3	100	$CH_3CH(Cl)CH_2COOCH_3$	27
1-Butene	10	60	$CH_3CH_2CH(Cl)CH_2COOCH_3$	11
1-Pentene	10	60	$CH_3CH_2CH_2CH(Cl)CH_2COOCH_3$	10
1-Hexene	10	50	$CH_3CH_2CH_2CH_2CH(Cl)CH_2COOCH_3$ and other chloroesters	16
2-Butene (cis)	10	50	$CH_3CH(Cl)CH(CH_3)COOCH_3$	13
2-Butene (trans)	10	50		6
Isobutene	10	60	$CH_3C(CH_3)(Cl)CH_2COOCH_3$	12
Vinyl chloride	10	50	$Cl_2CHCH_2COOCH_3$	5
Allyl chloride	12	40	$ClCH_2CH(Cl)CH_2COOCH_3$	5
Cyclohexene	Complex 5.2	50	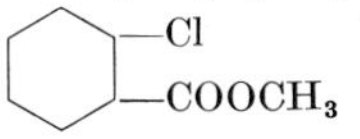 ⌬—Cl, —COOCH$_3$	36[b]

[a] Based on $PdCl_2$ used.
[b] Based on cyclohexene-palladium chloride complex prepared by the Kharasch method.

chloride. Some of the experimental results obtained with various olefins are shown in Table VII.

The mechanism in eq. (60) was proposed. The first step of the carbonylation reaction is the coordination of carbon monoxide to form **31**. Then insertion of the coordinated olefin at the chlorine–palladium bond follows to form the β-chloroalkyl palladium complex **(33)**. This complex undergoes carbon monoxide insertion to form the acyl-palladium complex **(34)** as is assumed in many metal carbonyl catalyzed carbonylation reactions. The final step is the formation of the chloroacyl chloride by the combination of the acyl group with chlorine.

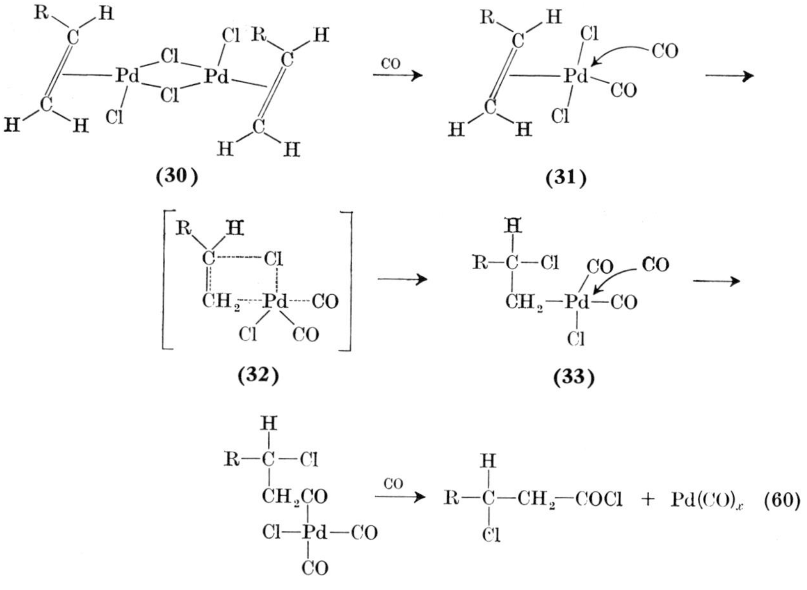

$$R-\overset{H}{\underset{Cl}{C}}-CH_2-COCl + Pd(CO)_x \quad (60)$$

In this reaction, palladium chloride is reduced to the zerovalent state. If the reduced palladium can be reoxidized to palladium chloride in the reaction system, as is done in the Wacker process, this carbonylation reaction will be quite useful for the production of α,β unsaturated acids. In a recent patent (114), it was claimed that acrylic acid was produced from ethylene by the catalytic action of palladium chloride in acetic acid. Reduced palladium is reoxidized with cupric chloride as in the Wacker process.

Cyclopropane is considered to have some double-bond character in certain reactions. It was found that cyclopropane can be carbonylated in the presence of palladium chloride. But the products actually isolated were a mixture of α-, β-, and γ-chlorobutyryl chlorides and the main product was α-chlorobutyryl chloride (115) [eq. (61)].

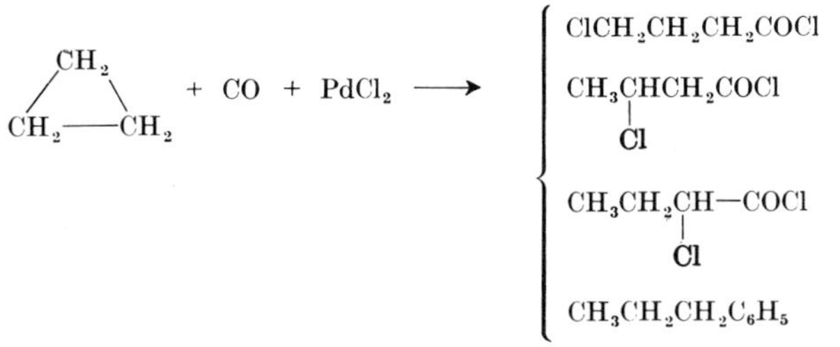

$$\triangle + CO + PdCl_2 \longrightarrow \begin{cases} ClCH_2CH_2CH_2COCl \\ CH_3CHCH_2COCl \\ \quad\quad | \\ \quad\quad Cl \\ CH_3CH_2CH-COCl \\ \quad\quad\quad | \\ \quad\quad\quad Cl \\ CH_3CH_2CH_2C_6H_5 \end{cases} \quad (61)$$

Recently, complex formation between cyclopropane and platinum chloride was studied and two complexes (35 and 36) were isolated after treatment with pyridine (116,117). If the same type of complex formation is possible with palladium chloride, α-chlorobutyryl chloride might be obtained from the complex (35), and γ-chlorobutyryl chloride

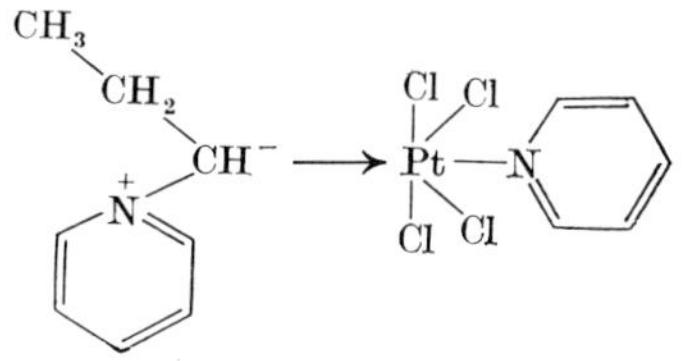

(35) 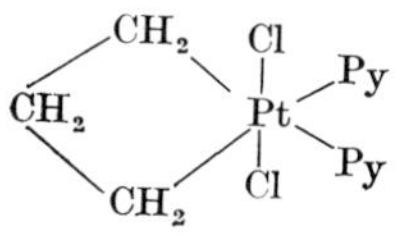   (36)   (62)

should be formed from the complex (36). The nature of the complex formation between cyclopropane and palladium chloride should be clarified before any reasonable mechanism is given for this carbonylation reaction. β-Chlorobutyryl chloride might be formed from propylene generated by the reaction of palladium chloride on cyclopropane. This is the first example of carbonylation of cyclopropane by the action of transition metal compounds. In addition to the above acyl chloride n-propylbenzene was obtained by the Friedel-Crafts reaction.

2. *Catalytic Carbonylation of Olefins*

Carbonylation of simple olefins to form carboxylic acid derivatives catalyzed by noble metal compounds was reported sometime ago in a patent (118). For example, an acid chloride was reported to be formed by the reaction of an olefin, carbon monoxide, and hydrogen chloride in benzene in the presence of palladium chloride.

Later it was found that the carbonylation of olefinic compounds can be carried out more smoothly in alcohol; the product is a saturated ester. In this carbonylation reaction, only a catalytic amount of palladium chloride is necessary. Tsuji, Morikawa, and Kiji found that the presence of metallic palladium and hydrogen halides is essential. This is a new catalytic system for the carbonylation of an olefin to form a carboxylic ester. Thus, by the reaction of ethylene with carbon monoxide (above 50 kg/cm^2) in ethanol containing hydrogen chloride (10–30%) at 100°, ethyl propionate was obtained in moderate yield. In addition, ethyl 4-oxohexanoate was obtained as a minor product (119). By the carbonylation of ethylene in dioxane catalyzed by

$$CH_2=CH_2 + CO + ROH \xrightarrow{Pd/HCl} CH_3CH_2CO_2R + CH_3CH_2COCH_2CH_2CO_2R \quad (63)$$

palladium and hydrogen iodide at 170°, the unsaturated lactones in eq. (64) were isolated (120,121). Also, the carbonylation can be carried

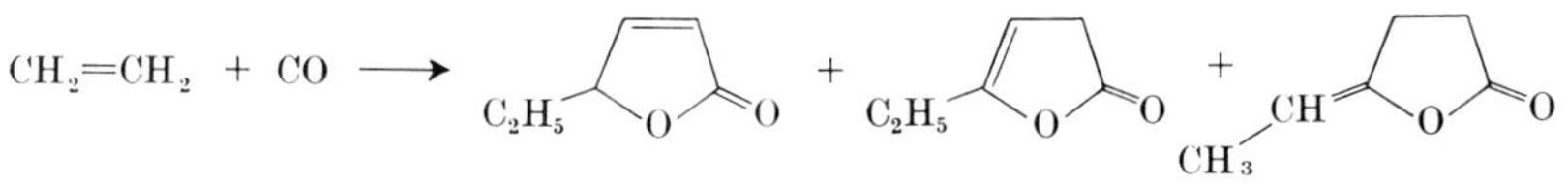

$$CH_2=CH_2 + CO \longrightarrow \text{(lactone products)} \quad (64)$$

out by using palladium complexes with phosphines as the catalyst, and comparable results are obtained (122,123). When olefins other than ethylene are carbonylated, the product is a mixture of normal and iso esters, and in general the iso ester is the predominant product.

$$RCH=CH_2 + CO + ROH \longrightarrow R-\underset{\underset{CO_2R}{|}}{CH}-CH_3 + RCH_2CH_2CO_2R \quad (65)$$

The carbonylation of olefins catalyzed by palladium seems to be quite useful as a new method of carboxylic acid preparation because of the mild reaction conditions and ease in handling the catalyst. However, it should be mentioned that the yield of the carbonylation reaction varies greatly depending on the reaction conditions and the structure of the olefin used. Metallic palladium is recovered after the reaction and recycled.

1,5-Cyclooctadiene (1,5-COD), behaving as a bidentate ligand, forms a very stable complex with palladium chloride. The complex cannot be carbonylated at room temperature in benzene, but it is carbonylated in alcohols at 100° to give a 4-cyclooctenecarboxylate (124), eq. (66).

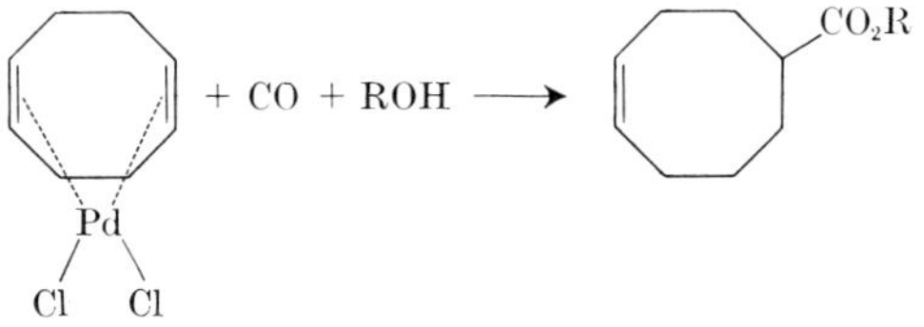

$$\text{[Pd(COD)Cl}_2\text{]} + \text{CO} + \text{ROH} \longrightarrow \text{cyclooctene-CO}_2\text{R} \tag{66}$$

Also, the carbonylation of 1,5-COD can be carried out in the presence of a catalytic amount of palladium chloride, or metallic palladium together with hydrogen halide in alcohol at 100° and 100 atm (124), or under more drastic conditions (150°, 1000 atm) using diiodobis(tributylphosphine)palladium (125). At first, 1,5-COD is carbonylated to form a 4-cyclooctenecarboxylate. Further carbonylation of the mono ester gives rise to a cyclooctanedicarboxylate. As shown in Table VIII, the mono ester can be obtained selectively by controlling the reaction conditions. This carbonylation of 1,5-COD seems to be the best method

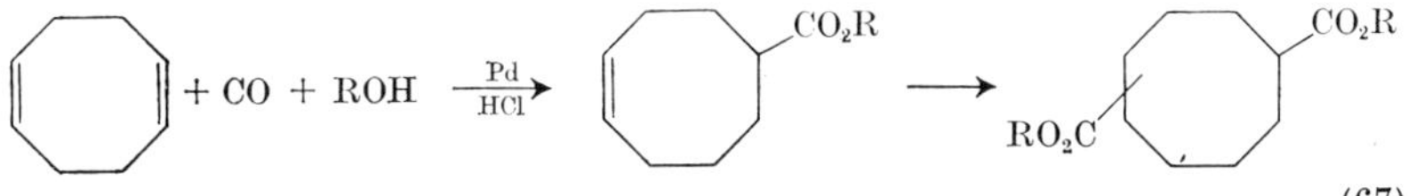

$$\text{1,5-COD} + \text{CO} + \text{ROH} \xrightarrow{\text{Pd}/\text{HCl}} \text{cyclooctene-CO}_2\text{R} \longrightarrow \text{RO}_2\text{C-cyclooctane-CO}_2\text{R} \tag{67}$$

of cyclooctanecarboxylate synthesis. Cyclooctanedicarboxylates obtained by the carbonylation are mixtures of 1,4 and 1,5 isomers. The isomers have not been separated. Cyclooctenecarboxylic acid can be converted into azelaic acid by heating in aqueous alkali hydroxide at 330–375° (126), eq. (68).

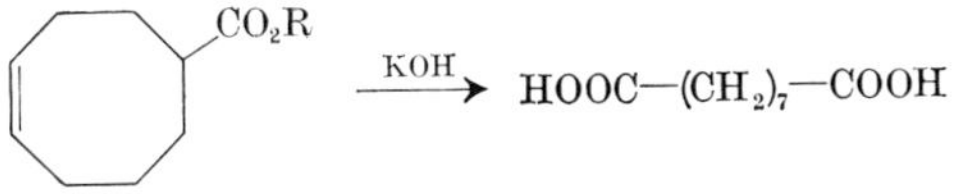

$$\text{cyclooctene-CO}_2\text{R} \xrightarrow{\text{KOH}} \text{HOOC-(CH}_2)_7\text{-COOH} \tag{68}$$

Under certain conditions, the carbonylation of 1,5-COD gives rise to transannular addition of carbon monoxide (127). Thus, 1,5-COD in tetrahydrofuran reacted with carbon monoxide at 150° and 1000 atm in the presence of 1% diiodobis(tributylphosphine)palladium to give bicyclo(3,3,1)nonen-2-one-9 in 40–45% yield. This reaction indicates that the double bond can interact with the acyl complex formed as the

TABLE VIII

Reaction of 1,5-Cyclooctadiene (COD) with Carbon Monoxide[a] (124)

Expt.	1,5-COD, ml	Solvent, ml	Catalyst, g	Reaction Temp., °C	Time, hr	Yield, %[b] Mono-ester	Diester
1	20	EtOH 30	$PdCl_2$ 3	100	3	58.4	19.8
2	20	EtOH 30	$PdCl_2$ 0.5	100	24	16.8	Trace
3	20	EtOH 30	$PdCl_2$ 3	200–250	4	58.0	0.8
4	8	EtOH 12	$PdBr_2$ 1.2	100	1.5	52.2	45.5
5	8	EtOH 12	PdI_2 1.2	100	3.5	5.0	95.0
6	20	10% HCl/EtOH 30[c]	$Pd(acac)_2$[d] 1	100	2	75.0	3.8
7	20	30% HCl/EtOH 30	$Pd(acac)_2$[d] 1	100	1	37.5	59.0
8	20	10% HCl/EtOH 30	Pd-black 0.5	100	24	18.6	Trace
9	20	10% HCl/EtOH 30	10% Pd on charcoal 5	100	24	31.0	31.0

[a] Carbon monoxide pressure was 100 kg/cm² in all cases.
[b] Yield based on 1,5-COD.
[c] 10% hydrogen chloride in absolute ethanol.
[d] Palladium acetylacetonate.

intermediate in the carbonylation reaction as shown in the mechanism in eq. (69) (compare the mechanism of the carbonylation reaction discussed later). The same cyclic ketone was synthesized by Foote and Woodward via several steps (128); the carbonylation method is apparently simple.

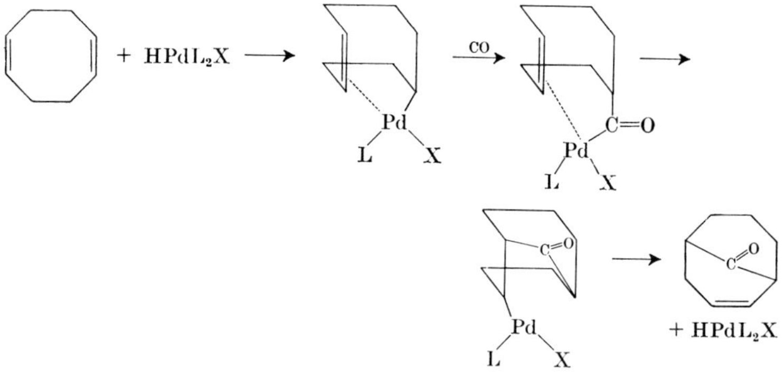

$$\text{(69)}$$

L = ligand

This type of cyclic ketone formation was also observed with α,ω-dienes. For example, the carbonylation of 1,4-pentadiene gave, in 5–10% yield, 2-oxocyclopentylacetate (37) as well as the expected ester product (125). 1,5-Hexadiene produced the cyclic γ-keto-ester

(40) in 40–50% yield, whereas 1,6-heptadiene afforded only a trace of the ketonic product. The mechanism in eq. (70) was given for the γ-keto-ester formation. At first, a palladium–carbon σ bond is formed by the insertion of one of the double bonds into the palladium–hydrogen bond. Then carbon monoxide insertion gives the acyl–palladium product (38). The next step is the insertion of the other double bond into the palladium–acyl bond to form the keto–alkyl–palladium complex (39). Finally, carbon monoxide insertion is repeated to form the keto ester (40).

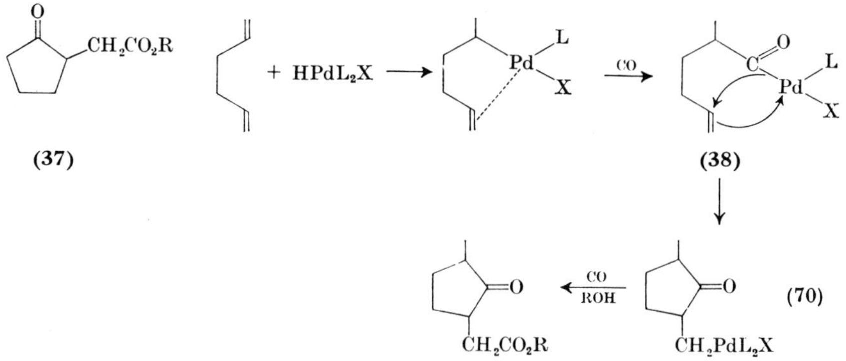

$$\text{(37)} \quad + \text{HPdL}_2\text{X} \longrightarrow \text{(38)} \xrightarrow{\text{CO}} \text{(39)} \xrightarrow[\text{ROH}]{\text{CO}} \text{(40)} \quad (70)$$

The formation of a 1,5,9-cyclododecatriene complex with palladium chloride was reported (129,130), but the structure of the complex is not exactly known. 1,5,9-Cyclododecatriene(1,5,9-CDT) was found to be carbonylated smoothly in alcohol in the presence of a catalytic amount of metallic palladium and hydrogen halide (131). In this carbonylation reaction, carbon monoxide is introduced stepwise and the first attack is mainly at the *trans* double bonds when *cis,trans,trans*-1,5,9-CDT is used. The product is cyclododecadienecarboxylate. Further, carbonylation occurs randomly at either the remaining *cis* or *trans* double bond, giving cyclododecenedicarboxylate. This diester is a mixture of several possible isomers. The last double bond cannot be carbonylated under any conditions. This is due to steric hindrance by the two ester groups which hinders the attachment of metallic palladium essential for the carbonylation. On the other hand, carbonylation of cyclododecene can be carried out smoothly to give cyclododecanecarboxylate. The results of the carbonylation of 1,5,9-CDT are shown in Table IX.

The carbonylation of 1,5,9-CDT has also been accomplished by the

TABLE IX

Carbonylation of 1,5,9-CDT[a] (131)

Catalyst[b]	HCl/EtOH[c], wt.%	Reaction		CO, kg/cm²	Yield, %[d]	
		Temp., °C	Time, hr		Monoester	Diester
PdCl₂	0	100	24	100	20	0
PdCl₂	7.5	100	1	100	54	37
PdCl₂	15	100	1	100	50	41
PdCl₂	15	100	15	100	0	0
PdCl₂	7.5	100	⅓	100	30	0
PdCl₂	7.5	100	½	100	64	3
PdCl₂	7.5	100	10	100	Trace	85
PdCl₂	7.5	100	5	50	33	45
PdCl₂	7.5	100	1	150	60	25
Pd–C	0	100	24	100	0	0
Pd–C	7.5	100	1	100	50	30

[a] Amount of 1,5,9-CDT, 10 g.
[b] Amount of PdCl₂, 1 g Pd–C (10%), 3 g.
[c] Volume of ethanol, 20 ml.
[d] Yield based on 1,5,9-CDT, 10 g.

catalytic action of cobalt carbonyl. In this case, however, monocarbonylation was observed with reduction of the remaining double bonds (132). Also, Lewis acid-catalyzed carbonylations of 1,5,9-CDT and

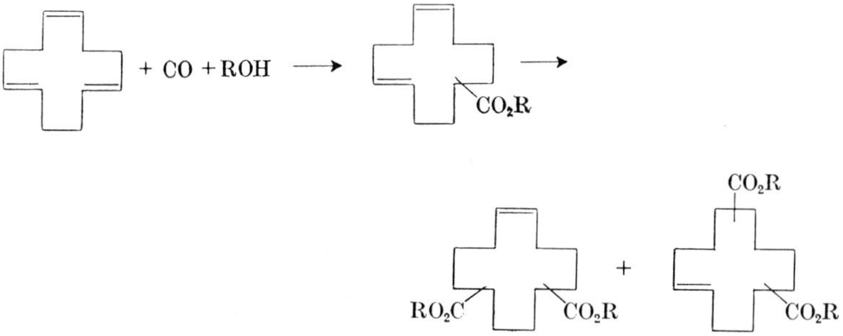

)71)

1,5-COD have been reported, but in this case, extensive ring contraction was observed as well (133,134). These complications make the palladium-catalyzed carbonylation the preferred method for the preparation of the 12- and 8-membered ring acid derivatives, because carbon monoxide is introduced stepwise without ring contraction under rather mild conditions.

Like 1,5-COD, norbornadiene forms a very stable palladium chloride

complex. Carbonylation of the complex has been carried out in benzene and a chloroacyl chloride with a nortricyclene structure was the product (135). The exact stereochemistry of the product is not

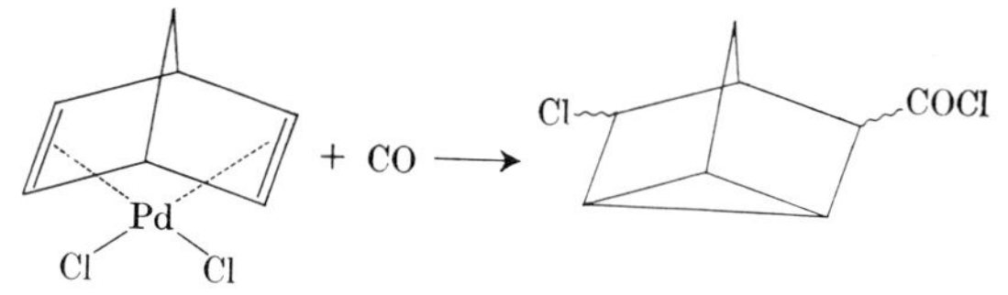

$$\text{[norbornadiene-PdCl}_2\text{ complex]} + \text{CO} \longrightarrow \text{[Cl, COCl-substituted nortricyclene]} \quad (72)$$

known. Carbonylation of norbornadiene itself in ethanol in the presence of a catalytic amount of palladium chloride was attempted with the hope of obtaining an ester, but none was formed (136). The product was found to be a polyketone, formed by 1:1 copolymerization of carbon monoxide and norbornadiene. The polymer has a molecular weight of about 3000 and a strong infrared absorption at 1695 cm^{-1}. From NMR studies, the following *cis* structure was assigned to the

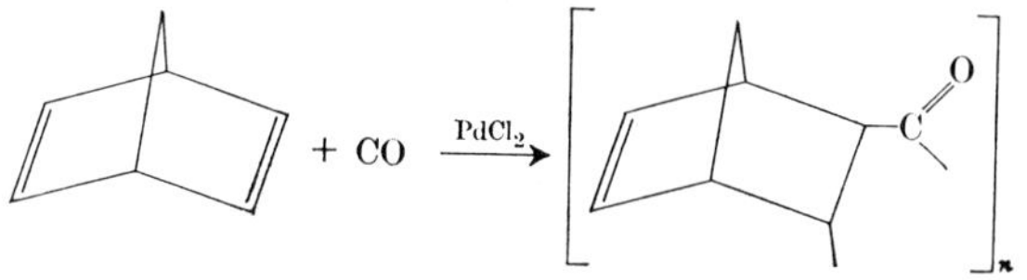

$$\text{[norbornadiene]} + \text{CO} \xrightarrow{\text{PdCl}_2} \text{[polyketone structure]}_n \quad (73)$$

polymer. This is a rare example of polyketone formation by 1:1 copolymerization of carbon monoxide and an olefinic compound with a transition metal catalyst.

C. ALDEHYDE FORMATION

In the metallic palladium-catalyzed carbonylation reactions so far described, the presence of hydrogen halide is essential for the catalysis. In addition to hydrogen halide, hydrogen itself instead of hydrogen halide was found to be effective for the carbonylation catalyzed by metallic palladium (137). In the absence of hydrogen halide, the reaction of an olefin, carbon monoxide, and hydrogen is catalyzed by metallic palladium to give an aldehyde. The aldehyde formation is generally called the oxo reaction, and cobalt carbonyl is the most commonly used catalyst. The yield of the aldehyde in the palladium-catalyzed reaction, however, is not high and a considerable amount of olefin is hydrogenated to saturated hydrocarbon.

$$\text{CH}_2\text{=CH}_2 + \text{CO} + \text{H}_2 \longrightarrow \text{CH}_3\text{CH}_2\text{CHO} \quad (+\text{CH}_3\text{CH}_3) \quad (74)$$

D. MECHANISM OF THE PALLADIUM-CATALYZED CARBONYLATION REACTIONS

Two types of carbonylation reactions catalyzed by palladium were described in the preceding sections. The first one proceeds in the presence of palladium chloride to give a β-chloroacyl chloride. In this carbonylation reaction, palladium chloride is reduced to metallic palladium; a mechanism has been suggested. The second type of carbonylation reaction is catalyzed by metallic palladium, and the presence of some hydrogen source is essential; hydrogen halides and hydrogen are both effective. The following mechanism has been proposed for the second type of carbonylation of olefinic compounds catalyzed by metallic palladium and hydrogen sources (138).

The first step is oxidative addition of hydrogen halide to give a palladium-hydride complex. Then insertion of the coordinated olefin into the palladium-hydrogen bond follows to give an alkyl-palladium complex **(41)**. The alkyl-palladium complex is converted into the acyl-palladium complex **(42)** by carbon monoxide insertion. The final process is cleavage of the acyl-palladium bond by combination of the acyl group with the coordinated chlorine to form an acyl chloride and metallic palladium. The acyl chloride then reacts with alcohol to give

$$Pd + HCl \rightleftharpoons H-Pd-Cl$$

$$\left. \begin{array}{l} H-Pd-Cl \\ RCH=CH_2 \end{array} \right\} \rightleftharpoons R-CH_2CH_2PdClL_n \underset{-CO}{\overset{CO}{\rightleftharpoons}}$$

$$(41)$$

$$RCH_2CH_2COPdClL_n \rightleftharpoons RCH_2CH_2COCl + Pd \quad (75a)$$
$$(42) \qquad \qquad \downarrow ROH$$
$$\qquad \qquad RCH_2CH_2CO_2R + HCl$$

$$Pd + H_2 \rightleftharpoons H-Pd-H$$

$$\left. \begin{array}{l} H-Pd-H \\ RCH=CH_2 \end{array} \right\} \rightleftharpoons RCH_2CH_2PdHL_n \underset{-CO}{\overset{CO}{\rightleftharpoons}}$$

$$(43)$$

$$RCH_2CH_2COPdHL_n \rightleftharpoons RCH_2CH_2CHO + Pd \quad (75b)$$
$$(44)$$
$$(L = \text{ligand})$$

ester and hydrogen halide. Thus the regeneration of metallic palladium and hydrogen halide makes the whole reaction a catalytic cycle. In the same way, in the aldehyde formation the reaction of hydrogen with metallic palladium forms a hydrogen–palladium bond. The alkyl-complex **(43)** formation is followed by carbon monoxide insertion to form the acyl bond **(44)**. Finally the acyl-complex collapses with the formation of an aldehyde and metallic palladium. The formation of a hydride complex by oxidative addition of hydrogen chloride or hydrogen to a metal complex is well known (139,140). Also the formation of an alkyl–metal complex by the addition of a metal hydride to an olefin is an established reaction.

The similarity of the two types of carbonylations which form β-chloroacyl chlorides or saturated esters is apparent. In the β-chloroacyl halide formation, the first step is the insertion of olefin into the palladium–chlorine bond. On the other hand, in the second case, the insertion of olefin takes place into the palladium–hydrogen bond, formed by oxidative addition of hydrogen halide or molecular hydrogen to metallic palladium. The divalent palladium in both cases is reduced after the carbonylation step and the reaction can be regarded as an oxidation reaction in certain respects.

E. DECARBONYLATION REACTIONS

It has been shown by several workers by using some transition metal complexes that the insertion reaction of carbon monoxide to form an acyl-complex is reversible depending on the pressure of carbon monoxide and temperature (141,142). For example, the reversible reaction in eq. (76) is well established.

$$\begin{array}{c} CH_3 \\ \backslash CO CO \\ Mn \\ / | \backslash \\ CO CO CO \end{array} \xrightleftharpoons[-CO]{+CO} \begin{array}{c} CH_3 \\ | \\ CO CO CO \\ \backslash | / \\ Mn \\ / | \backslash \\ CO CO CO \end{array} \quad (76)$$

Also, it is known that the alkyl–palladium phosphine complexes with β-hydrogens in the alkyl groups are unstable (143), and decompose by

$$\begin{array}{c} H L \\ | | \\ R\overset{\frown}{CH}\text{—}CH_2\text{—}Pd\text{—}Cl \\ | \\ L \end{array} \longrightarrow RCH\text{=}CH_2 + Pd + HCl + 2L \quad (77)$$

$$(L = \text{phosphine})$$

β-hydrogen elimination to give an olefin and palladium hydride, which then decomposes to give zerovalent palladium and H^+. Moiseev and Vargaftik studied the decomposition of the alkyl–palladium bond by reacting ethyl magnesium bromide with palladium chloride in ether (64). Equal amounts of ethylene and ethane were formed by the reactions in eqs. (78).

$$C_2H_5MgBr + PdCl_2 \rightarrow C_2H_5PdCl + MgBrCl \qquad (78a)$$

$$C_2H_5PdCl \rightarrow CH_2{=}CH_2 + HCl + Pd \qquad (78b)$$

$$C_2H_5MgBr + HCl \rightarrow CH_3{-}CH_3 + MgBrCl \qquad (78c)$$

If the mechanism in eqs. (78) is correct and the acyl–palladium bond (**42** or **44**) is formed reversibly, it is expected that acyl halides or aldehydes might be decarbonylated to olefins in the absence of carbon monoxide at certain temperatures. It is reasonable to expect that the acyl bond, once formed, can be converted easily to the alkyl complex. In other words, it is expected that an aldehyde or an acyl halide should be decarbonylated when it is heated with metallic palladium in the absence of carbon monoxide. Actually it has been known for some time that some specific aldehydes can be decarbonylated when heated above 180° in the presence of a catalytic amount of palladium and other hydrogenation catalysts (144–153). For example, in the ionone synthesis from α-pinene, *cis*-pinonic aldehyde was decarbonylated to give pinonone in 80% yield by heating with metallic palladium [eq. (79)] at

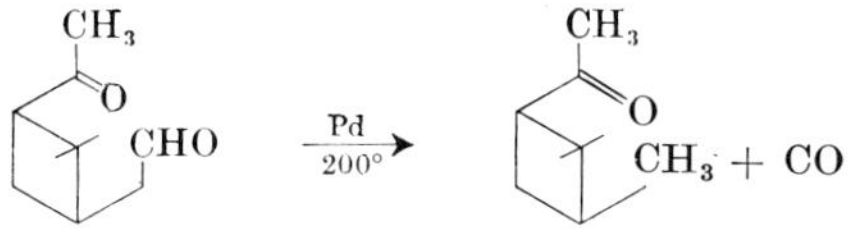

(79)

220° (149). *Trans*-α-substituted cinnamaldehydes can be decarbonylated to give *cis*-styrene derivatives as a main product [eq. (80)], when the product is distilled out as formed. Clearly, the initial product is largely, if not completely, the *cis* styrene (146). From the mechanism of

(80)

the palladium-catalyzed carbonylation of olefins to form aldehydes, it seems clear that aldehydes can be decarbonylated as the reverse process of the carbonylation. Further studies have shown that the decarbonylation of aldehydes using metallic palladium is a common reaction applicable to many aldehydes when they are heated above 180° (138). The product of the decarbonylation is an olefin and the corresponding saturated hydrocarbon. The latter is formed by hydrogenation of the olefin by the action of metallic palladium.

$$RCH_2CH_2CHO \xrightarrow{Pd} RCH=CH_2 + RCH_2CH_3 + CO + H_2 \quad (81)$$
$$\downarrow \text{isomerization}$$

In view of the fact that aldehydes can be decarbonylated smoothly by the catalytic action of metallic palladium, it is expected that acyl halides should also be decarbonylated by the catalytic action of palladium. When heated with a catalytic amount of metallic palladium

TABLE X

Decarbonylation of Acyl Halides (138)

Acyl halide, g	Catalyst, g	Reaction Time, hr	Temp., °C	CO + HCl, ml	Product	Yield, %
$CH_3(CH_2)_8COCl$, 20	1% Pd/C 1	10	200	2960	Nonenes	58
$CH_3(CH_2)_8COCl$, 5	$PdCl_2$ 0.1	1.5	200	1050	Nonenes	90
$CH_3(CH_2)_6COBr$, 5	$PdCl_2$ 0.2	1.5	200	750	Heptenes	80
$C_6H_5(CH_2)_2COCl$, 10	$PdCl_2$ 0.2	1.0	210	1780	Styrene	53
$C_6H_5CH_2COCl$, 20	1% Pd/C 1	3	220	2283	Benzyl-chloride	42
C_6H_5COCl, 10	1% Pd/C 1	24	200	100	Chloro-benzene	5

above 200°, acyl halides are decarbonylated to form olefins, carbon monoxide, and hydrogen halide. The most effective catalyst was found to be palladium chloride, which is readily reduced to metallic palladium by the action of the acyl halide at high temperature, eq. (82)

$$RCH_2CH_2COCl \xrightarrow[200°]{Pd} RCH=CH_2 + CO + HCl \quad (82)$$

(138). Some experimental results are shown in Table X. For example, when decanoyl chloride is heated with palladium chloride at 200° in a distilling flask, rapid evolution of carbon monoxide and hydrogen halide stops after one hour, during which time a mixture of nonene isomers is distilled off. The isomerization of the double bond is very fast and a mixture of isomeric olefins is always obtained. When it is impossible to form an olefin, the product is an alkyl halide. For example, phenylacetyl chloride is converted into benzyl chloride. Benzoyl chloride forms chlorobenzene, but the yield of the decarbonylation reaction with aromatic acid halides is very low. As will be described later, the decarbonylation of aromatic acid halides can be

$$C_6H_5CH_2COCl \rightarrow C_6H_5CH_2Cl + CO \qquad (83)$$

carried out smoothly with a rhodium complex. These smooth decarbonylations of aldehydes and acyl halides catalyzed by metallic palladium support the mechanism given above.

From these experimental results and the reaction mechanism, a mechanism for the well-known Rosenmund reduction was proposed (138,154). The Rosenmund reduction is the conversion of acyl halides into aldehydes by refluxing acyl halides in toluene or xylene in the presence of metallic palladium catalyst and hydrogen gas (155,156). The first step of the reduction is the formation of an acyl–palladium bond by oxidative addition of an acyl halide to metallic palladium. The acyl–palladium complex does not decarbonylate at the temperature of toluene or xylene reflux; instead it reacts with hydrogen to form an aldehyde and metallic palladium. For the decarbonylation, heating to 200° is necessary. It has been reported that the decisive factor in the Rosenmund reduction is the temperature (157). For the optimal yield of aldehydes, it is important to keep the temperature near the lowest point at which hydrogen chloride is evolved. Thus the mechanism of the Rosenmund reduction can be expressed by eq. (84).

$$R\text{—}COCl + Pd \longrightarrow RCO\text{—}Pd\text{—}Cl \xrightarrow{H_2}$$

$$RCO\text{—}\underset{\underset{H}{|}}{\overset{\overset{H}{|}}{Pd}}\text{—}Cl \longrightarrow RCHO + HCl + Pd \qquad (84)$$

For the mechanism of the Rosenmund reduction proposed here, the oxidative addition of acyl halide to metallic palladium to form the acyl–palladium complex is essential. Concerning the addition of an acyl halide to metallic palladium, Chiusoli and Agnes made an interesting observation (154). On an attempted Rosenmund reduction of 2,5-hexadienoyl chloride, they obtained phenol in high yield. In this facile cyclization reaction, the first step must be the addition of the acyl chloride to form an acyl–palladium bond. The coordination of the terminal double bond to the palladium, followed by cyclization through insertion of the double bond at the palladium–acyl bond is the probable mechanism, see eq. (85). In this case the formation of a stable product, i.e., phenol, is certainly the main driving force of the facile cyclization. The same type of cyclization to form cyclic ketones in the carbonylation of 1,5-cyclooctadiene and some α,ω-dienes was previously described.

$$\underset{\substack{\text{Cl}\\ \text{C=O}}}{\bigcirc} \xrightarrow{\text{Pd}} \underset{\substack{\text{Cl-Pd}\\ \text{C=O}}}{\bigcirc} \longrightarrow \underset{\substack{\text{O}\\ \text{ClPd}\ \text{H}}}{\bigcirc} \longrightarrow \underset{\text{OH}}{\bigcirc} + \text{Pd} + \text{HCl} \qquad (85)$$

The isolation of any of the intermediate complexes postulated in the carbonylation and decarbonylation reaction discussed above has been impossible, and it is difficult to determine whether these reactions proceed homogeneously through formation of soluble complexes or heterogeneously by absorption on the metal surface.

In the above mechanistic discussion, "oxidative additions" are assumed to occur with palladium complexes. Like the insertion reactions, oxidative addition is a common reaction of noble metal complexes and it plays a very important role in noble metal-catalyzed reactions. Oxidative addition reactions have become a topic of intensive study only in recent years. In these reactions, A-B type molecules add to an unsaturated four-coordinate square complex, whereupon an octahedral complex is formed with concomitant formal oxidation of the metal by two units. Both polar and nonpolar compounds such as hydrogen, halogens, hydrogen halides, nonmetal hydrides, reactive alkyl halides, acyl halides, and sulfonyl halides, participate in the reactions [see eq. (86)] (158). Also, saturated five-coordinate complexes undergo oxi-

$$\text{Me} + \text{A-B} \longrightarrow \underset{\substack{\text{A}\ \text{B}\\ \text{Me}}}{} \qquad (86)$$

dative addition to form six-coordinate complexes with loss of a neutral ligand.

$$\underset{\text{L}}{\text{Me}} + \text{A-B} \longrightarrow \underset{\substack{\text{A}\ \text{B}\\ \text{Me}}}{} + \text{L} \qquad (87)$$

Oxidative addition reactions are also observed with nontransition metals. Famous examples are the formation of Grignard reagents and Reformatsky reactions. But oxidative additions of noble metals and nontransition metals are quite different in several respects.

$$R—X + Mg^0 \to R—Mg^2—X \tag{88}$$

Several homogeneous catalytic processes involve reversible oxidative additions as an essential step. It should be noted that there is a parallelism between the oxidative addition of noble metal complexes and chemisorption on the transition metal surface.

F. CARBONYLATIONS OF ALLYLIC COMPOUNDS

π-Allyl–palladium chloride can be carbonylated in alcohol at about 100° to form 3-butenoate [eq. (89)]. When the reaction is carried out in benzene, 3-butenoyl chloride is the product (159,160). The carbonylation of a π-allyl–palladium complex is accompanied by reduction

$$\begin{array}{c} \text{CH}_2 \\ \parallel \\ \text{CH} \cdots \text{Pd} \\ \diagdown \\ \text{CH}_2 \\ \text{(5)} \end{array} \diagup \begin{array}{c} \text{Cl} \\ \diagup \\ \end{array} \begin{array}{c} \text{CO} + \text{ROH} \\ \diagup \\ \diagdown \\ \text{CO} \\ \text{in benzene} \end{array} \begin{array}{c} \text{CH}_2=\text{CH}—\text{CH}_2\text{CO}_2\text{R} + \text{Pd} + \text{HCl} \\ \\ \\ \text{CH}_2=\text{CH}—\text{CH}_2\text{COCl} + \text{Pd} \end{array} \tag{89}$$

of divalent to zerovalent palladium. However, the carbonylation of allylic compounds can be carried out in the presence of a catalytic amount of palladium chloride (161). In this reaction, carbon monoxide is inserted into the allylic position. Various types of allylic compounds, such as allylic halides, alcohols, ethers, or esters can be carbonylated in the presence of a catalytic amount of palladium chloride. When the reaction is carried out in an alcohol, the product is a β,γ-unsaturated ester. Some α,β-unsaturated esters and saturated esters are formed in the carbonylation of allylic halides with the influence of the hydrogen halide formed by the carbonylation. In order to avoid these side reactions, the carbonylation of allylic halides can be best carried out in tetrahydrofuran; the formation of free hydrogen halide is suppressed by the ring-opening reaction of tetrahydrofuran in eq. (90).

$$\text{CH}_2=\text{CH}—\text{CH}_2\text{Cl} + \text{CO} + \underset{\text{O}}{\bigcirc} \xrightarrow{\text{Pd}} \text{CH}_2=\text{CH}—\text{CH}_2\text{CO}_2(\text{CH}_2)_4\text{Cl}$$
$$\downarrow \text{ROH}$$
$$\text{CH}_2=\text{CH}—\text{CH}_2—\text{CO}_2\text{R} \tag{90}$$

When the carbonylation reaction is carried out in an aprotic solvent such as benzene or cyclohexane, with palladium chloride as the catalyst, carbon monoxide is inserted at the allylic position of various allylic compounds. Thus allyl chloride gives 3-butenoyl chloride. Allyl ethers form the corresponding ester. Allyl acetate gives the mixed anhydride of 3-butenoic and acetic acid, as in eqs. (91). In the carbonylation of biallyl ether, allyl 3-butenoate is formed as a result of

$$CH_2=CH-CH_2Cl \xrightarrow{CO} CH_2=CH-CH_2COCl \quad (91a)$$

$$CH_2=CH-CH_2OR \xrightarrow{CO} CH_2=CH-CH_2CO_2R \quad (91b)$$

$$CH_2=CH-CH_2OCOCH_3 \xrightarrow{CO} CH_2=CH-CH_2CO_2COCH_3 \quad (91c)$$

the first addition of carbon monoxide. This ester still has an allylic function to be carbonylated, and the second carbon monoxide insertion gives the anhydride of 3-butenoic acid.

$$CH_2=CH-CH_2OCH_2-CH=CH_2 \xrightarrow{CO}$$
$$CH_2=CH-CH_2CO_2CH_2-CH=CH_2 \xrightarrow{CO} (CH_2=CH-CH_2CO)_2O \quad (92)$$

Allylic rearrangement is observed in this carbonylation. Thus from both 2-buten-1-ol and 1-buten-3-ol, only ethyl 3-pentenoate is obtained. This result is explained by assuming that the same complex is formed as an intermediate in the carbonylation reaction from the two allylic alcohols because of delocalization of the double bonds. The complex gives 3-pentenoate as the sole product; see eq. (93).

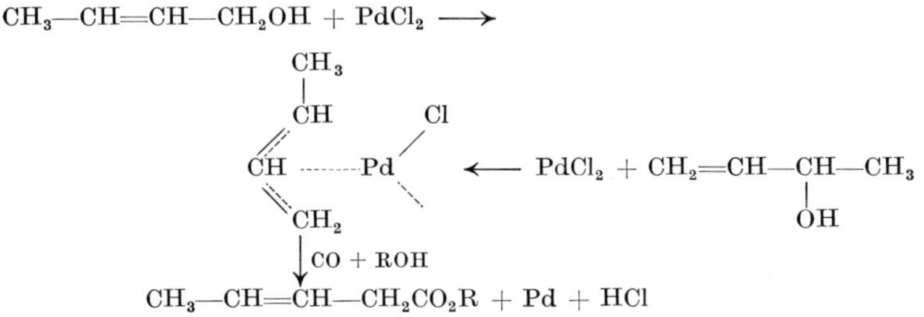

$$CH_3-CH=CH-CH_2OH + PdCl_2 \longrightarrow$$

$$\begin{array}{c} CH_3 \\ | \\ CH \\ \diagup\!\!\!\diagup \\ CH\cdots\cdots Pd\diagup^{Cl} \\ \diagdown \\ CH_2 \\ \downarrow CO + ROH \end{array} \longleftarrow PdCl_2 + CH_2=CH-CH-CH_3 \quad (93)$$
$$\hspace{6cm} \underset{OH}{|}$$

$$CH_3-CH=CH-CH_2CO_2R + Pd + HCl$$

Not only palladium chloride, but also metallic palladium catalyzes the carbonylation of allyl halides. In the metallic palladium-catalyzed carbonylation of allyl halides, the first step seems to be the formation of the π-allyl complex by oxidative addition of allyl chloride to metallic palladium [eq. (94)]. Actually, Fischer and Burger reported the formation of the π-allyl complex from metallic palladium and allyl bromide

$$CH_2=CH-CH_2Cl + Pd \longrightarrow \begin{array}{c} CH_2-Pd-Cl \\ | \\ CH \\ \diagdown \\ CH_2 \end{array} \longrightarrow \begin{array}{c} CH_2 \\ \diagup \\ CH \cdots \cdots Pd \\ \diagdown \\ CH_2 \end{array} \diagdown Cl$$

$$\xrightarrow{CO} CH_2=CH-CH_2COPd-Cl \longrightarrow CH_2=CH-CH_2COCl + Pd \quad (94)$$
$$\downarrow ROH$$
$$CH_2=CH-CH_2-CO_2R + HCl$$

(162). When allylic compounds other than halides are carbonylated, palladium chloride is used as the catalyst. It seems likely that metallic palladium and hydrogen halide formed from palladium chloride in the reaction medium are the catalytic species [eq. (95)]. Therefore, it is probable that these allylic compounds are first converted into allylic halides which then form the π-allylic complexes.

$$CH_2=CH-CH_2-Y + HX \longrightarrow CH_2=CH-CH_2-X \xrightarrow{Pd}$$

$$\begin{array}{c} CH_2 \\ \diagup \\ CH \cdots \cdots Pd \\ \diagdown \\ CH_2 \end{array} \diagdown X \xrightarrow{CO}$$

$$\qquad (95)$$

$$CH_2=CH-CH_2COX \xrightarrow{Y} CH_2=CH-CH_2COY + HX$$

X-halogen   Y-OR, OCOR, etc.

The products obtained by these carbonylations of allylic compounds are β,γ-unsaturated esters. Tsuji, Imamura, and Kiji discovered that a new type of π-allylic complex can be formed from β,γ-unsaturated esters and palladium chloride by elimination of hydrogen chloride as in eq. (96) (24,163). Corresponding α,β-unsaturated esters give the same complexes. This complex formation is a common reaction with α,β- and β,γ-unsaturated carbonyl compounds. In other words, any compounds having allylic hydrogens activated by an electron-attracting group should undergo this type of complex formation. For example, the esters of crotonic acid, 3-butenoic acid, and 3-pentenoic acid form the complexes. In addition to these compounds, some cyclohexenone derivatives also form the complexes (164).

When the complex prepared from 3-butenoate is carbonylated, the product is glutaconate, which has allylic hydrogens activated by two ester groups. Therefore, facile complex formation of glutaconate is

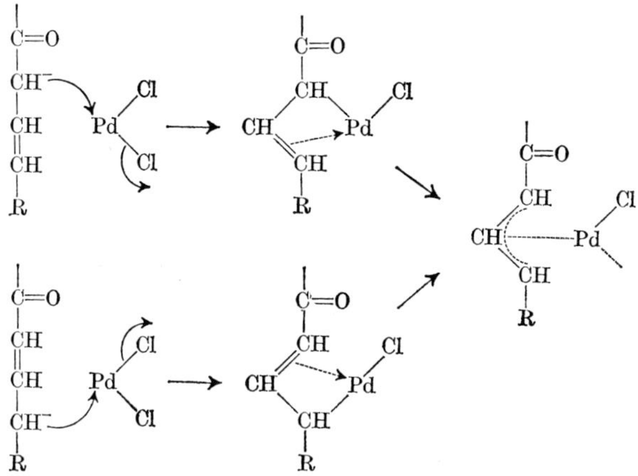

(96)

observed. The sequence of complex formation and carbonylation in eq. (97) was thus established. In this sequence of complex formation and carbonylation reactions, the introduction of carbon monoxide

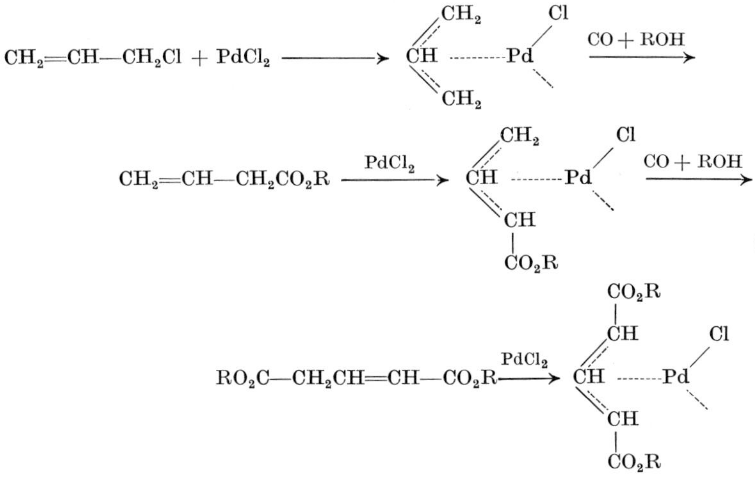

$$CH_2=CH-CH_2Cl + PdCl_2 \longrightarrow$$

$$CH_2=CH-CH_2CO_2R \xrightarrow{PdCl_2}$$

(97)

$$RO_2C-CH_2CH=CH-CO_2R \xrightarrow{PdCl_2}$$

molecules, one after another, starting from allylic compounds is possible. These reactions can be applied to olefinic compounds in the following way for the preparation of unsaturated mono- and diesters. At first a simple olefinic compound is treated with N-bromosuccinimide, lead tetraacetate, or other appropriate reagents to give an allylic compound and then the allylic compound is carbonylated at the allylic position to give a β,γ-unsaturated ester. This ester forms a π-allylic complex on reaction with palladium chloride, thus making introduction of the second carbon monoxide possible. Finally, an unsaturated diester can be obtained, as in eq. (98).

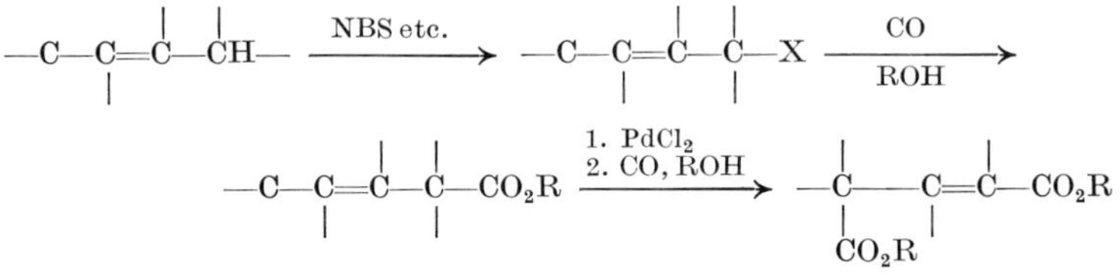

$$-\overset{|}{\underset{|}{C}}-\overset{}{C}=\overset{|}{C}-\overset{|}{C}H- \xrightarrow{\text{NBS etc.}} -\overset{|}{\underset{|}{C}}-\overset{}{C}=\overset{|}{C}-\overset{|}{C}-X \xrightarrow[\text{ROH}]{CO}$$

$$-\overset{|}{\underset{|}{C}}-\overset{}{C}=\overset{|}{C}-\overset{|}{C}-CO_2R \xrightarrow[\text{2. CO, ROH}]{\text{1. PdCl}_2} -\overset{|}{\underset{|}{\underset{CO_2R}{C}}}-\overset{}{C}=\overset{|}{C}-CO_2R \quad (98)$$

Another interesting application of these reactions was shown by the reaction of the complex from ethyl 3-hexenedioate (163). Ethyl 3-hexenedioate can be obtained in low yield by the carbonylation of the butadiene–palladium chloride complex. The hexenedioate has active hydrogens activated by two ester groups and forms the π-allylic complex easily. The complex has an active methylene group in the position conjugated with the π-allylic system. Treatment of this complex with a base forms an anion from which palladium is reductively removed as in eq. (99) forming muconate. This sequence of reactions

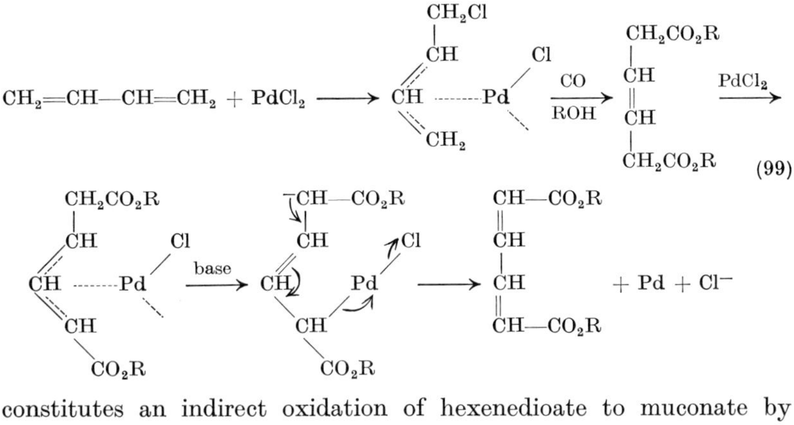

[Reaction scheme (99) showing conversion of $CH_2=CH-CH=CH_2 + PdCl_2$ through π-allyl palladium intermediates with CO, ROH, PdCl$_2$, and base to give $CH(CO_2R)=CH-CH=CH(CO_2R) + Pd + Cl^-$]

constitutes an indirect oxidation of hexenedioate to muconate by palladium chloride. In other words, palladium chloride is utilized for the abstraction of two hydrogens in a unique way. By this method, the terminal hydrogens of butadiene can be replaced with 2 moles of carbon monoxide to form muconic acid through a series of complex formation and carbonylation reactions, although the first step of the series, namely the carbonylation of the butadiene complex to form hexenedioate, proceeds in low yield. This sequence of reactions is a typical example of the combination of the two principal properties of palladium chloride, namely carbonylation and abstraction of two hydrogens through π-allylic complex formation.

Diene formation from the monoolefin shown above is certainly facilitated by the presence of two carbonyl groups located favorably for the activation of hydrogen. Diene formation from a simple monoolefin has also been reported. A simple olefin forms a π-allylic complex when heated between 80–100° with palladium chloride. Then the complex is decomposed to form conjugated diene by heating under high vacuum without solvent. For example, when the π-allylic 2-octenyl-palladium chloride formed from 1-octene was heated to 160° under 10^{-2} mm Hg, metallic palladium, hydrogen chloride, and a mixture of unsaturated hydrocarbons were obtained [eq. (100)]. In addition to a small amount of 2-octene, the main product was found to be a mixture of 1,3- and 2,4-dienes (165).

$$R'-CH=CH-CH_2CH_2R + PdCl_2 \longrightarrow$$

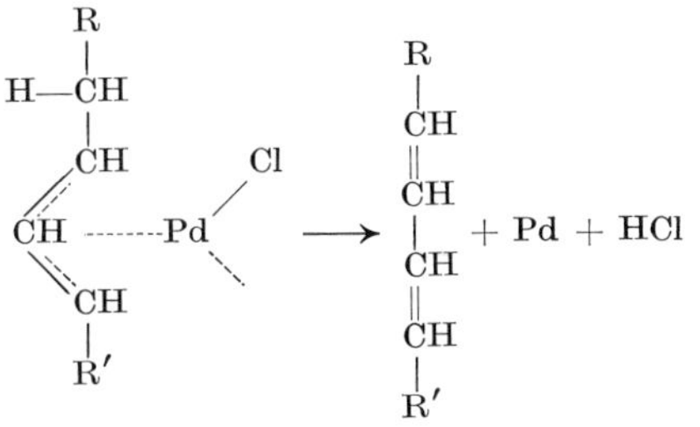

$$\begin{array}{c} R \\ | \\ H-CH \\ | \\ CH \\ \diagup \\ CH\text{------}Pd \\ \diagdown \\ CH \\ | \\ R' \end{array} \begin{array}{c} Cl \\ \diagup \\ \diagdown \end{array} \longrightarrow \begin{array}{c} R \\ | \\ CH \\ \| \\ CH \\ | \\ CH \\ \| \\ CH \\ | \\ R' \end{array} + Pd + HCl \quad (100)$$

G. CARBONYLATIONS OF CONJUGATED DIENES

Conjugated dienes form π-allylic complexes when treated with palladium chloride (20,21). The allylic complex formed from butadiene is a chloromethyl-substituted π-allyl-palladium chloride **(45)**, and a reaction similar to that of π-allyl-palladium chloride with carbon monoxide attacking at C-1 is possible. In addition, it is known that the chlorine of the complex at C-4 is reactive (like the chlorine of benzyl or allyl chloride) and can be replaced easily with a nucleophile such as an alkoxy group (21). It seems likely that allyl carbonium ions of the type shown here have considerable stability. Therefore, carbon monoxide attack at C-4 is expected. There are thus two possible sites of carbon monoxide attack in the diene complex.

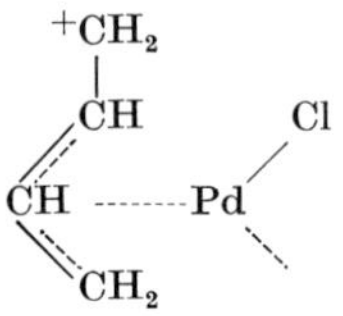

$$\begin{array}{c} {}^+CH_2 \\ | \\ CH \\ \diagup \quad \diagdown \\ CH \text{------} Pd \text{------} Cl \\ \diagdown \\ CH_2 \end{array}$$

The carbonylation of the butadiene complex was carried out in ethanol and benzene and the products shown in eq. (101) were obtained (166).

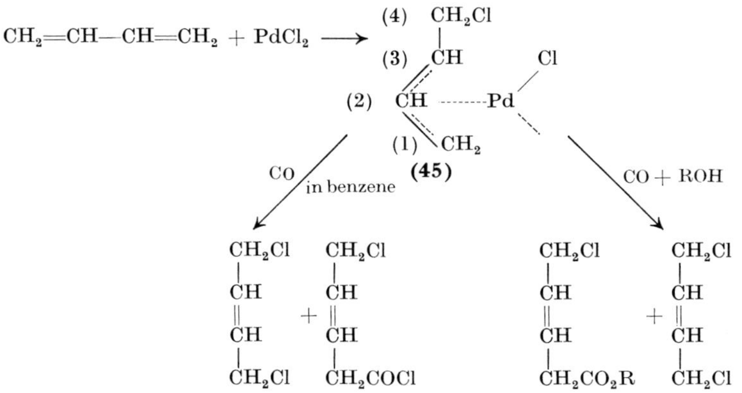

$$CH_2=CH-CH=CH_2 + PdCl_2 \longrightarrow \begin{array}{c} (4)\ CH_2Cl \\ | \\ (3)\ CH \\ \diagup \quad \diagdown Cl \\ (2)\ CH \text{------} Pd \\ (1)\ CH_2 \end{array}$$

Scheme branches: CO in benzene from (45); CO + ROH from the other side.

Products (101):

$$\begin{array}{cccc}
CH_2Cl & CH_2Cl & CH_2Cl & CH_2Cl \\
| & | & | & | \\
CH & CH & CH & CH \\
\| & + \ \| & \| & + \ \| \\
CH & CH & CH & CH \\
| & | & | & | \\
CH_2Cl & CH_2COCl & CH_2CO_2R & CH_2Cl
\end{array} \quad (101)$$

Further studies on the carbonylation of the isoprene complex (46) which has an ethoxy group instead of chlorine at C-4 have been carried out and different products were obtained depending on the reaction conditions, Scheme 4, (167). The carbonylation reaction in benzene at room temperature affords a mixture of acid chlorides and esters. After esterification, ethyl 5-ethoxy-3-methyl-3-pentenoate formed by C-1 attack is obtained as a main product. In addition, ethyl 4-methyl-3-pentenoate, ethyl 3-methyl-3-hexenedioate, and ethyl 4-ethoxy-4-methylvalerate are obtained as minor products. These minor products are formed by attack at C-4. When the reaction is carried out at 100°, ethyl 3-methyl-3-hexenedioate, formed by attack at C-1 and C-4, is the main product accompanied by γ,γ-dimethylbutyrolactone and ethyl 4-ethoxy-4-methylvalerate.

The carbonylation in ethanol at room temperature gives C-1 products

In Benzene

$$\text{(46)} \quad \begin{array}{c} \text{(2) } CH_3-C \\ \text{(1) } \diagdown CH_2 \end{array} \diagup\!\!\!\!\! \begin{array}{c} \text{(4) } CH_2OC_2H_5 \\ \text{(3) } CH \\ \end{array} \!\!\!\!\!\diagdown \!\!\text{-----Pd} \begin{array}{c} \\ Cl \\ \end{array}$$

room temp. →

$$\begin{cases} H_5C_2O-CH_2CH=C-CH_2CO_2C_2H_5 \\ \quad\quad\quad\quad\quad\quad\quad | \\ \quad\quad\quad\quad\quad\quad\quad CH_3 \\ CH_3-C=CH-CH_2-CO_2C_2H_5 \\ \quad\quad | \\ \quad\quad CH_3 \\ H_5C_2O_2C-CH_2CH=C-CH_2-CO_2C_2H_5 \\ \quad\quad\quad\quad\quad\quad\quad\quad\quad | \\ \quad\quad\quad\quad\quad\quad\quad\quad\quad CH_3 \\ \quad\quad CH_3 \\ \quad\quad | \\ CH_3-C-CH_2CH_2CO_2C_2H_5 \\ \quad\quad | \\ \quad\quad OC_2H_5 \end{cases}$$

at 100° ↘

$$\begin{cases} H_5C_2O_2C-CH_2CH=C-CH_2CO_2C_2H_5 \\ \quad\quad\quad\quad\quad\quad\quad\quad | \\ \quad\quad\quad\quad\quad\quad\quad\quad CH_3 \\ \\ \quad\quad CH_3 \diagup\!\!\!\!\!\diagdown\!\!\!CH_3 \\ \quad\quad\quad\quad\diagdown\!\!\!O\!\!\!\diagup \\ \quad\quad\quad\quad\quad\| \\ \quad\quad\quad\quad\quad O \\ \\ \quad\quad CH_3 \\ \quad\quad | \\ CH_3-CCH_2CH_2CO_2C_2H_5 \\ \quad\quad | \\ \quad\quad OC_2H_5 \end{cases}$$

(Scheme 4)

predominantly. The main product is ethyl 5-ethoxy-3-methyl-3-pentenoate, accompanied by a small amount of γ,γ-dimethylbutyrolactone. At 100°, the lactone is the main product, accompanied by C-4 product and the diester formed by C-1 and C-4 attack, indicating that the C-4 attack is predominant at high temperature. When hydrogen chloride is added to the reaction medium, exclusive attack at C-4 and hydrogenolysis are observed. Thus, at room temperature in ethanol containing hydrogen chloride, ethyl 4-methyl-3-pentenoate, ethyl 4-methyl-4-pentenoate and γ,γ-dimethylbutyrolactone are obtained. At 100°, only the lactone is obtained. From these experimental results, it can be concluded that the diene complex can be carbonylated at the two sites, giving different products depending on the reaction conditions. Under the conditions favorable for carbonium ion formation, C-4 attack is preferred. In a nonpolar solvent at lower temperatures, C-1 attack is predominant. Dicarbonylation is possible using the intermediate conditions; see Scheme 5.

In Ethanol

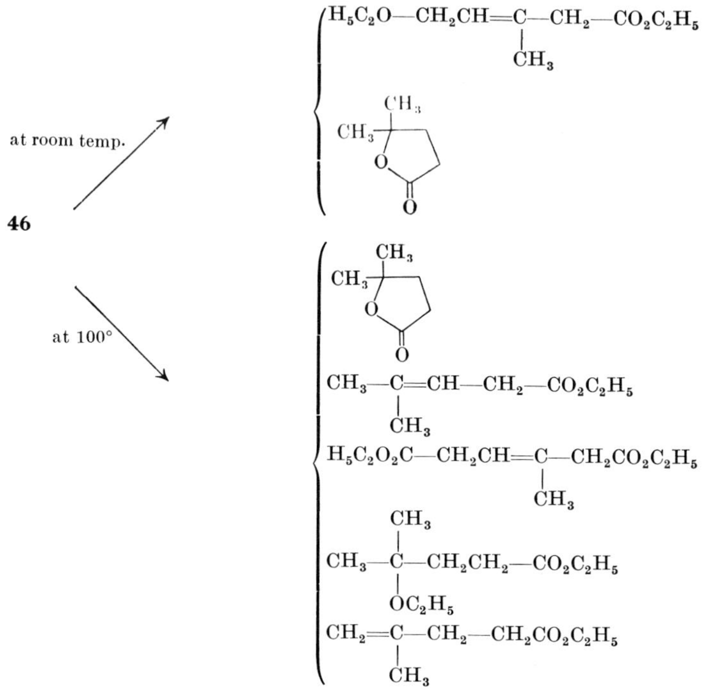

46
- at room temp. →
  - $H_5C_2O-CH_2CH=C(CH_3)-CH_2-CO_2C_2H_5$
  - γ-butyrolactone with two CH$_3$ at α-position (dimethyl-γ-butyrolactone)
- at 100° →
  - dimethyl-γ-butyrolactone
  - $CH_3-C(CH_3)=CH-CH_2-CO_2C_2H_5$
  - $H_5C_2O_2C-CH_2CH=C(CH_3)-CH_2CO_2C_2H_5$
  - $CH_3-C(CH_3)(OC_2H_5)-CH_2CH_2-CO_2C_2H_5$
  - $CH_2=C(CH_3)-CH_2-CH_2CO_2C_2H_5$

In Ethanol Containing Hydrogen Chloride

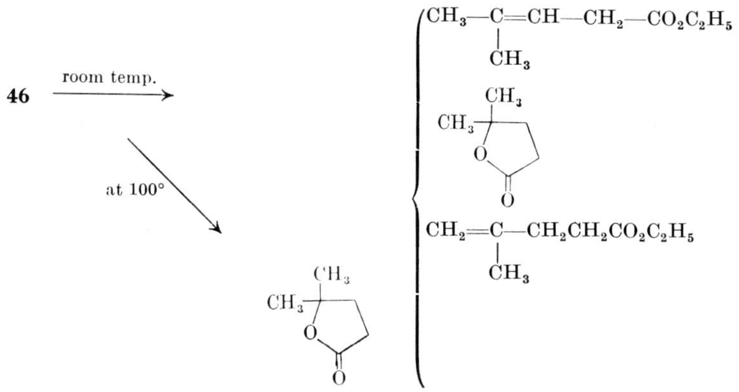

46
- room temp. →
  - $CH_3-C(CH_3)=CH-CH_2-CO_2C_2H_5$
  - dimethyl-γ-butyrolactone
  - $CH_2=C(CH_3)-CH_2CH_2CO_2C_2H_5$
- at 100° →
  - dimethyl-γ-butyrolactone

(Scheme 5)

Furthermore, carbonylation reaction of dienes can be carried out catalytically, giving different products (166). When a diene is carbonylated in alcohol containing hydrogen chloride in the presence of a catalytic amount of palladium chloride or metallic palladium, the product is a β,γ-unsaturated ester [eqs. (102)]. For example, butadiene

$$CH_2=CH-CH=CH_2 + CO + ROH \xrightarrow{PdCl_2} CH_3-CH=CH-CH_2CO_2R \quad (102a)$$

$$\underset{\underset{CH_3}{|}}{CH_2=CH-C=CH_2} + CO + ROH \xrightarrow{PdCl_2} \underset{\underset{CH_3}{|}}{CH_3-C=CH-CH_2-CO_2R} \quad (102b)$$

forms 3-pentenoate, but the yield of the ester varies greatly depending on the reaction conditions. Isoprene forms 4-methyl-3-pentenoate as a main product, and 4-methyl-4-pentenoate, γ,γ-dimethylbutyrolactone, and 4-ethoxy-4-methylvalerate are formed as minor products. Brewis and Hughes reported that the yield of 3-pentenoate varied greatly with the catalytic species (168). For example, dihalogenobis-(tributylphosphine)-μ,μ'-dihalogenodipalladium gave the product in 56% yield when the halogen was chlorine and in 73% yield when the halogen was bromine. With the same catalyst, isoprene gave methyl 3-methyl-3-pentenoate (15%), 4 methyl-3-pentenoate (38%), and 4-methyl-4-pentenoate (10%). 1,3-Pentadiene was carbonylated in methanol to form methyl 2-methyl-3-pentenoate (34%).

Cyclic conjugated dienes can also be carbonylated. 1,3-Cyclohexadiene was carbonylated to give ethyl 2-cyclohexenecarboxylate in 80% yield at 100° by the catalytic action of palladium chloride. The same ester was obtained by the carbonylation of 3-bromocyclohexene. 1,3-Cyclooctadiene was carbonylated to give 2-cyclooctenecarboxylate, but the yield was very low; probably the diene system is not coplanar and hence it cannot form the complex easily (124). Cyclopentadiene was carbonylated to give 2-cyclopentenecarboxylate [eqs. (103)] (73%) (168).

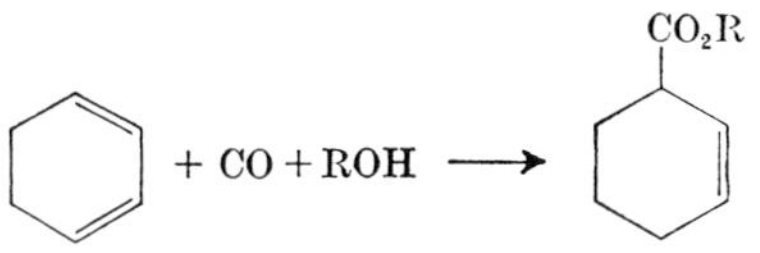

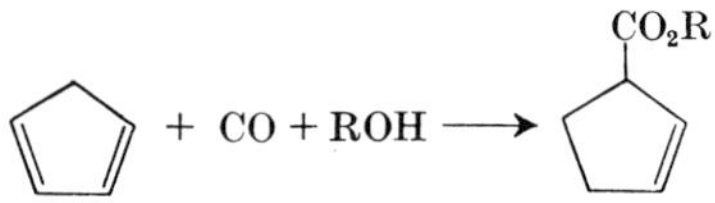

H. CARBONYLATIONS OF ALLENE COMPLEXES

Allene is known to form the following two types of allylic complexes (**47** and **48**) when treated with palladium chloride, depending on the solvents used (22,23). In a suggested mechanism of the complex formation, the center carbon atom of allene becomes cationic and either chlorine or another allene molecule attacks at that carbon giving the complexes, **47** and **48**; see eq. (104). When the complex formation

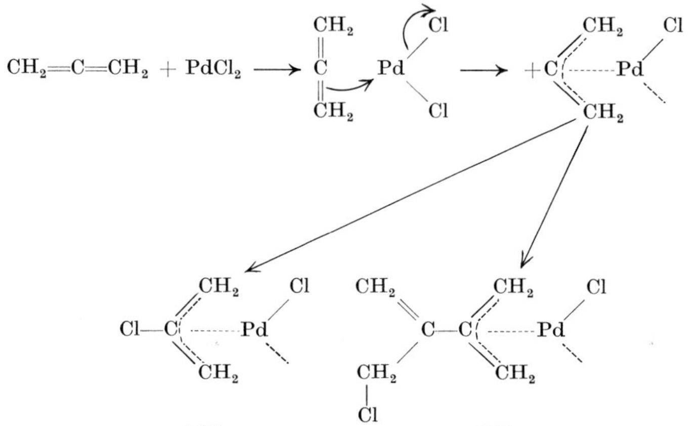

$$CH_2{=}C{=}CH_2 + PdCl_2 \longrightarrow \underset{CH_2}{\overset{CH_2}{C}}\hspace{-2pt}\diagdown\hspace{-8pt}Pd\hspace{-8pt}\diagup\hspace{-2pt}\underset{Cl}{\overset{Cl}{}} \longrightarrow +C\hspace{-2pt}\diagdown\hspace{-8pt}\underset{CH_2}{\overset{CH_2}{}}\hspace{-2pt}{-}{-}{-}Pd\hspace{-8pt}\diagup\hspace{-2pt}\underset{Cl}{\overset{Cl}{}}$$

(104)

(**47**)   (**48**)

is carried out in the presence of carbon monoxide, attack of carbon monoxide at the center carbon gives a π-allylic complex having a chlorocarbonyl group at that position. The complex is then carbonylated at the terminal position and the product is an itaconate ester [eq. (105)] (169). The yield is not high.

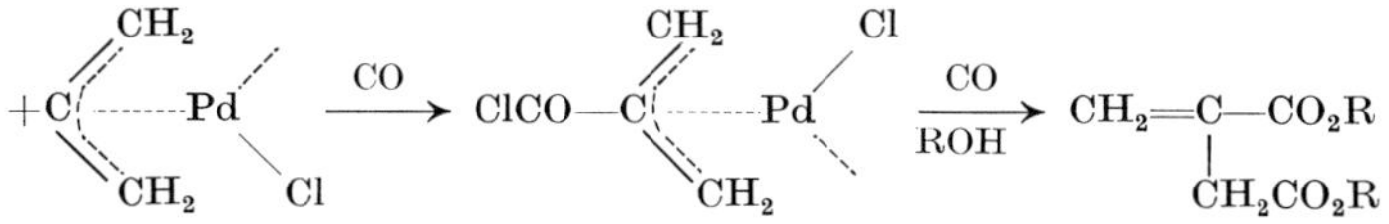

$$+C\cdots Pd \xrightarrow{CO} ClCO{-}C\cdots Pd \xrightarrow[ROH]{CO} CH_2{=}\underset{CH_2CO_2R}{\overset{\displaystyle CO_2R}{C}}$$

(105)

When the carbonylation of the complex **47** is carried out in ethanol, ethyl 3-chloro-3-butenoate is obtained. The carbonylation of the complex **48** has interesting possibilities, since this complex has several possible sites for carbon monoxide attack; see eqs. (106). Actually, the first attack of carbon monoxide gives rise to 4-hydroxy-3,4-dimethyl-2-pentenoic acid lactone (**49**). The product of the monocarbonylation has allylic lactone and diene systems both of which are

$$47 \longrightarrow CH_2=C-CH_2CO_2R \atop |\atop Cl \qquad (106a)$$

$$48 \longrightarrow \begin{cases} \text{(49)} \\ \text{(50)} \\ \text{(51)} \end{cases} \qquad (106b)$$

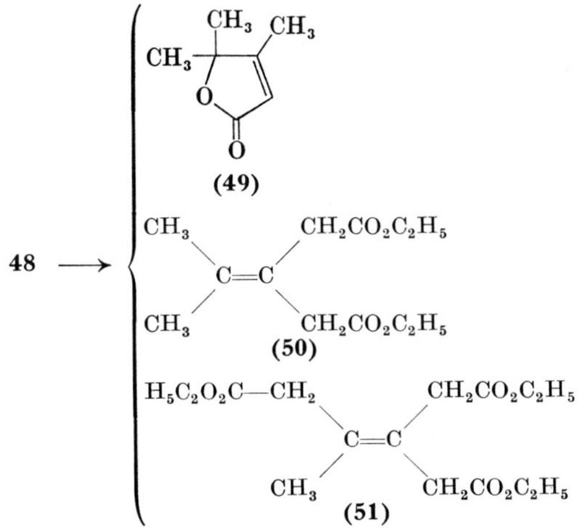

(49): 3,4,5-trimethyl-2(5H)-furanone-type structure with CH$_3$ groups

(50): $(CH_3)_2C=C(CH_2CO_2C_2H_5)_2$

(51): $H_5C_2O_2C-CH_2(CH_3)C=C(CH_2CO_2C_2H_5)_2$

available for π-allyl complex formation and further carbonylation. The dicarbonylation gives ethyl 3-isopropylideneglutarate **(50)**. This compound can react still further with carbon monoxide to give ethyl 3-ethoxycarbonylmethyl-4-methyl-3-hexenedioate **(51)**.

I. CARBONYLATIONS OF ACETYLENIC COMPOUNDS

Like olefinic compounds, acetylenic compounds can be carbonylated by the catalytic action of palladium. It should be noted that both palladium chloride and metallic palladium are known to be very active for the cyclization or oligomerization of acetylenic compounds. For example, diphenylacetylene cyclizes to give a tetraphenylcyclobutadiene complex when treated with palladium chloride (170). In addition, by the action of a catalytic amount of metallic palladium, diphenylacetylene and acetylenecarboxylate cyclize to form benzene derivatives in high yield (171). Therefore, it is rather surprising to find that the carbonylation of these acetylenic compounds can be easily carried out by the catalytic action of palladium chloride or metallic palladium without forming the above-mentioned cyclized products. Thus, it is apparent that in the competition between cyclization and carbonylation, the latter completely suppresses the former.

In contrast to olefinic compounds, a definite complex of palladium chloride with acetylenic compounds has not been reported until now with one exception (172). It is probable that the products of the interaction of palladium with triple bonds are too reactive to give an isolable complex.

Acetylenic compounds can be carbonylated using several metal carbonyls. The nickel carbonyl-catalyzed carbonylation of acetylene to form acrylic acid is the most famous example. Also cobalt carbonyl and iron carbonyl are known to be active for various types of carbonylation reactions of acetylenic compounds. It can be said that one of the specific features of the palladium-catalyzed carbonylation of acetylenic bonds is the extensive dicarbonylation rather than monocarbonylation. In other words, unlike the other metal carbonyl-catalyzed reactions, two moles of carbon monoxide are introduced as the main path of the carbonylation with a palladium catalyst.

Acetylene is carbonylated by the catalytic action of palladium chloride in alcohol containing iodine. The products are a mixture of esters of acrylic, propionic, succinic, fumaric, and maleic acids (173). When the carbonylation of acetylene is carried out in benzene in the presence of palladium chloride, fumaryl, maleyl, and muconyl chlorides are obtained in a stoichiometric reaction (174) [eq. (107)].

$$CH\equiv CH + CO + PdCl_2 \longrightarrow$$

$$\begin{array}{c} CH-COCl \\ \parallel \\ CH-COCl \end{array} + \begin{array}{c} CH-COCl \\ \parallel \\ ClOC-CH \end{array} + \begin{array}{c} CH-COCl \\ \parallel \\ CH \\ | \\ CH \\ \parallel \\ CH-COCl \end{array} + Pd \quad (107)$$

The carbonylation of acetylenic carboxylates by the use of metal carbonyls has not received sufficient study. Jones, Shen, and Whiting studied the nickel carbonyl-catalyzed carbonylation of certain acetylenic carboxylates, and they concluded that the carboxylate group deactivates the triple bond for carbonylation (175). On the other hand, Bryce-Smith reported that acetylenecarboxylate is easily trimerized to give a benzene derivative by heating with a small amount of metallic palladium, showing that metallic palladium and acetylenecarboxylate interact strongly (171).

Carbonylation of acetylenemono- and dicarboxylates can be carried out in the presence of metallic palladium and hydrogen chloride. Contrary to the Jones' observation, very smooth carbonylation is observed without giving a cyclized product (176). From acetylene-monocarboxylate, the products shown in eq. (108) are obtained.

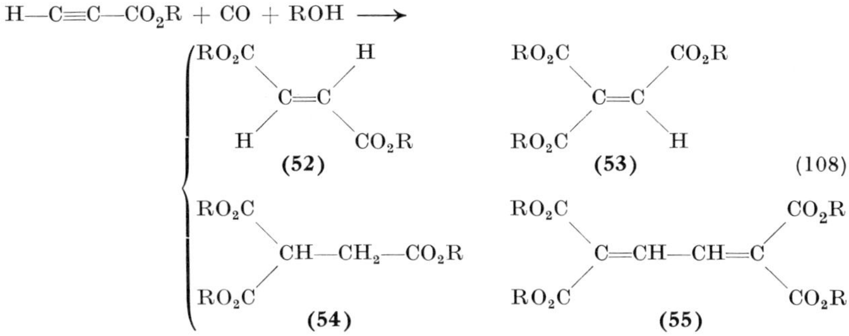

$$H-C\equiv C-CO_2R + CO + ROH \longrightarrow$$

$$\begin{cases} \begin{array}{cc} RO_2C\diagdown/H & RO_2C\diagdown/CO_2R \\ C=C & C=C \\ H/\diagdown CO_2R & RO_2C/\diagdown H \\ \textbf{(52)} & \textbf{(53)} \end{array} \\ \\ \begin{array}{cc} RO_2C\diagdown & RO_2C\diagdown/CO_2R \\ CH-CH_2-CO_2R & C=CH-CH=C \\ RO_2C/ & RO_2C/\diagdown CO_2R \\ \textbf{(54)} & \textbf{(55)} \end{array} \end{cases} \quad (108)$$

Acetylenedicarboxylate is also carbonylated smoothly even at room temperature, indicating that the ester groups facilitate the carbonylation reaction to a large extent. The products in eq. (109) are obtained.

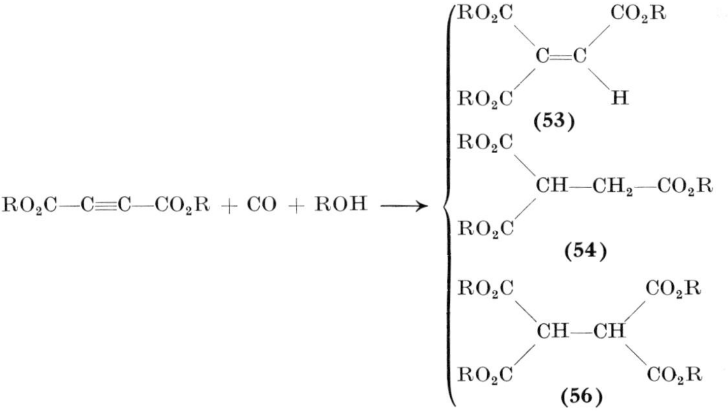

$$RO_2C-C\equiv C-CO_2R + CO + ROH \longrightarrow \begin{cases} \begin{array}{c} RO_2C\diagdown/CO_2R \\ C=C \\ RO_2C/\diagdown H \\ \textbf{(53)} \end{array} \\ \\ \begin{array}{c} RO_2C\diagdown \\ CH-CH_2-CO_2R \\ RO_2C/ \\ \textbf{(54)} \end{array} \\ \\ \begin{array}{c} RO_2C\diagdown/CO_2R \\ CH-CH \\ RO_2C/\diagdown CO_2R \\ \textbf{(56)} \end{array} \end{cases} \quad (109)$$

The characteristic point in these carbonylation reactions is that the product ratio is largely dependent on the concentration of hydrogen chloride in the reaction medium. Higher concentrations of hydrogen chloride tend to give dicarbonylation products rather than monocarbonylation products. Also, saturated esters, rather than unsaturated esters, are obtained when the concentration of hydrogen chloride is high. The results of the carbonylations are shown in Tables XI and XII.

As will be discussed later, the interaction of diphenylacetylene and palladium chloride or metallic palladium gives a variety of cyclized

TABLE XI

Carbonylation of Acetylenemonocarboxylate (176)

Catalyst, g	CH≡CCO$_2$Et, g	Solvent, ml	52, g (%)[a]	53 + 54, g (%)	55, g (%)
PdCl$_2$, 1	10	EtOH, 50	2.5 (14.3)	1.5 (6.0), 5:1	1.2 (3.4)
10% Pd/C, 2	10	10% HCl EtOH, 50	2.5 (14.3)	3.0 (12.0), 1:1	1.0 (2.8)
PdCl$_2$, 2	5	10% HCl EtOH, 50	1.7 (19.4)	5.0 (40), 1:4	1.7 (9.7)

[a] Yield based on ethyl acetylenemonocarboxylate.

TABLE XII

Carbonylation of Acetylenedicarboxylate (176)

Catalyst, g	EtO$_2$CC≡CCO$_2$Et, g (recovery, g)	Solvent, ml	53 + 54, g (%)	56, g (%)
PdCl$_2$, 1	5 (0.9)	EtOH, 50	2.5 (42.5)	0.5 (6.5)
PdCl$_2$, 2	5 (0.7)	10% HCl, EtOH, 50	1.5 (**54**) (24.3)	4.1 (**51**)

TABLE XIII

Carbonylation of Diphenylacetylene[a] (177)

Diphenyl-acetylene, g	Catalyst, g	Solvent, ml	Diphenyl-crotono-lactone, g (%)	Other products, g (%)
10	PdCl$_2$, 3	HCl (10%)/EtOH, 45	8.7 (66)	Diphenylmaleate, 4.7 (26)
10	PdCl$_2$, 2	EtOH, 50	2.7 (20)	2,3-Diphenyl-acrylate[b]
5	10% Pd–C, 2	HCl (10%)/EtOH, 50	2.3 (35)	2,3-Diphenyl-acrylate[b]
3.5	PdCl$_2$, 2	HCl (10%)/MeOH, 50	2.8 (60)	Diphenylmaleate, 2 (34)

[a] Reaction temperature 100°, CO pressure 100 kg/cm^2; reaction time 15 hr.
[b] Only a small amount, and the yield was not determined.

products under very mild conditions. In view of this fact, it is rather surprising to find that diphenylacetylene is carbonylated smoothly without side reactions by the catalytic action of metallic palladium and hydrogen chloride. Carbonylation of diphenylacetylene in alcohol containing hydrogen chloride proceeds smoothly, and extensive dicarbonylation is observed. The main product is diphenylcrotonolactone, accompanied by diphenylmaleate (177). At a lower concentration of hydrogen chloride, the yield of the lactone decreases drastically and a small amount of diphenylacrylate is obtained as shown in Table XIII. The lactone is formed by simultaneous *cis* attack of two moles of carbon monoxide on the triple bond, followed by reduction of one of the carbonyl functions; see eq. (110).

$$C_6H_5-C\equiv C-C_6H_5 + CO + ROH \longrightarrow \underset{O}{\overset{C_6H_5}{\underset{\diagup}{\diagdown}}}\!\!\!\!\!\!\!\!\!\!\!\!\!\!\!\!\!\!\! \underset{O}{\overset{C_6H_5}{\diagup}} + \underset{C_6H_5}{\overset{C_6H_5}{\diagdown}}\!\!\! C=C\!\!\! \underset{CO_2R}{\overset{CO_2R}{\diagup}} \quad (110)$$

$$+ C_6H_5CH=C\underset{CO_2R}{\overset{C_6H_5}{\diagdown}}$$

Carbonylation of propargyl alcohol was studied in the presence of palladium catalyst in methanol containing hydrogen chloride at 100° under carbon monoxide pressure (100 kg/cm^2) (178). Three molecules of carbon monoxide are introduced successively [see eq. (111)] and methyl 2-(methoxymethyl) acrylate (57) (small amount), methyl itaconate (58) (63%), and methyl aconitate (59) (10%) are obtained. The yields of these products change with the reaction conditions.

$$CH\equiv C-CH_2OH + CO + CH_3OH \longrightarrow$$

$$\underset{(57)}{CH_2=\underset{|}{\overset{CH_2OCH_3}{C}}-CO_2CH_3} + \underset{\underset{(58)}{CH_2CO_2CH_3}}{CH_2=\underset{|}{C}-CO_2CH_3} + \underset{\underset{(59)}{\underset{|}{CH_2CO_2CH_3}}}{\overset{CH-CO_2CH_3}{\underset{|}{\overset{\|}{C}-CO_2CH_3}}} \quad (111)$$

Probably, these products are formed by the paths in eqs. (112). Carbon monoxide attacks either C-1 or C-2 giving 2,3-butadienoate (60) and methoxymethylacrylate (57). These two esters are expected to be susceptible to further attack by carbon monoxide to give itaconate

(58). Methoxymethylacrylate **(57)** is an allylic ether and can be carbonylated. Also it was confirmed that 2,3-butadienoate **(60)** can

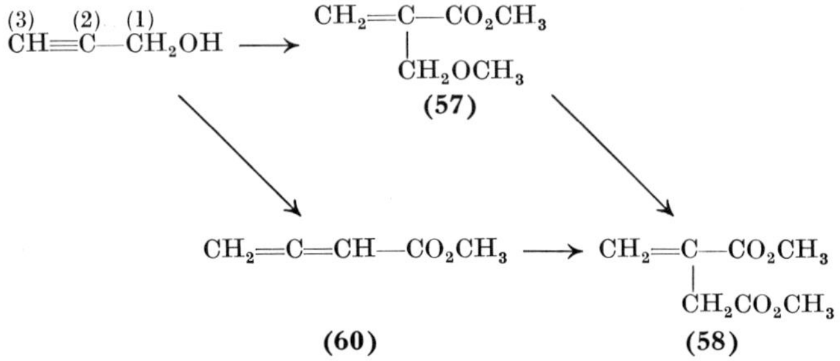

$$\overset{(3)}{CH}\equiv\overset{(2)}{C}-\overset{(1)}{CH_2OH} \longrightarrow \underset{\underset{(57)}{CH_2OCH_3}}{CH_2=C-CO_2CH_3}$$

$$\underset{(60)}{CH_2=C=CH-CO_2CH_3} \longrightarrow \underset{\underset{(58)}{CH_2CO_2CH_3}}{CH_2=C-CO_2CH_3}$$

(112)

be carbonylated to itaconate under the same conditions. It seems likely that aconitate **(59)** is formed by the simultaneous addition of two moles of carbon monoxide to the triple bond, followed by allylic carbonylation, eq. (113).

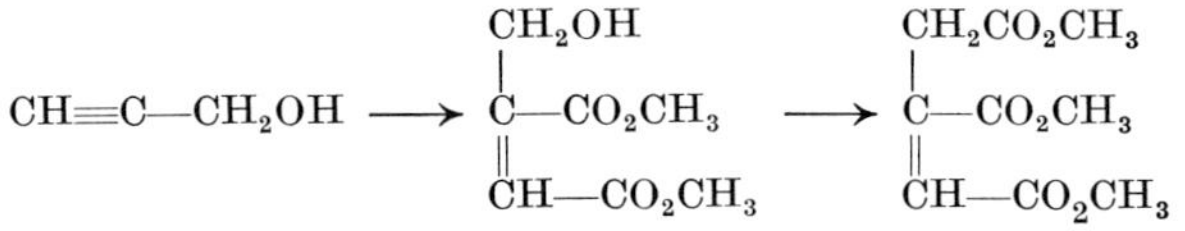

$$CH\equiv C-CH_2OH \longrightarrow \underset{\underset{CH-CO_2CH_3}{\parallel}}{\overset{CH_2OH}{\underset{|}{C}-CO_2CH_3}} \longrightarrow \underset{\underset{CH-CO_2CH_3}{\parallel}}{\overset{CH_2CO_2CH_3}{\underset{|}{C}-CO_2CH_3}}$$

(113)

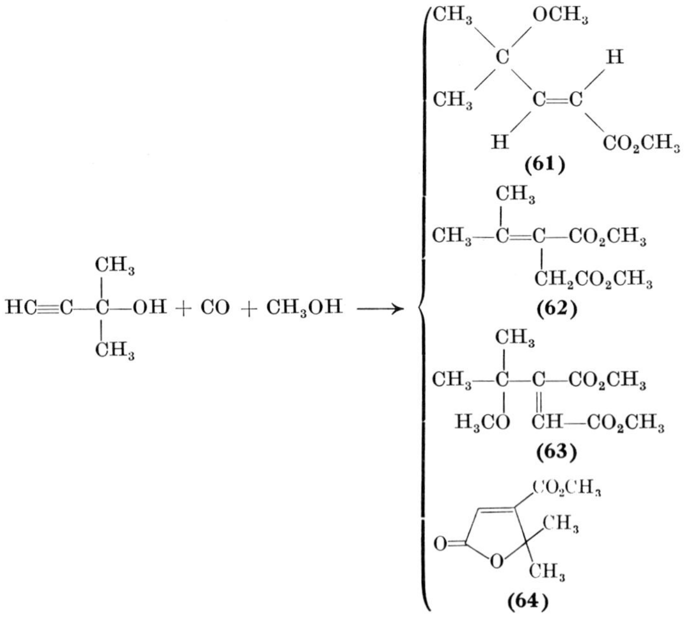

$$HC\equiv C-\underset{\underset{CH_3}{|}}{\overset{CH_3}{\underset{|}{C}}}-OH + CO + CH_3OH \longrightarrow \begin{cases} \text{(61)} \\ \text{(62)} \\ \text{(63)} \\ \text{(64)} \end{cases}$$

(114a)

(61): tetrasubstituted alkene with CH_3, CH_3, OCH_3 groups on one carbon of C=C and H, CO_2CH_3 on the other (with H also shown).

(62): $CH_3-\underset{\underset{CH_2CO_2CH_3}{|}}{\overset{CH_3}{\underset{|}{C}}}=C-CO_2CH_3$

(63): $CH_3-\underset{\underset{H_3CO}{|}}{\overset{CH_3}{\underset{|}{C}}}-\underset{\underset{CH-CO_2CH_3}{\parallel}}{C}-CO_2CH_3$

(64): furanone ring with CO_2CH_3, CH_3, CH_3 substituents.

Carbonylation of propargyl chloride in alcohol at room temperature gives 3-chloro-3-butenoate (small amount) and itaconate (66%). Substituted propargyl alcohols are also carbonylated. 2-Methyl-3-butyn-2-ol in methanol is attacked by one or 2 moles of carbon monoxide,

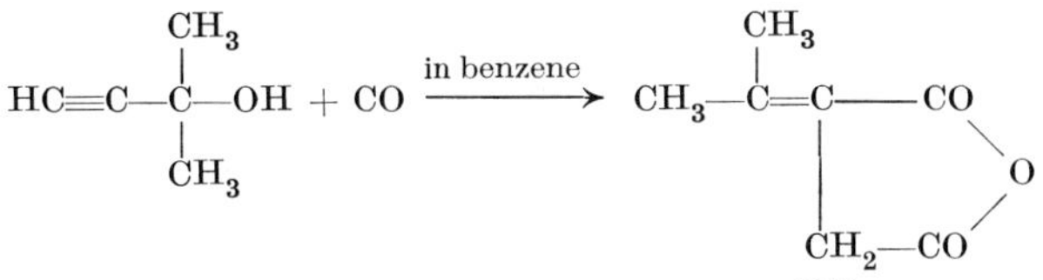

$$HC{\equiv}C-\underset{\underset{CH_3}{|}}{\overset{\overset{CH_3}{|}}{C}}-OH + CO \xrightarrow{\text{in benzene}} CH_3-\overset{\overset{CH_3}{|}}{C}{=}C-CO\diagdown O \diagup CH_2-CO \quad (114b)$$

(65)

giving 4-methoxy-4-methyl-2-pentenoate **(61)**, teraconate **(62)**, (1-methoxy-1-methylethyl)maleate **(63)** and terebate **(64)**. At higher concentrations of hydrogen chloride, terebate **(64)** and teraconate **(62)** are the main products. When the reaction is carried out in benzene in the presence of palladium chloride, teraconic anhydride **(65)** is obtained selectively in 42% yield; see eqs. (114).

J. CARBONYLATION OF THE AZOBENZENE COMPLEX

Complex formations of C=N and N=N bonds, conjugated with aromatic rings, with some transition metal compounds are known. Palladium chloride forms a stable complex **(66)** with azobenzene very easily (179). It is remarkable that the carbon–palladium bond is formed so easily in the substitution of the aromatic hydrogen by palladium. This complex is interesting for further use in aromatic substitution reactions because of its reactive palladium–carbon bond. Takahashi and Tsuji found that the complex reacts with carbon monoxide in alcohol or in water at 50° under pressure (100 atm) to give 2-phenyl-3-indazolinone in high yield [eq. (115)] (180).

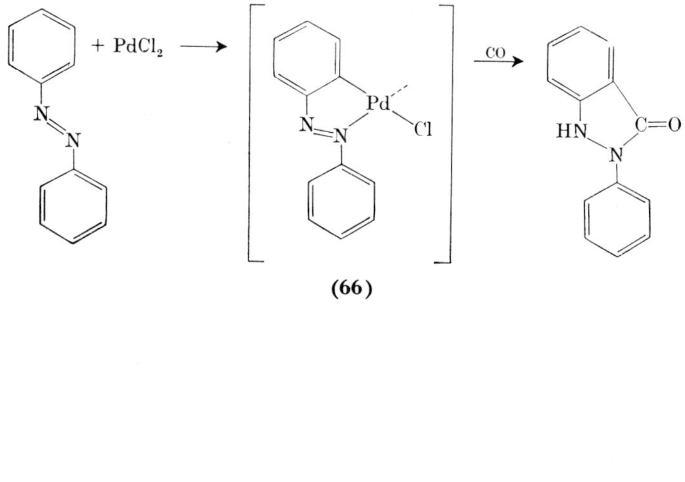

(66)

K. CARBONYLATIONS OF AMINES

Stern and Spector found that primary aliphatic and aromatic amines react with carbon monoxide in the presence of palladium chloride and disodium hydrogen phosphate (181). Divalent palladium is reduced to the zerovalent state abstracting two hydrogen atoms from the amine to form an isocyanate. It is remarkable that the reaction proceeds

$$R-NH_2 + CO + PdCl_2 \rightarrow R-N=C=O + Pd + 2HCl \quad (116)$$

even at atmospheric pressure of carbon monoxide, showing that the oxidative action of palladium chloride is very strong. Palladium chloride forms a stable complex with amines, and it seems likely that the amine complex reacts with carbon monoxide which is also coordinated with palladium. Isocyanate formation does not proceed through an intermediate formamide followed by dehydrogenation. It is also clear that isocyanate formation is not due to *in situ* formation of phosgene from palladium chloride and carbon monoxide.

Tsuji and Iwamoto carried out the reaction of an amine, carbon monoxide, palladium chloride and allyl chloride (182). By passing carbon monoxide into a mixture of allyl chloride, a primary amine and sodium palladous chloride at 60° in benzene, the formation of an isocyanate and π-allyl-palladium chloride was confirmed, eq. (117). The reaction can be explained by eq. (118). Palladium chloride and

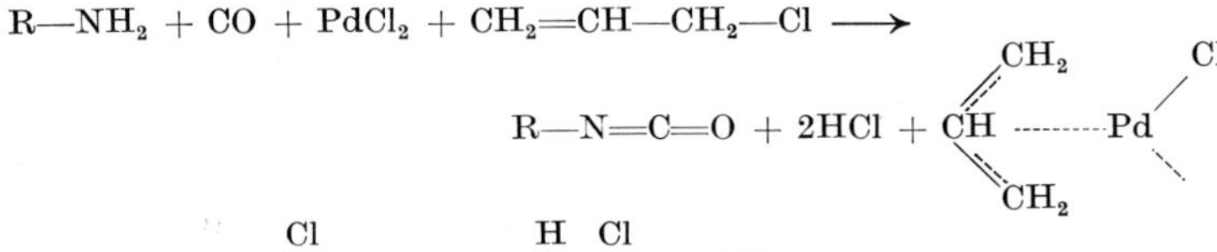

$$R-NH_2 + CO + PdCl_2 + CH_2=CH-CH_2-Cl \longrightarrow$$

$$R-N=C=O + 2HCl + \text{(π-allyl-Pd-Cl complex)} \quad (117)$$

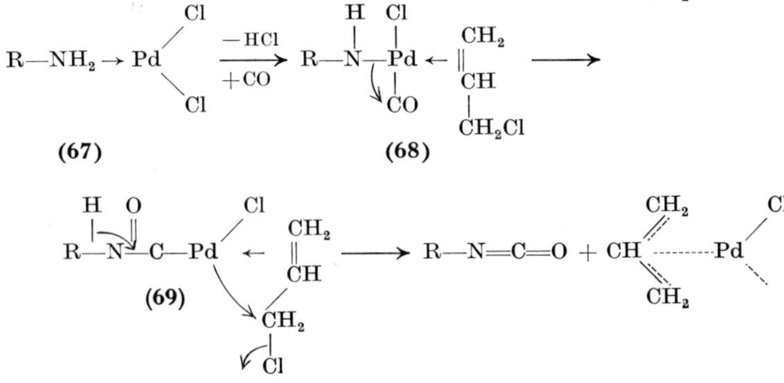

the amine form a complex (67), which is transformed into a new complex (68) by the action of carbon monoxide and allyl chloride. The next step is the insertion of carbon monoxide into the palladium–nitrogen bond to form the amide complex (69). Finally, the amide complex collapses to form isocyanate and π-allyl-palladium chloride. The net result is the abstraction of two hydrogen atoms from the amine by the oxidative action of palladium chloride. When the reaction is carried out in methanol at room temperature, a urethane is the product.

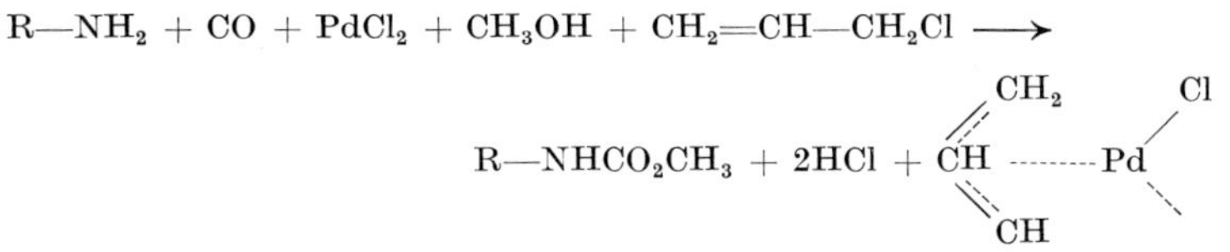

$$R-NH_2 + CO + PdCl_2 + CH_3OH + CH_2=CH-CH_2Cl \longrightarrow$$

$$R-NHCO_2CH_3 + 2HCl + \begin{array}{c} CH_2 \\ CH \\ CH \end{array} Pd \begin{array}{c} Cl \\ \end{array} \quad (119)$$

The formation of π-allyl complex from allyl chloride, carbon monoxide, water, and palladium chloride is explained by Nicholson, Powell and Shaw (183) as oxidative hydrolysis of carbon monoxide to form carbon dioxide and is shown in eq. (120). It is apparent that this

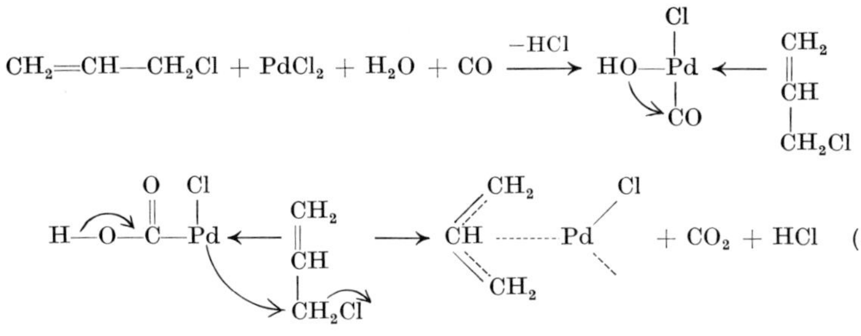

$$CH_2=CH-CH_2Cl + PdCl_2 + H_2O + CO \xrightarrow{-HCl} HO-Pd \begin{array}{c} Cl \\ | \\ CO \end{array} \longleftarrow \begin{array}{c} CH_2 \\ \| \\ CH \\ | \\ CH_2Cl \end{array}$$

$$H-O-\overset{O}{\underset{\|}{C}}-\overset{Cl}{\underset{|}{Pd}} \longleftarrow \begin{array}{c} CH_2 \\ \| \\ CH \\ | \\ CH_2Cl \end{array} \longrightarrow \begin{array}{c} CH_2 \\ CH \\ CH_2 \end{array} Pd \begin{array}{c} Cl \\ \end{array} + CO_2 + HCl \quad (120)$$

reaction and the above-mentioned isocyanate and π-allyl complex formations are closely related.

In the isocyanate formation, palladium chloride is reduced. On the other hand, Tsuji and Iwamoto found that the carbonylation of an amine can be carried out in the presence of metallic palladium (184). Thus from ammonia, urea was formed in poor yield. In the carbonylation of aliphatic amines, the products were a disubstituted urea, oxamide and formamide. Oxamide formation became predominant when a catalytic amount of palladium chloride was used. Aromatic amines formed only urea derivatives and no oxamide. Metallic palladium is strong enough to abstract hydrogen from the amine to give molecular hydrogen.

$$R\text{---}NH_2 + CO \xrightarrow{Pd} R\text{---}NHCONH\text{---}R$$
$$+ RNHCOCONHR + RNHCHO + H_2 \quad (121)$$

V. Carbonylation and Decarbonylation Reactions Catalyzed by Other Noble Metal Compounds

A. PLATINUM-CATALYZED CARBONYLATIONS

The formation of simple platinum carbonyls is not known, but some platinum compounds have been used for the carbonylation of olefins. The synthesis of α,β-unsaturated carboxylic esters from olefins and carbon monoxide in the presence of certain platinum carbonyl derivatives (185) was reported by Inoue and Tsutsumi using an electrochemical method. Anodic oxidation of methanol in the presence of styrene produced styrene glycol dimethyl ether and it seems likely that the reaction involved a methoxy radical as an intermediate (186). In the presence of carbon monoxide, the platinum used as a cathode quickly dissolved into the solution during the electrolysis of methanol containing sodium methoxide, giving a platinum carbonyl compound. It was found that this carbonyl compound of platinum reacts with olefins catalytically as well as electrochemically in the presence of carbon monoxide to give as a main product a methyl ester of the corresponding α,β-unsaturated carboxylic acid (187). For example, the electrolysis of a methanolic solution containing sodium methoxide and styrene (52 g) for 9 hr under carbon monoxide pressure (70 kg/cm²) gave rise to methyl *trans*-cinnamate as a main product (14% based on styrene). In addition, methyl β-methoxy-β-phenylpropionate (3.6%), methyl β-phenylpropionate (3.1%), dimethyl *meso*-3,4-diphenyladipate (trace), and styrene glycol dimethyl ether (5.6%) were obtained as minor products; see eq. (122). Although the mechanism of this

$$C_6H_5\text{---}CH\text{=}CH_2 + CO + CH_3O^- \xrightarrow[{[Pt_x(CO)_y]_n}]{} \begin{cases} C_6H_5CH\text{=}CH\text{---}CO_2CH_3 \\ C_6H_5CH\text{---}CH_2CO_2CH_3 \\ \quad | \\ \quad OCH_3 \\ C_6H_5CH_2CH_2CO_2CH_3 \\ C_6H_5CH\text{---}CH_2CO_2CH_3 \\ \quad | \\ C_6H_5CH\text{---}CH_2CO_2CH_3 \\ C_6H_5CH\text{---}CH_2\text{---}OCH_3 \\ \quad | \\ \quad OCH_3 \end{cases} \quad (122)$$

reaction was not elucidated, it seems probable that the carbomethoxy platinum carbonylate is formed from methoxy radicals and cathodically generated platinum carbonyl is the active species in the carbonylation reaction. The ester of the α,β-unsaturated acid is produced by the addition of the Pt-CO_2CH_3 group in the platinum carbonyl compound to the olefinic double bond via the electrode process, followed by further anodic oxidation or decomposition with sodium methoxide, eqs. (123). Although the reaction gives a mixture

$$CH_3O^- \xrightarrow[-e]{\text{anode}} CH_3O\cdot \qquad (123a)$$

$$[Pt_x(CO)_y]_n + CH_3O\cdot \longrightarrow Pt_x(CO)_{y-1}CO_2CH_3 \qquad (123b)$$

$$Pt_x(CO)_{y-1}CO_2CH_3 + C_6H_5\text{—}CH\text{=}CH_2 \longrightarrow C_6H_5CH\text{=}CHCO_2CH_3 \qquad (123c)$$

of products and seems to be quite complex, it is potentially interesting as an example of carbonylation under electrolytic conditions.

Other platinum complexes were reported to be active for carbonylation reactions. For example, the carbonylation of allyl alcohol was carried out by the catalytic action of tris[tri(p-fluorophenyl)phosphine]-platinum at 200°, and allyl-3-butenoate was obtained (188).

$$CH_2\text{=}CH\text{—}CH_2OH + CO \longrightarrow CH_2\text{=}CH\text{—}CH_2\text{—}CO_2CH_2\text{—}CH\text{=}CH_2 \qquad (124)$$

Platinum–tin chloride, prepared by dissolving stannous chloride dihydrate and chloroplatinic acid in methanol, has an interesting catalytic activity. For example, homogeneous hydrogenation of ethylene can be carried out with this complex (189). The complex was found to be active for the carbonylation of olefinic compounds. Thus, in methanolic solution, ethylene was converted into methyl propionate (190). Also, carbonylation of allene with this complex is known (191).

B. CARBONYLATION AND DECARBONYLATION REACTIONS BY USING RHODIUM COMPLEXES

1. *Carbonylation Reactions*

Rhodium carbonyl is one of the best-known carbonyls of noble metals. Like cobalt carbonyl, rhodium carbonyl catalyzes aldehyde formation from an olefin, carbon monoxide, and hydrogen. The rhodium catalyst is different from the cobalt in several respects (192,193). It was reported that the catalytic activity of rhodium carbonyl is 10^3 times higher than that of cobalt carbonyl and gives a

TABLE XIV

Aldehyde Formation by Co and Rh Carbonyls (193)

Olefin	Aldehyde			Reaction time, min
	Catalyst	Yield, %	B/U	
1-Hexene	Co	85	0.26	135
	Rh	87	0.83	60
1-Pentene	Co	84	0.27	125
	Rh	82	0.84	54
1-Butene	Co	89	0.23	140
	Rh	87	0.81	70
Propylene	Co	83	0.25	120
	Rh	83	0.88	55

higher yield of an aldehyde. The main product of the rhodium-catalyzed hydroformylation is a branched-chain aldehyde, rather than a normal aldehyde. Table XIV shows the results of comparative studies of the cobalt- and rhodium-catalyzed hydroformylation reactions. The ratios of the branched and unbranched aldehydes (B/U),

$$R-CH=CH_2 + CO + H_2 \longrightarrow R-\underset{\underset{CHO}{|}}{CH}-CH_3 + RCH_2CH_2CHO \quad (125)$$

in the cobalt- and rhodium-catalyzed reactions are clearly different. By the hydroformylation of methyl acrylate, cobalt carbonyl gives methyl β-formylpropionate and rhodium carbonyl gives α-formylpropionate, respectively, as the main products.

$$CH_3-\underset{\underset{CHO}{|}}{CH}-CO_2R \xleftarrow{\text{Rh carbonyl}} CH_2=CH-CO_2R \xrightarrow{\text{Co carbonyl}} CH_2-\underset{\underset{CHO}{|}}{CH_2}-CO_2R \quad (126)$$

In addition to rhodium carbonyl, some other rhodium complexes are known to be active for hydroformylation. For example, in the presence of tris(triphenylphosphine)trichlororhodium, 1-hexene was converted into n-heptaldehyde (70%) and 2-methylhexaldehyde (20%) in an ethanol–benzene solution at 55° using carbon monoxide and hydrogen (194). The reaction conditions were milder than the usual cobalt carbonyl-catalyzed hydroformylation. At 100°, when the H_2:CO ratio was larger than 1:1, further conversion of the aldehyde to alcohol was observed. With chlorotris(triphenylphosphine)rhodium in an ethanol–benzene solution, hexyne-1 reacted with a 1:4 mixture of

H_2 and CO at 110° to give heptaldehyde and 2-methylhexaldehyde, each in 15% yield (195).

Acetylenic compounds undergo carbonylation reactions with chlorocarbonyl rhodium dimer $[RhCl(CO)_2]_2$. The reaction of disubstituted acetylenes with this complex gives tetrasubstituted cyclopentadienones complexed with rhodium and tetrasubstituted p-benzoquinones (196).

2. Decarbonylation Reactions

In Section IV-E, the metallic palladium-catalyzed decarbonylation of aldehydes and acyl halides was described. Although the reaction is quite useful in certain cases, it has some disadvantages. For example, aromatic acid halides cannot be decarbonylated satisfactorily. Tsuji and Ohno found that chlorotris(triphenylphosphine)rhodium **(70)** is a better reagent for the decarbonylation.

The most characteristic property of this complex is its facile liberation of one mole of triphenylphosphine in solution to form a coordinately unsaturated, formally three-coordinate species **(71)** (197,229) [see eq. (127)]. This species has a vacant coordination site which can be

$$(PPh_3)_3RhCl \rightleftarrows (PPh_3)_2RhCl + PPh_3$$
$$\quad (70) \qquad\qquad\qquad (71)$$
$$\downarrow$$
$$(PPh_3)_2RhCl(S)$$
$$S = \text{solvent}$$
(127)

occupied either by weakly bound solvent molecules or by other ligands. **71** may also dimerize in solution. In particular, it can easily pick up one mole of carbon monoxide and form chlorocarbonylbis(triphenylphosphine)rhodium **(72)** which is a very stable complex [eq. (128)].

$$(PPh_3)_2RhCl + CO \longrightarrow \begin{array}{c} CO \quad\quad PPh_3 \\ \diagdown \ Rh \ \diagup \\ PPh_3 \quad\quad Cl \end{array}$$
$$\quad (71) \qquad\qquad\qquad (72)$$
(128)

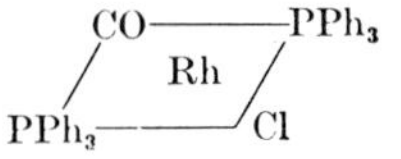

By using this property, the decarbonylation of carbonyl compounds was investigated. It was found that an aldehyde can be decarbonylated smoothly even at room temperature by the reaction in eq. (129) (198).

$$(PPh_3)_3RhCl + RCHO \longrightarrow (PPh_3)_2(CO)RhCl + RH + PPh_3$$
$$\quad (70) \qquad\qquad\qquad\qquad (72)$$
(129)

This is the most facile and selective method known for the decarbonylation of aldehydes. It can be said that the tendency to form **72** is so great that **70** can extract a carbonyl group from aldehydes. Some results of the decarbonylation of aldehydes are shown in Table XV. This selective removal of the aldehyde CO group may have wide

TABLE XV

Decarbonylation of Aldehydes Using $(PPh_3)_3RhCl$ (198)

Aldehyde	Solvent[a]	Reaction		Yield of complex, %	Product,[b] %
		Temp.	Time		
C_6H_5CHO	None	Reflux	5 min	80	Benzene
C_6H_5CHO	None	Room temp.	24 hr	77	Benzene
C_6H_5CHO	Toluene	Reflux	2 hr	92	Benzene (83)
$CH_3CH_2CH_2CHO$	Benzene	Room temp.	2 hr	65	Propane
$(CH_3)_2CHCHO$	Benzene	Room temp.	70 hr	83	Propane
$(CH_3)_2CHCHO$	Benzene	Reflux	30 min	40	Propane
$C_6H_5CH=CHCHO$	Benzene	Room temp.	12 hr	65	Styrene
$C_6H_5CH=CHCHO$	Benzene	Reflux	15 min	93	Styrene (77)
$C_6H_5CH=CHCHO$	CH_2Cl_2	Room temp.	8 hr	65	Styrene (60)
$p\text{-}ClC_6H_4CHO$	Benzene	Reflux	3 hr	90	Chlorobenzene (85)
$C_6H_5CH_2CH_2CHO$	Benzene	Reflux	10 min	90	Ethylbenzene (67)
$o\text{-}HOC_6H_4CHO$	Toluene	Reflux	20 min	76	Phenol (70)

[a] When no solvent was used, the reaction was carried out in an excess of aldehyde.
[b] Yields were determined by gas chromatography.

application. For example, the preparation of 1-dehydro-3-ketosteroids was carried out by the following sequence (199). Formylation of the 3-ketosteroid, followed by dehydrogenation with dichlorodicyanoquinone, gave an unsaturated formyl ketone. The formyl group was removed by use of the rhodium complex. This method can be applied to the introduction of a double bond in the methylene side of ketones of the type $R_2R_1CH\text{---}CH_2\text{---}CO\text{---}CHR_3CH_2R_4$.

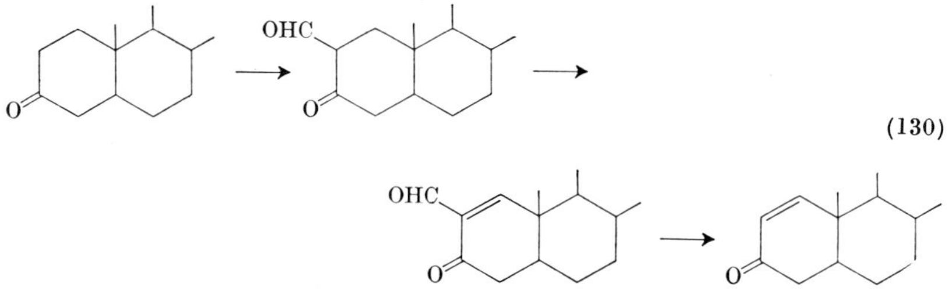

(130)

The decarbonylation of acyl halides with this complex proceeds smoothly, but it is necessary to warm up the solution for complete decarbonylation (200). Interestingly enough, a new complex was isolated by the reaction of an acyl halide with chlorotris(triphenylphosphine)rhodium. The acyl complex (73) is five-coordinated, and is formed by the oxidative addition of acyl halide to the rhodium

TABLE XVI

Acyl Rhodium Complexes, $RCORh(PPh_3)_2Cl_2$ (200)

R	Decomp. temp., °C	Yield, %	Molecular wt. Calcd.	Found
$CH_3(CH_2)_4-$	173–176	84	797	724
$CH_3(CH_2)_5-$	165–166	80	811	806
$CH_3(CH_2)_{14}-$	135–137	100	937	904
$CH_3(CH_2)_{16}-$	120–126	96	965	942
$C_6H_5CH_2CH_2-$	176–179	85		

complex (70) with the elimination of one mole of triphenylphosphine [see eqs. (131)]. This is the first example of an acyl complex formation

$$RCH_2CH_2COCl + (PPh_3)_3RhCl \xrightarrow{\Delta}$$
(70)
$$RCH{=}CH_2 + (PPh_3)_2(CO)RhCl + PPh_3 + HCl \quad (131a)$$
(72)

$$RCOCl + (PPh_3)_3RhCl \longrightarrow RCORhCl_2(PPh_3)_2 + PPh_3 \quad (131b)$$
(70) \qquad\qquad\qquad (73)

by the direct oxidative addition of an acyl halide to a metal complex. Some of the complexes isolated are shown in Table XVI. The acyl complex (73) is the intermediate in the decarbonylation and the complex can be converted into an olefin by heating. The product obtained is a mixture of isomeric olefins. 1-Olefins can be obtained selectively by treatment of the acyl complex with iodine; see eq. (132). Also, the complex is converted into the acyl halide and the complex 72 by treatment with carbon monoxide at 150° under pressure.

In the above-mentioned decarbonylation, chlorotris(triphenylphosphine)rhodium (70) is converted into chlorocarbonylbis(triphenylphosphine)rhodium (72). In other words, the reaction is stoichiometric with respect to the rhodium complex (70). On the other hand, a catalytic decarbonylation was found by using chlorocarbonylbis(triphenylphosphine)rhodium **(72)**. This complex is reasonably stable,

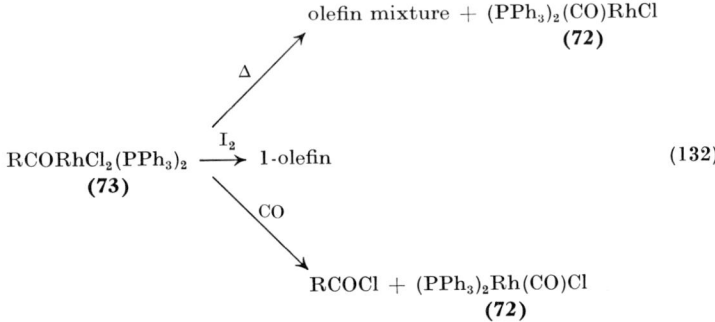

(132)

and more importantly, it is four-coordinated and coordinatively unsaturated, so that it can expand to a six-coordinated complex by the oxidative addition of an acyl halide or an aldehyde   The oxidative addition of methyl iodide to this complex was reported by Heck (201). In a related reaction, Chatt and Shaw reported the oxidative addition of acetyl bromide to $RhBr(CO)(PEt_2Ph)_2$ to give an acetylrhodium complex $[RhBr_2(CH_3CO)(CO)(PEt_2Ph)_2]$ (202). With this in mind, Tsuji and Ohno found that chlorocarbonylbis(triphenylphosphine)rhodium is actually active for the catalytic decarbonylation of aldehydes and acyl halides (203).   The complex is more efficient than palladium for decarbonylation, and the reaction proceeds homogeneously.

Acyl halides are decarbonylated to form olefins when heated to 200° in the presence of a catalytic amount of chlorocarbonylbis(triphenylphosphine)rhodium.   This complex has some advantages when compared with metallic palladium.   In the palladium-catalyzed decarbonylation reaction, the olefins obtained are a mixture of isomers,

TABLE XVII

Decarbonylation of Aliphatic Acid Halides (203)

Acyl halide, g	$(PPh_3)_2RhCOCl$, g	Temp., °C	Time, hr	Yield, %	Product
$CH_3(CH_2)_5COBr$, 4	0.1	200	0.5	80	Hexene
$CH_3(CH_2)_6COCl$, 8	0.1	190–200	1	91	Heptene
$CH_3(CH_2)_6COBr$, 8	0.1	200	1	90	Heptene

and inner olefins are the main products. On the other hand, in the rhodium complex-catalyzed decarbonylation of acyl halides, it is possible to isolate the 1-olefins as main products of the decarbonylation by selecting the proper reaction conditions. Some of the experimental results are shown in Table XVII. For example, when octanoyl bromide was decarbonylated by heating with a catalytic amount of either palladium chloride or the rhodium complex (72) at 200°, the results in eq. (133) were obtained.

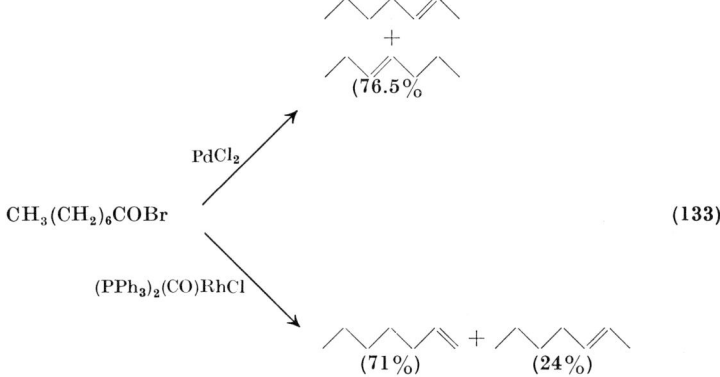

(133)

The most characteristic catalytic activity of the rhodium complex was observed in the reaction of aromatic acid halides (203). The decarbonylation of aromatic acid halides is not satisfactory with a palladium catalyst. On the other hand, aromatic acid halides can be decarbonylated smoothly by heating at 200° with the rhodium complex (72). Thus this is a new type of reaction which makes possible the introduction of a halogen on an aromatic ring. For example, when benzoyl chloride is heated with the complex at 200°, chlorobenzene distills off rapidly with the evolution of carbon monoxide. Benzoyl bromide reacts similarly to give bromobenzene. Phenylacetyl chloride

$$C_6H_5COX \xrightarrow{200°} C_6H_5X + CO \qquad (134)$$

is converted into benzyl chloride. Blum reported that chlorotris(triphenylphosphine)rhodium (70) is an active catalyst for the decarbonylation of aromatic acid halides and several examples were shown (204). But in this case too, the actual catalyst seems to be chlorocarbonylbis-(triphenylphosphine)rhodium (72) which is formed by a stoichiometric reaction with the acyl halide. The examples of catalytic decarbonylation are shown in Table XVIII. Formation of halides by decarbonylation of acyl halides can be accomplished by the Hunsdiecker reaction, but the reaction is unsatisfactory when applied to aromatic acid halides. Therefore, decarbonylation of aromatic acid halides by the rhodium complex is a very useful reaction.

TABLE XVIII

Decarbonylation of Aromatic Acid Halides (203,204)

Halide, g	Catalyst, g	Yield, %	Product
Phenylacetyl chloride, 8	$(PPh_3)_2RhCOCl$, 0.1	60	Benzyl chloride
Benzoyl chloride, 8	$(PPh_3)_2RhCOCl$, 0.2	85	Chlorobenzene
Benzoyl bromide, 8	$(PPh_3)_2RhCOCl$, 0.2	87	Bromobenzene
Benzoyl chloride, 12	$(PPh_3)_3RhCl$, 0.1	90	Chlorobenzene
p-Chlorobenzoyl chloride, 5	$(PPh_3)_3RhCl$, 0.1	79	p-Dichlorobenzene
o-Bromobenzoyl chloride, 5	$(PPh_3)_3RhCl$, 0.1	78	o-Bromochlorobenzene
2,4-Dichlorobenzoyl chloride, 30	$(PPh_3)_3RhCl$, 0.1	98	1,2,4-Trichlorobenzene
1-Naphthoyl chloride, 5	$(PPh_3)_3RhCl$, 0.1	96	1-Chloronaphthalene
2-Naphthoyl chloride, 4	$(PPh_3)_3RhCl$, 0.1	94	2-Chloronaphthalene
1-Naphthoylacetyl chloride, 4	$(PPh_3)_3RhCl$, 0.1	87	1-(Chloromethyl)-naphthalene

In addition to aromatic acid halides, Blum reported that aromatic sulfonyl halides can be converted into aromatic halides with the evolution of sulfur dioxide (205). In this case, the sulfonyl chloride should be purified very carefully, for otherwise it tends to polymerize easily. The liberation of sulfur dioxide is faster than the decarbonylation reaction. Examples are shown in Table XIX. Blum used chlorotris(triphenylphosphine)rhodium **(70)** as a catalyst, but it is possible to carry

$$Ar-SO_2Cl \longrightarrow Ar-Cl + SO_2 \qquad (135)$$

out the reaction by using chlorocarbonylbis(triphenylphosphine)-rhodium **(72)**. The removal of sulfur dioxide is easily conceivable in view of the fact that certain sulfonyl chlorides are known to add oxidatively to metallic complexes as shown in eq. (136) (46,206,207). The sulfur dioxide is removed from the complex by heating. In other

TABLE XIX

Decarbonylation of Sulfonyl Chlorides (205)

Sulfonyl chloride used, g	Product	Yield of pure product, %
Benzene, 17.6	Chlorobenzene	79
p-Toluene, 15.0	p-Chlorotoluene	72
p-Fluorobenzene, 15.5	p-Chlorofluorobenzene	61
p-Chlorobenzene, 10.0	p-Dichlorobenzene	85
2,5-Dichlorobenzene, 10.0	1,2,5-Trichlorobenzene	65
2-Naphthalene, 6.00	2-Chloronaphthalene	69
4-Fluoro-1-naphthalene, 5.0	1-Chloro-4-fluoronaphthalene	70
Benzene-1,3-di, 10.0	m-Dichlorobenzene	62

words, sulfonyl chlorides behave the same way as acyl halides towards metal complexes, and a sulfur dioxide insertion reaction, similar to the

$$\begin{array}{c} L \quad Cl \\ \diagdown \diagup \\ Ir \\ \diagup \diagdown \\ OC \quad L \end{array} \xrightarrow{R-SO_2Cl} \begin{array}{c} L \quad \overset{R}{\underset{|}{SO_2}} Cl \\ \diagdown |\diagup \\ Ir \\ \diagup |\diagdown \\ OC \quad Cl \quad L \end{array} \xrightarrow[-SO_2]{110°} \begin{array}{c} L \quad R \quad Cl \\ \diagdown |\diagup \\ Ir \\ \diagup |\diagdown \\ OC \quad Cl \quad L \end{array} \quad (136)$$

$$R = p\text{-}CH_3C_6H_4\text{-}$$

carbon monoxide insertion, is possible. Thus, Vaska and Bath reported the reversible addition of sulfur dioxide to a four-coordinated iridium complex (45).

$$IrCl(CO)(PPh_3)_2 + SO_2 \underset{\Delta}{\overset{25°}{\rightleftarrows}} (SO_2)IrCl(CO)(PPh_3)_2 \quad (137)$$

In view of the fact that oxidative additions of alkyl halides and acyl halides to chlorocarbonylbis(triphenylphosphine)rhodium **(72)** is possible, it is expected that the carbonylation of alkyl halides could be carried out catalytically with this complex (203). For example, benzyl chloride is carbonylated to form phenylacetyl chloride in the presence of a catalytic amount of this rhodium complex in benzene. It

$$C_6H_5CH_2Cl + CO \xrightarrow{72} C_6H_5CH_2COCl \quad (138)$$

can be said that chlorocarbonylbis(triphenylphosphine)rhodium **(72)** is active for decarbonylation of acyl halides in the absence of carbon monoxide and for carbonylation of reactive alkyl halides in the presence of carbon monoxide.

Thus, from these experimental results, the probable course of the decarbonylation and carbonylation reactions catalyzed by chlorotris(triphenylphosphine)rhodium and chlorocarbonylbis(triphenylphosphine)rhodium may be depicted as in Scheme 6. It appears that:

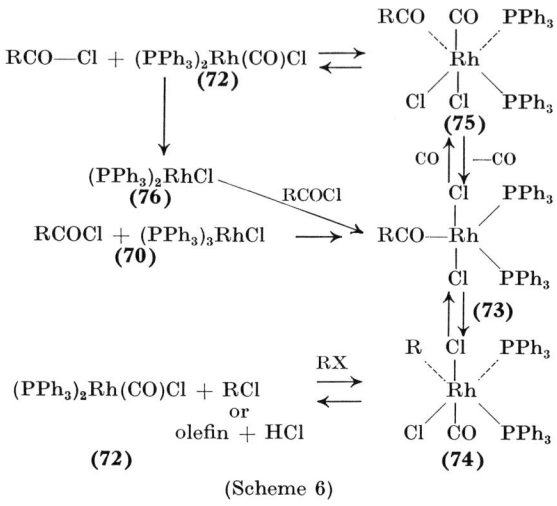

(Scheme 6)

1. The reaction of acyl halides with the complex **70** is irreversible and the complex **70** is not recovered under any conditions. Therefore, decarbonylation using the complex **70** is stoichiometric.

2. The course of the decarbonylation reaction catalyzed by the complex **72** is **72** + RCOCl → **75** → **73** → **74** → **72** + olefin or RCl. Another possible, but less likely path is through **72** → **76** → **73**, but no definite experimental evidence is available to decide which one is the real path.

3. The course of the carbonylation reaction of RCl is: **72** + RCl → **74** → **73** → **75** → **72** + RCOCl. Here, the most important point is that the complex **72** is formed after carbonylation and decarbonylation, and this complex plays the key role in the reactions.

It is known that there is a close analogy between a transition metal complex and a transition metal surface with respect to their reaction with hydrogen, hydrogen halides, carbon monoxide, and some other reagents. Thus, the carbonylation and decarbonylation reactions using metallic palladium and the rhodium complexes have great significance.

Rusina and Vlcek observed that $RhCl(CO)(PPh_3)_2$ is formed from rhodium trichloride and triphenylphosphine when they are heated in several oxygenated solvents (208). For example, rhodium trichloride and triphenylphosphine were converted into $RhCl(CO)(PPh_3)_2$ when heated in solvents such as alcohols, dimethylformamide, tetrahydrofuran, cyclohexanone, dioxane, and acetophenone. Although no attempt was made by Rusina and Vlcek to isolate the organic products, certainly these compounds are the source of carbon monoxide and the reaction seems to be interesting.

In connection with the decarbonylation of carbonyl compounds, the following interesting results of Chatt and of Vaska should be mentioned. It was found that certain noble metal compounds can be converted into carbonyl complexes by reaction with an alcohol. Detailed studies on this carbon monoxide abstracting ability of certain noble metal complexes have been made by Chatt and by Vaska. Chatt, Shaw, and Field (209) observed that $[Ru_2Cl_3(PEt_2Ph)_6]Cl$ reacts with ethanol in the presence of potassium hydroxide to give the hydridocarbonylruthenium complex. Hydrogen and carbon monoxide are derived from the ethanol, which by this reaction is converted into methane.

$$[Ru_2Cl_3(PEt_2Ph)_6]Cl + 2KOH + 2C_2H_5OH \longrightarrow$$
$$2[RuHCl(CO)(PEt_2Ph)_3] + 2CH_4 + 2KCl + 2H_2O \quad (139)$$

This type of reaction, namely the decomposition of ethanol into methane, hydrogen, and carbon monoxide, has never been realized by

$$CH_3CH_2OH \longrightarrow CH_3H + H^+ + [H^-, CO](\text{metal complex}) \quad (140)$$

ordinary organic chemistry. This example shows the interesting possibility of complex-catalyzed reactions. The mechanism in eq. (141) was

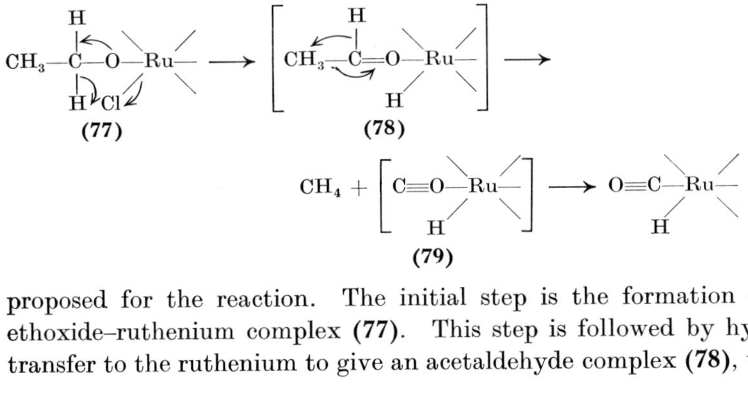

proposed for the reaction. The initial step is the formation of an ethoxide–ruthenium complex **(77)**. This step is followed by hydride transfer to the ruthenium to give an acetaldehyde complex **(78)**, which then breaks down to give methane and the carbonyl complex (**79**). Also Chatt and Shaw reported the formation of [RhCl(CO)(PEt$_2$Ph)$_2$] by the reaction of [RhCl$_3$(PEt$_2$Ph)$_3$] with ethanol (202). A similar reaction was observed by Vaska using an osmium complex. The reaction observed is eq. 142 (210). Again, RCH$_2$OH was converted

$$(NH_4)_2OsBr_6 + 4Ph_3P + RCH_2OH \longrightarrow$$
$$[OsHBr(CO)(PPh_3)_3] + RH + HBr + Ph_3PBr_2 + 2NH_4Br \quad (142)$$

into RH by donation of hydrogen and carbon monoxide to the osmium complex.

Although at present these reactions of noble metal complexes do not have much direct application to organic chemistry, it may be possible that in the future, noble metal complexes will become specific reagents in organic chemistry for other unique reactions. The ability of the complexes to abstract hydride and carbon monoxide from some oxygenated compounds to form stable hydride carbonyl complexes has no parallel in organic reactions. The smooth decarbonylation reaction with the rhodium complexes discussed in this chapter is a first and a most useful example. Certainly this is a field for future development.

Prince and Raspin reported briefly their studies on the reaction of phosphine complexes of ruthenium and rhodium with alcohols and aldehydes (211). Although more detailed studies are necessary, they observed the formation of ethylene by refluxing propionic acid with RhCl$_3$(Et$_2$PhP)$_3$.

C. RUTHENIUM-CATALYZED CARBONYLATIONS

The first conclusive report of a hydroformylation reaction catalyzed by a ruthenium complex was given by Wilkinson and co-workers (212). They found that Ru(CO)$_3$(Ph$_3$P)$_2$ catalyzes the hydroformylation of 1-pentene in benzene at 100° to give hexaldehyde in more than 80% yield.

It was found that diruthenium nonacarbonyl and ruthenium chloride can be used for the carbonylation of allene (213). Several reaction products were obtained depending on the reaction conditions. Methyl methacrylate (50%) was obtained by carbonylation in methanol at

$$CH_2{=}C{=}CH_2 + CO + CH_3OH \longrightarrow$$

$$CH_2{=}\underset{\underset{CH_3}{|}}{C}{-}CO_2CH_3 + CH_3O_2C{-}\underset{\underset{CH_3}{|}}{\overset{\overset{CH_3}{|}}{C}}{-}CH_2\overset{\overset{CH_2}{\|}}{C}{-}CO_2CH_3 \quad (143)$$

140° in the presence of diruthenium nonacarbonyl. At 190°, α,α-dimethyl-α'-methyleneglutarate (23%) was obtained in addition to methyl methacrylate (18%). Carbonylation carried out in water in the presence of ruthenium chloride yielded methacrylic acid and 3-hydroxy-1,3,4-trimethylcyclohexanecarboxylic acid lactone. It was suggested that the lactone was formed by the sequence in eq. (144).

$$
\begin{array}{c}
\text{CH}_3 \\
\text{CH}_2\!=\!\overset{|}{\text{C}}\!-\!\text{CO}_2\text{H}
\end{array}
+
\begin{array}{c}
\text{CH}_2\!-\!\text{C}\!=\!\text{CH}_2 \\
| \quad\quad | \\
\text{CH}_2\!-\!\text{C}\!=\!\text{CH}_2
\end{array}
\longrightarrow
\underset{\text{CO}_2\text{H}}{\overset{\text{CH}_3}{\bigodot}}
\longrightarrow
$$

$$
\underset{\text{CO}_2\text{H}}{\overset{\text{CH}_3}{\underset{\text{H}_3\text{C}}{\overset{\text{H}_3\text{C}}{\bigodot}}}}
\longrightarrow
\underset{\text{O}\quad\quad\text{O}}{\overset{\text{CH}_3}{\underset{\text{H}_3\text{C}}{\overset{\text{H}_3\text{C}}{\bigodot}}\text{CH}_3}}
\quad (144)
$$

The formation of hydroquinone from acetylene, carbon monoxide, and hydrogen was reported using ruthenium catalysts such as trimeric ruthenium tetracarbonyl (214,215).

Preparation of higher hydrocarbons or alcohols from carbon monoxide and hydrogen is known as the Fischer-Tropsch reaction, and a cobalt or iron catalyst is commonly used. It was found that metallic ruthenium or certain ruthenium compounds are active in the Fischer-Tropsch-type reaction. Very active ruthenium catalysts were discovered and the reaction can be carried out at relatively low temperatures. Guyer and co-workers studied the formation of long chain hydrocarbons at 100 atm from hydrogen and carbon monoxide (216). Pichler and co-workers discovered that ruthenium oxide, irradiated by ^{60}Co, is a very active catalyst. Polymethylene, very similar to low-pressure polyethylene, having molecular weights up to 100,000 was produced by the reaction of carbon monoxide and hydrogen at high pressure and at temperatures below 140° (217). Kölbel, Müller and Hammer reported that hydrogen can be replaced with water (218). Thus high-melting paraffin waxes (melting range about 131°, molecular weight up to 7000) were synthesized by feeding carbon monoxide into a suspension of finely divided metallic ruthenium in water at pressures from 75 to 200 atm, and temperatures from 150–260°.

VI. Homogeneous Hydrogenations

Several noble metals are widely used for the heterogeneous hydrogenation of various unsaturated compounds. In the past few years, several noble metal complexes have been found to act as catalysts for the homogeneous hydrogenation of olefinic and acetylenic compounds (4,219). Catalytic hydrogenation of unsaturated substrates involves the following three steps: (*1*) hydrogen activation, (*2*) substrate activation, and (*3*) hydrogen transfer. Several noble metal complexes are capable of facilitating these steps by coordinating both hydrogen and substrates. Until now, few studies have been made from the standpoint of organic synthesis on homogeneous hydrogenation with noble metal complexes, and this method has limited use at present. However, the method may be an important technique in organic chemistry in the future, if its scope and usefulness are established. In addition, it can be expected that a study of the mechanism of homogeneous reaction should contribute to an understanding of heterogeneous catalysis. In homogeneous hydrogenation, H_2 is split by catalysts with the formation of reactive metal hydride complexes as intermediates.

Homogeneous hydrogenations of several olefinic compounds, including maleic, fumaric, and acrylic acids, were carried out using a chlororuthenate complex as a catalyst (220,221). In an aqueous solution ($3M$ HCl), $RuCl_2$ forms a 1:1 complex with many olefins such as ethylene, propylene, or fumaric acid. The ruthenium complexes of unsaturated acids (maleic, fumaric, acrylic acids) react with hydrogen homogeneously, which adds to the olefinic bond. Thus fumaric acid is homogeneously hydrogenated to give succinic acid. However, ethylene and propylene are not hydrogenated. Reduction of fumaric acid with

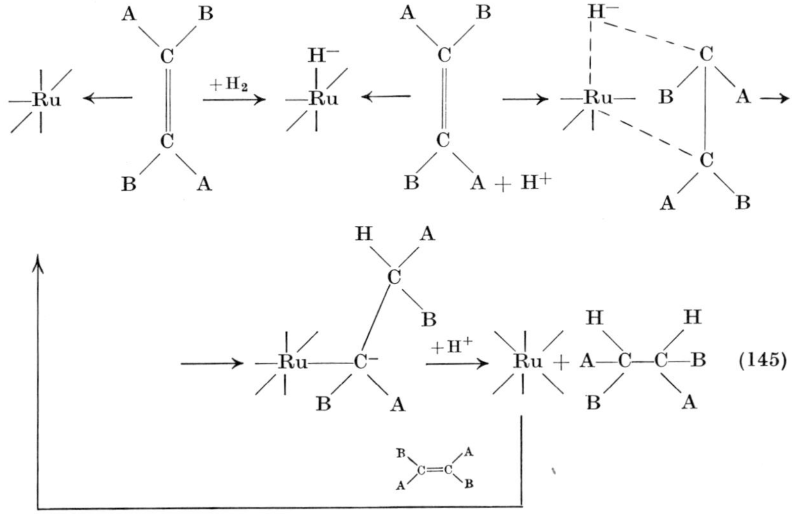

(145)

D_2 in H_2O solution gives undeuterated succinic acid, whereas reduction with H_2 in D_2O produces predominantly 2,3-dideuterated succinic acid, indicating that the hydrogen added to the double bond originated predominantly from water. To account for these observations, the mechanism in eq. (145) was proposed. The rate-determining step is the reaction of the ruthenium–olefin complex with H_2 to form a hydrido-π-olefin-ruthenium complex by heterolytic splitting of molecular hydrogen. Then rearrangement of the hydrido-π-olefin complex to a σ-alkyl complex by insertion of the olefin into the metal hydride bond follows. The final step is an electrophilic attack on the metal-bonded carbon atom by a proton to complete the hydrogenation and regenerate the catalyst. In this mechanism, the hydride ligand exchanges rapidly with water. It is significant to compare this mechanism with that proposed by Burwell (222) for the heterogeneous hydrogenation by a chromia catalyst shown in eq. (146). Other ruthenium complexes may

$$\text{Cr}\cdots\text{O} \xrightarrow{H_2} \overset{H}{\underset{|}{\text{Cr}}}\cdots\overset{H}{\underset{|}{\text{O}}} \xrightarrow{C_2H_4} \overset{\overset{CH_3}{|}}{\underset{|}{\text{Cr}}}\overset{CH_2}{\cdots}\overset{H}{\underset{|}{\text{O}}} \longrightarrow \text{Cr}\cdots\text{O} + C_2H_6 \quad (146)$$

be used for hydrogenations in organic solvents. $RuCl_2(Ph_3P)_4$ and $RuCl_2(Ph_3P)_3$ are active hydrogenation catalysts for olefins and acetylenes in benzene–ethanol (212). Treatment of the complexes in benzene–ethanol with hydrogen gives a hydrido complex $RuClH(Ph_3P)_3$ (IR absorption ν_{Ru-H} = ca. 2000 cm^{-1} and NMR τ = 28.6), and this hydrido species was confirmed as a hydrogenation intermediate. Diphenylacetylene is reduced to *cis*-stilbene by $RuClH(Ph_3P)_3$ and it was found that the added hydrogen came from molecular hydrogen and not from the alcohol. The mechanism shown in eq. (147) was proposed (223).

$$(PPh_3)_3Ru\begin{matrix}H\\ \\ Cl\end{matrix} \xrightarrow{R-C\equiv C-R} (PPh_3)_3Ru\begin{matrix}H\\ \\ Cl\end{matrix} \leftarrow \begin{matrix}R\\|\\C\\\|\\C\\|\\R\end{matrix} \longrightarrow$$

$$(PPh_3)_3Ru\begin{matrix}R\\ \diagdown\\ C\\ \diagup\\ Cl\end{matrix}\begin{matrix}\\ =\\ \\ \end{matrix}\begin{matrix}R\\ \diagup\\ C\\ \diagdown\\ H\end{matrix} \longrightarrow (PPh_3)_3RuHCl + \begin{matrix}R\\ \diagdown\\ H\end{matrix}C=C\begin{matrix}R\\ \diagup\\ H\end{matrix} \quad (147)$$

Cramer and co-workers found that ethylene and acetylene can be hydrogenated homogeneously by using a platinum–tin chloride complex as catalyst (189). The catalyst is prepared by dissolving stannous chloride dihydrate and chloroplatinic acid in methanol. Although the exact structure of the complex is not known, the catalyst is very active. When a 1:1 mixture of ethylene and hydrogen is admitted at 1 atm to a stirred solution of the catalyst, rapid and quantitative hydrogenation is observed. Similarly a 1:1 mixture of acetylene and hydrogen gives a mixture of ethane and ethylene (3:1). Stannous chloride has a strong ability to promote the coordination of ethylene to platinum. Also the function of stannous chloride is to stabilize the platinum against reduction to metallic platinum by hydrogen.

Jardine and McQuillin studied hydrogenation with the use of the phosphine complex of platinum in combination with stannous chloride, and found that the hydridochloride of platinum, [(Ph$_3$P)$_2$PtHCl], in the presence of stannous chloride in alcohol, is an effective catalyst for hydrogenation of norbornadiene to norbornane and 2,5-dimethyl-3-hexyn-2,5-diol to 2,5-dimethylhexane-2,5-diol (223). Hydrogenation of soy bean oil methyl ester with a similar catalyst was reported (224).

Vaska and Rhodes reported that square-planar carbonyl complexes, trans-[MX(CO)(Ph$_3$P)$_2$] (M = Ir, Rh, X = halogen), catalyze reactions of ethylene, propylene, and acetylene with molecular hydrogen in benzene at 40–60° (225,226). It was found that the iridium complex reversibly reacts with hydrogen and actually the hydrogen adducts, [H$_2$IrX(CO)(Ph$_3$P)$_2$], were isolated [see eq. (148)]. In addition, the complex reacts with ethylene, acetylene, and other unsaturated substrates at room temperature.

$$\begin{array}{c} X\diagdown\quad\diagup CH_2 \\ Ir \\ OC\diagup\quad\diagdown CH_2 \end{array} \xleftarrow{CH_2=CH_2} \begin{array}{c} X \\ | \\ Ir \\ | \\ C \\ \parallel \\ O \end{array} \xrightarrow{H-H} \begin{array}{c} X\diagdown\quad\diagup H \\ Ir \\ OC\diagup\quad\diagdown H \end{array} \quad (148)$$

(two trans-Ph$_3$P are normal to the plane of the page)

A significant observation was made in relating homogeneous and heterogeneous systems. Infrared bands (ν_{Ir-H} and ν_{Ir-D}) observed with the iridium complex after H$_2$ and D$_2$ addition are similar to the bands (ν_{Pt-H} and ν_{Pt-D}) of the chemisorbed hydrogen and deuterium on γ-alumina supported platinum metal (227). The observation shows a close analogy between a transition metal compound and a transition metal surface with respect to their reactions with H_2 and D_2.

Wilkinson and co-workers found that rhodium complexes such as $(PPh_3)_3RhCl_3$ are very active for homogeneous hydrogenation of olefins and acetylenes. Thus hexyne-1 was hydrogenated in an ethanol–benzene solution of $(PPh_3)_3RhCl_3$ rapidly and quantitatively to hexane with hydrogen at less than 1 atm pressure and 20°. Acetylenes were reduced faster than olefins (195).

The most useful and well-studied homogeneous hydrogenation catalyst so far discovered is chlorotris(triphenylphosphine)rhodium **(70)**. Some of the interesting properties of this complex and its use in the decarbonylation of aldehydes and acyl halides were described before. Extensive studies on this complex have been carried out by Wilkinson and co-workers (195,228,229). This complex is an extremely efficient catalyst for homogeneous hydrogenation of nonconjugated olefins and acetylenes at room temperature and 1 atm or below in benzene or similar solvents. Functional groups such as keto, hydroxy, cyano, nitro, chloro, azo, ether, ester, or carboxylic acids are not reduced by this catalyst. The characteristic features of the catalysis are the following: (1) terminal olefins are reduced more rapidly than inner olefins, (2) *cis* olefins are reduced faster than *trans* olefins, (3) conjugated diolefins such as butadiene or 1,3-cyclohexadiene are not hydrogenated at 1 atm [they are reduced at a higher pressure of ca. 60 atm], (4) chelating nonconjugated diolefins, e.g., 1,5-cyclooctadiene may be reduced very slowly at 1 atm but rapidly under pressure, (5) although propylene, butene, and higher olefins are reduced easily, ethylene is not hydrogenated. It was found that the hydrogenation of olefins proceeds through *cis* addition. When maleic acid is reduced with deuterium, the product is *meso*-1,2-dideuterosuccinic acid, indicating that predominantly *cis* deuteration of the double bond occurred. Therefore, this complex is very useful in organic chemistry for stereospecific deuteration, as will be shown by examples later.

The mechanism of the hydrogenation was studied with $(PPh_3)RhCl$ **(70)** by using NMR spectroscopy. In solution (chloroform or benzene), the complex **70** dissociates to form a coordinately unsaturated, formally three-coordinate species **(71)**. A solution of the complex in benzene or deuterochloroform takes up molecular hydrogen and the NMR spectrum shows high field lines at τ 28.2, 21.5, and 18.8. This spectrum indicates the presence of isomeric species containing Rh—H bonds

(IR band at ca. 2000 cm^{-1}). On sweeping the solution with nitrogen, the high-field lines disappear. The cycle can be repeated, showing the presence of a reversible equilibrium of the type in eq. (149). Also the

$$RhCl(PPh_3)_2 + H_2 \rightleftarrows RhCl(PPh_3)_2H_2 \qquad (149)$$
(71)

addition of an olefin caused instantaneous disappearance of the high field lines, and the NMR spectrum and gas chromatography showed the presence of paraffin. Resaturation of the solution with hydrogen again developed the high field bands. (PPh$_3$)$_3$RhCl dissociates in solvent (S) to give PPh$_3$ and **71**, which exists as a weakly solvated species, (PPh$_3$)$_2$RhCl(S) **(80)**, so that a site for olefin coordination is provided by displacement of the solvent. The solvated species reacts with hydrogen to give an octahedral *cis*-dihydrido-complex **(81)**. Attack of an olefin on the dihydrido-complex gives a transition state **(82)** in which both hydrogen and olefin are bound to the rhodium. Then the two hydrides are transferred to the olefin, see eq. (150).

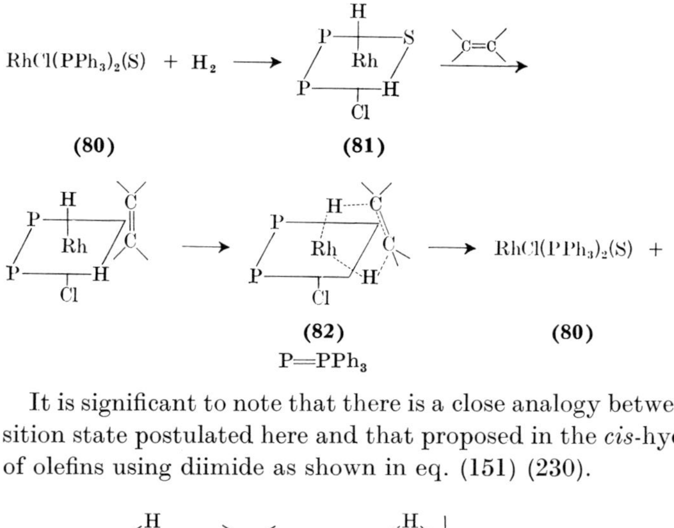

$$\text{RhCl(PPh}_3)_2(S) + H_2 \longrightarrow \underset{\textbf{(81)}}{\text{[Rh complex]}} \xrightarrow{C=C} \qquad$$

(80)

$$\longrightarrow \underset{\textbf{(82)}}{\text{[Rh complex]}} \longrightarrow \text{RhCl(PPh}_3)_2(S) + \underset{\textbf{(80)}}{\text{[alkane]}} \qquad (150)$$

P=PPh$_3$

It is significant to note that there is a close analogy between the transition state postulated here and that proposed in the *cis*-hydrogenation of olefins using diimide as shown in eq. (151) (230).

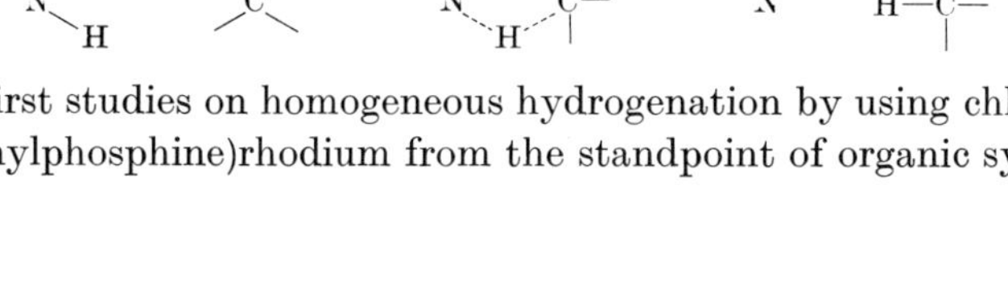

$$(151)$$

The first studies on homogeneous hydrogenation by using chlorotris(triphenylphosphine)rhodium from the standpoint of organic synthesis have been carried out by two groups (Birch and Djerassi). Djerassi and Gutzwiller (231) studied the hydrogenation of unsaturated steroidal ketones. The complex showed significant stereoselectivity. For example, Δ^1-3-ketosteroids are readily reduced, while Δ^4-3-ketosteroids are recovered unchanged. Then, the selective reduction of the following dienones was carried out: $\Delta^{1,4}$-androstadiene-3,17-dione **(83)** and $\Delta^{4,6}$-androstadiene-3,17-dione **(84)** were converted into the Δ^4-3-ketone **(85)** in 75–85% yield, [eq. (152)].

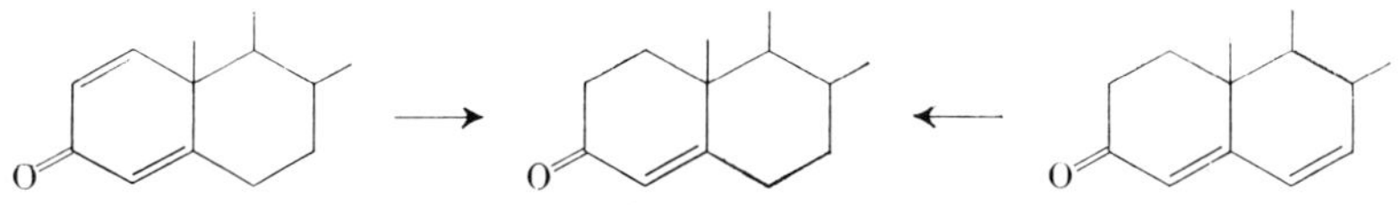

(83)　　　　　　　　(85)　　　　　　　　(84)　(152)

This method is also useful for deuterium labeling. Birch and Walker have shown that stereospecific *cis* addition of deuterium to a double bond is possible (232). For example, 22-dihydroergosteryl acetate is

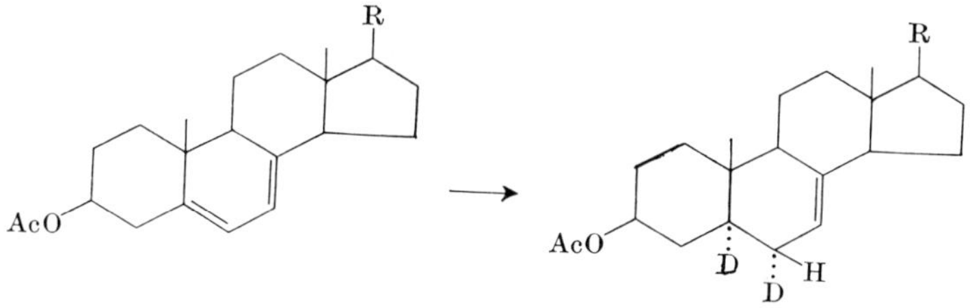

(153)

converted into 5α,6-d_2-ergost-7-en-3β-ol; see eq. (153). Hydrogenation of several types of compounds was studied to find the scope of this method (233). (+) Carvone is rapidly and specifically hydrogenated on the isopropenyl group. Thebaine is hydrogenated selectively to

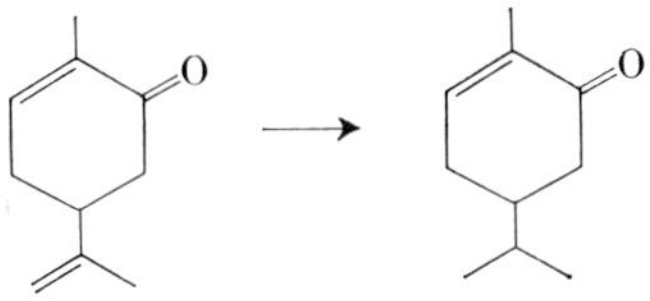

(154)

8,14-dihydrothebaine. It should be noted that the usual hydrogenation conditions give a mixture containing tetrahydro- and dihydrothebaine [eq. (155)]. Nitrostyrene was converted into phenylnitroethane without reduction of the nitro group [eq. (156)].

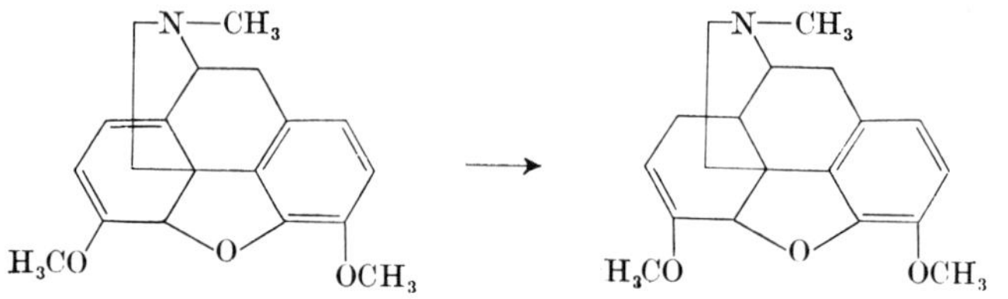

(155)

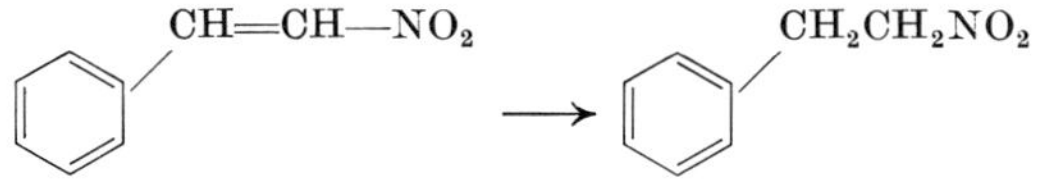

(156)

Homogeneous catalytic reduction of ketones by hydrogen transfer from isopropyl alcohol was carried out in the presence of an iridium trichloride–dimethyl sulfoxide complex. This reaction is formally analogous to the Meerwein Ponndorf reduction. In the presence of dimethyl sulfoxide, 78% of the axial alcohol was obtained from 4-t-butylcyclohexanone with the formation of isopropyl ether as a by-product. When a phosphite was used as a ligand, 100% of the axial alcohol was obtained from 3-t-butylcyclohexanone (234). The catalytic species was isolated and characterized as isomers of the octahedral complex $[(CH_3)_2SO]_3Ir_3Cl_3$.

VII. Hydrosilation Reactions Catalyzed by Noble Metal Compounds

It is known that silicon hydride behaves somewhat like hydrogen in the presence of transition metal compounds. It has been known that, like the hydrogenation reaction, the addition of a silicon hydride bond to an unsaturated bond is catalyzed by some noble metals, especially by platinum. Later it was found that platinum compounds are better catalysts and chloroplatinic acid is widely used (235). It was believed that the true catalyst is metallic platinum and not chloroplatinic acid. However, Ryan and Speier noted that the addition of trichlorosilane to olefins proceeds in a homogeneous system, showing that a soluble platinum complex is a catalytic species (236). From recent studies, it has become more and more apparent that there is a remarkable similarity between homogeneous hydrogenation and hydrosilation. Many studies have been made on hydrosilation catalyzed by noble metal compounds, and several reviews have been published (237–239). Therefore, it is not necessary or possible to cover all the results in this review. Only typical reactions and recent progress are treated.

Various types of silanes undergo the hydrosilation reaction but, in general, silanes having electron-attracting groups are most reactive. Chlorosilanes are extensively used. On the other hand, alkylsilanes are not very reactive (240). Silanes add to various types of unsaturated compounds. Simple and conjugated olefins and acetylenic compounds undergo facile reaction.

Simple olefins react with silanes easily with a suitable catalyst. The reaction is quite unique and useful because, with few exceptions, the silicon atom adds to the terminal carbon, regardless of the original position of the double bond in the olefins, to form primary alkylsilicons from nonterminal olefins. This reaction is very different from peroxide-initiated hydrosilation. At the same time, extensive isomerization of internal olefins accompanies the hydrosilation. When silicon deuteride is used, wide distribution of deuterium throughout the olefin and the hydrosilation product is observed, showing a prior equilibration between the olefin and the silicon hydrogen bond (236).

For example, while in the addition of trichlorosilane to 3-heptene catalyzed by acetyl peroxide, the trichlorosilyl group attacks the 3- or 4-positions (241), the reaction catalyzed by chloroplatinic acid gives

$$\underset{\underset{SiCl_3}{|}}{CH_3CH_2CH_2CH_2CHCH_2CH_3} \xleftarrow{peroxide} CH_3CH_2CH_2CH=CHCH_2CH_3 \xrightarrow{H_2PtCl_6} CH_3(CH_2)_5CH_2-SiCl_3 \qquad (157)$$

the n-heptyl derivative as a sole product [eq. (157)]. Also, the addition of trichlorosilane to 1-methylcyclohexene catalyzed by chloroplatinic acid gives, after reduction with lithium aluminum hydride, nearly pure (cyclohexylmethyl)silane, with a trace of the isomeric 1,2- and 1,3-methylsilylcyclohexane (242,243); see eq. (158).

$$HSiCl_3 + \underset{}{\text{(1-methylcyclohexene)}} \xrightarrow{H_2PtCl_6} \underset{}{\text{(CH_2SiCl_3-cyclohexane)}} \qquad (158)$$

On the other hand, the addition of symmetrical tetramethyldisiloxane to either 2- or 3-hexene in the presence of chloroplatinic acid gives mainly the terminal product but also the 2- and 3-positions of the hexyl group are attacked. According to Bank, Saam, and Speier (244), symmetrical tetramethyldisiloxane behaves somewhat differently from chlorosilane in being able to form secondary alkylsilicon derivatives from internal olefins.

Certain substituted olefins form more than one adduct when the olefinic double bond is conjugated with another multiple bond. Thus styrene reacts with methyldichlorosilane [eq. (159)] giving a mixture

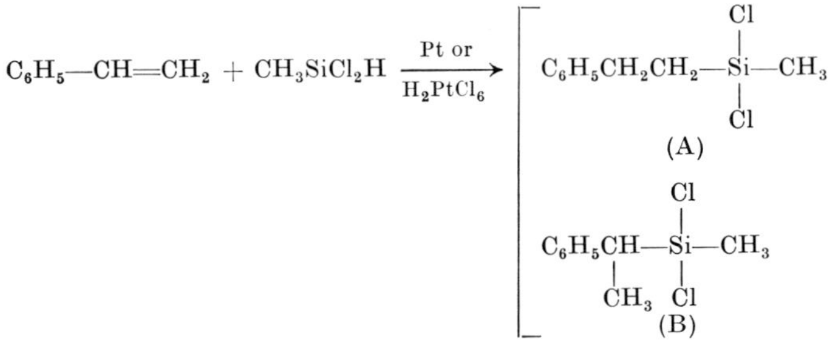

$$C_6H_5-CH=CH_2 + CH_3SiCl_2H \xrightarrow[H_2PtCl_6]{Pt \text{ or}} \begin{bmatrix} C_6H_5CH_2CH_2-\underset{\underset{Cl}{|}}{\overset{\overset{Cl}{|}}{Si}}-CH_3 \\ (A) \\ \\ C_6H_5CH-\underset{\underset{Cl}{|}}{\overset{\overset{Cl}{|}}{Si}}-CH_3 \\ CH_3 \\ (B) \end{bmatrix} \quad (159)$$

of addition products (ratio A:B = 33:55) (245–247). The effect of the phenyl group is also apparent from the following results. The addition of silanes to phenylalkenes of the formula $C_6H_5(CH_2)_nCH=CH_2$ in the presence of chloroplatinic acid gives two products. The silyl group adds at the terminal carbon (A) and in a position α to the phenyl (C). The A/C ratio was dependent upon the silanes used (248,249). Similar results were obtained in the chloroplatinic acid-catalyzed hydrosilation of 4-*o*-, *m*- and *p*- chlorophenyl-1-butene [eq. (160)] (250). The expected straight-chain compound was the main product, accompanied by the benzylsilicon compound.

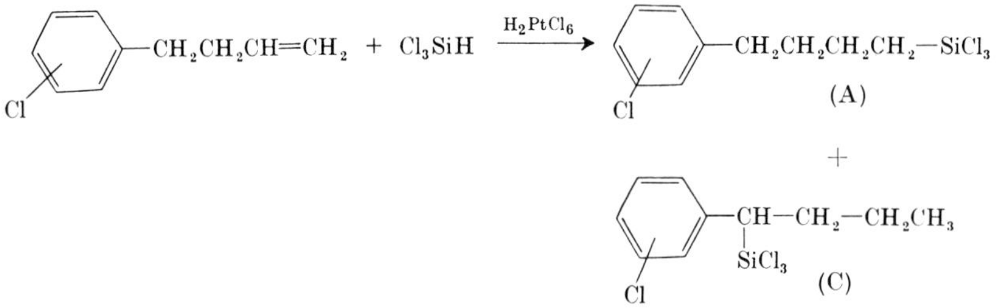

$$\underset{Cl}{\bigcirc}-CH_2CH_2CH=CH_2 + Cl_3SiH \xrightarrow{H_2PtCl_6} \underset{Cl}{\bigcirc}-CH_2CH_2CH_2CH_2-SiCl_3 \quad (A)$$

$$+$$

$$\underset{Cl}{\bigcirc}-\underset{SiCl_3}{\overset{|}{CH}}-CH_2-CH_2CH_3 \quad (C)$$

$$(160)$$

Carbonyl conjugated double bonds also react with silane in the presence of noble metal catalysts. For example, trichlorosilane reacts with methyl acrylate *via* 1,2-addition as shown in eq. (161) (251–253)

$$Cl_3SiH + CH_2=CH-CO_2CH_3 \xrightarrow{H_2PtCl_6} Cl_3Si\underset{\underset{CH_3}{|}}{C}H-CO_2CH_3 \quad (161)$$

On the other hand, a trialkylsilane adds 1,4 to methyl acrylate to give the unsaturated acetal, and acrylic acid gives the saturated ester (251); see eqs. (162). Unsaturated aldehydes and ketones react by

$$R_3SiH + CH_2=CH-CO_2CH_3 \longrightarrow CH_3-CH=C\begin{matrix}OSiR_3\\ \\OCH_3\end{matrix} \quad (162a)$$

$$R_3SiH + CH_2=CH-CO_2H \longrightarrow$$

$$\left(CH_3-CH=C\begin{matrix}OSiR_3\\ \\OH\end{matrix}\right) \longrightarrow CH_3CH_2CO_2SiR_3 \quad (162b)$$

1,4-addition to form silyl vinyl ethers; eqs. (163).

$$R_3SiH + CH_2=CH-CHO \longrightarrow CH_3CH=CH-OSiR_3 \quad (163a)$$

$$R_3SiH + CH_2=CH-COR \longrightarrow CH_3-CH=\underset{\underset{R}{|}}{C}-OSiR_3 \quad (163b)$$

Reactions with conjugated dienes proceed smoothly. 1,4-Addition was reported with butadiene (254). Various silanes, except trimethylsilane, also add 1,4 to isoprene in the presence of chloroplatinic acid (255), eq. (164). Additions to cyclooctene, 1,5-cyclo-

$$CH_2=CH-\underset{\underset{CH_3}{|}}{C}=CH_2 + SiHCl_3 \longrightarrow CH_3-CH=\underset{\underset{CH_3}{|}}{C}-CH_2SiCl_3 \quad (164)$$

octadiene (256,257), cyclododecatriene (258), and cyclooctatetraene (259) have been reported.

With allyl halides, hydrosilation proceeds with some hydrogenolysis of the halogen (260–263), eq. (165).

$$Cl-CH_2CH=CH_2 + H-\overset{|}{\underset{|}{Si}}- \longrightarrow$$

$$CH_3CH=CH_2 + CH_3CH_2CH_2\overset{|}{\underset{|}{Si}}- + ClCH_2CH_2CH_2-\overset{|}{\underset{|}{Si}}- \quad (165)$$

Also, skeletal rearrangement accompanying the formation of a terminally substituted product from an internal olefin is known. Benkeser and Cunico reported an interesting skeletal rearrangement in the addition reaction of trichlorosilane to 1- and 4-*t*-butylcyclohexene catalyzed by dichlorobis(ethylene)-μ,μ'-dichlorodiplatinum. The products of the reaction are 1-trichlorosilyl-2-(1-methylcyclohexyl)propane and a ring substituted derivative (264). The former is also synthesized by the addition of trichlorosilane to 1-methyl-1-isopropenylcyclohexane; see eqs. (166).

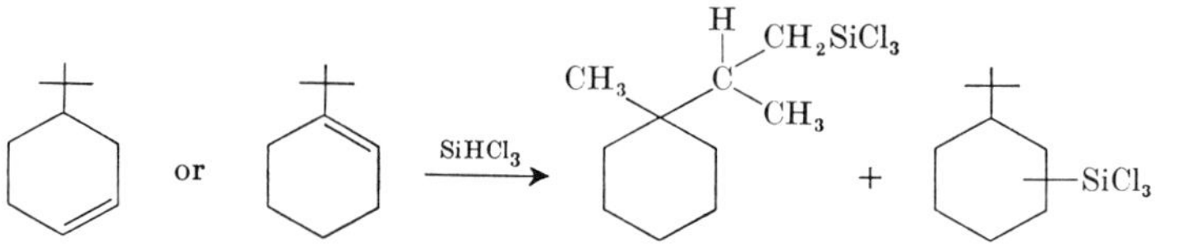

$$\text{(166a)}$$

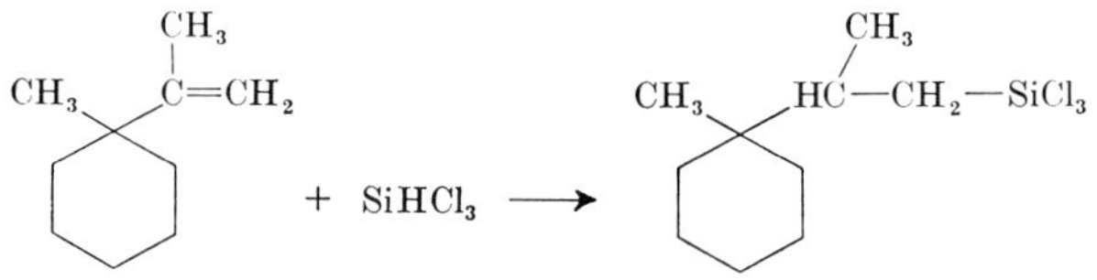

$$\text{(166b)}$$

The addition of trichlorosilane to substituted acetylenes was found to be a stereoselective *cis* addition to form *trans* olefinic compounds when the reaction was catalyzed by platinized charcoal, in contrast to the *trans* addition reaction catalyzed by peroxide (265). Also chloro-

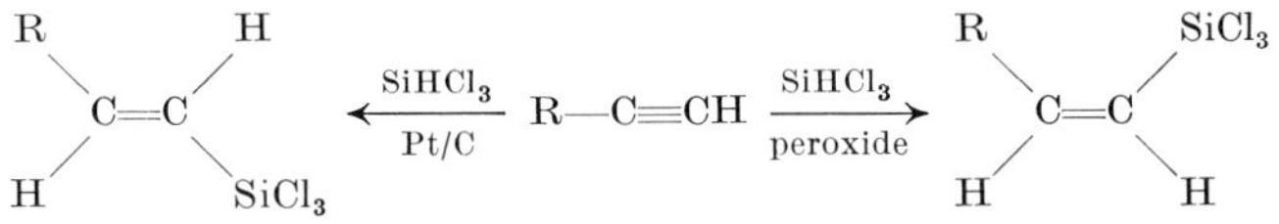

$$\text{(167)}$$

platinic acid catalyzes *cis* addition to acetylenes (266). With 2-butyne, addition of methyldichlorosilane proceeds stereospecifically in a *cis* manner at the original position of the triple bond without rearrangement to give *cis*-2-methyldichlorosilyl-2-butene (267). However, sometimes

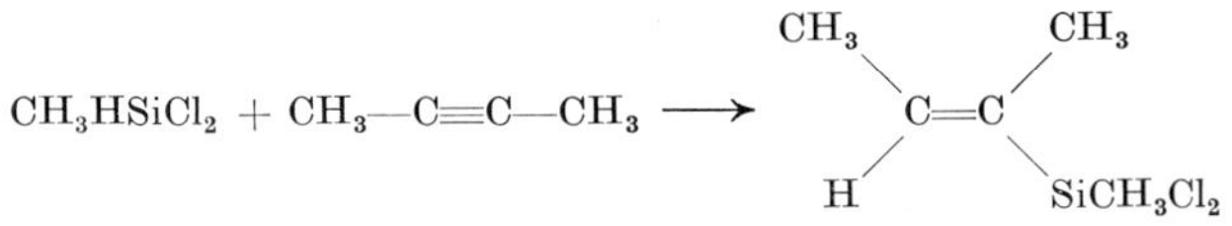

$$\text{(168)}$$

the addition reaction to a triple bond is not completely selective. For example, with propargyl alcohol or chloride, addition takes place in both directions [eqs. (169)], the ratios depending on the silanes (268–275). In general, triple bonds are more reactive than double bonds

$$HC{\equiv}C{-}CH_2OH \xrightarrow[HSiR_3]{H_2PtCl_6} R_3SiCH{=}CH{-}CH_2OH + R_3SiCH{=}CH{-}CH_2OSiR_3 \quad (169a)$$

$$R_3SiH + CH{\equiv}C{-}CH_2X \longrightarrow R_3SiCH{=}CH{-}CH_2X \quad (169b)$$
$$X = \text{halogen}$$

$$R_3SiH + CH{\equiv}C{-}CH_2OH \longrightarrow CH_2{=}\underset{SiR_3}{C}{-}CH_2OH \quad (169c)$$

and with enyl compounds, the triple bond is attacked preferentially by silanes, eqs. (170) (276–278).

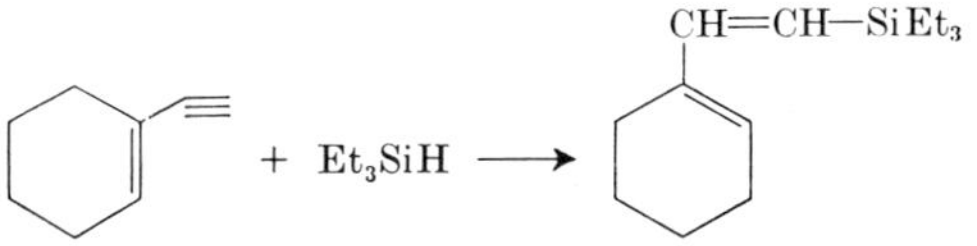

[cyclohexenyl-C≡CH] + Et$_3$SiH ⟶ [cyclohexenyl-CH=CH-SiEt$_3$] (170a)

$$CH_2{=}CH{-}C{\equiv}CH + CH_3SiHCl_2 \longrightarrow Cl_2\underset{CH_3}{Si}{-}CH{=}CH{-}CH{=}CH_2 \quad (170b)$$

Another interesting and useful reaction is the hydrosilation of a pyridine ring catalyzed by palladium, found by Cook and Lyons (279). They found that trimethylsilane adds to pyridine and picolines in the presence of palladium and other noble metal catalysts under very mild conditions to yield a variety of 1,2- and 1,4-dihydropyridine derivatives. Palladium causes isomerization of the products, and the products isolated vary considerably with reaction time, temperature, and other reaction conditions. For example, the compounds in eq. (171) were

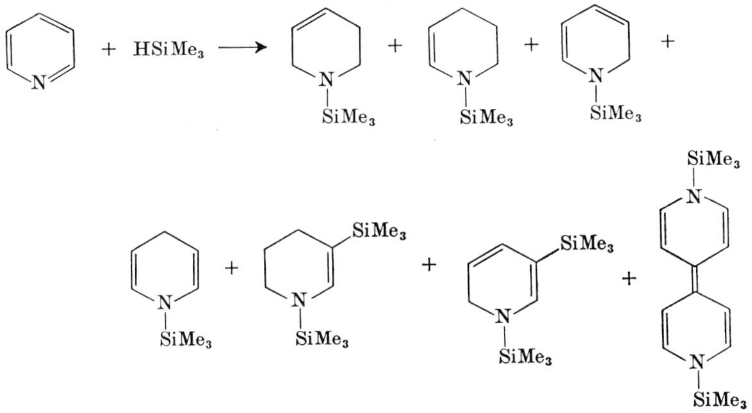

[pyridine] + HSiMe$_3$ ⟶ [N-SiMe$_3$ dihydropyridine] + [N-SiMe$_3$ dihydropyridine] + [N-SiMe$_3$ dihydropyridine] +

[N-SiMe$_3$ dihydropyridine] + [N-SiMe$_3$, 3-SiMe$_3$ tetrahydropyridine] + [N-SiMe$_3$, 3-SiMe$_3$ dihydropyridine] + [4,4'-bis(N-SiMe$_3$)-bipyridine with SiMe$_3$ groups] (171) obtained from pyridine. The main product was the 1,4-dihydropyridine derivative. Unsubstituted 1,4-dihydropyridine has been prepared and isolated by this procedure for the first time (280). Treatment of 1-trimethylsilyl-1,4-dihydropyridine with methanol containing a small amount of potassium hydroxide yielded 1,4-dihydropyridine, eq. (172). It seems likely that palladium catalyzes the reaction by

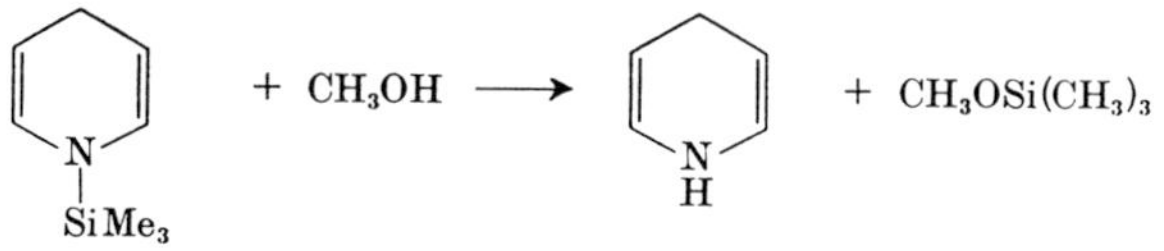

$$\text{(pyridine-SiMe}_3) + CH_3OH \longrightarrow \text{(1,4-dihydropyridine-H)} + CH_3OSi(CH_3)_3 \qquad (172)$$

splitting the silane homolytically. Rhodium was found to be active, but gave a lower rate than palladium. The metallic palladium-catalyzed reaction is interesting in view of the fact that metallic palladium or palladium complexes are not active for the hydrosilation of olefinic compounds. The mechanism of the reaction is not known at present. This is a type of hydrogenation, and silicon hydride is the hydrogen source.

The mechanism of hydrosilation catalyzed by noble metal compounds is not completely clear. Simple addition of H^- and R_3Si^+, or a radical mechanism, cannot account for the experimental results. The most probable mechanism is coordination of the double bond and homolytic splitting of the silane by metallic compounds. Harrod and Chalk (281) studied the hydrosilation reaction from the standpoint of homogeneous catalysis by using noble metal complexes, and concluded that the catalyst functions are: (1) activation of the silane, or Si—H bond cleavage, (2) activation of the olefin by coordination to the metal, and (3) resistance to destructive reduction of the metal ion. Thus, palladium complexes are generally easily reduced to the metallic state and cannot be used for the hydrosilation reaction. The mechanism in eq. (173) was proposed in which a transformation from square planar to

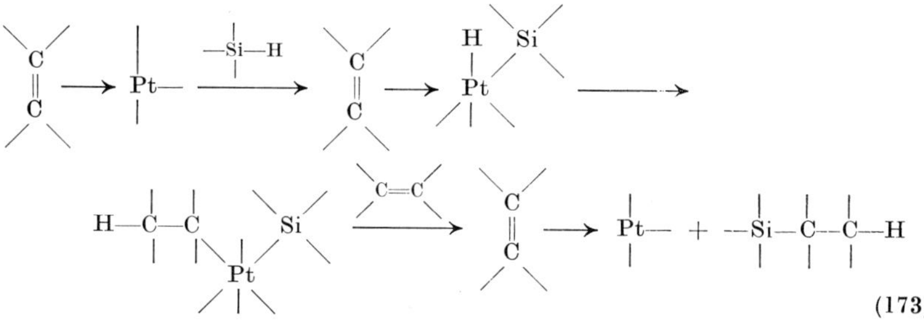

$$(173)$$

octahedral is required. For this requirement, platinum and rhodium complexes are most suitable. The oxidative addition of silane is an important step in this mechanism. Actually, oxidative addition of chlorosilane to bis(triphenylphosphine)carbonylchloroiridium was confirmed [eq. (174)], but this complex is too stable and cannot catalyze

$$\begin{array}{c}\text{PPh}_3\diagdown\diagup\text{CO}\\ \text{Ir}\\ \text{PPh}_3\diagup\diagdown\text{Cl}\end{array}\xrightarrow{-\overset{|}{\underset{|}{\text{Si}}}-\text{H}}\begin{array}{c}\text{PPh}_3\diagdown\overset{-\overset{|}{\text{Si}}-}{|}\diagup\text{H}\\ \text{Ir}\\ \text{OC}\diagup\underset{\text{Cl}}{|}\diagdown\text{PPh}_3\end{array} \qquad (174)$$

hydrosilation. The analogous platinum complex, however, was not isolated as a stable complex. In this mechanism of hydrosilation, the transformation of a π-complexed olefin into a σ-complex takes place, and the similarity between the homogeneous hydrogenation and hydrosilation is apparent. Also this step is certainly responsible for the easy isomerization of the olefinic bonds before hydrosilation which places silicon on the terminal carbon.

VIII. Addition Reactions of Olefinic and Acetylenic Compounds

One of the essential catalytic actions of noble metal compounds is in the addition or polymerization of olefinic and acetylenic compounds. There have been many reports treating noble metal-catalyzed polymerization reactions. For example, butadiene can be polymerized stereospecifically by rhodium or palladium chloride (282–286). It does not seem appropriate, however, to attempt to treat them all, and here only a few selected examples, interesting from the standpoint of organic syntheses, are described. Rhodium and ruthenium salt-catalyzed reactions seem to be the most interesting and useful. It is said that salts of the 8th group noble metals in protic solvents (e.g., water or alcohol) act analogously to the Ziegler catalyst through an anionic coordinated mechanism (287), and several examples support this assumption. Different from the Ziegler type catalyst, which has to be handled in aprotic solvents and in the complete absence of oxygen, noble metal salts can be handled easily without exact exclusion of oxygen.

Alderson, Jenner, and Lindsey (288) found that addition reactions of various terminal double bonds take place in the presence of ruthenium or rhodium chloride. These reactions involve an intermolecular hydrogen shift. They are effected at temperatures of 30–150° under moderate pressure in alcoholic media containing low concentrations of soluble chlorides of rhodium or ruthenium. These addition reactions differ from the known acid-catalyzed and Friedel-Crafts reactions in that the acidity is low and ethylene shows a high reactivity compared with higher olefins. They carried out the reaction of ethylene at 40° in alcohol with 0.1 mole % of rhodium chloride trihydrate, based on ethylene. Ethylene was supplied at one to several hundred atmospheric pressures and a mixture of 1- and 2-butenes was obtained.

$$CH_2{=}CH_2 + CH_2{=}CH_2 \longrightarrow CH_2{=}CH-CH_2CH_3 \longrightarrow CH_3-CH{=}CH-CH_3$$
(cis and trans)
(175)

Although the primary product seems to be 1-butene, the butenes obtained were a mixture of isomers, the composition of which was somewhat variable depending on the reaction conditions. Usually trans-2-butene was the main product. Ruthenium chloride is also an effective catalyst of ethylene dimerization. Platinum chloride and palladium chloride–ethylene complexes are said to be active for the reaction also (289).

Rhodium trichloride combined with potassium acetate catalyzed, in 54% conversion, the dimerization of butadiene at 100°. The main product was 2,4,6-octatriene, which was presumably formed by double bond migration in the initially formed 1,3,6-octatriene (288).

$$2CH_2{=}CH-CH{=}CH_2 \rightarrow CH_2{=}CH-CH{=}CH-CH_2-CH{=}CH-CH_3 \rightarrow$$
$$CH_3-CH{=}CH-CH{=}CH-CH{=}CH-CH_3 \quad (175)$$

An interesting and useful reaction is the dimerization of methyl acrylate. Dimethyl 2-hexenedioate was obtained by heating a solution of methyl acrylate in methanol to 140° in the presence of rhodium chloride. The conversion was not very high. On the other hand, ruthenium chloride gave the dimer in 56% yield at 150° in the presence of a small amount of ethylene. This is a remarkable reaction.

$$2CH_2{=}CH-CO_2CH_3 \rightarrow H_3CO_2C-CH{=}CH-CH_2CH_2CO_2CH_3 \quad (176)$$

The addition of ethylene to butadiene with rhodium chloride catalyst occurs with great facility and, interestingly, to the almost complete exclusion of dimerization of either component. The reaction proceeds rapidly at 50° in high conversion to give in over 90% yield a mixture of 1,4- and 2,4-hexadienes. It seems likely that 1,4-hexadiene is the primary product of the addition and 2,4-hexadiene is formed by a subsequent isomerization. The effect of the structure of the diene on

$$CH_2=CH_2 + CH_2=CH-CH=CH_2 \rightarrow CH_2=CH-CH_2CH=CH-CH_3 \rightarrow$$
$$CH_3CH=CH-CH=CH-CH_3 \quad (177)$$

its reactivity in the addition reaction is very large. Thus the most facile addition was found to be the reaction of ethylene with 1,3-pentadiene, and a conversion of over 95% was achieved at 50° in the presence of 0.2% rhodium trichloride trihydrate. The product was 3-methyl-1,4-hexadiene. The reaction of ethylene with isoprene was slower than that with butadiene, and 4-methyl-1,4-hexadiene was obtained in low yield, eqs. (178). Styrene reacted with ethylene at 50°

$$CH_2=CH_2 + CH_3CH=CH-CH=CH_2 \longrightarrow CH_2=CH-\underset{\underset{CH_3}{|}}{CH}-CH=CH-CH_3 \quad (178a)$$

$$CH_2=CH_2 + CH_2=\underset{\underset{CH_3}{|}}{C}-CH=CH_2 \longrightarrow CH_2=CH-CH_2-\underset{\underset{CH_3}{|}}{C}=CH-CH_3 \quad (178b)$$

to give 2-phenyl-2-butene in 40% yield. The addition of ethylene to

$$CH_2=CH_2 + C_6H_5CH=CH_2 \longrightarrow$$
$$CH_2=CH-\underset{\underset{C_6H_5}{|}}{CH}-CH_3 \longrightarrow CH_3CH=\underset{\underset{C_6H_5}{|}}{C}-CH_3 \quad (179)$$

methyl acrylate was catalyzed by ruthenium chloride and the principal product was methyl 3-pentenoate (47%). Other examples of addition

$$CH_2=CH_2 + CH_2=CH-CO_2CH_3 \rightarrow CH_3-CH=CH-CH_2CO_2CH_3 \quad (180)$$

reactions and their products are listed here.

Olefin	Diene or olefin	Product
$CH_2=CH_2$	1,3-Hexadiene	3-Ethyl-1,4-hexadiene
	2,4-Hexadiene	3-Methyl-1,4-heptadiene
	Chloroprene	2- or 3-Chloro-2,4-hexadiene
$CH_3-CH=CH_2$	Propylene	C_6 Olefin mixture
	Butadiene	2-Methyl-1,4-hexadiene
	Isoprene	2,4-Dimethyl-1,4-hexadiene

Cramer studied these noble metal-catalyzed addition reactions of ethylene and proposed the mechanism in eq. (181) (290). It was ob-

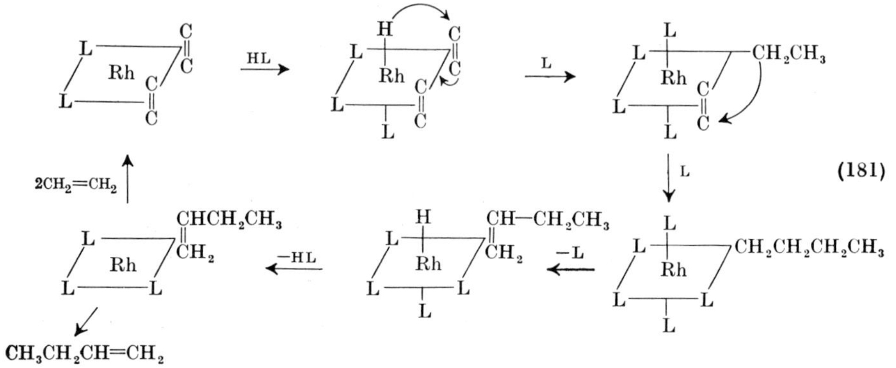

(181)

L = Cl or solvent

served that the presence of Cl^-, Br^-, or I^- is essential for butene formation. At first rhodium chloride trihydrate seems to be reduced to form a bisethylene–rhodium complex. Protonation of the ethylene-complex gives an ethyl-rhodium complex. Then the rate-determining step of ethylene insertion to give a butyl–rhodium complex follows. The final step is the release of the π-complexed butene and regeneration of the catalyst by coordination with ethylene.

Acrylonitrile cannot be dimerized by ruthenium chloride, but hydrodimerization of acrylonitrile to give adiponitrile by the catalytic action of some ruthenium compounds was claimed in a patent (291). Thus ruthenium acetylacetonate catalyzes the hydrodimerization of acrylonitrile in about 50% conversion at 110° under hydrogen pressure, eq. (182). In this reaction, acrylonitrile is also reduced to propionitrile.

$$CH_2=CH-CN \xrightarrow[H_2]{Ru\ compound} \begin{cases} NC(CH_2)_4CN \\ NCCH=CHCH_2CH_2CN \\ CH_3CH_2CN \end{cases} \quad (182)$$

Nicholson and Shaw found that ruthenium trichloride reacts with butadiene in 2-methoxyethanol at 90° to give a complex which was found to be dichloro(dodeca-2,6,10-triene-1,12-diyl)ruthenium, $RuCl_2$-$(C_4H_6)_3$ (292,293). The complex was formed by the catalytic trimerization of butadiene. It should be noted that the effect of the solvent on the course of the ruthenium-catalyzed reaction is remarkable. On pyrolysis, the complex gives *cis,trans,trans-* and *trans,trans,trans-*1,5,9-cyclododecatriene. It is rather surprising, in view of the fact that the corresponding complex of nickel is extremely unstable and difficult to handle, that the intermediate complex of the butadiene

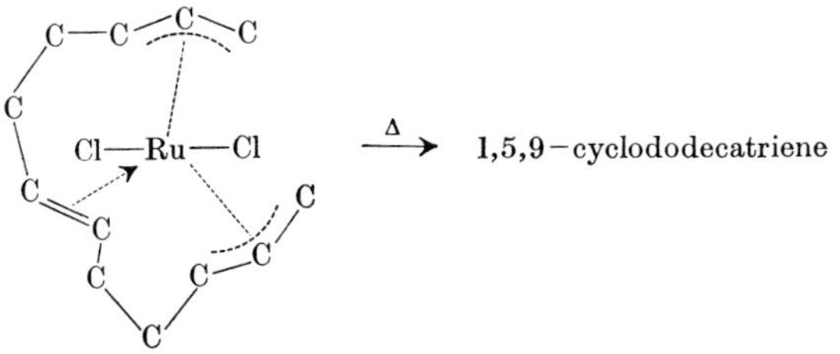

$$\text{[Ru complex with butadiene ligands]} \xrightarrow{\Delta} 1,5,9\text{-cyclododecatriene} \tag{183}$$

trimerization is obtained so easily as a stable complex by using such a simple compound as ruthenium trichloride.

Another example of a noble metal-catalyzed reaction which is worth noting is the polymerization of some unsaturated cyclic olefins. It was found that some cyclic olefins undergo ring-opening polymerization rather than vinyl polymerization at the expense of the double bond. For example, the bicyclo(2,2,1)heptene-2 ring system undergoes the polymerization in eq. (184) by the catalytic action of hydrated ruthenium, osmium, and iridium salts in alcohol (294,295).

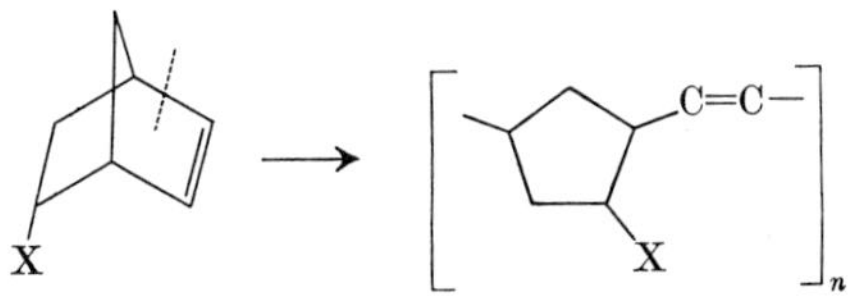

$$\text{norbornene} \longrightarrow \left[\text{ring-opened polymer} \right]_n \tag{184}$$

Natta, Dall'asta, and Porri found that cyclobutene and 3-methylcyclobutene polymerize exclusively by ring opening under the catalytic action of ruthenium trichloride in polar media to form polybutadiene and polypentadiene, respectively (296), eq. (185).

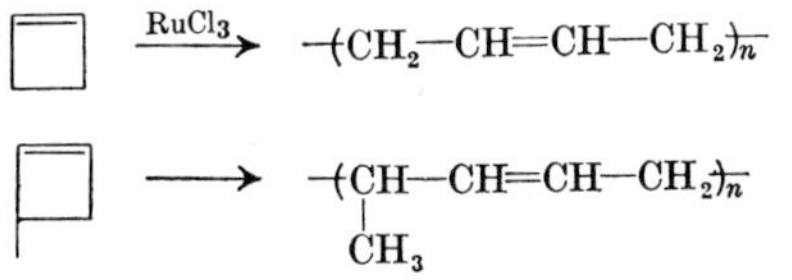

$$\square \xrightarrow{RuCl_3} -(CH_2-CH=CH-CH_2)_n-$$

$$\square \longrightarrow -(CH-CH=CH-CH_2)_n- \atop {\overset{|}{CH_3}} \tag{185}$$

It is explained that these ring openings are possible because the original cyclic systems are strained molecules; however, it is rather remarkable from the standpoint of organic chemistry that these ring systems can be opened under such mild conditions. Such ring opening reactions are quite difficult by usual organic chemical techniques. The reactions involved in the above-mentioned dimerizations and polymerizations are unique, showing the very characteristic catalytic activity of noble metal compounds. It is expected that further useful applications of these unique reactions will be found by additional careful studies of the reactions of noble metal compounds.

Based on the assumption that some hydrogenation catalysts should interact with olefinic compounds, Katz and Mrowca studied addition reactions of norbornadiene in the presence of rhodium metal on carbon. They found that norbornadiene dimerizes readily in the presence of metallic rhodium at 90° to give the compounds **86** and **87** as main products (297).

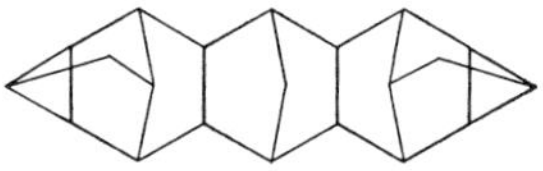

(86) 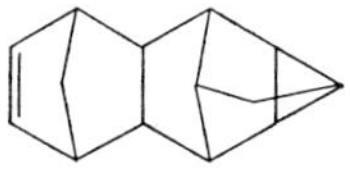   (87)

One of the interesting catalytic activities of palladium is cyclization and polymerization of acetylenic compounds. Various acetylenes react under nitrogen in the presence of catalytic amounts of palladium. The products are dimer, trimer, or polymer depending on the nature of the acetylenes. For example, dimethyl acetylenedicarboxylate in benzene trimerized to give hexamethyl mellitate in 93% yield (171). Phenylacetylene dimerizes to 1-phenylnaphthalene at 100° by the catalytic action of metallic palladium produced by the reduction of palladium chloride with sodium borohydride [eq. (186)], and no tri-

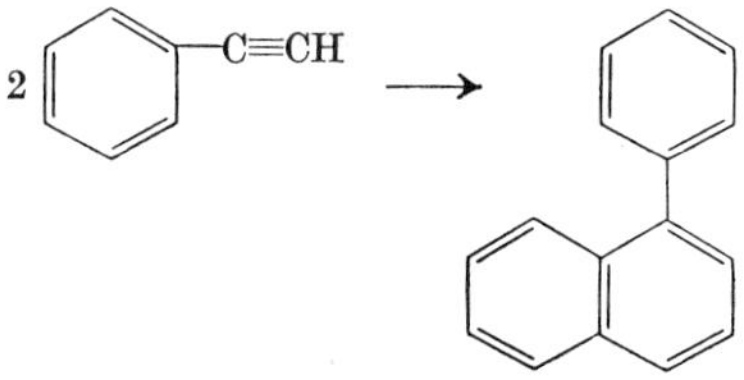

(186)

phenylbenzene is formed. Acetylenemonocarboxylic acid and its ester, propargyl alcohol, propargyl bromide, butyndiol, and 1-octyne react with palladium vigorously, but only yellow polymers are obtained.

The catalytic activity of palladium chloride on diphenylacetylene has been studied extensively. Bis-benzonitrile–palladium chloride, in a catalytic amount in nonhydroxylic solvents such as benzene, chloroform, and acetone, effects the smooth trimerization of diphenylacetylene to form hexaphenylbenzene and this seems to be the best method for the preparation of this compound (298). Other disubstituted acetylenes were also trimerized to benzene derivatives (299).

The most interesting reaction of palladium chloride and diphenylacetylene is the formation of the tetraphenylcyclobutadiene complex. The first report of the reaction was given briefly by Malatesta and co-workers (300,301). Because of the facile formation of the cyclobutadiene system, the reaction has attracted much attention and extensive studies on this reaction have been carried out (170,302–304). When diphenylacetylene is allowed to react with the benzonitrile complex of palladium chloride in ethanol, or better with sodium chloropalladate in aqueous ethanol (305), the complex (88) is obtained. When the complex (88) is treated with hydrogen chloride, it is converted into the tetraphenylcyclobutadiene–palladium chloride complex (89). The complex (89) is very stable and does not change even in hot hydrochloric acid. Several chemical transformations of the complexes (88 and 89) have been carried out. 89 is converted by the action of a base in ethanol into a dimeric complex (90) which is isomeric with 88.

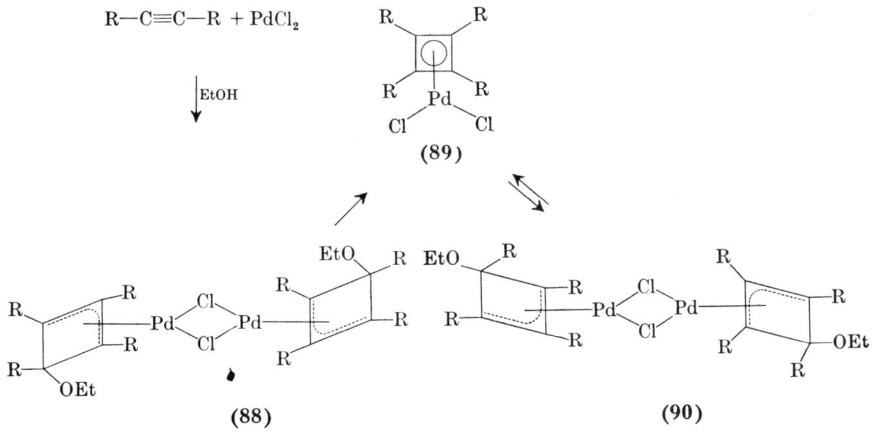

88 and 90 differ only in the orientation of the ethoxy and phenyl groups.

An interesting reaction of the complex (89) is a smooth ligand transfer (306,307). Maitlis and co-workers found that tetraphenylbutadiene can be transferred from palladium chloride to other metallic compounds such as nickel or iron carbonyl. For example, reaction of tetraphenylbutadiene–palladium bromide with iron or nickel carbonyl gave tetraphenylcyclobutadiene-iron tricarbonyl and the corresponding nickel bromide, respectively [eq. (188)]. It is remarkable that the

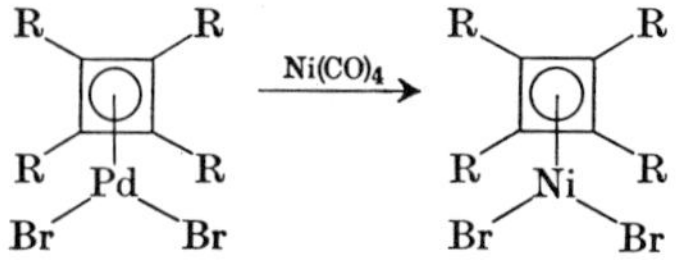

$$\begin{array}{c}\text{R-□-R} \\ \text{R-Pd-R} \\ \text{Br Br}\end{array} \xrightarrow{\text{Ni(CO)}_4} \begin{array}{c}\text{R-□-R} \\ \text{R-Ni-R} \\ \text{Br Br}\end{array} \quad (188)$$

cyclobutadiene ring, which cannot exist free, can be transferred without decomposition from one metal to the other.

IX. Resolution of Diastereoisomers by Complex Formation with Platinum Compounds

Platinum compounds form stable olefin complexes, from which the olefin can be recovered under very mild conditions. An ingenious application of this complex-forming property of platinum compounds was discovered by Cope and co-workers, and then extended elegantly by Paiaro and Panunzi for the resolution of enantiomers. It has been suggested by Blomquist, Liu and Bohrer (308) that *trans* cyclic olefins of intermediate size (8–10 membered rings) should be capable of existence in stable enantiomorphic conformations, and *trans*-cyclooctene is a typical example. Resolution of *trans*-cyclooctene, however, cannot be done by the usual methods, because it has no group suitable for the direct formation of diastereoisomeric pairs of compounds with an optically active compound. This problem has now been overcome by virtue of the strong complex-forming ability of *trans*-cyclooctene

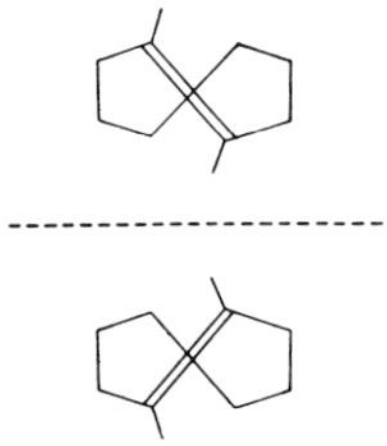

(91)

with platinum complexes **(91)**. *trans*-Cyclooctene has molecular asymmetry due to restriction of rotation **(91)**. Cope and co-workers succeeded in resolving cyclooctene as in eqs. (189) (309,310). At first the Zeise salt was formed from ethylene and potassium tetrachloroplatinate [eq. (189a)]. This salt was converted into *trans*-dichloro(ethylene)

[(+)α-methylbenzylamine]platinum by reaction with (+)α-methylbenzylamine [eq. (189b)]. The ethylene in the complex was then readily displaced by *trans*-cyclooctene [eq. (189c)]. The resulting complex is a mixture of diastereoisomers, *trans*-dichloro[(−)*trans*-cyclooctene][(+)α-methylbenzylamine]platinum, which is dextrorotatory, and *trans*-dichloro[(+)*trans*-cyclooctene][(+)α-methylbenzylamine]platinum, which is levorotatory. The difference in solubility of the diastereoisomers makes their separation by fractional crystallization possible. Decomposition of the resolved complexes with an aqueous solution of potassium cyanide [eq. (189d)], followed

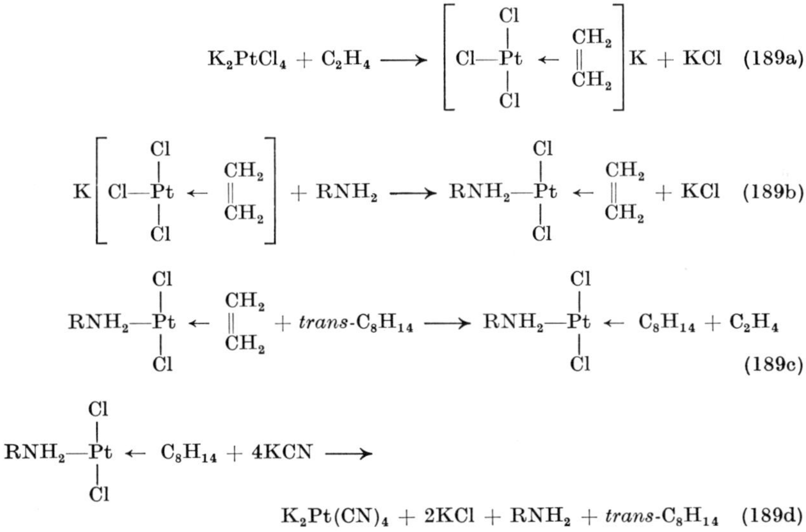

$$K_2PtCl_4 + C_2H_4 \longrightarrow \begin{bmatrix} Cl \\ | \\ Cl-Pt \leftarrow \| \begin{array}{c} CH_2 \\ CH_2 \end{array} \\ | \\ Cl \end{bmatrix} K + KCl \quad (189a)$$

$$K \begin{bmatrix} Cl \\ | \\ Cl-Pt \leftarrow \| \begin{array}{c} CH_2 \\ CH_2 \end{array} \\ | \\ Cl \end{bmatrix} + RNH_2 \longrightarrow \begin{array}{c} Cl \\ | \\ RNH_2-Pt \leftarrow \| \begin{array}{c} CH_2 \\ CH_2 \end{array} \\ | \\ Cl \end{array} + KCl \quad (189b)$$

$$\begin{array}{c} Cl \\ | \\ RNH_2-Pt \leftarrow \| \begin{array}{c} CH_2 \\ CH_2 \end{array} \\ | \\ Cl \end{array} + trans\text{-}C_8H_{14} \longrightarrow \begin{array}{c} Cl \\ | \\ RNH_2-Pt \leftarrow C_8H_{14} \\ | \\ Cl \end{array} + C_2H_4 \quad (189c)$$

$$\begin{array}{c} Cl \\ | \\ RNH_2-Pt \leftarrow C_8H_{14} \\ | \\ Cl \end{array} + 4KCN \longrightarrow$$

$$K_2Pt(CN)_4 + 2KCl + RNH_2 + trans\text{-}C_8H_{14} \quad (189d)$$

by distillation at room temperature under reduced pressure gave resolved enantiomorphs of *trans*-cyclooctene, $[\alpha]_D^{25}$ −458° and $[\alpha]_D^{25}$ +440°.

Also the resolution of *cis,trans*-1,5-cyclooctadiene formed by two successive Hofmann degradations of *N*-methylgranatamine was done with the platinum complex containing optically active (+)α-methylbenzylamine (311). Displacement of ethylene in the complex *trans*-dichloro (ethylene)[(+)α-methylbenzylamine]platinum by *cis–trans*-1,5-cyclooctadiene gave *trans*-dichloro(*cis,trans*-1,5-cyclooctadiene) [(+)α-methylbenzylamine]platinum **(92)**. Complex formation occurred at the *trans* double bond as shown below. Fractional crystallization of this complex to constant rotation and decomposition with sodium cyanide gave optically active $(-)cis,trans$-1,5-cyclo-

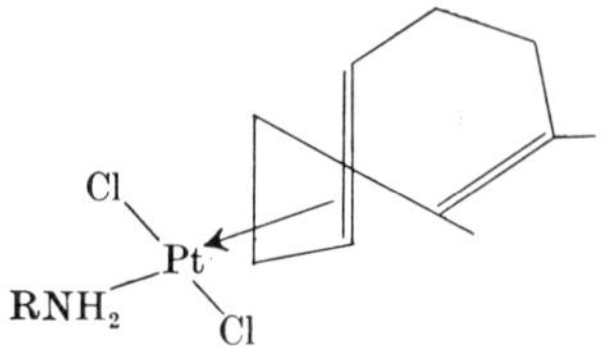

(92)

octadiene $[\alpha]_D^0 - 152°$. This method of resolution should be general for olefins which form sufficiently stable π-complexes with platinum compounds.

As another example, optically active *endo*-dicyclopentadiene was obtained by Paiaro, Panunzi, and Renzi by the following sequence of reactions (312). The monomeric complex of platinum (93) with *endo*-dicyclopentadiene was converted by stereospecific oxyplatination with methanol into a methoxy complex (94) which has a dimeric structure. It was proved by Stille and co-workers that the methoxy group takes the *exo* position and the platinum the *endo* position in this complex (313–315). These complexes (93 and 94) can be resolved

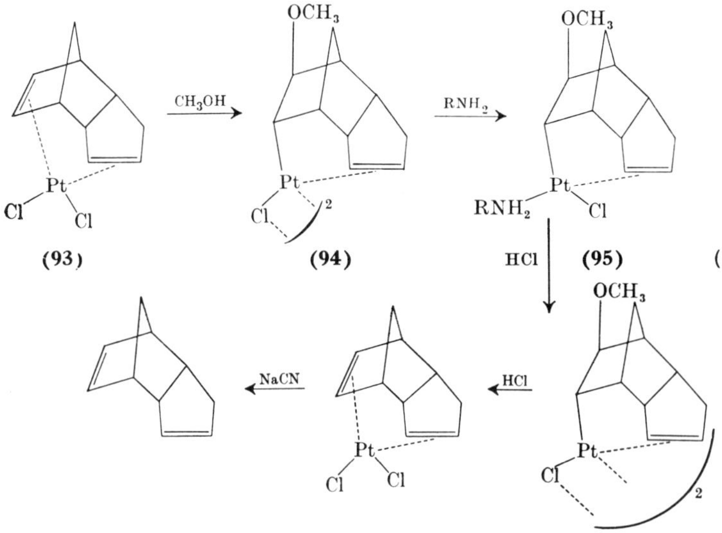

(93) (94) (95) (190)

(96)

into optical antipodes. The reaction of optically active (S)-α-methylbenzylamine with the complex (94) formed a new diastereoisomeric pair of amine complexes of the type [diene-OR, [(S)-α-methylbenzylamine)PtCl] (95) (for the nomenclature of R and S, see ref. 316). Recrystallization from a carbon tetrachloride–cyclohexane mixture separated the pair to constant optical rotation, and two fractions were obtained having $[\alpha]_D^{25} - 114°$ and $[\alpha]_D^{25} + 100°$. Treatment of the optically active complex with hydrochloric acid removed the amine and then the methoxy group to form the complex of *endo*-dicyclopentadiene (96). Finally, optically active dicyclopentadiene ($[\alpha]_D^{25} +$ 60°) was obtained for the first time in carbon disulfide solution by shaking with an aqueous solution of sodium cyanide.

The following elegant work concerning the molecular asymmetry of a simple olefin has been reported by Paiaro and Panunzi (317,318). An olefinic compound which has no asymmetric group and does not have symmetry planes perpendicular to the plane of the double bond, possesses two enantiomorphic faces. When the double bond of the olefin linked to two different substituent groups, $\begin{matrix} R \\ \diagdown \\ C= \\ \diagup \\ R' \end{matrix}$, is π-complexed with transition metal compounds, each of the unsaturated carbon atoms becomes asymmetric. Thus Paiaro and Panunzi predicted that a pair of enantiomorphs should be obtained if an olefinic compound with nonsuperimposable faces is π-bonded to transition metals, and if the olefin and an optically active ligand such as an optically active amine, are coordinated to the transition metal, two different diastereoisomers are possible as shown in structures **97a** and **97b**.

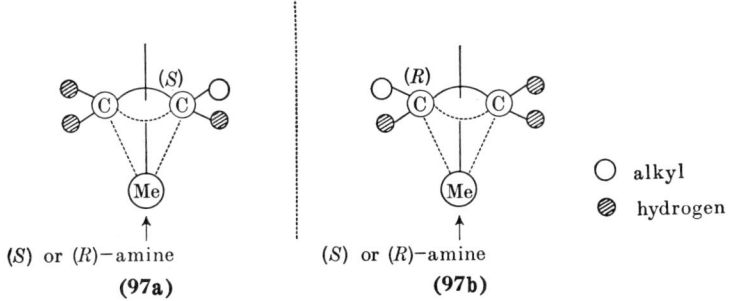

They actually prepared and resolved the diastereoisomeric pairs of propylene, *trans*-2-butene, and styrene, coordinated to platinum and containing optically active (R and S) α-methylbenzylamine of the general type *trans*-dichloro(olefin)(amine)platinum. The resolution was done by preferential recrystallization from suitable solvents.

The diastereoisomeric mixtures were prepared by the following two methods:

A. The exchange of the ethylene of *trans*-dichloro(ethylene)(amine)platinum with corresponding olefinic compounds.

$$\textit{trans-}\text{Pt(ethylene–amine)Cl}_2 + \text{olefin} \rightarrow \textit{trans-}\text{Pt(olefin–amine)Cl}_2 + \text{C}_2\text{H}_4 \tag{191}$$

B. The exchange of ethylene in bis[chloro(ethylene)-μ,μ'-dichloroplatinum] with olefin and the successive formation of the diastereoisomeric pairs with the optically active amine.

It was found that pure diastereoisomers epimerize in solution and hence preferential crystallization of the diastereoisomers is possible by using a suitable solvent–nonsolvent mixture. For example, from the diastereoisomeric pair propylene-(S)-α-methylbenzylamine, only the (−)-(S) diastereoisomer was obtained. From the styrene complex, the (+)-(S) diastereoisomer was obtained from all solvents. Interestingly, from the *trans*-2-butene-(S)-α-methylbenzylamine complex, (−)-(S) was obtained by using a solvent mixture containing cyclohexane, and (+)-(S) diastereoisomer was obtained by using the solvent mixture without cyclohexane.

In addition, it is possible to obtain complex anions of the type $(\text{PtCl}_3\text{-olefin})^-$ containing the resolved coordinated olefin by treating the diastereoisomers with hydrogen chloride and subsequently with $\text{Pt}(\text{NH}_3)_4\text{Cl}_2$ according to the eq. (192).

$$\textit{trans-}\text{Pt(olefin–amine)Cl}_2 + \text{HCl} \rightarrow [\text{H–amine}][\text{Pt(olefin)Cl}_3]$$
$$2[\text{H–amine}][\text{Pt(olefin)Cl}_3] + \text{Pt}(\text{NH}_3)_4\text{Cl}_2 \rightarrow$$
$$2\text{amine-HCl} + [\text{Pt}(\text{NH}_3)_4][\text{Pt(olefin)Cl}_3]_2 \tag{192}$$

In addition to the molecular asymmetry of olefin π-complexes, the same kind of molecular asymmetry has been recognized with π-allylic complexes. For example, in a 1-substituted π-allylic complex, C-1 becomes asymmetric by complexation and can be designated as (R) or (S) (319). The π-allylic complex of palladium was prepared from mesityl oxide and palladium chloride (25), from which a diastereoisomeric mixture was prepared by splitting the chloride bridge with

(S)-α-methylbenzylamine as shown by structures **98a** and **98b**. The resolution was achieved by crystallizing the crude diastereoisomeric mixture from carbon tetrachloride to give chloro-(1-acetyl-2-methylallyl) [(S)-α-methylbenzylamine]palladium. The optical activity

<pre>
        CH₃   CH₃
        | |
      O=C   C=O
         \   /
          C—H   H—C
H₃C—C   C—CH₃
          CH₂   H₂C
           \   /
           Pd   Pd
          / \   / \
        Cl   *amine   *amine Cl

        (98a)   (98b)
</pre>

measurement showed that only one of the two possible diastereoisomers was quantitatively obtained by a second-order asymmetric transformation in the carbon tetrachloride crystallization. The epimerization of the pure (−)diastereoisomer took place very quickly at temperatures higher than −20°. Furthermore, they discovered that asymmetric induction is possible when an olefin is complexed *cis* to an optically active amine in a platinum complex (320–322). In other words, for *cis*-coordinated complexes, the equilibrium constant of eq. (193) is generally different from unity.

$$\begin{array}{c} \text{Cl} \\ | \\ \text{amine }(S)\text{—Pt—Cl} \\ | \\ \text{olefin }(R) \end{array} \rightleftarrows \begin{array}{c} \text{Cl} \\ | \\ \text{amine }(S)\text{—Pt—Cl} \\ | \\ \text{olefin }(S) \end{array} \qquad (193)$$

The deviation of the molecular rotation of an olefin complex from that of the corresponding ethylene complex was observed with olefins of the type *trans*-RCH=CH—R. For example, for the *cis* complexes of *trans*-2-butene, *trans*-3-hexene, and *trans*-1,4-dichlorobutene, 25% or more excesses of the (−)diastereoisomers in acetone at room temperature were formed. This observation indicates that asymmetric induction occurs in the coordination of the olefin. Also, when the ethylene complex was allowed to react with 2 moles of (R and S) racemic *trans*-cyclooctene at room temperature until complete exchange was observed, the unreacted cyclooctene was found to be (−)cyclooctene with an enantiomeric purity of about 30%. Treatment of the mixture of the diastereoisomers with potassium cyanide yielded

(+)-cyclooctene with the same degree of optical purity. The origin of the asymmetric induction seems to be the steric interaction between the optically active amine and the *cis*-coordinated olefin. For the *trans*-coordinated complex, no effective asymmetric induction was observed. Also, an interesting observation of asymmetric induction was made with the levorotatory enantiomer of *endo*-dicyclopentadiene described before (312). The complex **(99)** was allowed to react with an excess of *d,l*-sec-butanol to give a butoxydicyclopentadiene complex, and unreacted butanol was recovered [eq. (194)]. Interestingly

$$\text{(99)} \; (l) + CH_3CH_2\overset{H}{\underset{OH}{C}}-CH_3 \; (d,l) \longrightarrow \left[\text{complex with } O\text{-Bu} \right]_2 + CH_3CH_2\underset{CH_3}{CH}-OH \; (d) \quad (194)$$

enough, the recovered butanol was found to be dextrorotatory. The results show the existence of asymmetric induction, and are very important in connection with the mechanism of stereospecific polymerization of olefins. Asymmetric syntheses by means of metal complexes seem to be a promising field for future study.

Another example of resolution by means of noble metal complexes is the resolution of optically active sulfoxides (323). The formation of dimethyl sulfoxide transition metal complexes is well known, and this property of sulfoxides was ingeniously applied to the resolution of an optically active sulfoxide. Cope and Caress carried out the resolution of ethyl *p*-tolyl sulfoxide by forming the complex (+ or —)-*trans*-dichloro(ethyl *p*-tolyl sulfoxide)(α-methylbenzylamine)platinum. The complex was prepared by displacement of the ethylene in (+ or —)-*trans*-dichloro(ethylene)(α-methylbenzylamine)platinum with ethyl *p*-tolyl sulfoxide. When (+)-α-methylbenzylamine was used, the complex contained the diastereomers *trans*-dichloro[(—)-ethyl *p*-tolyl sulfoxide][(+)-α-methylbenzylamine]platinum and *trans*-dichloro[(+)-ethyl *p*-tolyl sulfoxide] [(+)-α-methylbenzylamine]platinum. Fractional crystallization of these complexes from methylene chloride-benzene-pentane afforded the less soluble isomer, structure **100**,

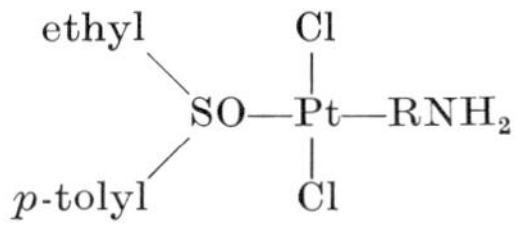

```
      ethyl      Cl
           \     |
           SO—Pt—RNH₂
           /     |
     p-tolyl    Cl
         (100)
```

$[\alpha]_D^{25} + 84.7°$. A similar pair of diastereoisomers was obtained with (−)-α-methylbenzylamine. The less soluble isomer was *trans*-dichloro-[(+)-ethyl *p*-tolyl sulfoxide][(−)-α-methylbenzylamine]platinum, $[\alpha]_D^{25} - 84.6°$. These resolved complexes were decomposed with an aqueous sodium cyanide solution and distillation of the sulfoxide obtained gave (−)-ethyl *p*-tolyl sulfoxide, $[\alpha]_D^{25} - 203.6°$, and (+)-ethyl *p*-tolyl sulfoxide, $[\alpha]_D^{25} + 203.2°$.

The examples above show that a new field of chemistry has been explored by the elegant application of π-complex formation with noble metal compounds.

X. Miscellaneous Reactions

Several other reactions which can be carried out in the presence of noble metal compounds are described in this section.

It is well known that noble metal compounds catalyze olefin isomerizations very efficiently (1). In addition, some skeletal rearrangements are possible. Frye, Kuljian, and Viebrock found that the 4-vinylcyclohexene–palladium chloride complex is converted into the 1,5-cyclooctadiene–palladium chloride complex on standing overnight at room temperature in 35% conversion (324). It is remarkable that the skeletal rearrangement proceeds under very mild conditions and certainly palladium chloride plays an important role.

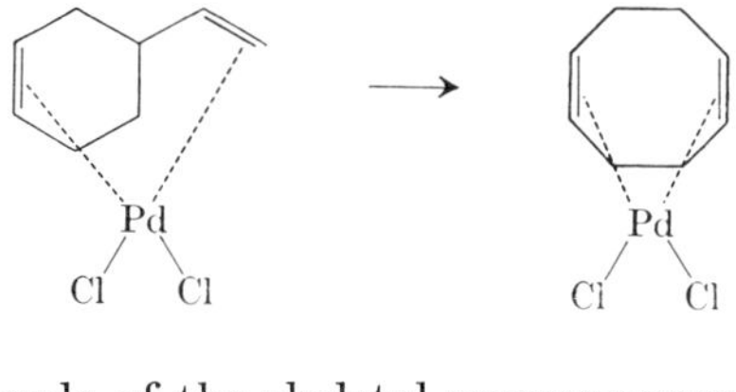

(195)

As another example of the skeletal rearrangement of a cyclic compound catalyzed by noble metal compounds, Trebellas, Olechowski, and Jonassen found that the reaction of the palladium chloride–benzonitrile complex in benzene with *cis,trans*-1,5-cyclododecadiene resulted in the formation of the *cis*-1,2-divinylcyclohexane–palladium chloride complex (325). Sodium chloroplatinate also formed the divinylcyclohexane complex from 1,5-cyclododecadiene. The Cope rearrangement of 1,5-cyclododecadiene to divinylcyclohexane can be carried out by heating to 150° (326,327). On the other hand, the catalytically activated Cope rearrangement can be carried out at room temperature.

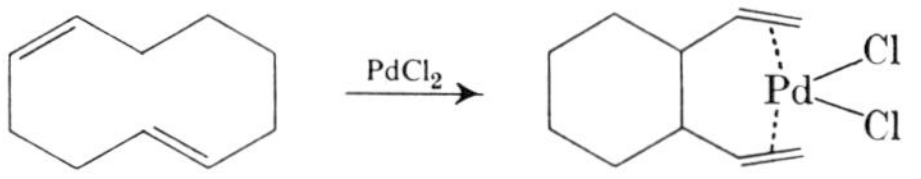

(196)

It is well known that the reaction of allyl alcohol with palladium chloride affords π-allyl-palladium chloride in addition to acrolein and propylene. But the yield of the complex is not high and by-products are formed. The side reaction was studied by Hafner, Prigge, and Smidt and the products were shown to be propylene and unsaturated cyclic alcohols having the formula $C_6H_{10}O_2$ (328). They are formed by disproportionation. The formation of these products is catalyzed by

$$3C_3H_5OH \rightarrow C_3H_6 + C_6H_{10}O_2 + H_2O \qquad (197)$$

palladium chloride as long as it is not consumed by π-allyl-palladium chloride formation. The structures of the cyclic alcohols were determined by chemical and spectroscopic studies to be 4-methylenetetrahydrofurfuryl alcohol and 4-methyl-2,5-dihydrofurfuryl alcohol. The mechanism of the formation shown in eq. (198) was given.

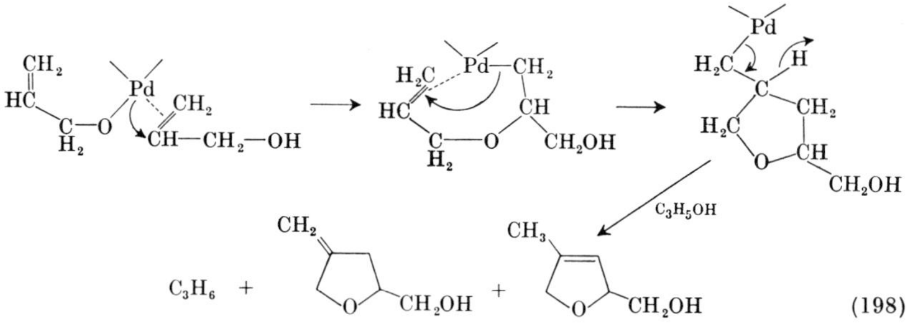

(198)

Several other noble metal compounds react with allylic alcohols in interesting ways. Milgram and Urry found that chloroplatinic acid is a very efficient catalyst for the formation of allyl ether. In the presence of 0.002 mole of chloroplatinic acid per mole of allyl alcohol, allyl alcohol is converted into allyl ether at 70–90°. In the presence of a saturated alcohol, both alkyl allyl and diallyl ethers are formed, but no dialkyl ether is formed [eqs. (199)]. The real catalytic species

$$CH_2=CH-CH_2OH \rightarrow CH_2=CH-CH_2-O-CH_2-CH=CH_2 \quad (199a)$$
$$CH_2=CH-CH_2OH + ROH \rightarrow$$
$$CH_2=CH-CH_2-O-R + CH_2=CH-CH_2-O-CH_2-CH=CH_2 \quad (199b)$$

seems to be a divalent platinum complex (329). On the other hand, a chlororuthenium complex was found to be a very efficient catalyst for hydrogen transfer with allyl alcohols. Boiling a $2 \times 10^{-3}M$ solution of ruthenium trichloride in 50% aqueous allyl alcohol causes reduction to the divalent state. The intramolecular and intermolecular hydrogen transfer reactions in eqs.(200) proceed smoothly in the presence of the

$$2CH_2=CH-CH_2OH \rightarrow CH_2=CH-CH_3 + CH_2=CH-CHO + H_2O \quad (200a)$$
$$CH_2=CH-CH_2OH \rightarrow CH_3CH_2CHO \quad (200b)$$

ruthenium catalyst, and the products are propylene, acrolein, and propionaldehyde (330). 2-Buten-1-ol is converted into ethyl methyl ketone and a mixture of n-butenes. Propargyl alcohol is transformed into a 1:1 mixture of ethylene and carbon monoxide. Rhodium chloride was found to be active, but less efficient.

Rinehart and Fuest studied the reaction of allyl alcohol in the presence of ruthenium and rhodium catalysts and proposed the π-allyl route [see eq. (201)] in order to explain the rearrangement of the

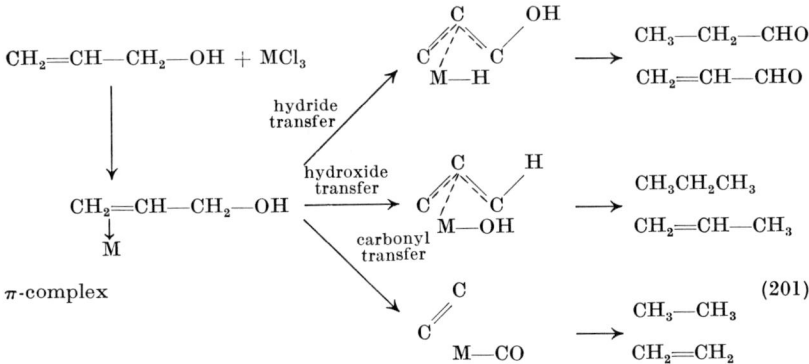

alcohols (331). The reaction mechanism involves competitive loss of hydride or hydroxide to the metal atom to form a π-allylic complex intermediate. The metal first forms a π-complex with allyl alcohol.

Then three different π-allylic complexes are formed from the π-complex. Hydride can migrate to the metal to produce a hydroxy π-allyl complex which leads to aldehyde products. Hydroxide may be lost to the metal to form a π-allyl complex which produces propane and propylene. As a side reaction, loss of carbonyl to the metal can lead to the formation of ethylene, metal carbonyl, and ethane as decarbonylation products.

Osmium tetroxide is used for the hydroxylation of olefins. Djerassi and Engle reported that ruthenium tetroxide is a more powerful oxidizing agent than osmium tetroxide (332). Ruthenium tetroxide is less toxic, less volatile, and less expensive than osmium tetroxide. It can oxidize sulfides to sulfoxides and sulfones (332). Secondary alcohols are oxidized to ketones and primary alcohols to aldehydes and acids (333,338–340). Unlike osmium tetroxide, ruthenum tetroxide causes olefinic carbon–carbon bond cleavage (333,341–346). An interesting reaction is the oxidation of an ether to an ester (333,334). Thus

$$\text{cyclohexene} + \text{RuO}_4 \longrightarrow \text{cyclohexane-CHO-CHO} \tag{202}$$

tetrahydrofuran can be oxidized to butyrolactone smoothly in nearly quantitative yield, eq. (203). The ruthenium tetroxide oxidation was

$$\text{THF} + \text{RuO}_4 \longrightarrow \text{butyrolactone} \tag{203}$$

applied to a steroidal alcohol (335). Oxidation to a ketone was complete in a few minutes at room temperature. Ruthenium dioxide produced during the oxidation can be reconverted into tetroxide when sodium metaperiodate is present in the reaction mixture. Therefore, the oxidation can be carried out in the presence of a catalytic amount of ruthenium tetroxide by using sodium metaperiodate.

π-Allylpalladium chloride was used for the decomposition of some azo compounds. Armstrong found that π-allylpalladium chloride is an efficient catalyst for the reaction of 2-butyne and ethyl diazoacetate at 0–10° to give ethyl 1,2-dimethyl-1-cyclopropene-3-carboxylate. Usually copper or copper salts are used for the decomposition of diazo compounds, but in contrast, they are effective only at higher temperatures. The mechanism shown in eq. (204) was given (336).

Reactions of 1,2,3,4-tetrachlorodiazocyclopentadiene with acetylene catalyzed by copper salts or π-allyl-palladium chloride were carried

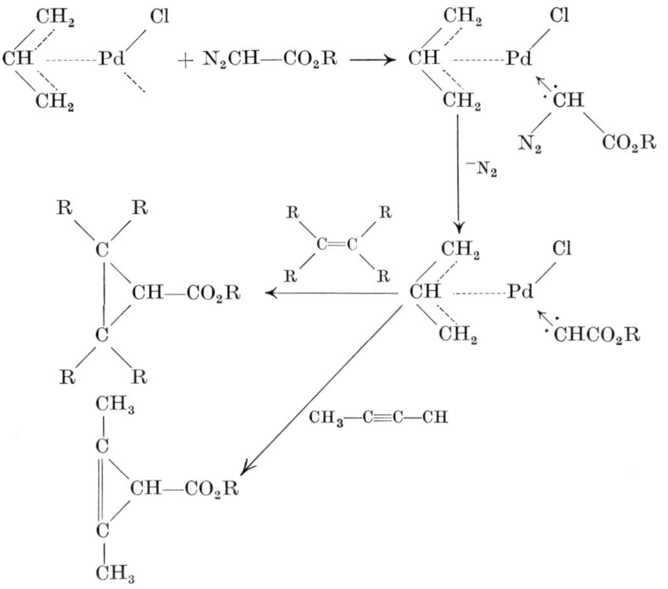

(204)

out by McBee, Calundann, and Hodgins, eq. (205). In the copper-catalyzed reaction, spiro(2,4)heptatriene was obtained. On the other

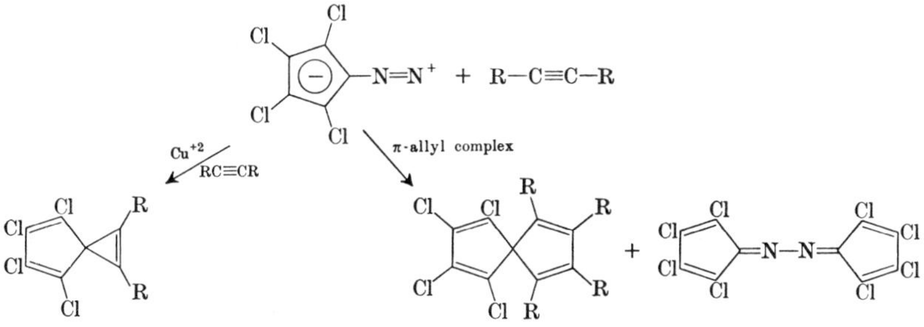

(205)

hand, in the π-allyl-palladium chloride-catalyzed reaction, no cyclopropene derivative was formed. The products were 1,3,6,8-spiro(4,4)-nonatetraene and tetrachlorocyclopentadienone azine (337). Probably spirononatetraene was formed by the insertion of tetrachlorocyclopentadiene carbene–palladium complex on the tetraalkylcyclobutadiene–palladium π-complex as shown in eq. (206).

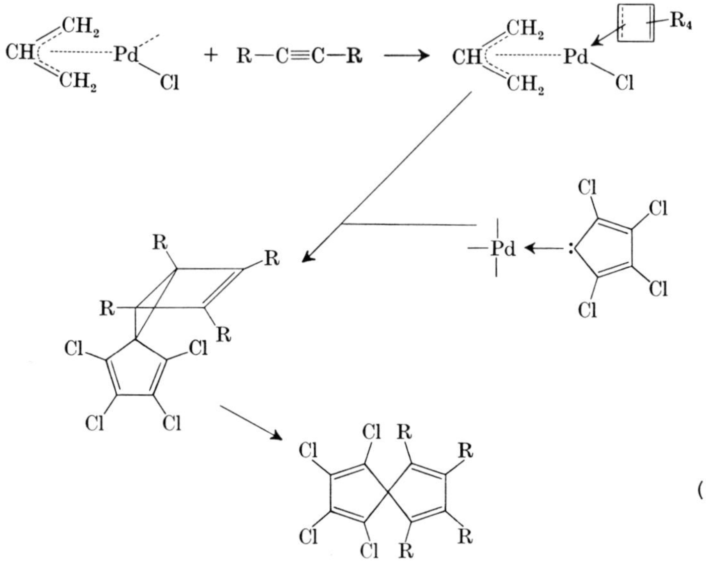

$$\text{(206)}$$

XI. Experimental

A. PREPARATION OF PALLADIUM CHLORIDE COMPLEXES

1. *Palladium Chloride–Benzonitrile Complex and Olefin Complexes* (12)

The palladium chloride–benzonitrile complex is soluble in benzene and is very useful for the preparation of various olefinic complexes of palladium and for reactions of palladium chloride in solution. The complex can be prepared easily in the following way. About 2 g of palladium chloride is dissolved in 30 ml of purified benzonitrile by heating to 100° in an oil bath. The solution is filtered while hot and left to cool until crystallization of the yellowish orange product is complete. The crystals are collected by filtration. More precipitate can be obtained by adding petroleum ether. The complex is dried in a desiccator. Various olefinic complexes can be prepared by adding an olefin to a benzene solution of the palladium chloride–benzonitrile complex. The olefin complexes are mostly insoluble in benzene and precipitate rapidly.

2. π-Allyl Palladium Chloride Complex (18)

Palladium chloride (4.44 g) and sodium chloride (2.95 g) are dissolved by warming in methanol (150 ml) containing 2.25 g of water. Then allyl chloride (about 10 g or more) is added. Carbon monoxide is passed into the solution at room temperature with stirring until the brown color disappears. Most of the methanol is removed under reduced pressure and the concentrated solution is poured into water. Repeated extraction with chloroform or methylene chloride, followed by evaporation of the solvent, gives yellowish crystals of π-allylpalladium chloride. The yield is almost quantitative.

3. Reaction of 1,5-Cyclooctadiene–Palladium Chloride Complex with Diethyl Malonate (108)

1,5-Cyclooctadiene complex (0.5 g), anhydrous sodium carbonate (0.5 g), and diethyl malonate (1 g) are mixed in ether (5 ml). The mixture is stirred at room temperature for 15 hr, during which time the yellowish complex gradually turns white. The white complex is collected by filtration and washed with water and ether. The complex is dried and recrystallized from ethyl acetate–hexane mixture. The mp is 155–156° and the yield is quantitative.

B. PREPARATION OF 2-DODECANONE FROM 1-DODECENE ON A LABORATORY SCALE (57)

Palladium chloride (0.02 mole) and cupric chloride dihydrate (0.02 mole) are dissolved in a mixture of dimethylformamide (50 ml) and water (7 ml). The stirred solution is maintained between 60–70° during the reaction. 1-Dodecene is added dropwise over a period of 2.5 hr while oxygen is bubbled through the solution (3.3 liters/hr). After the reaction, the solution is washed several times with water and 2-dodecanone is collected by fractional distillation. The yield is 87%.

C. PREPARATION OF exo-2-CHLORO-syn-7-ACETOXYNORBORNANE (90)

Norbornene (20 g), anhydrous sodium acetate (16 g), anhydrous cupric chloride (50 g), and palladium chloride (1 g) are mixed in 200 ml of acetic acid. The mixture is heated and stirred at 80° for 7 hr, during which time the color of the cupric salt gradually turns to that of the cuprous salt. After the reaction, the mixture is filtered and the filter cake is washed with ether. The washing and the filtrate are combined and poured into water. The product is extracted several times with hexane. After the usual work-up of the extract, *exo*-2-chloro-*syn*-7-acetoxynorbornane is obtained by distillation under vacuum at 63–65° (0.1 mm). The yield is 29.3 g (84%).

D. CARBONYLATION OF ALLYL CHLORIDE (161)

Allyl chloride (5 g), tetrahydrofuran (5 g), benzene (20 ml), and palladium chloride (0.9 g) are placed in an autoclave (100 ml) which is then charged with carbon monoxide (100 kg/cm^2). When heated to 80° with stirring, a rapid pressure drop is observed. After 5 hr, the autoclave is cooled and opened. Precipitated palladium is collected by filtration and the filtrate is subjected to fractional distillation to give 10.2 g (89%) of 4-chlorobutyl 3-butenoate; bp 103–104°/13 mm.

E. DECARBONYLATION OF OCTANOYL BROMIDE WITH CHLOROCARBONYLBIS(TRIPHENYLPHOSPHINE)RHODIUM (203)

Octanoyl bromide (8 g) and chlorocarbonylbis(triphenylphosphine)-rhodium (0.1 g) are mixed in a distilling flask and kept at 200° in an oil bath. Rapid evolution of hydrogen bromide and carbon monoxide is observed and heptene is distilled off. After 1 hr, the flask becomes almost empty. The distillate is redistilled to give 3.3 g of a heptene mixture. Gas chromatographic analysis showed that the mixture consists of 1-heptene (71%), *trans*-2-heptene (24%), *cis*-2-heptene (5%), and 3-heptene (small amount).

F. REACTION OF BENZENESULFONYL CHLORIDE WITH CHLOROTRIS(TRIPHENYLPHOSPHINE)RHODIUM (205)

A mixture of benzenesulfonyl chloride (17.6 g, should be purified carefully before the reaction to prevent polymerization) and chlorotris-(triphenylphosphine)rhodium (0.07 g) is heated in a Claisen flask equipped with a 25 cm long Vigreux column. The temperature at the top of the column is controlled by the rate of heating and is not allowed to exceed 132°. The evolution of sulfur dioxide decreases gradually. After 75 min, no more chlorobenzene distills over, and a polymer remains in the flask. The distillate is extracted with methylene chloride, washed with 10% sodium hydroxide solution and water, and dried. Redistillation at 131° gives 8.8 g (79%) of pure chlorobenzene.

G. DIMERIZATION OF METHYL ACRYLATE BY USING RUTHENIUM CHLORIDE (288)

A mixture of methanol (40 g), methyl acrylate (144 g), ruthenium chloride (2 g), and hydroquinone (2 g) is placed in a pressure vessel. The mixture is heated to 210° for 10 hr. Fractional distillation of the product gives a mixture of methyl acrylate and methyl propionate (65 g), dimethyl α-dihydromuconate (35 g, 44%), and a nonvolatile residue (38 g).

ACKNOWLEDGMENTS

The author expresses his sincere appreciation to Dr. P. M. Henry (Hercules Co.), Prof. R. Hüttel (University of München), Dr. R. Jira (Consortium für Elektrochem. Ind., München), Prof. M. Kumada (Kyoto University), Prof. G. Paiaro (University of Napoli), Dr. R. G. Schulz (Monsanto Co.), and Dr. H. G. Tennent (Hercules Co.) for their kind help.

References

1. M. Orchin, "The Homogeneous Catalytic Isomerization of Olefins by Transition Metal Compounds," in *Advan. Catalysis*, **16**, 1 (1966).
2. W. A. Waters, "Oxidation Processes," in *Organic Chemistry, Advanced Treatise*, Vol. 4, Wiley, New York, 1953, p. 1180.
3. P. A. Plattner, "Dehydrogenation with Sulfur, Selenium, and Platinum Metals," in *Newer Methods in Organic Chemistry*, Interscience, New York, 1948, p. 21.
4. J. Halpern, *Chem. Eng. News*, Oct. 31, 1966, p. 68.
5. G. E. Coates, *Organometallic Compounds*, Wiley, New York, 1960.
6. R. S. Nyholm, "Structure and Reactivity of Transition Metal Complexes," *Proceedings of the Third International Congress on Catalysis*, Vol. 1, North-Holland, Amsterdam, 1965, p. 25.
7. J. P. Collman, "Reactions of Ligands Coordinated with Transition Metals," in *Transition Metal Chemistry*, Vol. 2, Dekker, New York, 1966, p. 1.
8. E. O. Fischer and H. Werner, *π-Complexes*, Vol. 1, Elsevier, Amsterdam, 1966.
9. W. C. Zeise, *Pogg. Ann.*, **9**, 632 (1827); **21**, 497 (1831).
10. J. Chatt and L. A. Duncanson, *J. Chem. Soc.*, **1953**, 2939.
11. K. Birnbaum, *Ann.*, **145**, 67 (1868).
12. M. S. Kharasch, R. C. Seyler, and C. Mayo, *J. Am. Chem. Soc.*, **60**, 882 (1938).
13. N. Nakamura and N. Gunji, *J. Japan Petrol. Inst.*, **6**, 695 (1963).
14. W. M. MacNevin and S. A. Giddings, *Chem. Ind. (London)*, **1960**, 1191.
15. G. F. Pregaglia, M. Donati, and F. Conti, *Chem. Ind. (London)*, **1966**, 1923.

16. M. L. H. Green and P. L. I. Nagy, *Advan. Organomet. Chem.*, **2**, 325 (1964). Review article on π-allyl complexes.
17. R. Hüttel and J. Kratzer, *Angew. Chem.*, **71**, 456 (1959).
18. W. T. Dent, R. Long, and A. J. Wilkinson, *J. Chem. Soc.*, **1964**, 1585.
19. J. Smdit and W. Hafner, *Angew. Chem.*, **71**, 284 (1959).
20. B. L. Shaw, *Chem. Ind. (London)*, **1962**, 1190.
21. S. D. Robinson and B. L. Shaw, *J. Chem. Soc.*, **1963**, 4806.
22. R. G. Schultz, *Tetrahedron Letters*, **1964**, 301; *Tetrahedron*, **20**, 2809 (1964).
23. M. S. Lupin and B. L. Shaw, *Tetrahedron Letters*, **1964**, 883.
24. J. Tsuji, S. Imamura, and J. Kiji, *J. Am. Chem. Soc.*, **86**, 4491 (1964).
25. G. W. Parshall and G. Wilkinson, *Chem. Ind. (London)*, **1962**, 261.
26. R. Hüttel and H. Christ, *Chem. Ber.*, **96**, 3101 (1963).
27. R. Hüttel, J. Kratzer, and M. Bechter, *Chem. Ber.*, **94**, 766 (1961).
28. R. Hüttel and H. Christ, *Chem. Ber.*, **97**, 1439 (1964).
29. R. Hüttel, H. Christ, and K. Herzog, *Chem. Ber.*, **97**, 2710 (1964).
30. R. Hüttel and H. Dietl, *Chem. Ber.*, **98**, 1753 (1965).
31. R. Hüttel, H. Dietl, and H. Christ, *Chem. Ber.*, **97**, 2037 (1964).
32. G. E. Coates and F. Glocking, "Transition Metal Alkyls and Aryls," in *Organometallic Chemistry*, Reinhold, New York, 1960, p. 426.
33. R. F. Heck, "Insertion Reactions of Metal Complexes," in *Mechanism of Inorganic Reactions*, American Chemical Society, Advances in Chemistry Series, No. 49, 1965, p. 181.
34. P. Cossee, *Rec. Trav. Chim.*, **85**, 1151 (1966).
35. J. Chatt, P. L. Pauson, and L. M. Venanzi, "Metal Carbonyls and Related Compounds," in *Organometallic Chemistry*, Reinhold, New York, 1960, p. 468.
36. E. W. Abel, *Quart. Rev.*, **17**, 133 (1963).
37. (a) A. P. Ginsberg, "Hydride Complexes of the Transition Metals," in *Transition Metal Chemistry*, Vol. 1, Dekker, New York, 1965, p. 112. (b) M. L. H. Green and D. J. Jones, "Hydride Complexes of the Transition Metals," in *Advan. Inorg. Radiochem.*, **7**, 115 (1965).
38. J. Chatt and B. L. Shaw, *J. Chem. Soc.*, **1962**, 5075.
39. J. P. Collman and J. W. Kang, *J. Am. Chem. Soc.*, **88**, 3459 (1966).
40. A. D. Allen and C. V. Senoff, *Chem. Commun.*, **1965**, 621.
41. L. Vaska, *Science*, **140**, 809 (1963).
41a. L. Vaska and D. L. Catone, *J. Am. Chem. Soc.*, **88**, 5324 (1966).
42. S. Takahashi, K. Sonogashira, and N. Hagihara, *Nippon Kagaku Zasshi*, **87**, 610 (1966).
43. M. C. Baird, D. N. Lawson, J. T. Mague, J. A. Osborn, and G. W. Wilkinson, *Chem. Commun.*, **1966**, 129.
44. S. J. La Placa and J. A. Ibers, *Inorg. Chem.*, **5**, 405 (1966).

45. L. Vaska and S. S. Bath, *J. Am. Chem. Soc.*, **88**, 1333 (1966).
46. J. P. Collman and W. R. Roper, *J. Am. Chem. Soc.*, **88**, 180 (1966).
47. F. D. Mango and I. Dovoretzky, *J. Am. Chem. Soc.*, **88**, 1654 (1966).
48. J. S. Anderson, *J. Chem. Soc.*, **1934**, 971.
49. F. C. Phillips, *Z. Anorg. Chem.*, **6**, 213 (1894); *Am. Chem. J.*, **16**, 225 (1894).
50. S. C. Ogburn and W. C. Brastow, *J. Am. Chem. Soc.*, **55**, 1307 (1933).
51. J. Smidt, W. Hafner, R. Jira, J. Sedlmeier, R. Sieber, R. Ruttinger, and H. Kojer, *Angew. Chem.*, **71**, 176 (1959).
52. J. Smidt, W. Hafner, R. Jira, R. Sieber, J. Sedlmeier, and A. Sabel, *Angew. Chem.*, **74**, 93 (1962); *Intern. Ed.*, **1**, 80 (1962); *Chem. Ind. (London)*, **1962**, 54.
53. J. Jira and W. Freiesleben, "Oxidation of Olefins to Carbonyl Compounds and Related Reactions with Noble Metal Salts," in *Organometallic Reactions*, Wiley, New York, in press.
54. I. I. Moiseev, M. N. Vargaftik, and Ya. K. Syrkin, *Dokl. Akad. Nauk SSSR*, **130**, 820 (1960).
55. W. Hafner, R. Jira, J. Sedlmeier, and J. Smidt, *Chem. Ber.*, **95**, 1575 (1962).
56. E. Kopp and J. Smidt, *Ann.*, **693**, 117 (1966).
57. W. H. Clement and C. M. Selwitz, *J. Org. Chem.*, **29**, 241 (1964).
58. J. Smidt and R. Sieber, *Angew. Chem.*, **71**, 626 (1959).
59. M. N. Vargaftik, I. I. Moiseev, and Ya. K. Syrkin, *Dokl. Akad. Nauk SSSR*, **147**, 399 (1962).
60. K. Teramoto, T. Oga, S. Kikuchi, and M. Ito, *Yuki Gosei Kagaku Kyokaishi*, **21**, 298 (1963).
61. M. N. Varagaftik, I. I. Moiseev, and Ya. K. Syrkin, *Izv. Akad. Nauk SSSR Ser. Khim.*, **1963**, 1147.
62. I. I. Moiseev, M. N. Vargaftik, and Ya. K. Syrkin, *Izv. Akad. Nauk SSSR Ser. Khim.*, **1963**, 1144; *Chem. Abstr.*, **59**, 5837 (1963).
63. M. N. Vargaftik, I. I. Moiseev, and Ya. K. Syrkin, *Dokl. Akad. Nauk SSSR*, **153**, 140 (1963).
64. I. I. Moiseev and M. N. Vargaftik, *Dokl. Akad. Nauk SSSR*, **166**, 370 (1966); *Chem. Abstr.*, **64**, 11248 (1966).
65. P. M. Henry, *J. Am. Chem. Soc.*, **86**, 3246 (1964).
66. P. M. Henry, *J. Am. Chem. Soc.*, **88**, 1595 (1966).
67. P. M. Henry, "Homogeneous Catalysis," *Advan. Chem. Ser.*, in press.
68. R. Jira, J. Sedlmeier, and J. Smidt, *Ann.*, **693**, 99 (1966).
69. R. Hüttel and J. Kratzer, *Angew. Chem.*, **71**, 456 (1959).
70. R. Hüttel and M. Bechter, *Angew. Chem.*, **71**, 456 (1959).
71. A. V. Nikiforova, I. I. Moiseev, and Ya. K. Syrkin, *Zh. Obshch. Khim.*, **33**, 3239 (1963); *Chem. Abstr.*, **60**, 3995 (1964).
72. Imperial Chemical Industries, Ltd., French Patent, 1,372,946 (1964); *Chem. Abstr.*, **62**, 452 (1965).

73. I. I. Moiseev, M. N. Vargaftik, and Ya. K. Syrkin, *Dokl. Akad. Nauk SSSR*, **133**, 377 (1960).
74. E. W. Stern and M. L. Spector, *Proc. Chem. Soc.*, **1961**, 370.
75. D. Clark and P. Hayden, The Symposium of New Chemistry of Ethylene, preprint, Division of Petroleum Chemistry, Am. Chem. Soc., 1966, p. D-5.
76. Imperial Chemical Industries, Ltd., Belg. Pat., 628,733 (1963); *Chem. Abstr.*, **60**, 1574 (1964).
77. W. H. Clement and C. M. Selwitz, *Tetrahedron Letters*, **1962**, 1081.
78. I. I. Moiseev and M. N. Vargaftik, *Izv. Akad. Nauk SSSR Ser. Khim.*, **1965**, 759.
79. E. W. Stern and M. L. Spector, *Proc. Chem. Soc.*, **1963**, 111.
80. R. Cramer and R. V. Lindsey, *J. Am. Chem. Soc.*, **88**, 3534 (1966).
81. J. F. Harrod and A. J. Chalk, *J. Am. Chem. Soc.*, **88**, 3491 (1966).
82. D. R. Bryant, J. E. Mckeon and P. S. Starchar, Abstr. 2nd International Symposium in Organometallic Chemistry, 1965, Madison, p. 94.
83. W. Kitching, Z. Rappoport, S. Winstein, and W. C. Young, *J. Am. Chem. Soc.*, **88**, 2054 (1966).
84. A. D. Belov, G. Yu. Pek, and I. I. Moiseev, *Izv. Akad. Nauk SSSR Ser. Khim.*, **1965**, 2204.
85. I. I. Moiseev, A. D. Belov, and Y. K. Syrkin, *Izv. Akad. Nauk SSSR Ser. Khim.*, **1963**, 1527.
86. M. N. Vargaftik, I. I. Moiseev, and Ya. K. Syrkin, *Izv. Akad. Nauk SSSR Ser. Khim.*, **1962**, 930.
87. R. G. Schultz and D. E. Gross, "Homogeneous Catalysis," *Advan. Chem. Ser.*, American Chemical Society, in press.
88. C. B. Anderson and S. Winstein, *J. Org. Chem.*, **28**, 605 (1963).
89. N. Green, R. N. Haszeldine, and J. Lindley, *J. Organomet. Chem.*, **6**, 107 (1966).
90. W. C. Baird, *J. Org. Chem.*, **31**, 2411 (1966).
91. H. Hirai, H. Sawai, and S. Makishima, 20th Annual Meeting, Japan Chemical Society, 1967, Tokyo.
92. E. W. Stern, M. L. Spector, and H. P. Leftin, *J. Catalysis*, **6**, 152 (1966).
93. Y. Odaira, T. Oishi, T. Yukawa, and S. Tsutsumi, *J. Am. Chem. Soc.*, **88**, 4105 (1966).
94. Farbwerke Hoechst, Belgian Pat., 663,698; Netherland Application 6,505,608; *Chem. Abstr.*, **64**, 12557 (1966).
95. Distillers Co. Ltd., British Pat., 918,062 (1963); *Chem. Abstr.*, **59**, 5021 (1963).
96. Farbwerke Hoechst, Neth. Appl., 6,504,213; Belgian Pat., 662,098; *Chem. Abstr.*, **64**, 8030 (1966).
97. I. Moritani and Y. Fujiwara, Abstr. Symp. on Organometallic Chem., Osaka, Japan, 1966, p. 220; *Tetrahedron Letters*, **1967**, 1119.

98. R. van Helden and G. Verberg, *Rec. Trav. Chim.*, **84**, 1263 (1965).
99. E. J. Corey and M. F. Semmelhack, *Tetrahedron Letters*, **1966**, 6237.
100. J. M. Davidson and C. Trigg, *Chem. Ind. (London)*, **1966**, 457.
101. J. L. Garnett and W. A. Sollich, *Aust. J. Chem.*, **18**, 1003 (1965).
102. F. R. Mayo and M. D. Hurwitz, *J. Am. Chem. Soc.*, **71**, 776 (1949).
103. J. L. Garnett and W. A. Sollich, "π-Complex Absorption in Hydrogen Exchange in Group VIII Transition Metal Catalysis," in *Advan. Catalysis*, **16**, 95 (1966).
104. J. Tsuji, H. Takahashi, and M. Morikawa, *Tetrahedron Letters*, **1965**, 4387.
105. J. Tsuji, H. Takahashi, and M. Morikawa, *Kogyo Kagaku Zasshi*, **69**, 920 (1966).
106. J. Chatt, L. M. Vallarino, and L. M. Venanzi, *J. Chem. Soc.*, **1957**, 2496.
107. J. Chatt, L. M. Vallarino, and L. M. Venanzi, *J. Chem. Soc.*, **1957**, 3413.
108. J. Tsuji and H. Takahashi, *J. Am. Chem. Soc.*, **87**, 3275 (1965).
109. C. W. Bird, *Chem. Rev.*, **62**, 283 (1962).
110. E. O. Fischer and A. Volger, *J. Organometal. Chem.*, **3**, 161 (1965).
111. A. Treiber, *Tetrahedron Letters*, **1966**, 2831.
112. J. Tsuji, M. Morikawa, and J. Kiji, *Tetrahedron Letters*, **1963**, 1061.
113. J. Tsuji, M. Morikawa, and J. Kiji, *J. Am. Chem. Soc.*, **86**, 4851 (1964).
114. Union Oil Co. of California, Belgian Pat., 664,782 (1966).
115. J. Tsuji, M. Morikawa, and J. Kiji, *Tetrahedron Letters*, **1965**, 817.
116. N. A. Bailey, R. D. Gillard, M. Keeton, R. Mason, and D. R. Russel, *Chem. Commun.*, **1966**, 396, *Proc. 9th Intern. Conf. Coordination Chem.*, Birkhaeuser, Basel, 1966, p. 187.
117. D. M. Adams, J. Chatt, R. G. Guy, and N. Sheppard, *J. Chem. Soc.*, **1961**, 738.
118. T. Anderson and V. A. Engelhardt, U.S. Pat., 3,065,242 (1962).
119. J. Tsuji, M. Morikawa, and J. Kiji, *Tetrahedron Letters*, **1963**, 1437.
120. Imperial Chemical Industries, Ltd., Netherland Application, 6,511,995; *Chem. Abstr.*, **65**, 7064 (1966).
121. Badische Anilin Soda Fabrik A.G., Belgian Pat., 673,867 (1966).
122. Badische Anilin Soda Fabrik A. G., Belgian Pat., 651,532, Netherland Application 6,409,121; *Chem. Abstr.*, **63**, 14726 (1965), French Pat., 1,406,194 (1965).
123. Badische Anilin Soda Fabrik A. G., Netherland Application 6,516,439; *Chem. Abstr.*, **65**, 15,249 (1966).
124. J. Tsuji, S. Hosaka, T. Susuki, and J. Kiji, *Bull. Chem. Soc. (Japan)*, **39**, 141 (1966).
125. S. Brewis and P. R. Hughes, *Chem. Commun.*, **1965**, 489.
126. L. I. Zakharkin, SSSR, Pat., 179,758 (1966); *Chem. Abstr.*, **65**, 7062 (1966).
127. S. Brewis and P. R. Hughes, *Chem. Commun.*, **1966**, 6.
128. C. S. Foote and R. B. Woodward, *Tetrahedron*, **20**, 687 (1964).

129. E. Kuljian and H. Frye, *Z. Naturforsch.*, **19b**, 651 (1964).
130. G. Paiaro, N. Netto, A. Musco, and R. Palumbo, *Ric. Sci. Rend.*, **A3**, 1441 (1965); *Chem. Abstr.*, **65**, 2295 (1966).
131. J. Tsuji and T. Nogi. *Bull. Chem. Soc. (Japan)*, **39**, 146 (1966).
132. T. Rull, *Bull. Soc. Chim. France*, **1964**, 2680.
133. K. E. Moller, *Brennstoff Chem.*, **45**, 129 (1964); *Angew. Chem.*, **75**, 1122 (1963).
134. M. Genas and T. Rull, *Bull. Soc. Chim. France*, **1962**, 1837.
135. J. Tsuji and J. Kiji, unpublished work.
136. J. Tsuji and S. Hosaka, *Polymer Letters*, **3**, 703 (1965).
137. J. Tsuji, N. Iwamoto, and M. Morikawa, *Bull. Chem. Soc. (Japan)*, **38**, 2213 (1965).
138. J. Tsuji, K. Ohno, and T. Kajimoto, *Tetrahedron Letters*, **1965**, 4565.
139. A. Sacco and R. Ugo, *J. Chem. Soc.*, **1964**, 3274.
140. L. Vaska and J. W. DiLuzio, *J. Am. Chem. Soc.*, **84**, 679 (1962).
141. T. H. Coffield, J. Kozikowski, and R. D. Closson, *J. Org. Chem.*, **22**, 598 (1957).
142. R. J. Mawby, F. Basolo, and R. G. Pearson, *J. Am. Chem. Soc.*, **86**, 3994, 5043 (1964).
143. G. Calvin and G. E. Coates, *J. Chem. Soc.*, **1960**, 2008.
144. J. F. Hemidy and F. G. Gault, *Bull. Soc. Chim. France*, **1965**, 1710.
145. N. E. Hoffman and T. Puthenpurackal, *J. Org. Chem.*, **30**, 420 (1965).
146. N. E. Hoffman, A. T. Kanakkanatt, and R. F. Schneider, *J. Org. Chem.*, **27**, 2687 (1962).
147. H. E. Eschinazi, *Bull. Soc. Chim. France*, **1952**, 967.
148. H. E. Eschinazi and H. Pines, *J. Org. Chem.*, **24**, 1369 (1959).
149. H. E. Eschinazi, *J. Am. Chem. Soc.*, **81**, 2905 (1959).
150. J. O. Hawthone and M. H. Wilt, *J. Org. Chem.*, **25**, 2215 (1960).
151. J. M. Conia and C. Faget, *Bull. Soc. Chim. France*, **1964**, 1963.
152. W. M. Schubert and R. R. Kintner, in *Chemistry of the Carbonyl Group*, S. Patai, Ed., Interscience, New York, 1966, p. 747.
153. M. S. Newman and J. R. Mangham, *J. Am. Chem. Soc.*, **71**, 3342 (1949).
154. G. P. Chiusoli and G. Agnes, *Chim. Ind (Milan)*, **46**, 548 (1964).
155. E. Mosettig and R. Mozingo, Vol. 4, Wiley, New York, 1948, p. 362.
156. O. Bayer, *Methoden der Organischen Chemie Band VII*, Georg Thieme, Verlag, Stuttgart, 1954, p. 285.
157. T. Boehm and G. Schuman, *Arch. Pharm.*, **271**, 490 (1933); *Chem. Abstr.*, **28**, 1033 (1934).
158. J. P. Collman and W. R. Roper, *J. Am. Chem. Soc.*, **88**, 3504 (1966).
159. J. Tsuji, J. Kiji, and M. Morikawa, *Tetrahedron Letters*, **1963**, 1811.
160. W. T. Dent, R. Long, and G. H. Whitfield, *J. Chem. Soc.*, **1964**, 1588.

161. J. Tsuji, J. Kiji, S. Imamura, and M. Morikawa, *J. Am. Chem. Soc.*, **86**, 4359 (1964).
162. E. O. Fischer and G. Burger, *Z. Naturforsch.*, **16b**, 702 (1961).
163. J. Tsuji and S. Imamura, *Bull. Chem. Soc. (Japan)*, **40**, 197 (1967).
164. A. Kasahara, T. Tanaka, and K. Asamiya, *Bull. Chem. Soc. Japan*, **40**, 351 (1967).
165. M. Donati and F. Conti, *Tetrahedron Letters*, **1966**, 4953.
166. J. Tsuji, J. Kiji, and S. Hosaka, *Tetrahedron Letters*, **1964**, 605.
167. J. Tsuji and S. Hosaka, *J. Am. Chem. Soc.*, **87**, 4075 (1965).
168. S. Brewis and P. R. Hughes, *Chem. Commun.*, **1965**, 157.
169. J. Tsuji and T. Susuki, *Tetrahedron Letters*, **1965**, 3027.
170. For review, P. M. Maitlis, *Advan. Organometal. Chem.*, **4**, 95 (1966).
171. D. Bryce-Smith, *Chem. Ind. (London)*, **1964**, 239.
172. E. O. Greaves and P. M. Maitlis, *J. Organometal. Chem.*, **6**, 104 (1966).
173. G. Jacobsen and H. Spathe, German Pat., 1,138,760 (1962); *Chem. Abstr.*, **58**, 6699 (1963).
174. J. Tsuji, M. Morikawa, and N. Iwamoto, *J. Am. Chem. Soc.*, **86**, 2095 (1964).
175. E. R. H. Jones, T. Y. Shen, and M. C. Whiting, *J. Chem. Soc.*, **1951**, 48.
176. J. Tsuji and T. Nogi, *J. Org. Chem.*, **31**, 2641 (1966).
177. J. Tsuji and T. Nogi, *J. Am. Chem. Soc.*, **88**, 1289 (1966).
178. J. Tsuji and T. Nogi, *Tetrahedron Letters*, **1966**, 1801.
179. A. C. Cope and R. W. Siekman, *J. Am. Chem. Soc.*, **87**, 3272 (1965).
180. H. Takahashi and J. Tsuji, *J. Organometal. Chem.*, **10**, 571 (1967).
181. E. W. Stern and M. L. Spector, *J. Org. Chem.*, **31**, 596 (1966).
182. J. Tsuji and N. Iwamoto, *Chem. Commun.*, **1966**, 828.
183. J. K. Nicholson, J. Powell, and B. L. Shaw, *Chem. Commun.*, **1966**, 174.
184. J. Tsuji and N. Iwamoto, *Chem. Commun.*, **1966**, 380.
185. T. Inoue and S. Tsutsumi, *Bull. Chem. Soc. (Japan)*, **38**, 2122 (1965).
186. T. Inoue and S. Tsutsumi, *Bull. Chem. Soc. (Japan)*, **38**, 661 (1965).
187. T. Inoue and S. Tsutsumi, *J. Am. Chem. Soc.*, **87**, 3525 (1965).
188. G. W. Parshall, *Z. Naturforsch.*, **18b**, 772 (1963).
189. R. D. Cramer, E. L. Jenner, R. V. Lindsey, Jr., and U. G. Stolberg, *J. Am. Chem. Soc.*, **85**, 1691 (1963).
190. E. L. Jenner and R. V. Lindsey, Jr., U.S. Pat., 2,876,254 (1959); *Chem. Abstr.*, **53**, 17,906 (1959).
191. R. E. Benson, U.S. Pat., 2,871,262 (1959); *Chem. Abstr.*, **53**, 14,008 (1959).
192. H. Wakamatsu, *Nippon Kagaku Zasshi*, **85**, 227 (1964).
193. H. Wakamatsu, *Yuki Gosei Kagaku Kyokai Shi*, **22**, 1038 (1964).
194. J. A. Osborn, G. Wilkinson, and J. F. Young, *Chem. Commun.*, **1965**, 17.

195. F. H. Jardine, J. A. Osborn, G. Wilkinson, and J. F. Young, *Chem. Ind. (London)*, **1965**, 560.
196. P. M. Maitlis and S. McVey, *J. Organometal. Chem.*, **4**, 254 (1965).
197. M. A. Bennett and P. A. Longstaff, *Chem. Ind. (London)*, **1965**, 846.
198. J. Tsuji and K. Ohno, *Tetrahedron Letters*, **1965**, 3969.
199. Y. Shimizu, H. Mitsuhashi, and E. Capri, *Tetrahedron Letters*, **1966**, 4113.
200. J. Tsuji and K. Ohno, *J. Am. Chem. Soc.*, **88**, 3452 (1966).
201. R. F. Heck, *J. Am. Chem. Soc.*, **86**, 2796 (1964).
202. J. Chatt and B. L. Shaw, *J. Chem. Soc. A.*, **1966**, 1437.
203. J. Tsuji and K. Ohno, *Tetrahedron Letters*, **1966**, 4713.
204. J. Blum, *Tetrahedron Letters*, **1966**, 1605.
205. J. Blum, *Tetrahedron Letters*, **1966**, 3041.
206. J. P. Bibler and A. Wojcicki, *J. Am. Chem. Soc.*, **86**, 505 (1964).
207. J. P. Bibler and A. Wojcicki, *J. Am. Chem. Soc.*, **88**, 4862 (1966).
208. A. Rusina and A. A. Vlcek, *Nature*, **206**, No. 4981, 295 (1965).
209. J. Chatt, B. L. Shaw, and A. E. Field, *J. Chem. Soc.*, **1964**, 3466.
210. L. Vaska, *J. Am. Chem. Soc.*, **86**, 1943 (1964).
211. R. H. Prince and K. A. Raspin, *Chem. Commun.*, **1966**, 156.
212. D. Evans, J. A. Osborn, F. H. Jardine, and G. Wilkinson, *Nature*, **208**, 1203 (1965).
213. T. J. Kealy and R. E. Benson, *J. Org. Chem.*, **26**, 3126 (1961).
214. P. Pino, private communication.
215. E. I. du Pont de Nemours & Co., British Pat., 850,433 (1960); *Chem. Abstr.*, **56**, 419 (1962).
216. P. Guyer, D. Thomas, and A. Guyer, *Helv. Chim. Acta*, **52**, 481 (1959), and preceding papers.
217. H. Pichler, B. Firnhaber, D. Kioussis, and A. Dawallu, *Makromol. Chem.*, **70**, 12 (1964), and preceding papers.
218. H. Kölbel, W. H. Müller, and H. Hammer, *Makromol. Chem.*, **70**, 1 (1964), and preceding papers.
219. J. Halpern, Development in Homogeneous Catalysis, *Proc. 3rd Intern. Congress on Catalysis*, Vol. 1, North Holland, Amsterdam, 1965, p. 146.
220. J. Halpern, J. F. Harrod, and B. R. James, *J. Am. Chem. Soc.*, **83**, 753 (1961).
221. J. Halpern, J. F. Harrod, and B. R. James, *J. Am. Chem. Soc.*, **88**, 5150 (1966).
222. R. L. Burwell, *Chem. Eng. News*, Aug. 22, 1966, p. 56.
223. I. Jardine and F. J. McQuillin, *Tetrahedron Letters*, **1966**, 4871.
224. J. C. Bailor, Jr. and H. Itatani, *Inorg. Chem.*, **4**, 1618 (1965).
225. L. Vaska, *Inorg. Nuclear Chem. Letters*, **1**, 89 (1965).
226. I. Vaska and and R. E. Rhodes, *J. Am. Chem. Soc.*, **87**, 4970 (1965).

227. W. A. Pliskin and R. P. Eischens, *Z. Physik. Chem. N.F.*, **24**, 11 (1960).
228. J. F. Young, J. A. Osborn, F. H. Jardine and G. Wilkinson, *Chem. Commun.*, **1965**, 131.
229. J. A. Osborn, F. H. Jardine, J. F. Young, and G. Wilkinson, *J. Chem. Soc. A*, **1966**, 1711.
230. S. Hünig, H. R. Müller, and W. Thier, *Angew. Chem.*, **77**, 368 (1965).
231. C. Djerassi and J. Gutzwiller, *J. Am. Chem. Soc.*, **88**, 4537 (1966).
232. A. J. Birch and K. A. M. Walker, *Tetrahedron Letters*, **1966**, 4939.
233. A. J. Birch and K. A. M. Walker, *J. Chem. Soc. C*, **1966**, 1894.
234. Y. M. Y. Haddad, H. B. Henbest, J. Husband, and T. R. B. Mitchell, *Proc. Chem. Soc.*, **1964**, 361.
235. J. L. Speier, J. A. Webster, and G. H. Barnes, *J. Am. Chem. Soc.*, **79**, 974 (1957).
236. J. W. Ryan and J. L. Speier, *J. Am. Chem. Soc.*, **86**, 895 (1964).
237. C. Eaborn, *Organosilicon Compounds*, Butterworths, London, 1960, p. 45.
238. V. Bazant, V. Chvalovsky, and J. Rathousky, *Organosilicon Compounds*, Academic Press, New York, 1965, p. 139.
239. M. Kumada and R. Okawara, *Yukikeisokagaku*, Maki Shoten, Tokyo, 1959.
240. A. D. Petrov, V. A. Ponomarenko, B. A. Sokolov, and G. V. Odabashyan, *Izv. Akad. Nauk SSSR Ser. Khim.*, **1957**, 1206.
241. J. L. Speier, R. Zimmerman, and J. A. Webster, *J. Am. Chem. Soc.*, **78**, 2278 (1956).
242. T. G. Selin and R. West, *J. Am. Chem. Soc.*, **84**, 1863 (1962).
243. J. C. Saam and J. L. Speier, *J. Am. Chem. Soc.*, **83**, 1351 (1961).
244. H. M. Bank, J. C. Saam, and J. L. Speier, *J. Org. Chem.*, **29**, 792 (1964).
245. J. W. Ryan and J. L. Speier, *J. Org. Chem.*, **24**, 2052 (1959).
246. M. F. Shostakovskii, B. A. Sokolov, A. N. Grishko, K. F. Lavriva, and G. I. Kagan, *Zh. Obshch. Khim.*, **32**, 3882 (1962); *Chem. Abstr.*, **58**, 12,591 (1963).
247. E. A. Chernyshev, M. E. Dolgaya, and E. D. Lubuzh, *Izv. Akad. Nauk SSSR Ser. Khim.*, **1965**, 650; *Chem. Abstr.*, **63**, 2296 (1965).
248. M. C. Musolf and J. L. Speier, *J. Org. Chem.*, **29**, 2519 (1964).
249. A. D. Petrov, E. A. Chernyshev, M. E. Dolgaya, Yu. P. Egorov, and L. A. Leites, *Zh. Obshch. Khim.*, **30**, 376 (1960); *Chem. Abstr.*, **54**, 22,435 (1960).
250. R. W. Bott, S. Eaborn, and K. Leyshon, *J. Chem. Soc.*, **1964**, 1548.
251. A. D. Petrov and S. I. Sadykh-Zade, *Bull. Soc. Chim. France*, **1959**, 1932; *Dokl. Akad. Nauk SSSR*, **121**, 1 (1958).
252. A. D. Petrov, S. I. Sadykh-Zade, and E. I. Filatova, *Zh. Obshch. Khim.*, **29**, 2936 (1959); *Chem. Abstr.*, **54**, 11,984 (1960).
253. L. Goodman, R. M. Silverstein, and A. Benitez, *J. Am. Chem. Soc.*, **79**, 3073 (1957).
254. D. L. Bailey and A. N. Pines, *Ind. Eng. Chem.*, **46**, 2363 (1954).

255. I. Shiihara, W. F. Hoskyns, and H. W. Post, *J. Org. Chem.*, **26**, 4000 (1961).
256. R. M. Pike and P. M. McDonagh, *J. Chem. Soc.*, **1963**, 2831.
257. C. R. Kruger, *Inorg. Nucl. Chem. Letters*, **1**, 85 (1965).
258. H. Takahashi, H. Okita, M. Yamaguchi, and I. Shiihara, *J. Org. Chem.*, **28**, 3353 (1963).
259. P. M. Pike and P. M. McDonagh, *J. Chem. Soc.*, **1963**, 1058.
260. J. W. Ryan, G. K. Menzie, and J. L. Speier, *J. Am. Chem. Soc.*, **82**, 3601 (1960).
261. V. A. Ponomarenko, B. A. Sokolov, Kh. M. Minachev, and A. D. Petrov, *Dokl. Akad. Nauk SSSR*, **106**, 76 (1956); *Chem. Abstr.*, **50**, 13,726 (1956).
262. A. D. Petrov, V. A. Ponomarenko, B. A. Sokolov, and G. V. Odabashyan, *Izv. Akad. Nauk SSSR;* **1957**, 1206; *Chem. Abstr.*, **52**, 6160 (1958).
263. M. A. Mamedov, I. M. Akhmedov, M. M. Guseinov, and S. I. Sadykh-Zade, *Zh. Obshch. Khim.*, **35**, 461 (1965); *Chem. Abstr.*, **63**, 626 (1965).
264. R. A. Benkeser and R. F. Cunico, *J. Organometal. Chem.*, **6**, 441 (1966).
265. R. A. Benkeser and R. A. Hickner, *J. Am. Chem. Soc.*, **80**, 5298 (1958).
266. R. A. Benkeser, M. L. Burrous, L. E. Nelson, and J. V. Swisher, *J. Am. Chem. Soc.*, **83**, 4385 (1961).
267. J. W. Ryan and J. L. Speier, *J. Org. Chem.*, **31**, 2698 (1966).
268. V. F. Mironov, *Dokl. Akad. Nauk SSSR*, **153**, 848 (1963); *Chem. Abstr.*, **60**, 8056 (1964).
269. L. L. Shchukovskaya and R. I. Palchik, *Zh. Obshch. Khim.*, **35**, 1122 (1965); *Chem. Abstr.*, **63**, 9876 (1965).
270. B. A. Sokolov, A. N. Grishko, K. F. Lavrova, and G. I. Kagan, *Zh. Obshch. Khim.*, **34**, 3610 (1964); *Chem. Abstr.*, **62**, 9166 (1965).
271. V. F. Mironov and N. G. Maksimova, *Izv. Akad. Nauk SSSR*, **1960**, 2059; *Chem. Abstr.*, **55**, 14,297 (1961).
272. L. L. Shchukovskaya, R. I. Palchik, and A. D. Petrov, *Dokl. Akad. Nauk SSSR*, **160**, 621 (1965); *Chem. Abstr.*, **62**, 14,717 (1965).
273. Z. V. Belyakova, M. G. Pomerantseva, and S. A. Golubtsov, *Zh. Obshch. Khim.*, **35**, 1048 (1965); *Chem. Abstr.*, **63**, 9978 (1965).
274. R. Sultanov, E. M. Khalilova, and S. I. Sadykh-Zade, *Azerb. Khim. Zh.*, **1964**, 97; *Chem. Abstr.*, **62**, 10,456 (1965).
275. S. I. Sadykh-Zade, I. A. Shikhiev, and E. M. Khalilova, *Zh. Obshch. Khim.*, **34**, 1393 (1964); *Chem. Abstr.*, **61**, 5683 (1964).
276. A. D. Petrov and S. I. Sadykh-Zade, *Izv. Akad. Nauk SSSR*, **1958**, 513; *Dokl. Akad. Nauk SSSR*, **129**, 584 (1959).
277. M. D. Stadnichuk and A. A. Petrov, *Zh. Obshch. Khim.*, **33**, 3563 (1963).
278. M. D. Stadnichuk, *Zh. Obshch. Khim.*, **34**, 2931 (1964); *Chem. Abstr.*, **61**, 16,088 (1964).
279. N. C. Cook and J. E. Lyons, *J. Am. Chem. Soc.*, **88**, 3396 (1966).
280. N. C. Cook and J. E. Lyons, *J. Am. Chem. Soc.*, **87**, 3283 (1965).

281. A. J. Chalk and J. F. Harrod, *J. Am. Chem. Soc.*, **87**, 16 (1965).
282. A. J. Canale and W. A. Hewett, *J. Polymer Sci. B.*, **2**, 1041 (1964).
283. U. Giannini, E. Ciampelli, and G. Bruckner, *Makromol. Chem.*, **66**, 209 (1963).
284. P. Teyssie and R. Dauby, *Bull. Soc. Chim. France*, **1965**, 2842.
285. R. E. Rinehart, H. P. Smidt, H. S. Witt, and H. Romeyn, *J. Am. Chem. Soc.*, **83**, 4864 (1961); *ibid.*, **84**, 4145 (1962).
286. A. G. Canale, W. H. Hewett, T. M. Shryne, and E. A. Youngman, *Chem. Ind. (London)*, **1962**, 1054.
287. G. Natta, G. Dall'asta, and G. Motroni, *J. Polymer Sci. B*, **2**, 349 (1964).
288. T. Alderson, E. L. Jenner, and R. V. Lindsey, Jr., *J. Am. Chem. Soc.*, **87**, 5638 (1965).
289. J. T. van Gemert and P. R. Wilkinson, *J. Phys. Chem.*, **68**, 645 (1964).
290. R. Cramer, *J. Am. Chem. Soc.*, **87**, 4717 (1965).
291. S. A. Rhone-Poulenc, French Pat., 1,451,443 (1966); Belgian Pat., 677,989 (1966).
292. J. K. Nicholson and B. L. Shaw, *J. Chem. Soc. A*, **1966**, 807.
293. J. E. Lydon, J. K. Nicholson, B. L. Shaw, and M. R. Truter, *Proc. Chem. Soc.*, **1964**, 421.
294. F. W. Michelotti and W. P. Keaveney, *J. Polymer Sci. A*, **3**, 895 (1965).
295. R. E. Rinehart and H. P. Smith, *Polymer Letters*, **3**, 1049 (1965).
296. G. Natta, G. Dall'asta, and L. Porri, *Makromol. Chem.*, **81**, 253 (1965).
297. T. Katz and J. J. Mrowca, *J. Am. Chem. Soc.*, **88**, 4012 (1966).
298. A. T. Blomquist and P. M. Maitlis, *J. Am. Chem. Soc.*, **84**, 2329 (1962).
299. F. Zingales, *Ann. Chim. (Rome)*, **52**, 1174 (1962); *Chem. Abstr.*, **59**, 3794 (1963).
300. L. Malatesta, G. Santarella, L. Vallarino, and F. Zingales, *Angew. Chem.*, **72**, 34 (1960).
301. L. Malatesta, G. Santarella, L. Vallarino and F. Zingales, *Atti. Accad. Naz. Lincei Rend. Classe Sci. Fis. Mat. Nat.*, **27**, 230 (1959).
302. L. M. Vallarino and G. Santarella, *Gazz. Chim. Ital.*, **94**, 252 (1964).
303. P. M. Maitlis, D. Pollock, M. L. Games, and W. J. Pryde, *Can. J. Chem.*, **43**, 470 (1965).
304. R. C. Cookson and D. W. Jones, *J. Chem. Soc.*, **1965**, 1881.
305. P. M. Maitlis and M. L. Games, *Can. J. Chem.*, **42**, 183 (1964).
306. P. M. Maitlis and M. L. Games, *J. Am. Chem. Soc.*, **85**, 1887 (1963).
307. P. M. Maitlis, A. Efraty, and M. L. Games, *J. Am. Chem. Soc.*, **87**, 719 (1965).
308. A. T. Blomquist, L. H. Liu, and J. C. Bohrer, *J. Am. Chem. Soc.*, **74**, 3643 (1952).
309. A. C. Cope, C. R. Ganellin, and H. W. Johnson, *J. Am. Chem. Soc.*, **84**, 3191 (1962).

310. A. C. Cope, A. R. Ganellin, H. W. Johnson, T. V. vanAuken, and H. J. S. Winkler, *J. Am. Chem. Soc.*, **85**, 3276 (1963).
311. A. C. Cope, J. K. Hecht, H. W. Johnson, H. Keller, and H. J. S. Winkler, *J. Am. Chem. Soc.*, **88**, 761 (1966).
312. G. Paiaro, A. Panunzi, and A. De Renzi, *Tetrahedron Letters*, **1966**, 3905.
313. J. K. Stille, R. A. Morgan, D. D. Whitehurst, and J. R. Doyle, *J. Am. Chem. Soc.*, **87**, 3232 (1965).
314. J. K. Stille and R. A. Morgan, *J. Am. Chem. Soc.*, **88**, 5135 (1966).
315. W. A. White, H. M. Powell, and L. M. Venanzi, *Chem. Commun.*, **1966**, 310.
316. R. S. Cahn, C. K. Ingold, and V. Prelog., *Experientia*, **12**, 93 (1956).
317. G. Paiaor, P. Corradini, P. Palumbo, and A. Panunzi, *Makromol. Chem.*, **71**, 184 (1964).
318. G. Paiaro and A. Panunzi, *J. Am. Chem. Soc.*, **86**, 5148 (1964).
319. P. Corradini, G. Maglio, A. Musco, and G. Paiaro, *Chem. Commun.*, **1966**, 618.
320. P. Corradini, G. Paiaro, A. Panunzi, S. F. Mason, and G. H. Searle, *J. Am. Chem. Soc.*, **88**, 2863 (1966).
321. G. Paiaro and A. Panunzi, *Tetrahedron Letters*, **1965**, 441.
322. A. Panunzi and G. Paiaro, *J. Am. Chem. Soc.*, **88**, 4841 (1966).
323. A. C. Cope and E. A. Caress, *J. Am. Chem. Soc.*, **88**, 1711 (1966).
324. H. Frye, E. Kuljian, and J. Viebrock, *Inorg. Nuclear Chem. Letters*, **2**, 119 (1966).
325. J. C. Trebellas, J. R. Olechowski, and H. B. Jonassen, *J. Organometal. Chem.*, **6**, 412 (1966).
326. C. A. Grob, H. Link, and P. W. Scheiss, *Helv. Chim. Acta*, **46**, 483 (1963).
327. P. Heimbach, *Angew. Chem.*, **76**, 859 (1964).
328. W. Hafner, H. Prigge, and J. Smidt, *Ann.*, **693**, 109 (1966).
329. J. Milgram and W. H. Urry, Proc. 7th International Conference on Coordination Chemistry, Stockholm, 1962, p. 265.
330. J. K. Nicholson and B. L. Shaw, *Proc. Chem. Soc.*, **1963**, 282.
331. R. E. Rinehart and R. W. Fuest, *Chem. Eng. News*, Feb. 15, 1965, p. 40.
332. C. Djerassi and R. R. Engle, *J. Am. Chem. Soc.*, **75**, 3838 (1953).
333. L. M. Berkowitz and P. N. Rylander, *J. Am. Chem. Soc.*, **80**, 6682 (1958).
334. M. E. Wolff, J. F. Kerwin, F. F. Owings, B. B. Lewis, B. Blank, A. Magnani, and V. Georgian, *J. Am. Chem. Soc.*, **82**, 4117 (1960); *J. Org. Chem.*, **28**, 2729 (1963).
335. H. Nakata, *Tetrahedron*, **19**, 1959 (1963).
336. R. K. Armstrong, **31**, 618 (1966).
337. E. T. McBee, G. W. Calundann, and T. Hodgins, *J. Org. Chem.*, **31**, 4260 (1966).
338. F. M. Dean and J. C. Knight, *J. Chem. Soc.*, **1962**, 4745.

339. E. J. Corey, J. Casanova, P. A. Vatakencherry, and R. Winter, *J. Am. Chem. Soc.*, **85**, 169 (1963).
340. V. M. Parikh and J. K. N. Jones, *Can. J. Chem.*, **43**, 3452 (1965).
341. R. Pappo and A. Becker, *Bull. Res. Council Israel*, **5A**, 300 (1956).
342. G. Snatke and H. W. Fehlhaber, *Ann.*, **663**, 123 (1963).
343. G. Stork, A. Meisels, and J. E. Davis, *J. Am. Chem. Soc.*, **85**, 3419 (1963).
344. F. Sondheimer, R. Mechoulam, and M. Sprecher, *Tetrahedron*, **20**, 2473 (1964).
345. S. Sarel and Y. Yanuka, *J. Org. Chem.*, **24**, 2018 (1959).
346. F. G. Oberender and J. A. Dixon, *J. Org. Chem.*, **24**, 1226 (1959).

SUPPLEMENTARY REFERENCES

Literature available to the end of 1966 in Japan has been covered in the preceding sections. The following papers have appeared since this review was written; additional papers published before, which were not covered, have also been included. The sections of the review to which these references are relevant are indicated. Many papers have been published on the formation of complexes and only typical ones are cited.

Section II

CS_2, COS and alkyl and aryl isothiocyanate and perfluorothioacetone complexes of nickel, palladium, platinum, rhodium and iridium. M. C. Baird and G. Wilkinson, *J. Chem. Soc.*, *A*, **1967**, 865.
Acetylene complexes of iridium and rhodium. J. P. Collman and J W. Kang, *J. Am. Chem. Soc.*, **89**, 844 (1967).
The coordination of small molecules by bistriphenylphosphineplatinum(O); The reaction with H_2S, H_2Se and H_2Te. D. Morelli, A. Serge, R. Ugo, G. LaMonica, S. Cenini, F. Conti, and F. Bonati, *Chem. Commun.*, **1967**, 524.
The mechanism of the formation of an iridium complex of molecular nitrogen via organic azide. J. P. Collman, *J. Am. Chem. Soc.*, **89**, 169 (1967).
Nonaromatization reactions of bicyclo(2,2,0)hexa-2,5-diene. E. E. van Tamelen and D. Carty, *J. Am. Chem. Soc.*, **89**, 3922 (1967).
Dewar hexamethylbenzene palladium chloride. H. Dietl and P. M. Maitlis, *Chem. Commun.*, **1967**, 759.
The formation of π-allylic palladium complexes from allene and palladium chloride and the reverse reactions. M. S. Lupin, J. Powell, and B. L. Shaw, *J. Chem. Soc.*, *A*, **1966**, 1687.
The role of DMF in the interaction of olefins with palladium chloride; a new method of synthesis in mild conditions of π-allyl palladium. D. Morelli, R. Ugo, F. Conti, and M. Donati, *Chem. Commun.*, **1967**, 801.
A novel hexamethylbenzene rhodium chloride complex. B. L. Booth, R. N. Haszeldine, and M. Hill, *Chem. Commun.*, **1967**, 1118.

Section II (continued)

Oxygen Complexes von Nullwertigen Nickel, Palladium und Platinum. G. Wilke, H. Schott, and P. Heimbach, *Angew. Chem.*, **79**, 62 (1967).

Oxidation of alkylbenzenes catalyzed by rhodium complexes. J. Blum, H. Rosenman, and E. D. Bergmann, *Tetrahedron Letters*, **1967**, 3665.

Metal ion facilitation of atom-transfer oxidation–reduction reactions. J. P. Collman, M. Kubota, and J. W. Hosking, *J. Am. Chem. Soc.*, **89**, 4809 (1967).

Oxidation of coordinated ligands; sulfato and nitrato complexes of platinum. C. D. Cook and G. S. Jauhal, *J. Am. Chem. Soc.*, **89**, 3066 (1967).

Synthesis and structure of the dichloro-1,5-diene palladium. I. A. Zakharova, G. A. Kukina, T. S. Kuli-Zade, I. I. Moiseev, G. Ya. Pek, and M. A. Porai-Koshits, *Zh. Neorgan. Khim.*, **11**, 2543 (1966); *Chem. Abstr.*, **66**, 38036s (1967).

Ruthenium complexes containing molecular nitrogen. A. D. Allen, F. Bottomley, R. O. Harris, V. P. Reinsalu, and C. V. Senoff, *J. Am. Chem. Soc.*, **89**, 5595 (1967).

The formation of $Ru(NH_3)_5N_2^{2+}$ in aqueous solution by direct action of molecular nitrogen. D. E. Harrison and H. Taube, *J. Am. Chem. Soc.*, **89**, 5906 (1967).

π-Complexes of palladium chloride with straight-chain olefins. G. F. Pregaglia, M. Donati, and F. Conti, *Chem. Ind.*, **1966**, 1923.

New hydrido and oxygen complexes of rhodium. M. Takesada, H. Yamazaki, and N. Hagihara, *Bull. Chem. Soc. Japan*, **41**, 270 (1968).

Olefin complexes of platinum and palladium. S. Takahashi and N. Hagihara, *Nippon Kagaku Zasshi*, **88**, 1306 (1967).

Addition of some simple molecules to transition metal phosphine complexes and the crystal and molecular structure of Pd $[(PPh_3)]_2(CS_2)$. T. Kashiwagi, N. Yasuoka, T. Ueki, N. Kasai, M. Kakudo, S. Takahashi, and N. Hagihara, *Bull. Chem. Soc. Japan*, **41**, 296 (1968).

π-Allyl ligand transfer reactions between cobalt and palladium complexes. R. F. Heck, *J. Am. Chem. Soc.*, **90**, 317 (1968).

π-Allylic palladium complexes from methyl sorbate. A. Kasahara and T. Izumi, *Bull. Chem. Soc. Japan*, **41**, 516 (1968).

π-Allyl-Komplexe durch Decarboxylierung von ungesättigten Malonsaurederivate. R. Hüttel und H. Schmid, *Chem. Ber.*, **101**, 252 (1968).

The formation of a π-allylic palladium chloride complex from vinylcyclopropane derivatives. T. Shono, T. Yoshimiura, Y. Matsumura, and R. Oda, *J. Org. Chem.*, **33**, 876 (1968).

Triphenylphosphine complexes of ruthenium and rhodium. Reversible combinations of molecular nitrogen and hydrogen with the ruthenium complex. A. Yamamoto, S. Kitazume, and S. Ikeda, *J. Am. Chem. Soc.*, **90**, 1089 (1968).

Electrophilic aromatic substitution reactions by platinum and palladium chlorides on N,N-dimethylbenzylamine. A. C. Cope and E. C. Friedrich, *J. Am. Chem. Soc.*, **90**, 909 (1968).

Reduktive Zerlegung von π-Allyl-Palladiumchloride-Komplexen. R. Hüttel and P. Kochs, *Chem. Ber.*, **101**, 1043 (1968).

Section III-B

Olefin oxidation with palladium(II) in solution (review). A. Aguilo, *Advan. Organomet. Chem.*, **5**, 321 (1967).

Homogeneous oxidation of alcohols with palladium(II) salts. W. G. Lloyd, *J. Org. Chem.*, **39**, 2575 (1967).

Hydride transfer reactions catalyzed by metal complexes. H. F. Charman, *J. Chem. Soc., B*, **1967**, 629.

Oxidation of styrene with palladium salts in aqueous tetrahydrofuran. H. Okada and H. Hashimoto, *Kogyo Kagaku Zasshi*, **69**, 2137 (1966).

Section III-C

Oxidation of olefins by combination of palladium chloride and copper chloride in acetic acid. P. M. Henry, *J. Org. Chem.*, **32**, 2575 (1967).

Aromatic substitution of styrene–palladium chloride complex. II. Effect of metal acetate. Y. Fujiwara, I. Moritani, M. Matsuda, and S. Teranishi, *Tetrahedron Letters*, **1968**, 633.

The oxidative coupling of vinyl acetate with palladium acetate; synthesis of 1,4-diacetoxy-1,3-butadiene. C. F. Kohll and R. van Helden, *Rec. Trav. Chim.*, **86**, 193 (1967).

Oxidative dimerization of β-substituted α-olefins by palladium acetate. H. C. Volger, *Rec. Trav. Chim.*, **86**, 677 (1967).

Stereochemistry of the reaction of bicyclo(2,2,1)heptadiene palladium chloride with methoxide anions. M. Green and R. I. Hancock, *J. Chem. Soc., A*, **1967**, 2054.

Reactions of primary amines and acetate ion with platinum and palladium alkadiene halide complexes. G. Paiaro, A. De Renzi, and R. Palumbo, *Chem. Commun.*, **1967**, 1150.

Esters of substituted acids from olefins. W. C. Baird, French Pat. 1437262, *Chem. Abstr.*, **66**, 10594 (1967).

One-step preparation of vinyl acetate from acetaldehyde and acetic anhydride. Kurashiki Rayon Co., French Pat., 1442980, *Chem. Abstr.*, **66**, 104707g (1967).

The preparation of ethylene glycol acetate. Du Pont, British Pat., 1058995, *Chem. Abstr.*, **66**, 94702t (1967).

The mechanism of ethylene oxidation by palladium salt in acetic acid. I. I. Moiseev, A. P. Belov, V. A. Igoshin, and Ya. K. Syrkin, *Dokl. Akad. Nauk*, **173**, 863 (1967); *Chem. Abstr.*, **67**, 53332z (1967).

Aliphatic unsaturated nitriles. Asahi Kasei Co., Belgian Pat., 670276, *Chem. Abstr.*, **65**, 15241 (1966).

Reaction of styrene with palladium salts. Effects of anion and copper salts on the products. S. Uemura and K. Ichikawa, *Nippon Kagaku Zasshi*, **88**, 893 (1967).

Effect of oxygen on the acetoxylation and other reactions of the acetato complexes of lead(IV) and palladium(II). J. M. Davidson and C. Trigg, *Chem. Ind.*, **1967**, 1361.

Section III-C (continued)

Homogeneous metal-catalyzed exchange of aromatic compounds; a new general isotopic hydrogen labelling procedure. J. L. Garnett and R. J. Hodges, *J. Am. Chem. Soc.*, **89**, 4546 (1967).

Specificity in the homogeneous metal-catalyzed isotopic hydrogen exchange of polycyclic aromatic hydrocarbons; evidence for complex formation between aromatic hydrocarbons and transition metals. J. L. Garnett and R. J. Hodges, *Chem. Commun.*, **1967**, 1220.

Palladium chloride for dimerizing aromatics. A. F. Ellis, U.S. Pat., 3294484, *Chem. Abstr.*, **66**, 104799w (1967).

Homogeneous metal-catalyzed isotopic hydrogen exchange in aromatic compounds; the labelling of nitro, bromobenzene, naphthalene and acetophenone. J. L. Garnett, *Chem. Commun.*, **1967**, 1001.

Section III-E

Palladium catalyzed reaction of ethylene, γ-butyrolactone and cupric chloride. T. Saegusa, T. Tsuda, and K. Isayama, *Tetrahedron Letters*, **1967**, 3599.

The reaction of acetylacetone with styrene in the presence of palladium chloride. S. Uemura and K. Ichikawa, *Bull. Chem. Soc. Japan*, **40**, 1016 (1967).

The reaction of acetylacetonato (π-allylic)palladium(II) complexes with carbon monoxide and conjugated dienes. Y. Takahashi, S. Sakai, and Y. Ishii, *Chem. Commun.*, **1967**, 1092.

Section IV-A

The direct conversion of aromatic nitro compounds to isocyanates by carbon monoxide. W. B. Hardy and R. F. Bennett, *Tetrahedron Letters*, **1967**, 961.

Preparation of aroyl halides. National Distillers & Chem. Corp., Netherland Application, 6614185, *Chem. Abstr.*, **67**, 64066s (1967).

Carbonylation and decarbonylation reactions catalyzed by palladium. J. Tsuji and K. Ohno, *J. Am. Chem. Soc.*, **90**, 94 (1968).

Section IV-B

Reaction of carbomethoxymercuric chloride with olefin and π-allylpalladium chloride complexes. T. Saegusa, T. Tsuda, and K. Nishijima, *Tetrahedron Letters* **1967**, 4255.

Section IV-C

Carbonylation of piperylene in the presence of palladium chloride. C. Bordence and W. E. Marsico, *Tetrahedron Letters*, **1967**, 1541.

Section IV-D

Stereochemistry of oxidative addition reaction of Ir(I) complexes. J. P. Collman, *Inorg. Chem.*, **7**, 27 (1968).

Section IV-E

A new method of introducing the neopentyl group. M. S. Newman and N. Gill, *J. Org. Chem.*, **31**, 3860 (1966).

The palladium catalyzed decarbonylation of β-phenylisovaleraldehydes. A notable diminution of the neophyl rearrangement. J. W. Wilt and V. P. Abegg, *J. Org. Chem.*, **33**, 923 (1968).

Section IV-J

2-(Phenylazo)phenyl complexes of the transition metals. R. F. Heck, *J. Am. Chem. Soc.*, **90**, 313 (1968).

Section V-B

Carbonylation reactions of Schiff bases and azobenzene by rhodium catalysts and preparation of azobenzene complexes of rhodium. T. Jo, N. Hagihara, and S. Murahashi, *Nippon Kagaku Zasshi*, **88**, 786 (1967).

Selective decarbonylation of α,β-unsaturated aldehydes using rhodium complexes. K. Ohno and J. Tsuji, *Tetrahedron Letters*, **1967**, 2173.

Decarbonylation of aromatic carbonyl compounds catalyzed by rhodium complexes. J. Blum, E. Oppenheimer, and E. D. Bergmann, *J. Am. Chem. Soc.*, **89**, 2338 (1967).

Formation of aryl fluorides via decarbonylation of aroyl fluorides. G. Olah and P. Kreienbuhl, *J. Org. Chem.*, **32**, 1614 (1967).

Rearrangement of 32-oxygenated lanostanes. J. Fried and J. W. Brown, *Tetrahedron Letters*, **1967**, 925.

Addition reaction of tris(triphenylphosphine)chlororhodium(I) hydridoalkyl, and acyl complexes; carbon monoxide insertion and decarbonylation reactions. M. C. Baird, J. T. Mague, J. A. Osborn, and G. Wilkinson, *J. Chem. Soc.*, A, **1967**, 1347.

Decarbonylation of diphenylketene with organometallic compounds. P. Hong, K. Sonogashira and N. Hagihara, *Nippon Kagaku Zasshi*, **89**, 74 (1968).

Oxoreaction of ethyl acrylate by rhodium carbonyl. Y. Takegami, Y. Watanabe, and H. Masada, *Bull. Chem. Soc. Japan*, **40**, 1459 (1967).

Novel decarbonylation reactions of aldehydes and acyl halides using rhodium complexes. K. Ohno and J. Tsuji, *J. Am. Chem. Soc.*, **90**, 99 (1968).

Section VI

Addition reaction of tris(triphenylphosphine)chlororhodium. M. C. Baird, J. T. Mague, J. A. Osborn, and G. Wilkinson, *J. Chem. Soc.*, A, **1967**, 1347.

Homogeneous catalytic hydrogenation of unsaturated aldehydes to form saturated aldehydes. F. H. Jardine and G. Wilkinson, *J. Chem. Soc.*, C, **1967**, 270.

Selective catalytic homogeneous hydrogenation of terminal olefins using tris-(triphenylphosphine)hydridochlororuthenium(II); hydrogen transfer in exchange and isomerization reactions of olefins. P. S. Hallman, D. Evans, J. A. Osborn and G. Wilkinson, *Chem. Commun.*, **1967**, 305.

Section VI (continued)

Homogeneous hydrogenation in the presence of sulfur compounds. A. J. Birch and K. A. M. Walker, *Tetrahedron Letters*, **1967**, 1935.

Hydrogenation en phase homogé; reduction de doubles liaisons par le deuterium et le chlorure de tris(triphenylphosphine)rhodium. J. F. Biellmann and H. Liesenfelt, *Bull. Soc. Chim. France*, **1966**, 4029.

Etude de l'hydrogenation en phase homogé. J. F. Biellmann and H. Liesenfelt, *Compt. Rend. Acad. Sci. Paris C*, **263**, 251 (1966).

Catalysis of the transfer of hydrogen from propan-2-ol to α,β-unsaturated ketones by organoiridium compounds. J. Trocha-Grimshaw and H. B. Henbest, *Chem. Commun.*, **1967**, 544.

Homogeneous catalysis with *trans*-chlorocarbonylbis(triphenylphosphine)iridium. G. C. Eberhardt and L. Vaska, *J. Catalysis*, **8**, 183 (1967).

Homogeneous catalysis in the reaction of olefinic substances; IX. Homogeneous catalysis of specific hydrogenation of polyolefins by some platinum and palladium complexes. M. A. Tayin and J. C. Bailar, *J. Am. Chem. Soc.*, **89**, 4330 (1967).

Selective hydrogenation of methyl linoleate and isomerization of methyl oleate by homogeneous catalysis with platinum complexes containing triphenylphosphine or triphenylstibine. J. C. Bailar and H. Itatani, *J. Am. Chem. Soc.*, **89**, 1592 (1967).

Homogeneous hydrogenation of methyl linolenate catalyzed by platinum-tin complexes. E. N. Frankel, E. A. Emken, H. Itatani, and J. C. Bailar, *J. Org. Chem.*, **32**, 1447 (1967).

Selective reduction using chlorotris(triphenylphosphine)rhodium. M. Brown and L. W. Piszkiewicz, *J. Org. Chem.*, **32**, 2013 (1967).

Catalyseurs d'hydrogenation homogené au rhodium. R. Stern, Y. Chevallier, and L. Sajus, *Compt. Rend. Acad. Sci. Paris C*, **264**, 1740 (1967).

A catalyst for the homogeneous hydrogenation of aldehydes under mild conditions. R. S. Coffey, *Chem. Commun.*, **1967**, 923.

Hydride transfer reactions catalyzed by metal complexes. H. B. Charman, *Nature*, **212**, 278 (1966).

Further studies on the homogeneous hydrogenation of olefins using tris(triphenylphosphine)halogenorhodium(I) catalysts. F. H. Jardine, J. A. Osborn, and G. Wilkinson, *J. Chem. Soc., A*, **1967**, 1574.

Homogeneous hydrogenation of olefins catalyzed by iridium complexes. M. Yamaguchi, *Kogyo Kagaku Zasshi*, **70**, 675 (1967); *Chem. Abstr.*, **67**, 99542w (1967).

Homogeneous hydrogenation with platinum-tin chloride complexes as catalysts. L. P. van't Hof and B. G. Linsen, *J. Catal.*, **7**, 295 (1967).

Kinetic study of iridium(I) complexes as homogeneous hydrogenation catalysts. B. R. James and N. A. Memon, *Can. J. Chem.*, **46**, 217 (1968).

Katalytische Hydrierungen und Deuterierungen von Steroiden in homogener Phase. W. Voelter and C. Djerassi, *Chem. Ber.*, **101**, 58 (1968).

Section VII

The formation of 1,6-bis(trichlorosilyl)hexane by the chloroplatinic acid catalyzed hydrosilation of 1-hexene. R. A. Benkeser, R. F. Cunico, S. Dunny, P. R. Jones, and P. G. Nerlekar, *J. Org. Chem.*, **32**, 2634 (1967).

Group VIII metal-catalyzed reactions of organosilicon hydrides with amines, hydrogen halides and hydrogen sulfides. L. H. Sommer and J. D. Citron, *J. Org. Chem.*, **32**, 2470 (1967).

Stereospecific platinum-catalyzed hydrosilation of 1-octene with optically active R_3SiH. L. H. Sommer, K. W. Michael, and H. Fujimoto, *J. Am. Chem. Soc.*, **89**, 1519 (1967).

Test for reversibility of platinum-catalyzed hydrosilation of olefins. L. Spialter and D. H. O'Brien, *J. Org. Chem.*, **32**, 222 (1967).

Stereospecific exchange of optically active R_3SiH catalyzed by group VIII metals. L. H. Sommer, J. E. Lyons, H. Fujimoto, and K. W. Michael, *J. Am. Chem. Soc.*, **89**, 5489 (1967).

Ionisierungsenergien von Silyl- und Alkyl-äthylenen. H. Bock und H. Seidel, *Angew. Chem.*, **79**, 1106 (1967).

Addition reactions of hydrosilanes to vinylpyridines. N. S. Nametkin, L. N. Lyashenko, T. I. Chernysheva, S. N. Borisov, and V. A. Pestunovich, *Dokl. Akad. Nauk SSSR*, **174**, 1105 (1967); *Chem. Abstr.*, **68**, 13051w (1968).

The addition of methyldichlorosilane to butyne-2. J. W. Ryon, J. L. Speier, *J. Org. Chem.*, **31**, 2698 (1966).

Synthesis and some conversions of ε-silicon containing ketones. N. V. Komarov and V. K. Roman, *Zh. Obshch. Khim.*, **35**, 2017 (1965); *Chem. Abstr.*, **64**, 6675 (1966).

Synthesis of unsaturated silicon-containing epoxy compounds. S. I. Sadykh-Zade, R. B. Babaeva, and A. Salimov, *Zh. Obshch. Khim.*, **36**, 695 (1966); *Chem. Abstr.*, **65**, 8948c (1966).

Acetylenic formals and their hydrosilation. I. A. Shikhiev, A. A. Vatankha, and B. M. Guseinzade, *Zh. Obshch. Khim.*, **36**, 1293 (1966).

Synthesis of (methoxymethylvinyl)triethylsilanes. E. G. Kagan, *Zh. Obshch. Khim.*, **37**, 1692 (1967).

Stereochemistry of asymmetric silicon. X. Solvent and reagent effects on stereochemistry crossover in alkoxy-alkoxy exchange reactions at silicon centers. L. H. Sommer and H. Fujimoto, *J. Am. Chem. Soc.*, **90**, 982 (1968).

Hydrosilation in the synthesis of organosilanes. R. N. Meals, *Pure Appl. Chem.*, **13**, 141 (1966).

Section VIII

Formation of dichloro(2,7-dimethylocta-2,6-diene-1,8-diyl)ruthenium(IV) from $RuCl_3$ and isoprene. L. Porri, M. C. Gallazzi, A. Colombo, and G. Allegra, *Tetrahedron Letters*, **1965**, 4187.

The reaction of rhodium chloride with dienes. K. C. Dewhirst, *J. Org. Chem.*, **32**, 1297 (1967).

Section VIII (continued)

The dimerization of butadiene by palladium complex catalysts. S. Takahashi, T. Shibano, and N. Hagihara, *Tetrahedron Letters*, **1967**, 2451.

The dimerization of butadiene by palladium complex catalysts. S. Takahashi, T. Shibano, and N. Hagihara, *Bull. Chem. Soc. Japan*, **41**, 454 (1958).

The dimerization of butadiene in methanol by a palladium complex catalyst. S. Takahashi, H. Yamazaki, and N. Hagihara, *Bull. Chem. Soc. Japan*, **41**, 254 (1968).

Oligomerization and dimerization of butadiene under homogeneous catalysis; reactions with nucleophiles and the synthesis of 1,3,7-octatriene. E. J. Smutny, *J. Am. Chem. Soc.*, **89**, 6793 (1967).

The dimerization of alkenes by palladium and rhodium chloride. A. D. Ketley, L. P. Fischer, A. J. Berlin, C. R. Morgan, E. H. German, and T. R. Steadman, *Inorg. Chem.*, **6**, 657 (1967).

Acrylonitrile complex of ruthenium trichloride which catalyzes the dimerization of acrylonitrile to 1,4-dicyanobut-1-ene. A. Misono, Y. Uchida, and M. Hidai, *Chem. Commun.*, **1967**, 357.

Dimerization of acrylonitrile by ruthenium chloride. A. Misono, Y. Uchida, M. Hidai, H. Shinohara, and Y. Watanabe, *Bull. Chem. Soc. Japan*, **41**, 396 (1968).

The dimerization of ethylene using palladium chloride as the catalyst. Y. Kusunoki, R. Katsuno, N. Hasegawa, S. Kurematsu, Y. Nagano, K. Ishii, and S. Tsutsumi, *Bull. Chem. Soc. Japan*, **39**, 2021 (1966).

The mechanism of the synthesis of 1,4-hexadiene from ethylene and butadiene and of its isomerization to 2,4-hexadiene. R. Cramer, *J. Am. Chem. Soc.*, **89**, 1633 (1967).

Butadiene from vinyl chloride; the platinum(II)-catalyzed coupling of vinyl halides. F. N. Jones, *J. Org. Chem.*, **32**, 1667 (1967).

Octatriene production. E. J. Smutny, U.S. Pat., 3267169, *Chem. Abstr.*, **65**, 18497 (1966).

Section IX

Molecular asymmetry, VII. *trans*-6,7,10,11-Tetrahydro-5H-benzocyclononene. A. C. Cope and M. W. Fordice, *J. Am. Chem. Soc.*, **89**, 6187 (1968).

Molecular asymmetry VIII. *trans*-Bicyclo(8,2,2)tetradeca-5,10,12,13-tetraene. A. C. Cope and B. A. Pawson, *J. Am. Chem. Soc.*, **90**, 636 (1968).

Section X

Valence isomerization of quadricyclene to norbornadiene catalyzed by transition metal complexes. H. Hogeveen and H. C. Volger, *J. Am. Chem. Soc.*, **89**, 2486 (1967).

Valence isomerization of hexamethyl Dewar benzene to hexamethylbenzene catalyzed by rhodium olefin complexes. H. C. Volger and H. Hogeveen, *Rec. Trav. Chim.*, **86**, 830 (1967).

Section X (continued)

Photolysis and stereochemistry of oxypalladation adduct of 1,5-cyclooctadiene. C. B. Anderson and B. J. Burreson, *Chem. Ind.*, **1967**, 620.

The stereochemical course of metal catalyzed cycloaddition reactions of norbornadiene. T. J. Katz and N. Acton, *Tetrahedron Letters*, **1967**, 2601.

The preparation of tetracyclo(4,3,0,0^{2,4},0^{3,7})non-8-ene and the dimerization of it and of benzonorbornadiene by rhodium on carbon. T. J. Katz, J. C. Carnaban, and R. Boecke, *J. Org. Chem.*, **32**, 1301 (1967).

Isomerization of 3,4-dichloro-1-butene catalyzed by various palladium compounds. A. Oshima, *Nippon Kagaku Zasshi*, **89**, 92 (1968).

New catalysts for olefin-formaldehyde condensations; palladium compounds. S. Sakai, Y. Kawashima, Y. Takahashi, and Y. Ishii, *Chem. Commun.*, **1967**, 1073.

Eine neue Synthese von Cyclooctatriene-1,3,5. W. Ziegenbein, *Chem. Ber.*, **98**, 1427 (1965).

The oxidation of cyclobutanols and aromatic rings with ruthenium tetroxide. J. A. Caputo and R. Fuchs, *Tetrahedron Letters*, **1967**, 4729.

The oxidation of carbohydrate derivatives with ruthenium tetroxide. P. J. Beynon, D. M. Collins, P. T. Doganges, and W. G. Overend, *J. Chem. Soc., C*, **1966**, 1131.

Synthesis of a new σ-bonded dimethyl rhodium derivative $C_5H_5Rh(CH_3)_2(PPh_3)$. A. Kasahara, T. Izumi, and K. Tanaka, *Bull. Chem. Soc. Japan*, **40**, 699 (1967).

ELECTROCHEMICAL PREPARATION OF CYCLIC COMPOUNDS

By J. D. ANDERSON, J. P. PETROVICH, AND M. M. BAIZER, *Central Research Department, Monsanto Company, St. Louis, Missouri*

CONTENTS

- I. Introduction 258
- II. Anodic Cyclizations 259
    - A. By Kolbe Reactions 259
        - 1. Carboxylate Radical Intermediates 259
        - 2. Hydrocarbyl Radical Intermediates 260
        - 3. Carbonium Ion Intermediates 261
    - B. By Methoxylation 262
- III. Cathodic Cyclizations Starting with Various Reagents 264
    - A. Carboxylic Acid Derivatives 264
    - B. Nitro Compounds 265
    - C. Oximes 266
    - D. Mercurials 266
    - E. Halides 267
    - F. Bis-Activated Olefins 269
    - G. Bicyclo Keto Amines 272
- IV. Electrochemical-plus-Chemical (EC) Cyclizations 274
    - A. Kolbe Reactions 274
    - B. Anodic Methoxylation 275
    - C. Cathodic Formation of Dichlorocarbene 276
    - D. Cathodic Formation of Benzyne 276
    - E. Anodic Formation of a Ketimine 276
    - F. Anodic Thiocyanation 277
- V. Experimental 278
    - A. *cis*-2,4-Dicarbomethoxybicyclobutane (Anodic) 278
    - B. 4-Phenyl-3,4-dihydrocoumarin (Anodic) 279
    - C. 1,3-Dimethylbicyclobutane (Cathodic) 279
    - D. 2,3-Bis(dicarbethoxymethyl)-1,2,3,4-tetrahydroquinoxaline (Cathodic) 279
    - E. Diethylcyclopentane-1,2-diacetate (Cathodic) 280
    - References 281

I. Introduction

The development of methods, particularly those of broad scope, for the synthesis of cyclic compounds by "conventional" *chemical* techniques has continued to engage the interest of organic chemists over the years. The enormous body of literature that has consequently resulted has recently been reviewed (1–5). By contrast, the literature on *electrochemical* syntheses of cyclic systems is sparse and scattered. It is the purpose of this chapter to assemble and review for the first time reports on the utilization of electrochemical techniques for effecting cyclization reactions. It will become obvious that many attractive synthetic and mechanistic research problems in this area remain to be investigated.

From a narrow point of view, perhaps only those reactions should be considered electrochemical cyclizations in which intramolecular ring closure occurs concomitantly with oxidation (anodic) or reduction (cathodic). We have attempted to achieve a fairly comprehensive coverage of the literature in this category. However, there are many instances in which the electrochemical preparation of an intermediate is followed by intermolecular reaction of the intermediate (*in situ* or subsequently) with a second component to form a cyclic compound. This class of electrochemical-plus-chemical reactions (EC reaction) is ill-defined and vast in scope; therefore, only a few nontrivial examples of it are included in this review. Finally, for practical reasons we can only mention but not adopt the broadest point of view concerning electrochemical cyclizations, namely, that all cyclizations in which an electron-transfer step is critically involved are in principle electrochemical in nature. If electron transfer is mediated by an agent other than an electrode (e.g., an alkali metal), we consider the reaction "pseudo-electrochemical" and do not include it in this review.

Historically it is seen that early attempts at electrochemical syntheses of cyclic compounds involved mainly the use of the Kolbe reaction (6). Electrolysis of the alkali metal salt of glutaric acid yielded propylene and not cyclopropane (7). Presumably, a hydrogen migration was involved. Electrolysis of β,β-dimethylglutaric acid salts gave no cyclopropane derivatives even though hydrogen migration was impossible (8). Instead, a structural rearrangement occurred leading

$$^-OOCCH_2(CH_2)_nCH_2COO^- \xrightarrow{-2e^-} \text{CH}_2\underset{(CH_2)_n}{\overset{}{\diagup\diagdown}}\text{CH}_2 \quad (1)$$

mainly to 2-methylbutene. A number of other dicarboxylic acids have been electrolyzed without forming cycloalkanes [eq. (1)] (9).

II. Anodic Cyclizations

A. BY KOLBE REACTIONS

Despite the earlier failures referred to above, the Kolbe reaction has in the last few years been successfully employed in the synthesis of cyclic compounds. It is currently recognized (6,10) that products may arise from intermediate carboxylate radicals (1), from hydrocarbyl radicals (2) or from carbonium ions (3), all of which are formed by anodic oxidation of carboxylates. The ability to generate a particular intermediate species depends upon electrolysis conditions (including the

$$RCOO^- \xrightarrow{-e^-} RCOO\cdot \xrightarrow{-CO_2} R\cdot \xrightarrow{-e^-} R^+$$
$$\quad\quad\quad\quad\quad (1) \quad\quad\quad (2) \quad\quad (3)$$

nature of the anode) and the structure of the starting carboxylic acid. It has often been very difficult to distinguish mechanistically between product formation via **2** and product formation via **3**.

1. Carboxylate Radical Intermediates

Koehl (11) has recently synthesized 4-phenylcoumarin by the Kolbe electrolysis of 3,3-diphenylacrylic acid. This product was formed by intramolecular attack of the acyloxy radical (**4**) on one of the phenyl groups, eq. (2).

$$Ph_2C=CHCOO^- \xrightarrow{-e^-} Ph_2C=CHCOO\cdot \longrightarrow \text{[4-phenylcoumarin]} \quad (2)$$
$$(4)$$

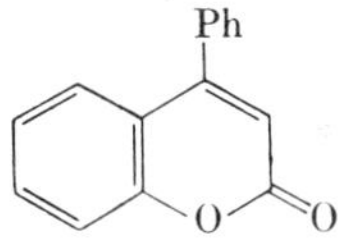

Bonner and Mango (12), in an earlier report, prepared the saturated analog presumably via the same type of intermediate, eq. (3).

$$Ph_2CHCH_2COO^- \xrightarrow{-e^-} \text{[4-phenylchroman-2-one]} \quad (3)$$

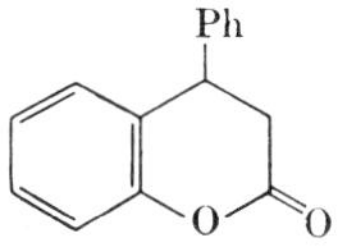

Phloretic acid (**5a**) and phloretylglycine (**5b**) have been oxidized anodically to a dienone lactone (**6**) in a study aimed at developing a selective chemical method for the cleavage of tyrosyl peptide bonds (13). A similar oxidation (14) of p-hydroxy-*cis*-cinnamic acid (**7**) gave the spirolactone (**8**) which on acid rearrangement yielded umbelliferone (**9**) and 6-hydroxycoumarin (**10**), eqs. (4) and (5). In the latter study,

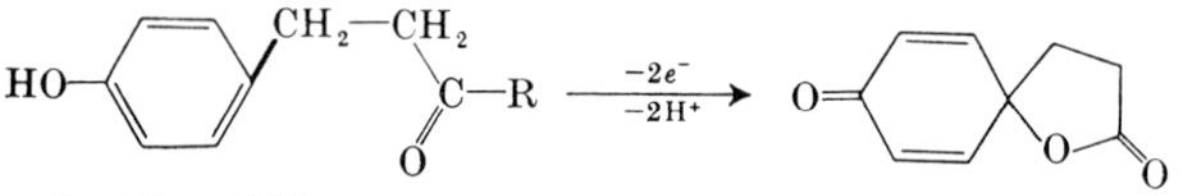

$$\text{(4)}$$

5a, R = OH
5b, R = —NHCH$_2$COOH

(6)

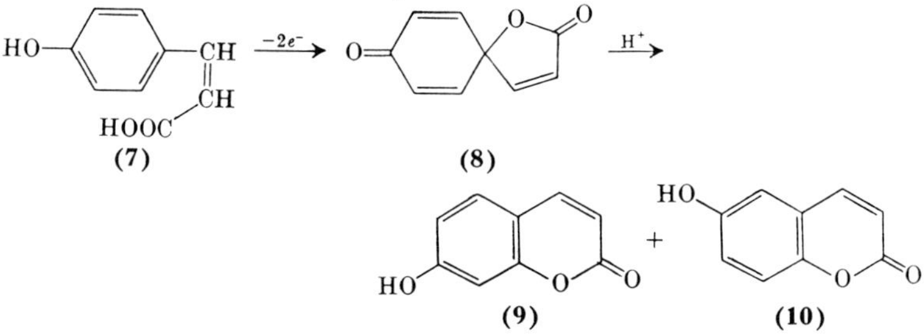

(7) (8) (9) (10)

$$\text{(5)}$$

N-carbomethoxytyrosine (**11**), a derivative of **5a**, was also oxidized to **12**, the corresponding derivative of **6**:

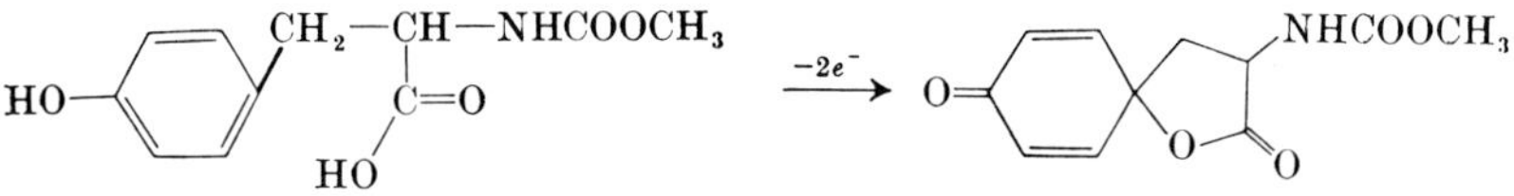

(11) (12) (6)

2. Hydrocarbyl Radical Intermediates

Vellturo and Griffin (15) haev synthesized a bicyclobutane structure using the Kolbe electrolysis of a 1,3-cyclobutanedicarboxylic acid.

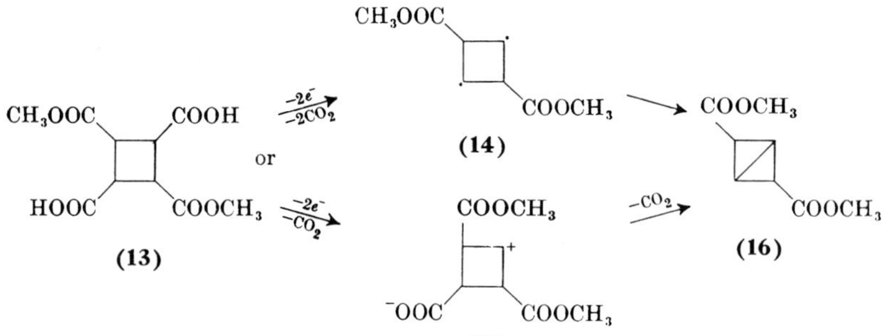

(13) (14) (15) (16) (7)

This anodic oxidation of *trans,trans,trans*-1,3-dicarboxy2,4-dicarbomethoxycyclobutane **(13)** gave 2,4-dicarbomethoxybicyclobutane **(16)**. The reactive intermediate could be the diradical **(14)**. However, the authors cited feel that a stepwise process consisting of oxidation and monodecarboxylation to a zwitterion **(15)** followed by further decarboxylation and collapse to the product is more probable.

3. *Carbonium Ion Intermediates*

Traynham and Dehn (16) have used the Kolbe reaction on a series of medium-ring cycloalkanecarboxylic acids. Bicyclic products, the products of transannular carbonium ion reactions, are formed. For example, the electrolysis of cyclooctanecarboxylic acid gave bicyclo-[5.1.0]octane **(17)** and bicyclo[3.3.0]octane **(18)**, eq. (8).

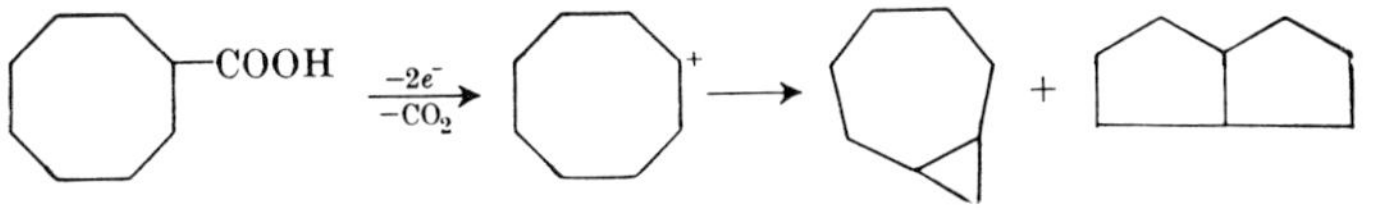

Other systems have been studied wherein a hydrocarbon carbonium ion has been generated via the Kolbe electrolysis; the ion then reacts to give ring enlargements and/or bicyclic products. Electrolysis (17) of 1-methylcyclohexaneacetic acid **(19)** in methanol gave 1-methylcycloheptene **(20)** and 1-methylcycloheptylmethyl ether **(21)**, eq. (9). Presumably, these products were formed as a result of an intermediate carbonium ion.

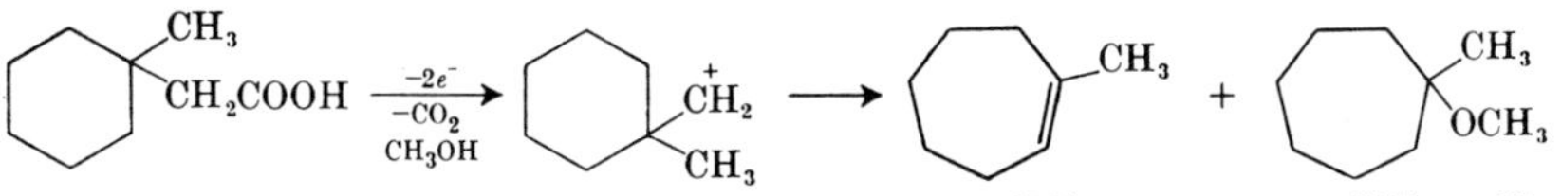

Corey et al. (10) have also observed carbonium ion behavior using the Kolbe electrolysis. Electrolysis of *exo*- or *endo*-5-norbornene-2-carboxylic acid **(22)** in methanol gave 3-methoxynortricyclene **(23)**, the "nonclassical" ion product.

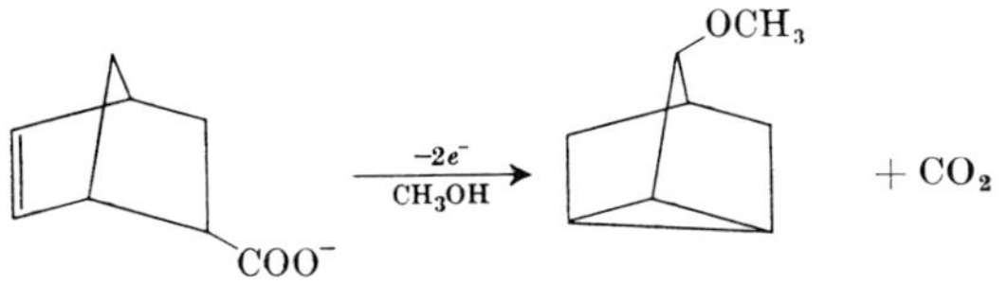

Bunyan and Hey (18,19) have shown that phenyl radicals can be produced by the Kolbe reaction at elevated temperatures. The high temperature is apparently required to break down the stable carboxylate radical which is the first-formed intermediate. This procedure has been used in electrolyses of a series of o-benzoyl benzoic acids **(24)** to give 3-substituted fluorenone derivatives **(25)**.

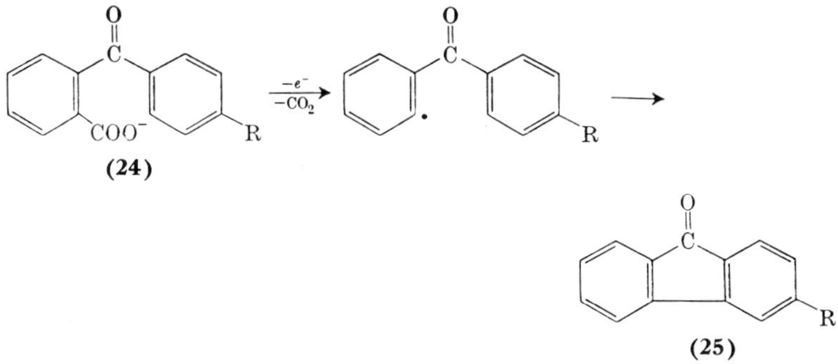

B. BY METHOXYLATION

Carwood, Scott, and Weedon (20) have oxidized a series of linear monocarboxylic acids which contain olefinic linkages in the chain. Depending on the site of unsaturation, the resultant free radical from the Kolbe electrolysis can react intramolecularly with the olefinic linkage to give cyclic products. Electrolysis of hept-6-enoic acid **(26)** gave two types of cyclopentane compounds which were produced by combination of the two radical intermediates **(27 and 28)**.

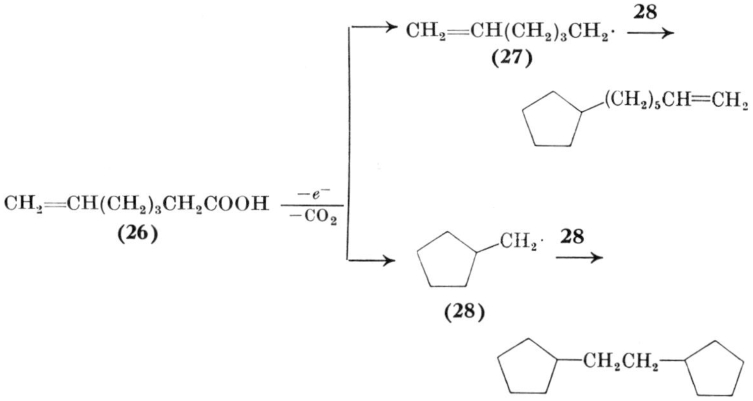

Overberger and Kabasakalian (21) have anodically oxidized various isomers of perhydrodiphenic acids **(29)**. These reactions yielded lactones of 2(1-hydroxycyclohexyl)cyclohexanecarboxylic acid **(30)**. The proposed mechanism involved a hydrogen radical transfer followed by an intramolecular coupling of the rearranged radical and the initial radical formed at the anode.

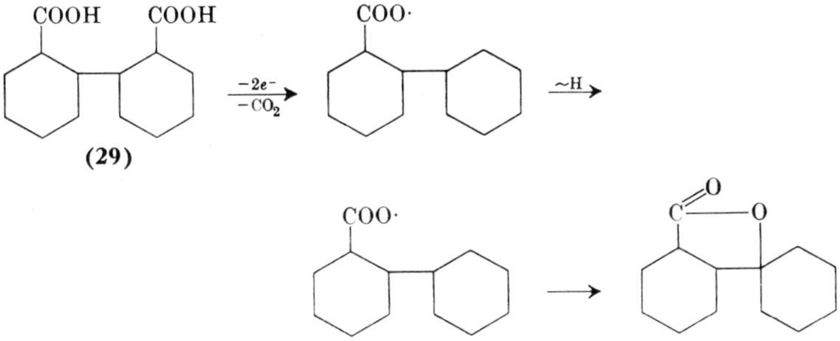

$$\text{(29)} \xrightarrow[-CO_2]{-2e^-} \quad \xrightarrow{\sim H}$$

$$\longrightarrow \quad \text{(30)} \qquad (14)$$

Pasquinelli (22) has synthesized benzene by the electrooxidation of *trans*-1,2-dihydrophthalic acid, eq. (15).

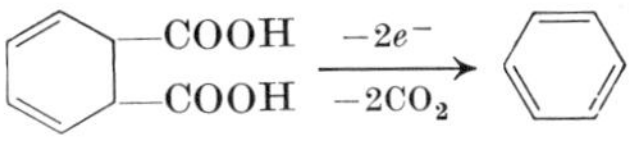

$$\text{(dihydrophthalic acid)} \xrightarrow[-2CO_2]{-2e^-} \text{(benzene)} \qquad (15)$$

Cyclopropanes were recently obtained, among other products, by Koehl (23) by anodic oxidation, preferably at graphite, of *n*-butanoic acid, 2-methylbutanoic acid, 3-methylbutanoic acid, and *n*-pentanoic acids. No discussion of mechanism has been presented.

$$CH_3(CH_2)_2COO^- \xrightarrow{-xe^-} \triangle \qquad (16)$$

In an anodic cyclization not involving a Kolbe reaction, Weinberg and Brown (24), establishing that methoxylation occurred at the alkyl rather than at the benzylic carbon in *N*-benzylamines, formed, e.g., 3-benzyloxazolidine **(32)** from *N*-benzyl-*N*-methylethanolamine **(31)**.

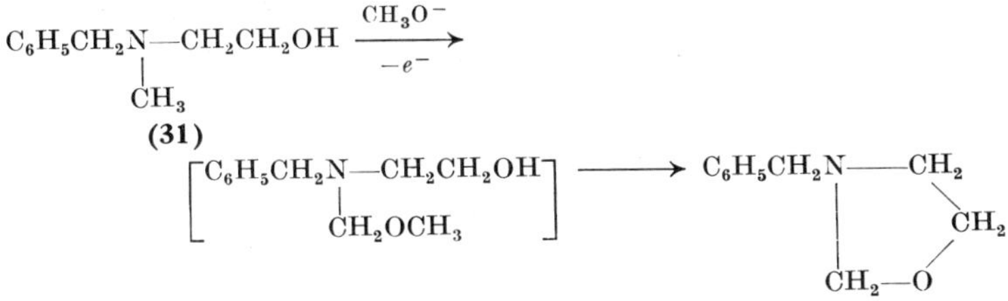

$$\underset{\underset{CH_3}{|}}{C_6H_5CH_2N}-CH_2CH_2OH \xrightarrow[-e^-]{CH_3O^-}$$

(31)

$$\left[\underset{\underset{CH_2OCH_3}{|}}{C_6H_5CH_2N}-CH_2CH_2OH \right] \longrightarrow \underset{\underset{CH_2-O}{|}}{\underset{\underset{}{|}}{C_6H_5CH_2N}}\underset{\underset{CH_2}{}}{\overset{\overset{CH_2}{}}{\diagdown}} \qquad (17)$$

(32)

III. Cathodic Cyclizations

The literature on electrolytic reductions of organic compounds (25) far exceeds that on oxidations. Many functional groups have been cathodically reduced with resultant formation of cyclic compounds: carbonyl functions (26–28), α-aminoketones (29,30), nitro compounds (31–34), organomercurials (35), halogen derivatives (36–38), and activated olefins (39–42).

A. CARBOXYLIC ACID DERIVATIVES

A keto acid of appropriate structure can be reduced electrochemically to yield a lactone. Bredt (26) has shown that 3-oxocamphononic acid (33) on reduction in aqueous sulfuric acid forms 3-hydroxycamphononic acid lactone (34) in good yield [eq. (18)].

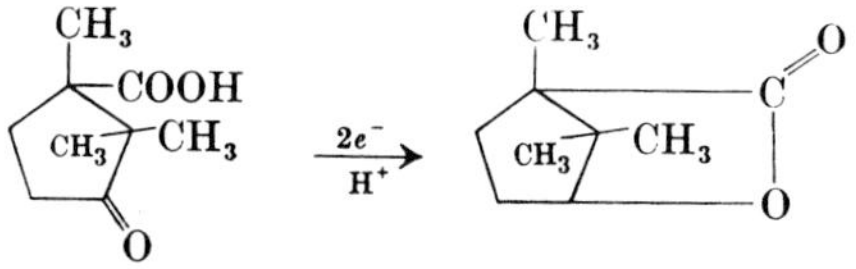

$$(33) \xrightarrow{2e^-, H^+} (34) \quad (18)$$

Similarly, Wawzonek, Laitinen, and Kwiatkowski (28) have found that the reduction of various esters of o-benzoylbenzoic acid gives 3-phenylphthalide, eq. (19).

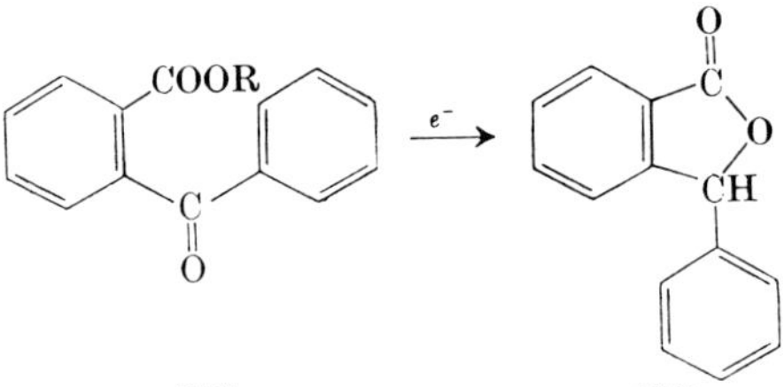

$$(35) \xrightarrow{e^-} (36) \quad (19)$$

The electrochemical reduction of the diammonium salt of an α,β-dicarboxylic acid yields a lactone. For example, (27), diammonium o-phthalate (37) gives the corresponding lactone (38) in almost quantitative yield [eq. (20)].

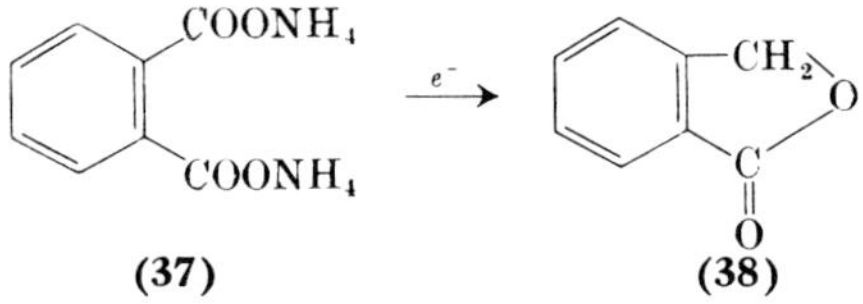

$$(37) \xrightarrow{e^-} (38) \quad (20)$$

B. NITRO COMPOUNDS

The electrochemical reduction of aromatic nitro compounds was shown (43) to yield coupled azo derivatives by Elbs and Kopp. The

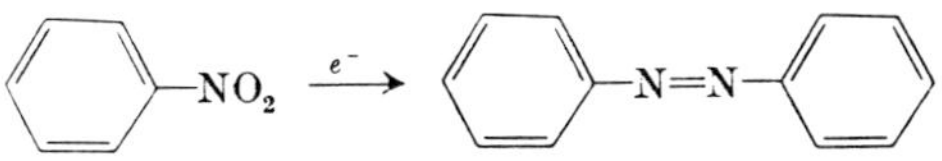

$$\text{Ph-NO}_2 \xrightarrow{e^-} \text{Ph-N=N-Ph} \tag{21}$$

application of this reaction [eq. (21)] to the synthesis of cyclic compounds was first accomplished by Wohlfahrt (33) who reduced 2,2'-dinitrobiphenyl **(39)** and obtained benzo[c]cinnoline **(40)** in 95% yield [eq. (22)]. Subsequently, Wittig and Stichnoth (32) obtained

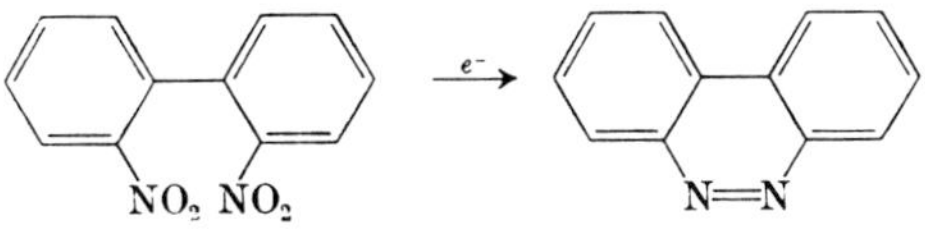

$$(39) \xrightarrow{e^-} (40) \tag{22}$$

1,10-dimethyl-3,4-benzo[c]cinnoline **(42)** from the electrochemical reduction of 6,6'-dinitro-2,2'-bitolyl **(41)** (6), eq. (23). The reduction of a nitro compound can be controlled electrochemically to yield the hydroxylamine. Gleu and Pfannstiel (31) used this fact to obtain

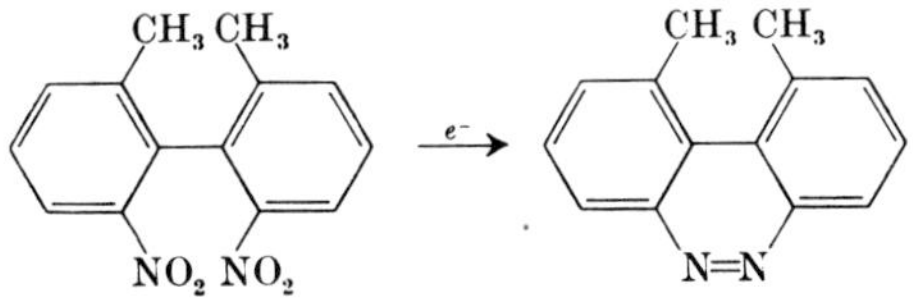

$$(41) \xrightarrow{e^-} (42) \tag{23}$$

benzisozoline-4-carboxylic acid **(44)** from the reduction of 3-nitrophthalic acid **(43)** [eq. (24)].

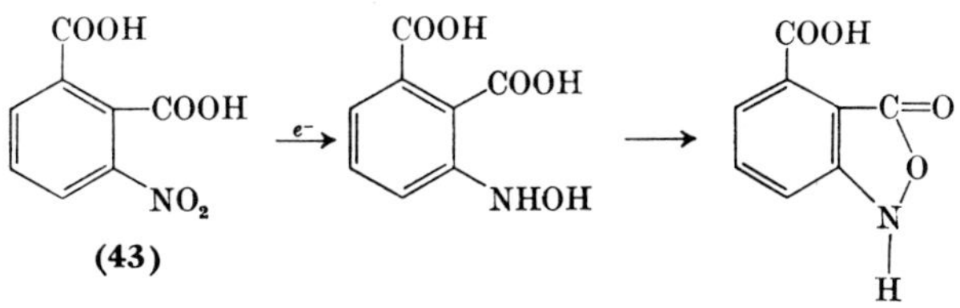

$$(43) \xrightarrow{e^-} \text{(NHOH intermediate)} \rightarrow (44) \tag{24}$$

C. OXIMES

Lund and co-workers (44,45) have found that the controlled electrolysis of "fluorescein oxime" **(45)** and "phenolphthalein oxime" **(47)** yields cyclic lactams as the major product, eqs. (25) and (26).

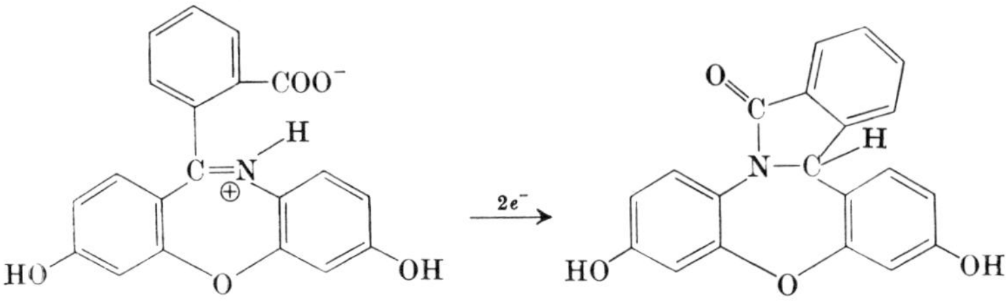

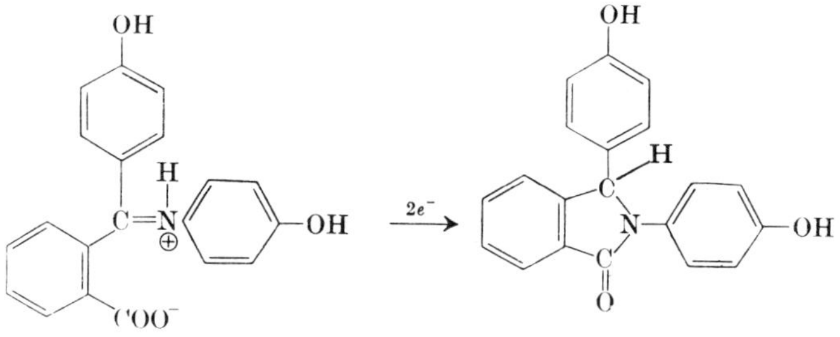

D. MERCURIALS

Only one example of the reduction of an organomercurial to yield cyclic products has been reported. Recently, Dessy and Kandil (35) have shown that 1-phenylethynyl-8-chloromercurynaphthalene **(49)** is converted electrochemically to 1-phenylacenaphthalene **(50)** presumably by way of an intramolecular anionic attack on the triple bond, eq. (27).

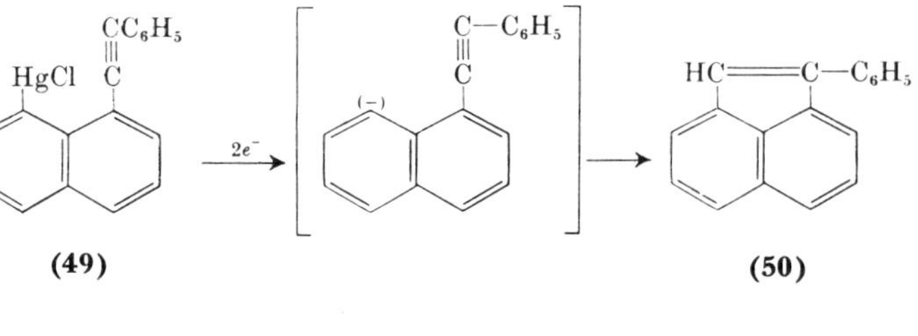

E. HALIDES

The reduction of vicinal dihalides has been shown to yield olefins. In the simplest case, 1,2-dibromomethane yields ethylene as well as ethane on electrochemical reduction (35). This reaction has been applied to the formation of cyclic products. Rifi (37) has shown that 1-chloro-3-bromobutane **(51)**, 1,3-dibromo-1,3-dimethylcyclobutane **(52)**, and 1,1,3,3-tetrachloro-2,2,4,4-tetramethylcyclobutane **(53)** all yield bicyclobutane derivatives on electrochemical reduction [eqs. (28)–(30)]. The reaction was extended to α,ω-dihaloalkanes with good

$$Cl\!\!-\!\!\diamondsuit\!\!-\!\!Br \longrightarrow \diamondsuit + \diamondsuit + \diamondsuit \qquad (28)$$
$$\text{(51)} \qquad (60\%) \quad (20\%) \quad (10\%)$$

$$\underset{\text{(52)}}{\overset{CH_3 \quad CH_3}{\underset{Br \quad Br}{\diamondsuit}}} \longrightarrow CH_3\!\!-\!\!\diamondsuit\!\!-\!\!CH_3 \qquad (29)$$

$$\underset{\text{(53)}}{\overset{CH_3 \ CH_3}{\underset{CH_3 \ CH_3}{\overset{Cl \quad Cl}{\underset{Cl \quad Cl}{\diamondsuit}}}}} \longrightarrow \underset{CH_3 \ CH_3}{\overset{CH_3 \ CH_3}{Cl\!\!-\!\!\diamondsuit\!\!-\!\!Cl}} \qquad (30)$$

success. The size of the rings, however, was limited to three and four members. The reduction of 1,3-dibromopropane **(53a)** and 1,4-dibromobutane **(55)** gave cyclopropane and cyclobutane, respectively [eqs. (31)–(32)]. Spiropentane **(58)** was obtained from the electrolysis

$$\underset{\text{(53a)}}{\overset{CH_2}{\underset{BrCH_2 \quad CH_2Br}{\diagdown}}} \xrightarrow{2e^-} \triangle \qquad (31)$$
$$\qquad \qquad \text{(54)}$$

$$\underset{\text{(55)}}{\overset{CH_2\!\!-\!\!CH_2}{\underset{BrCH_2 \quad CH_2Br}{\diagdown}}} \xrightarrow{2e^-} \square + \text{butane} \qquad (32)$$
$$\qquad \qquad (25\%) \ (75\%)$$
$$\qquad \qquad \text{(56)}$$

of 1,3-dibromo-2,2-bis(bromomethyl)propane **(57)** [eq. (33)]. Attempts to form cyclopentane from 1,5-dibromopentane were unsuccessful.

$$\underset{\text{(57)}}{\overset{BrCH_2 \quad CH_2Br}{\underset{BrCH_2 \quad CH_2Br}{\diagdown\!\!\diagup}}} \xrightarrow{4e^-} \bowtie \qquad (33)$$
$$\qquad \qquad \qquad \text{(58)}$$

Three possible mechanisms can be written for the reductive cyclization of dihalo compounds. The rate-determining step is probably a one-electron reduction which yields a radical and a halide anion. Of the three modes of decomposition of the intermediate A [eq. (34)],

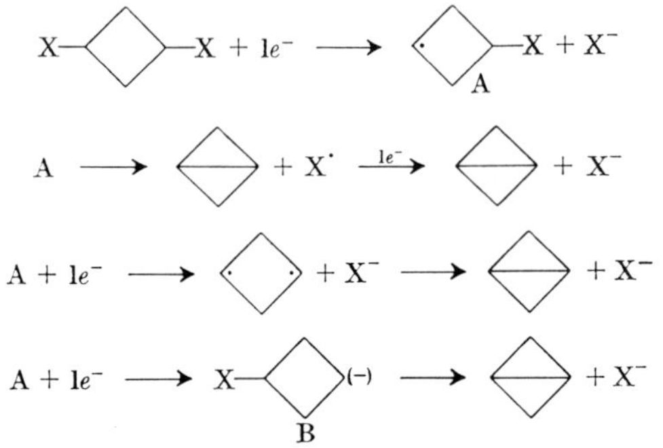

$$X-\square-X + 1e^- \longrightarrow \underset{A}{\square-X} + X^- \quad (34)$$

$$A \longrightarrow \square + X^{\cdot} \xrightarrow{1e^-} \square + X^- \quad (35)$$

$$A + 1e^- \longrightarrow \square + X^- \longrightarrow \square + X^- \quad (36)$$

$$A + 1e^- \longrightarrow \underset{B}{X-\square^{(-)}} \longrightarrow \square + X^- \quad (37)$$

Rifi indicates that the most likely is eq. (37), i.e., the further reduction of the radical to the anion B followed by the intramolecular displacement of the halogen yielding the observed cyclic products. To lend convincing support to this proposal, Rifi has shown that the electrochemical reduction of 3-bromopropyltriethylammonium bromide (59) yielded only cyclopropane and triethylamine [eq. (38)]. The displacement of triethylamine by the carbanion is clearly the most likely route in this system.

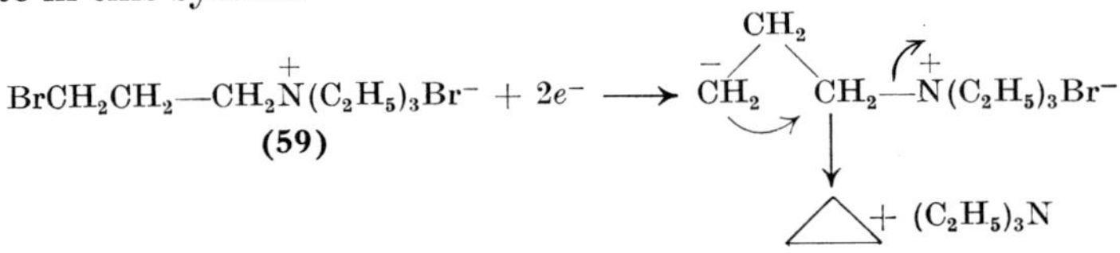

$$\underset{(59)}{BrCH_2CH_2-CH_2\overset{+}{N}(C_2H_5)_3Br^-} + 2e^- \longrightarrow \overset{CH_2}{\underset{CH_2}{\diagdown}}\overset{}{\underset{CH_2-\overset{+}{N}(C_2H_5)_3Br^-}{\diagup}} \longrightarrow \triangle + (C_2H_5)_3N \quad (38)$$

Another example of the formation of cyclic products from the electrochemical reduction of a dihalo compound (38) is the formation of (2,2)paracyclophane from α,α'-dibromo-*p*-xylene (60), eq. (39).

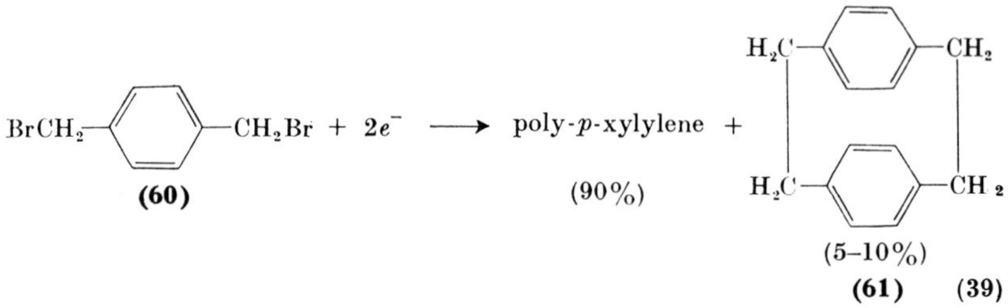

$$\underset{(60)}{BrCH_2-\bigcirc-CH_2Br} + 2e^- \longrightarrow \text{poly-}p\text{-xylylene} + \text{(61)} \quad (39)$$

(90%)   (5–10%)

The yield of (2,2)paracyclophane is only ~5–10%; the major product is poly-p-xylylene. Covitz (38) suggests that p-xylylene **(62)** is the major product of the electrochemical step [eq. (40)]; this step is probably concerted since its half-wave potential is considerably lower than that of model compounds. p-Xylylene does polymerize (46,47) and gives (2,2)paracyclophane by dimerization (48,49).

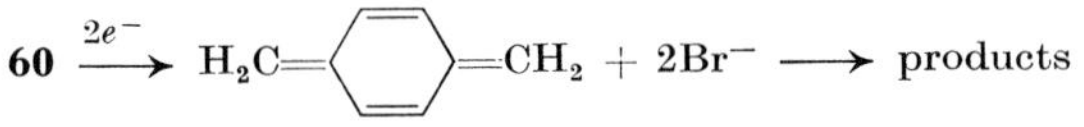

$$60 \xrightarrow{2e^-} H_2C=\langle\rangle=CH_2 + 2Br^- \longrightarrow \text{products} \quad (40)$$
$$(62)$$

F. BIS-ACTIVATED OLEFINS

To date the most widely explored electrochemical method for the formation of cyclic products is the reduction of bis-activated olefins (39–42), electrohydrocyclization (EHC). The method is applicable for the formation of heterocyclic as well as carbocyclic ring systems: o-bis(α-dicarbethoxyvinylamino)benzene **(63)** has been converted electrochemically to 2,3-bis(dicarbethoxymethyl)-1,2,3,4-tetrahydroquinoxaline **(64)** in 86% yield [eq. (41)]; 1,2-bis(2-ethoxycarbonylvinyloxy)ethane **(65)** gives 2,3-bis(ethoxycarbonylmethyl)-1,4-dioxane **(66)** in 89% yield, eq. (42). In the carbocyclic ring systems, the

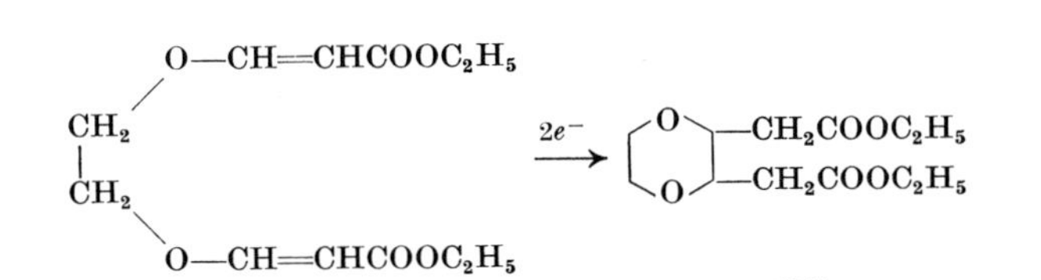

$$\text{(63)} \xrightarrow{2e^-} \text{(64)} \quad (41)$$

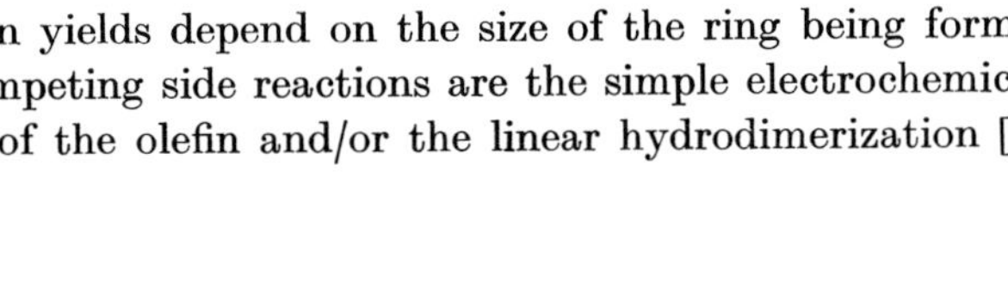

$$\text{(65)} \xrightarrow{2e^-} \text{(66)} \quad (42)$$

cyclization yields depend on the size of the ring being formed. The major competing side reactions are the simple electrochemical hydrogenation of the olefin and/or the linear hydrodimerization [eq. (43)].

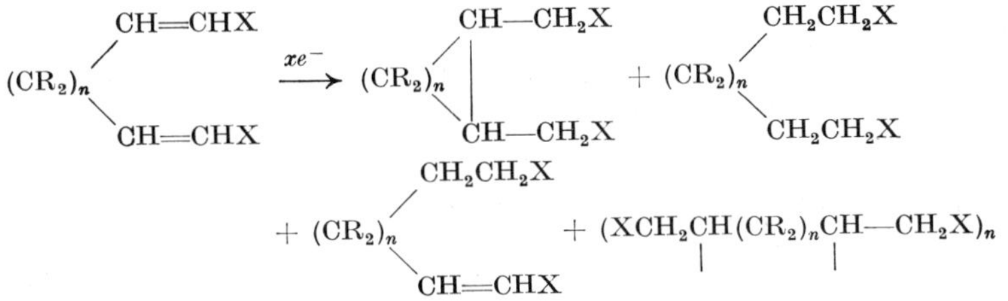

$$\underset{\text{CH=CHX}}{\overset{\text{CH=CHX}}{(CR_2)_n}} \xrightarrow{xe^-} \underset{\text{CH—CH}_2X}{\overset{\text{CH—CH}_2X}{(CR_2)_n|}} + \underset{\text{CH}_2\text{CH}_2X}{\overset{\text{CH}_2\text{CH}_2X}{(CR_2)_n}}$$

$$+ \underset{\text{CH=CHX}}{\overset{\text{CH}_2\text{CH}_2X}{(CR_2)_n}} + (XCH_2CH(CR_2)_nCH\text{—}CH_2X)_n \quad (43)$$

The cyclopropyl, cyclopentyl, and cyclohexyl rings were formed in yields of 90%, see Table I. In the case of the cyclobutyl and cycloheptyl rings, considerably poorer yields were obtained. All attempts to form 8-, 14-, and 18-membered rings failed.

TABLE I

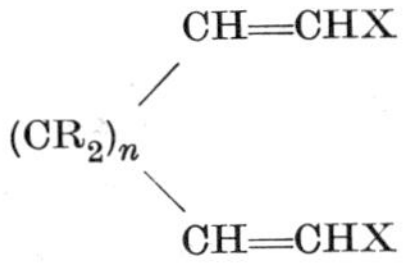

$$\underset{\text{CH=CHX}}{\overset{\text{CH=CHX}}{(CR_2)_n}}$$

n	Ring size	R	X	% Yield, cyclic product
1	3	C_2H_5	$CO_2C_2H_5$	98
2	4	H	$CO_2C_2H_5$	41
2	4	H	CN	15
3	5	H	$CO_2C_2H_5$	100
4	6	H	$CO_2C_2H_5$	90
5	7	H	$CO_2C_2H_5$	~10
6	8	H	$CO_2C_2H_5$	0

Substituents in the β-olefinic position militate against the formation of cyclic products. 2-Phenyl-2,7-nonadiene-1,9-dioate **(67)** gave 1-phenyl-1,2-cyclopentanediacetate **(68)** in 65% yield as compared to a nearly quantitative yield in the des-phenyl compound.

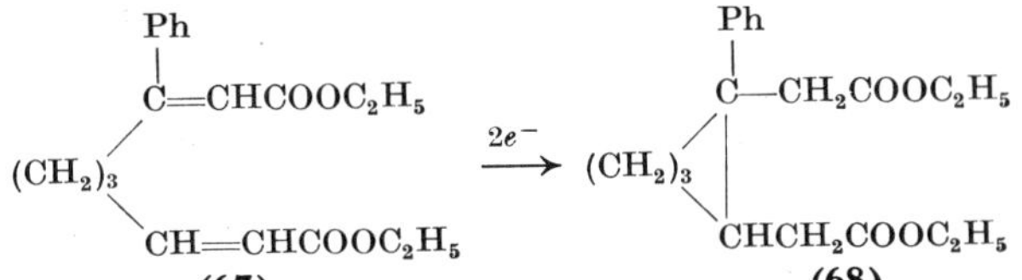

$$\underset{\underset{\text{CH=CHCOOC}_2H_5}{}}{\overset{\overset{\text{Ph}}{|}}{\underset{(CH_2)_3}{\overset{C=CHCOOC_2H_5}{}}}} \xrightarrow{2e^-} \underset{\underset{\text{CHCH}_2\text{COOC}_2H_5}{}}{\overset{\overset{\text{Ph}}{|}}{\underset{(CH_2)_3}{\overset{C\text{—}CH_2COOC_2H_5}{|}}}} \quad (44)$$

$$\text{(67)} \qquad\qquad \text{(68)}$$

The EHC reaction has been extended to the formation of the bicyclic norbornane ring system. The electrolysis of diethyl-cis-1,3-cyclopentanediacrylate (69) gave diethyl-trans-2,3-norbornanediacetate (70) in 37% yield. This example of a transannular cyclization gives a considerably lower yield than the formation of the simple five-membered ring. The angle strain in the bicyclic system is probably the cause of the lower yield.

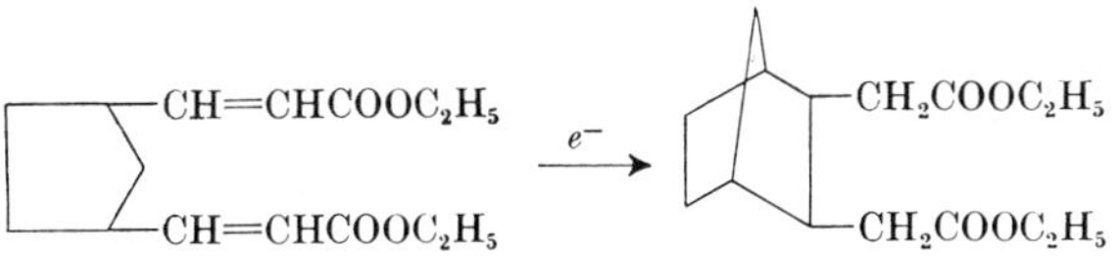

$$\text{(69)} \xrightarrow{e^-} \text{(70)} \qquad (45)$$

where (69) is diethyl-cis-1,3-cyclopentanediacrylate with two —CH=CHCOOC$_2$H$_5$ groups, and (70) is the norbornane bicyclic with two —CH$_2$COOC$_2$H$_5$ groups.

The mechanism of the electrochemical cyclization of bis-activated olefins has been studied intensively. From polarographic, coulometric, and controlled potential electrolysis data, a concerted reduction–cyclization mechanism has been proposed. The bis-activated olefin is reduced and cyclized in a single one-electron rate-determining step forming the anion radical (71). This anion radical is subsequently

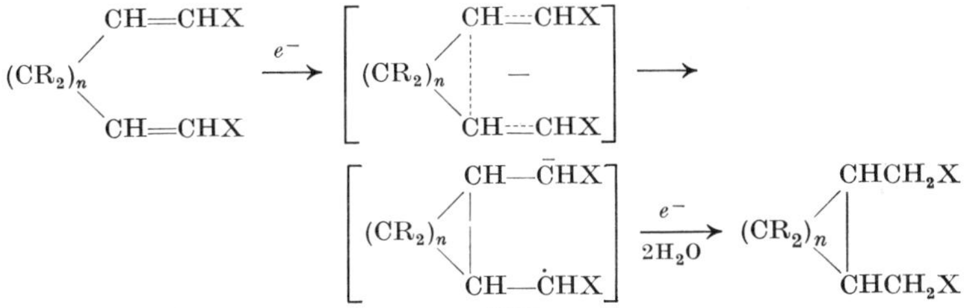

$$(CR_2)_n \begin{matrix} CH=CHX \\ \\ CH=CHX \end{matrix} \xrightarrow{e^-} \left[(CR_2)_n \begin{matrix} CH \cdots CHX \\ | \\ CH \cdots CHX \end{matrix} \right] \longrightarrow$$

$$\left[(CR_2)_n \begin{matrix} CH-\bar{C}HX \\ | \\ CH-\dot{C}HX \end{matrix} \right] \xrightarrow[2H_2O]{e^-} (CR_2)_n \begin{matrix} CHCH_2X \\ | \\ CHCH_2X \end{matrix} \qquad (46)$$

(71)

reduced in another one-electron step and then protonated to yield the observed cyclic products. The reaction is an overall two-electron process.

Two other examples of the use of activated olefins in the formation of cyclic products have been observed, one involving a reduction–displacement sequence and the other the apparent dimerization of two electrochemically-generated anion radicals. Dimethyl o-[(bis-β-ethoxycarbonyl)vinyl]phenethylsulfonium p-toluenesulfonate (72) gives diethyl-3-indanylmalonate **(73)** on electrochemical reduction [eq. (47)]. 1,4-*bis*-Dicyanomethyl-2,3,5,6-tetraphenylbenzene **(75)** is formed

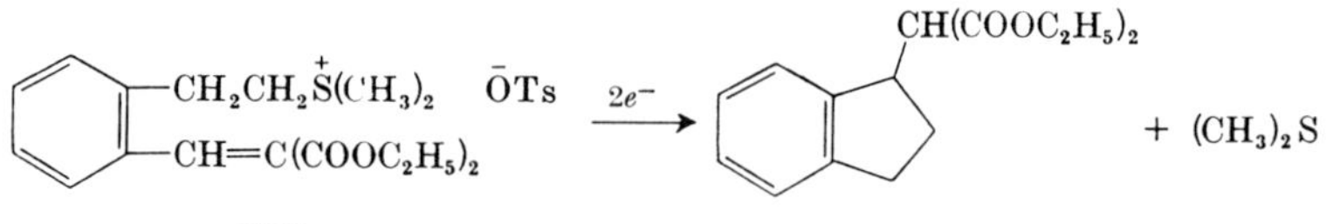

$$\text{(72)} \xrightarrow{2e^-} \text{(73)} + (CH_3)_2S \qquad (47)$$

where **(72)** is the o-substituted benzene with $-CH_2CH_2\overset{+}{S}(CH_3)_2\ \bar{O}Ts$ and $-CH=C(COOC_2H_5)_2$ groups, and **(73)** is the indane bearing $CH(COOC_2H_5)_2$.

from the electrochemical reduction of dicyanomethylene-diphenyl-cyclopropene **(74)** [eq. (48)].

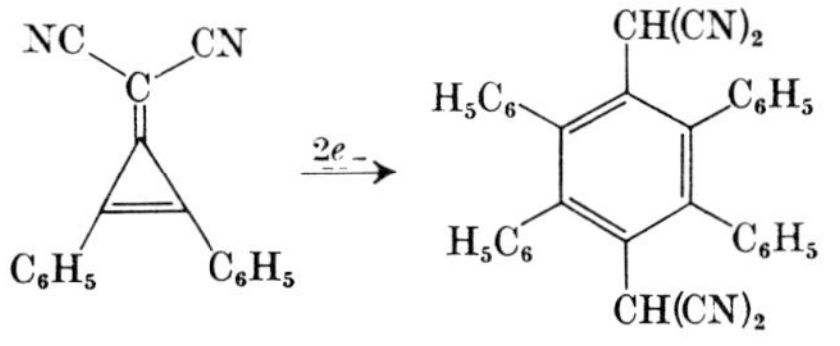

$$\text{(74)} \xrightarrow{2e^-} \text{(75)} \qquad (48)$$

where **(74)** is the cyclopropene with $=C(CN)_2$ and two C_6H_5 groups, and **(75)** is the benzene ring with four C_6H_5 substituents and two $CH(CN)_2$ groups in the 1,4-positions.

G. BICYCLIC KETO AMINES

Leonard, Swann, and co-workers (29,30) have employed electrochemical reduction in an intriguing way to prepare monocyclic systems from bicyclic ones. It had been reported (51) by the same senior authors that reduction of 1-methyl-2-ethyl-3-piperidone **(76)** at a lead cathode in 30% sulfuric acid yields N-methylheptylamine **(77)** as the major product [eq. (49)]. By incorporating the α-aminoketone

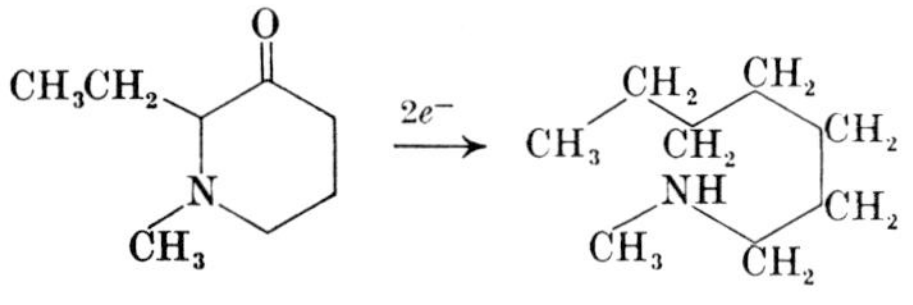

$$\text{(76)} \xrightarrow{2e^-} \text{(77)} \qquad (49)$$

structure in a bicyclic system it was possible by a similar technique to prepare medium-sized cyclic hydroxyamines (Table II).

Quite a variety of cyclic compounds can be prepared from the electrochemical reduction of organic compounds: lactams from keto acids and *o*-phthalic acids; cyclic azo compounds from dinitro compounds; bicyclobutanes, cyclopropanes, and cyclobutanes; and paracyclophanes from dihalo compounds, and heterocyclic as well as carbocyclic

TABLE II

Electrochemical Synthesis of Hydroxy-Substituted Cyclic Amines from Bicyclic α-Aminoketones

Compound	Product	Yield, %
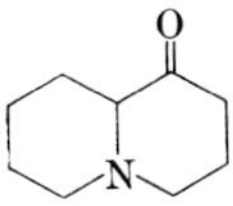 1-Ketoquinolizidine	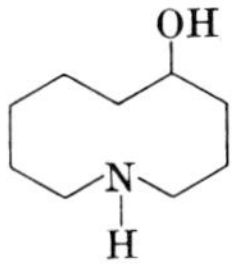 5-Hydroxyazacyclodecane	59
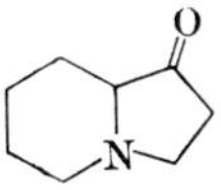 1-Keto-octahydropyrrocoline	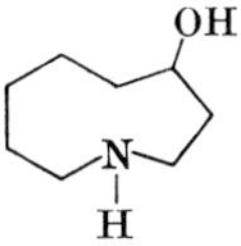 4-Hydroxyazacyclononane	48
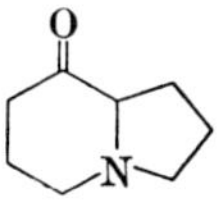 8-Keto-octahydropyrrocoline	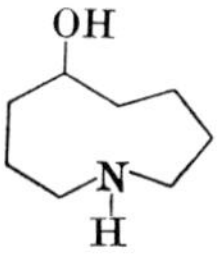 5-Hydroxyazacyclononane	47
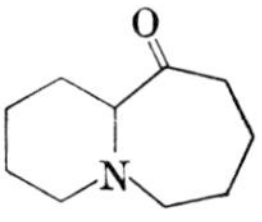 6-Keto-1-azabicyclo[5.4.0]hendecane	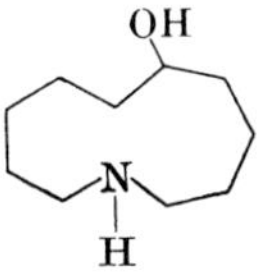 6-Hydroxyazacyclohendecane	71
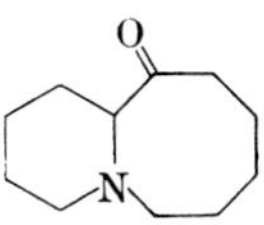 7-Keto-1-azabicyclo[6.4.0]dodecane	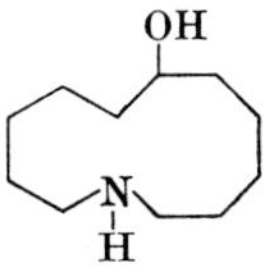 7-Hydroxyazacyclododecane	42

rings up to cycloheptane from bis-activated olefins. More work is necessary in these areas to define the further uses and limits of electrochemical cyclization reactions.

IV. EC Cyclizations

EC (electrochemical-plus-chemical) reactions are construed for our purposes to include those cyclization reactions in which (1) an intermediate is formed electrochemically and subsequently reacts intermolecularly with another substrate to produce a cyclic product or (2) a chemical cyclization reaction is preceded by an electrochemical reaction which was purposely designed to give a product capable of undergoing the chemical step. The literature on this category of reactions is rather diffuse and does not appear under a formal title or heading. As a result, it is almost impossible to be all-inclusive in reviewing this type of reaction. Therefore, only illustrative examples of the various types of reactions that have been carried out are given.

It is sometimes difficult to judge from the results reported whether cyclization occurred in the course of the electrolysis or in the course of the isolation of products.

A. KOLBE REACTIONS

Electrochemical steps have been used to synthesize large ring compounds. For example, Ställberg-Stenhagen (52) has synthesized ± muscone using the Kolbe electrolysis in the reaction sequence. A "crossed-Kolbe" electrolysis of the sodium salts of methyl hydrogen tridecanoate **(78)** and methyl hydrogen β-methylglutarate **(79)** yielded β-methyl thapsic acid **(80)**. This product was subsequently converted to the diacid chloride and then to the cyclic diketone followed by conversion to muscone **(81)**.

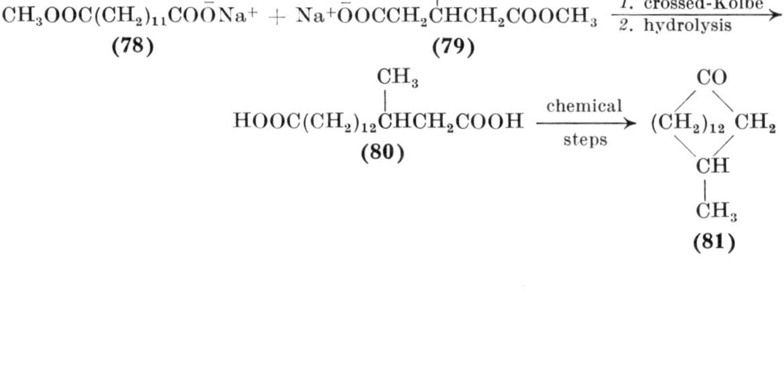

$$CH_3OOC(CH_2)_{11}COO^-Na^+ + Na^+\bar{O}OCCH_2\underset{|}{\overset{CH_3}{C}}HCH_2COOCH_3 \xrightarrow[\text{2. hydrolysis}]{\text{1. crossed-Kolbe}}$$
$$(78) \qquad\qquad (79)$$

$$HOOC(CH_2)_{12}\underset{|}{\overset{CH_3}{C}}HCH_2COOH \xrightarrow{\text{chemical steps}} \underset{\underset{CH_3}{\overset{|}{CH}}}{\overset{CO}{(CH_2)_{12}}}CH_2 \quad (50)$$
$$(80) \qquad\qquad\qquad (81)$$

ELECTROCHEMICAL CYCLIZATION REACTIONS 275

Another use of the Kolbe reaction is illustrated in the reaction sequence developed by Šorm et al. (53), for the synthesis of 1,1,4,8-tetramethylcycloundecane (humulane). These workers electrolyzed the salts of methyl hydrogen γ-methylglutarate (82) and benzyl hydrogen β,β-dimethylglutarate (83) and obtained the crossed-Kolbe product. Hydrogenolysis of this material gave the half-ester (84). Another crossed-Kolbe reaction involving 84 and the salt of methyl hydrogen β-methylglutarate (85) gave the diester (86). Acyloin cyclization of (86) followed by reduction gave humulane (87).

$$\underset{(82)}{CH_3OOCCH(CH_3)CH_2CH_2COOH} + \underset{(83)}{HOOCCH_2C(CH_3)_2CH_2COOCH_2Ph} \xrightarrow[2.\ \text{hydrogenolysis}]{1.\ -2e^-,\ -2CO_2}$$

$$\underset{(84)}{CH_3OOCCH(CH_3)(CH_2)_3C(CH_3)_2CH_2COOH} \quad (51)$$

$$84 + \underset{(85)}{HOOCCH_2CH(CH_3)CH_2COOCH_3} \xrightarrow[-2CO_2]{-2e^-} (86)$$

$$\xrightarrow{\text{acyloin}} \xrightarrow{[H]} (87) \quad (52)$$

B. ANODIC METHOXYLATION

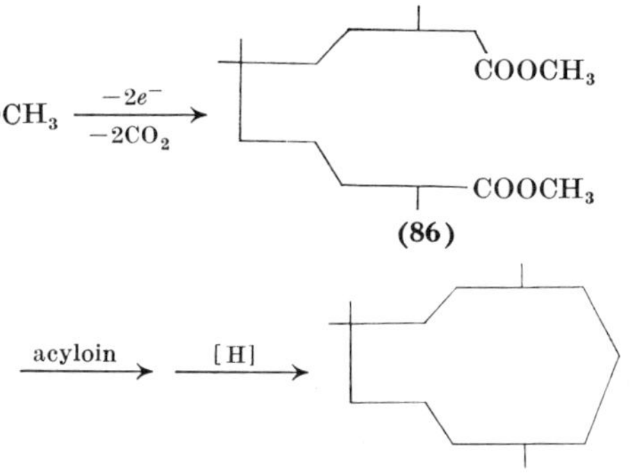

Ponomarev and Markushina (54) have synthesized a variety of spiro compounds of the 1,6-dioxaspiro-[4,4]-nonane type using electrochemical techniques. Electrooxidation of methoxide gave alkoxylation

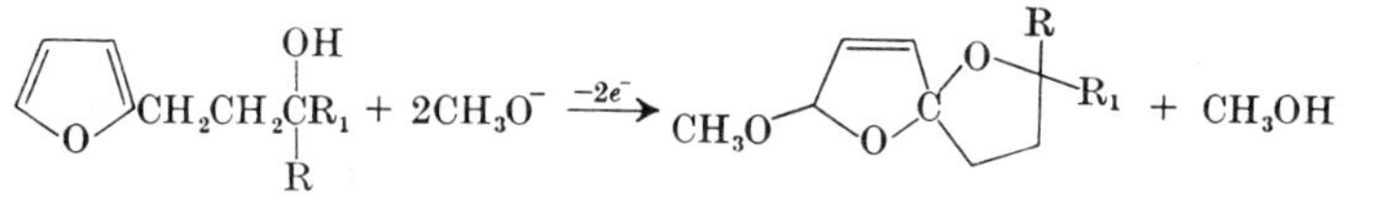

$$\underset{R}{\underset{|}{\text{furyl-}}CH_2CH_2CR_1(OH)} + 2CH_3O^- \xrightarrow{-2e^-} CH_3O-\text{(spiro)}-R_1 + CH_3OH \quad (53)$$

R = H, CH$_3$, (CH$_3$)$_2$CHCH$_2$, and CH$_3$CH$_2$ R$_1$ = H, H, H, and CH$_3$

of a variety of furylalkanols. At the same time the resultant methoxyl radicals effected a ring closure to give the above-mentioned spiro derivative, eq. (53).

C. CATHODIC FORMATION OF DICHLOROCARBENE

Wawzonek and Duty (55) have reported the electrochemical preparation of a carbene intermediate and the "trapping" of this intermediate with an olefin to give the corresponding cyclopropane derivative. Thus, electroreduction of carbon tetrachloride formed dichlorocarbene which, in the presence of tetramethylethylene, yielded 1,1-dichloro-2,2,3,3-tetramethylcyclopropane, eqs. (54).

$$CCl_4 + 2e^- \rightarrow CCl_3^- + Cl^- \tag{54a}$$

$$CCl_3^- \rightarrow CCl_2 + Cl^- \tag{54b}$$

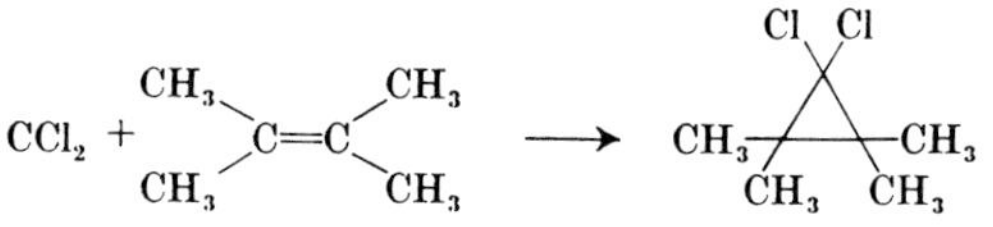

$$CCl_2 + \underset{CH_3}{\overset{CH_3}{>}}C=C\underset{CH_3}{\overset{CH_3}{<}} \longrightarrow \text{1,1-dichloro-2,2,3,3-tetramethylcyclopropane} \tag{54c}$$

D. CATHODIC FORMATION OF BENZYNE

In another study also involving electroreduction of an organohalogen compound, Wawzonek and Wagenknecht (56) have evidence for the production of the benzyne intermediate. (In a sense this reaction in itself is an electrochemical cyclization reaction.) The intermediate was trapped as the furan adduct.

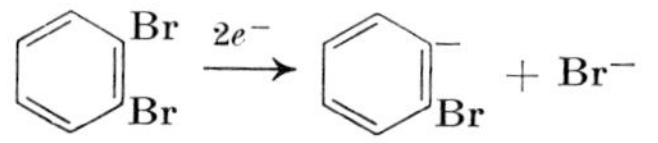

$$\text{o-dibromobenzene} \xrightarrow{2e^-} \text{bromobenzene anion} + Br^- \tag{55a}$$

$$\text{bromobenzene anion} \longrightarrow \text{benzyne} + Br^- \tag{55b}$$

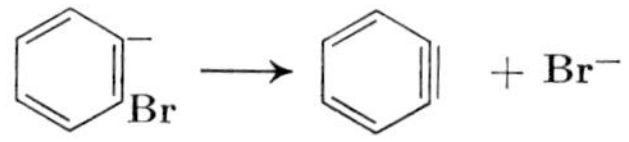

$$\text{benzyne} + \text{furan} \longrightarrow \text{furan adduct} \tag{55c}$$

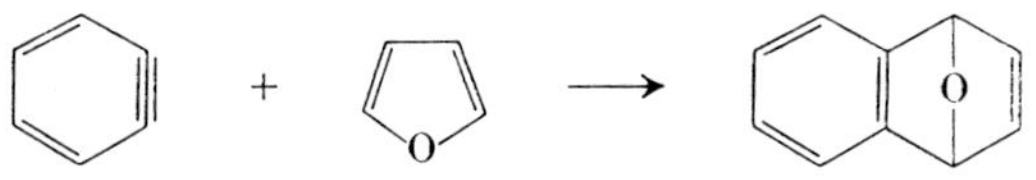

E. ANODIC FORMATION OF KETIMINE

Benkeser and co-workers (57) have noted a triazine synthesis from the electrooxidation of methylamine. Electrooxidation of methylamine using lithium chloride as the electrolyte resulted in a moderate yield of 1,3,5-trimethylhexahydro-*s*-triazine. Oxidation of the methylamine could have occurred in either of two ways: direct electrochemical oxidation or chemical oxidation via intermediately-formed atomic chlorine. Regardless of the oxidation pathway, the methylamine was presumably oxidized to methyleneimine. This intermediate then reacted with more methylamine followed by loss of ammonia and finally trimerization, eqs. (56).

$$CH_3NH_2 \xrightarrow{\text{electrooxidation}} CH_2=NH \underset{}{\overset{CH_3NH_2}{\rightleftarrows}} H_2NCH_2NHCH_3 \quad (56a)$$

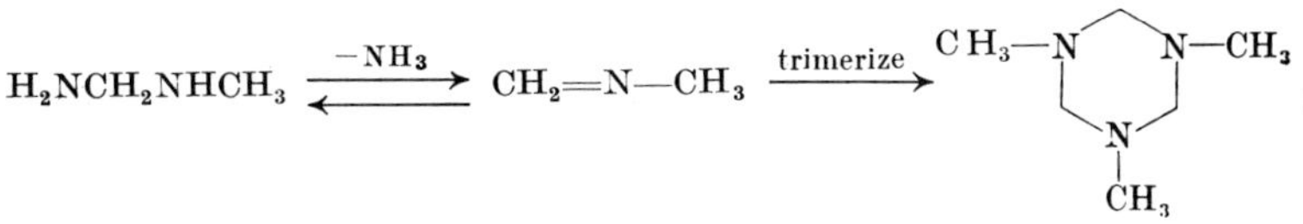

$$H_2NCH_2NHCH_3 \underset{}{\overset{-NH_3}{\rightleftarrows}} CH_2=N-CH_3 \xrightarrow{\text{trimerize}} \begin{array}{c} CH_3-N \quad N-CH_3 \\ \diagdown \quad \diagup \\ N \\ | \\ CH_3 \end{array} \quad (56b)$$

F. ANODIC THIOCYANATION

Melnikov and Cherkasova (58) have synthesized a series of benzothiazoles using electrochemical thiocyanation in the reaction sequence. These researchers electrooxidized thiocyanate ion in the presence of a variety of aromatic amines. The resulting products were then cyclized to the benzothiazoles. For example, *p*-phenetidine was thiocyanated to 2-amino-5-ethoxyphenyl thiocyanate. This product was then cyclized to 2-amino-6-ethoxybenzothiazole, eq. (57).

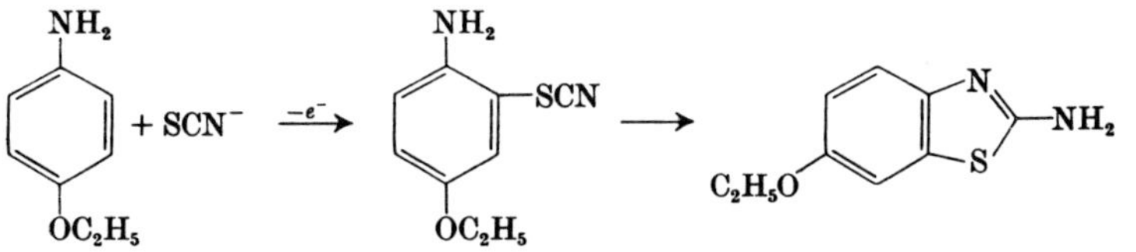

$$\underset{OC_2H_5}{\underset{|}{\bigcirc}}^{NH_2} + SCN^- \xrightarrow{-e^-} \underset{OC_2H_5}{\underset{|}{\bigcirc}}^{NH_2}\text{-SCN} \longrightarrow \underset{C_2H_5O}{\bigcirc}\overset{N}{\underset{S}{\diagup}}\text{-NH}_2 \quad (57)$$

Reductive coupling of acetone and acrylonitrile in 20% sulfuric acid (59) yielded a mixture of γ-hydroxy-γ-methylvaleronitrile **(88)** and γ,γ-dimethylbutyrolactone **(89)**, eq. (58).

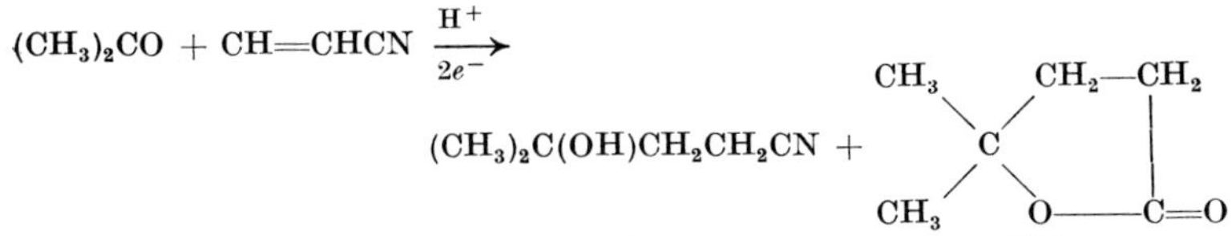

$$(CH_3)_2CO + CH=CHCN \xrightarrow[2e^-]{H^+}$$

$$(CH_3)_2C(OH)CH_2CH_2CN + \begin{array}{c} CH_3 \quad CH_2-CH_2 \\ \diagdown \diagup \quad | \\ C \quad | \\ \diagup \diagdown \quad | \\ CH_3 \quad O----C=O \end{array} \quad (58)$$

$$\quad\quad\quad\quad\quad\quad (88) \quad\quad\quad\quad (89)$$

Reductive coupling of benzalaniline and acrylonitrile yielded (60), among other products, 1,5-diphenyl-2-pyrrolidinone **(90)**; likewise

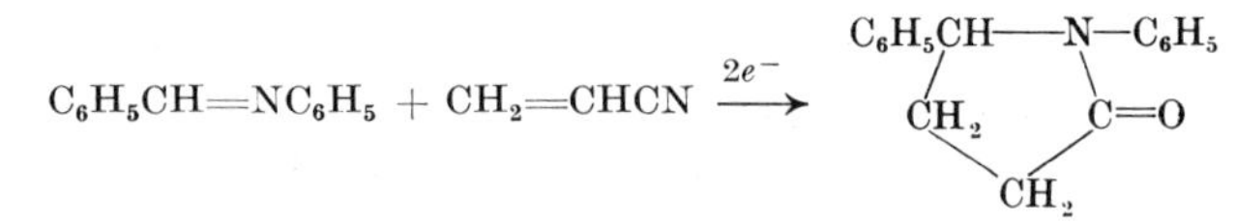

$$C_6H_5CH{=}NC_6H_5 + CH_2{=}CHCN \xrightarrow{2e^-} \underset{\textbf{(90)}}{\begin{array}{c} C_6H_5CH{-}\!\!-\!\!N{-}C_6H_5 \\ | \qquad\qquad | \\ CH_2 \qquad C{=}O \\ \diagdown \quad \diagup \\ CH_2 \end{array}} \qquad (59)$$

reductive coupling of azobenzene and ethyl acrylate formed 1,2-diphenyl-3-oxopyrazolidine **(91)**:

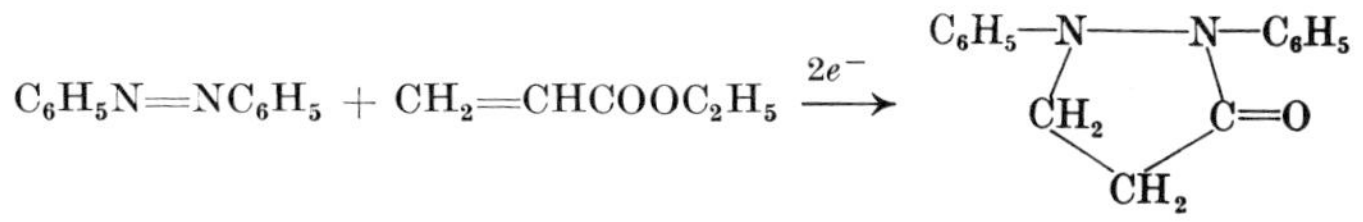

$$C_6H_5N{=}NC_6H_5 + CH_2{=}CHCOOC_2H_5 \xrightarrow{2e^-} \underset{\textbf{(91)}}{\begin{array}{c} C_6H_5{-}N{-}\!\!-\!\!N{-}C_6H_5 \\ | \qquad\qquad | \\ CH_2 \qquad C{=}O \\ \diagdown \quad \diagup \\ CH_2 \end{array}} \qquad (60)$$

V. Experimental

It cannot be emphasized too often that organic chemists who wish to carry out electrochemical syntheses will find that the necessary equipment is very simply assembled. The apparatus and procedures used, e.g., by B. C. L. Weedon in his studies of the Kolbe reaction have been described in a previous volume of this series (6). The "cell" used in the preparation of 1,14-tetradecanedioic acid (39) was a three-necked flask. Detailed discussions of techniques are presented by Swann (61) and by Allen (62).

A. *CIS*-2,4-DICARBOMETHOXYBICYCLOBUTANE (15)

trans,trans,trans-1,3-Dicarboxy-2,4-dicarbomethoxycyclobutane (1.0 g, 3.85 mmole) was dissolved in 40 ml of dry methanol. About 5% of the diacid diester was converted to the salt by the addition of sodium metal (0.01 g, 0.4 mmole). The system was purged with nitrogen and sealed. The gaseous products from the electrolysis were allowed to expand into a balloon. The solution was electrolyzed at a potential of 80–90 V between two smooth platinum electrodes until it became basic, ca. 4–5 hr at a current of 1.0–0.55 A. The electrolysis mixture was cooled by means of an ice bath. At the end of the reaction, the solvent was removed at reduced pressure while keeping the reaction mixture cold. The residual dark yellow solution was chromatographed on a

2 m × 6 mm column packed with 30% SE-30 on Chromosorb P at 220°. A white crystalline solid was collected. Repeated sublimation of this material gave cis-2,4-dicarbomethoxybicyclobutane, mp 83–85°.

B. 4-PHENYL-3,4-DIHYDROCOUMARIN (12)

A solution of 3,3-diphenylpropanoic acid (5.37 g) and sodium acetate (1.59 g) in 30 ml of acetic acid was electrolyzed for 38 hr using two platinum foil electrodes (1.25 cm × 1.25 cm) at a current of 0.2 A. The solution was stirred magnetically and maintained between 32–38° by external cooling. The majority of the solvent was removed by distillation at reduced pressure and the residue was dissolved in ether. The ether solution was washed twice with 5% aqueous ammonium hydroxide and water, dried over magnesium sulfate, and filtered and evaporated to yield 3.85 g of a thick, amber oil. 4-Phenyl-3,4-dihydrocoumarin was isolated by column chromatography on silicic acid with hexane–benzene mixtures as elutant. Recrystallization from ethanol gave a solid, mp 81.5–83.5°, undepressed on admixture with an authentic sample.

C. 1,3-DIMETHYLBICYCLOBUTANE (37)

A solution of 1,3-dibromo-1,3-dimethylcyclobutane (50 g, 0.2 mole) in 230 ml of dimethylformamide/lithium bromide solution* was introduced into the cathode chamber of an H cell. 150 ml of the same dimethylformamide/lithium bromide solution was placed in the anode chamber. The cathode was a mercury pool, the anode a platinum wire. The compartments were separated by a sintered disk. 40 V was applied across the cell resulting in a current of 0.5 A. These conditions were maintained for 16 hr. Distillation of the crude electrolysis solution gave 1,3-dimethylbicyclobutane, bp 54.5° in 55–94% yield from successive runs.

D. 2,3-BIS(DICARBETHOXYMETHYL)-
1,2,3,4-TETRAHYDROQUINOXALINE (39)

The divided cell used has been described (63). The catholyte consisted of o-bis(β-dicarbethoxyvinylamino)benzene (40.0 g; 0.089 mole), 28.0 g of tetraethylammonium p-toluenesulfonate, and 12.0 g of water dissolved in 104.0 g of acetonitrile. The anolyte was a saturated

* Concentration of salt, $0.1M$.

solution of tetraethylammonium p-toluenesulfonate in water. The electrolysis was carried out at a current of 2 A for 2.38 hr. The temperature of the solution was 25° and the cathode voltage -1.73 to -1.85 V (vs. SCE). The catholyte was poured into water and extracted two times with methylene chloride. The organic layers were combined, washed with water, and dried over anhydrous sodium sulfate. The solvent was removed by distillation at reduced pressure. The oily residue on crystallization from methanol gave 2,3-bis-(dicarbethoxymethyl)-1,2,3,4-tetrahydroquinoxaline (34.4 g, 0.077 mole), an 86% yield based on current input.

E. DIETHYL CYCLOPENTANE-1,2-DIACETATE (40)

The divided cell mentioned above was used. The catholyte consisted of diethyl 2,7-nonadiene-1,9-dioate (40.0 g), 26.9 g of tetraethylammonium p-toluenesulfonate, and 10.0 g of water dissolved in 70 g of acetonitrile. The anolyte was a saturated solution of tetraethylammonium p-toluenesulfonate in water. The electrolysis was carried out at a current of 2 A for 2.25 hr with a solution temperature of 25° and a cathode voltage of -1.98 V (vs. SCE). The catholyte was diluted with water and extracted several times with methylene chloride. The organic extracts were combined, washed with water, dried over anhydrous sodium sulfate, and the solvent was removed by distillation. Distillation at reduced pressure gave 20.7 g of a mixture of 78% diethyl *trans*-cyclopentane-1,2-diacetate and 22% diethyl *cis*-cyclopentane-1,2-diacetate, bp 108–114° at 0.5 mm.

Note added in proof

The formation of decalin from the electrochemical reduction of 1,6-dibromocyclodecane, as well as the formation of cyclopropane from 1,3-dibromopropane, has been implied by Zavoda, Krupicka, and Sicher (64) from polarographic results. However, no reaction products were isolated in these cases.

ACKNOWLEDGMENTS

We are grateful to Dr. F. H. Covitz and Dr. M. R. Rifi of Union Carbide Corporation for permitting us to read the manuscripts of their papers before publication.

References

1. E. H. Rodd, *Chemistry of Carbon Compounds*, Vol. 2A, Elsevier, New York, 1953.
2. L. I. Belinkii, *Russ. Chem. Rev. (Eng. Trans.)*, **1964**, 551.
3. M. Julia, *Record Chem. Progr. (Kresge-Hooker Sci. Lib.)*, **25**, 3 (1964).
4. E. Vogel, *Angew. Chem.*, **72**, 4 (1960).
5. K. T. Finley, *J. Chem. Educ.*, **42**, 536 (1965).
6. B. C. L. Weedon, in *Advances in Organic Chemistry*, R. A. Raphael, E. C. Taylor, and H. Wynberg, Eds., Interscience, New York, 1960, Vol. 1, pp. 1–34.
7. B. L. Vanzetti, *Gazz. Chim. Ital.*, **34**, II, 511 (1904).
8. J. Walker and J. K. Wood, *J. Chem. Soc.*, **1906**, 598.
9. G. E. Svadkovskya and S. A. Voitkevich, *Russ. Chem. Rev. (Eng. Trans.)*, **1960**, 161, and references cited therein.
10. E. J. Corey, N. L. Bauld, R. T. LaLonde, J. Casanova, and E. T. Kaiser, *J. Am. Chem. Soc.*, **82**, 2645 (1960).
11. W. J. Koehl, Jr., *J. Org. Chem.*, **32**, 614 (1967).
12. W. A. Bonner and F. D. Mango, *J. Org. Chem.*, **29**, 430 (1964).
13. H. Iwaski, L. A. Cohen, and B. Witkop, *J. Am. Chem. Soc.*, **85**, 3701 (1963).
14. A. I. Scott, P. A. Dodson, F. McCapra, and M. B. Meyers, *J. Am. Chem. Soc.*, **85**, 3702 (1963).
15. A. F. Vellturo and G. W. Griffin, *J. Org. Chem.*, **31**, 2241 (1966).
16. J. G. Traynham and J. S. Dehn, *J. Am. Chem. Soc.*, **89**, 2139 (1967).
17. C. Walling, *Free Radicals in Solution*, Wiley, New York, 1957, p. 581.
18. P. J. Bunyan and D. H. Hey, *J. Chem. Soc.*, **1962**, 324.
19. P. J. Bunyan and D. H. Hey, *J. Chem. Soc.*, **1962**, 2771.
20. R. F. Carwood, C. J. Scott, and B. C. L. Weedon, *Chem. Commun.*, **1965**, 14.
21. C. G. Overberger and P. Kabasakalian, *J. Am. Chem. Soc.*, **79**, 3182 (1957).
22. E. A. Pasquinelli, *Anales Assoc. Quim. Arg.*, **31**, 181 (1943).
23. W. J. Koehl, Jr., U.S. Pat., 3,321,387, May 23, 1967.
24. N. L. Weinberg and E. A. Brown, *J. Org. Chem.*, **31**, 4058 (1966).
25. F. D. Popp and H. P. Schultz, *Chem. Rev.*, **62**, 19 (1962).
26. J. Bredt, *J. Prakt. Chem.*, **84**, 786 (1911).
27. B. Sakurai, *Bull. Chem. Soc. (Japan)*, **1**, 127 (1932).
28. S. Wawzonek, H. A. Laitinen, and S. J. Kwiatkowski, *J. Am. Chem. Soc.*, **66**, 827 (1944).
29. N. J. Leonard, S. Swann, Jr., and J. Figueras, Jr., *J. Am. Chem. Soc.*, **74**, 4620 (1952).

30. N. J. Leonard, S. Swann, Jr., and E. H. Mottus, *J. Am. Chem. Soc.*, **74**, 6251 (1952).
31. K. Gleu and K. Pfannstiel, *J. Prakt. Chem.*, **146**, 129 (1936).
32. G. Wittig and B. Stichnoth, *Ber.*, **68B**, 928 (1935).
33. T. Wohlfahrt, *J. Prakt. Chem. (Ser. 2)*, **65**, 295 (1902).
34. C. Baezner and H. Gardiol, *Ber.*, **39**, 2512 (1906).
35. R. E. Dessy and S. A. Kandil, *J. Org. Chem.*, **30**, 3857 (1965).
36. M. von Stackelberg and W. Stracke, *Z. Elektrochem.*, **53**, 118 (1949).
37. M. R. Rifi, *J. Am. Chem. Soc.*, **89**, 4442 (1967).
38. F. H. Covitz, *J. Am. Chem. Soc.*, **89**, 5403 (1967).
39. J. D. Anderson and M. M. Baizer, *Tetrahedron Letters*, **1966**, 511.
40. J. D. Anderson, M. M. Baizer, and J. P. Petrovich, *J. Org. Chem.*, **31**, 3890 (1966).
41. J. P. Petrovich, J. D. Anderson, and M. M. Baizer, *J. Org. Chem.*, **31**, 3897 (1966).
42. S. Andreades and E. W. Zahnow, Extended Abstracts, Electrochemical Society Meeting, May 7–12, 1967, Dallas, Texas, p. 70.
43. K. Elbs and O. Kopp, *Z. Elektrochem.*, **5**, 108 (1898).
44. H. Lund, P. Lunde, and F. Kaufmann, *Acta Chem. Scand.*, **20**, 1631 (1963).
45. H. Lund, *Acta Chem. Scand.*, **14**, 359 (1960).
46. L. A. Errede and J. M. Hoyt, *J. Am. Chem. Soc.*, **82**, 436 (1960).
47. J. R. Schaefgen, *J. Polymer Sci.*, **15**, 203 (1965).
48. L. A. Errede, R. S. Gregorian, and J. M. Hoyt, *J. Am. Chem. Soc.*, **82**, 5218 (1960).
49. L. A. Errede and J. P. Cassidy, *J. Am. Chem. Soc.*, **82**, 3653 (1960).
50. M. M. Baizer, *Tetrahedron Letters*, **1963**, 973.
51. N. J. Leonard, S. Swann, Jr., and H. L. Drydon, Jr., *J. Am. Chem. Soc.*, **74**, 2871 (1952).
52. S. Ställberg-Stenhagen, *Arkiv. Kemi*, **3**, 273 (1951).
53. F. Šorm, M. Streibl, V. Jarolím, L. Novotný, L. Dolejs, and V. Heront, *Chem. Ind. (London)*, **1954**, 252.
54. A. A. Ponomarev and I. A. Markushina, *Dokl. Akad. Nauk SSSR*, **126**, 99 (1959).
55. S. Wawzonek and R. Duty, *J. Electrochem. Soc.*, **108**, 1135 (1961).
56. S. Wawzonek and J. H. Wagenknecht, *J. Electrochem. Soc.*, **110**, 429 (1963).
57. R. A. Benkeser, E. M. Kaiser, and R. F. Lambert, *J. Am. Chem. Soc.*, **86**, 5272 (1964).
58. N. N. Melnikov and E. M. Cherkasova, *Zh. Obshch. Khim.*, **14**, 13 (1944).
59. K. Sugino and T. Nonaka, *J. Electrochem. Soc.*, **112**, 1241 (1965).
60. M. M. Baizer, J. D. Anderson, J. H. Wagenknecht, M. R. Ort, and J. P. Petrovich, *Electrochim. Acta*, **12**, 1377 (1967).

61. S. Swann, Jr., in *Technique of Organic Chemistry*, A. Weissberger, Ed., Interscience, New York, 1956, Vol. 2, pp. 385–523.
62. M. J. Allen, *Organic Electrode Processes*, Reinhold, New York, 1958.
63. M. M. Baizer, *J. Electrochem. Soc.*, **111,** 215 (1964).
64. J. Závada, J. Krupica, and J. Sicher, *Coll. Czech. Chem. Commun.*, **28,** 1664 (1963).

DIMETHYLSULFOXIDE (DMSO) IN ORGANIC SYNTHESIS

By

T. DURST *Department of Chemistry, University of Ottawa, Ottawa, Canada*

CONTENTS

I.	Introduction	286
II.	Methylsulfinyl Carbanion	289
	A. Preparation	289
	B. Reactions of Methylsulfinyl Carbanion	290
	1. Reaction with Ketones and Aldehydes	291
	2. Reaction with Imines	295
	3. Reaction with Esters	296
	4. Reaction with Alkyl Halides and Tosylates	301
	5. Reaction with Aromatic Halides	307
	6. Reaction with Aromatic and Olefinic Systems	309
	7. Miscellaneous Reactions of Methylsulfinyl Carbanion . .	314
III.	Dimethyloxosulfonium Methylid	318
	A. Trimethyloxosulfonium Salts	318
	B. Preparation of Dimethyloxosulfonium Methylid	320
	C. Reactions of Dimethyloxosulfonium Methylid	321
	1. Reaction with Ketones and Aldehydes	321
	2. Reaction with Carboxylic Acid Derivatives	330
	3. Additions to Conjugated Olefinic Systems	338
	4. Reaction with Carbon–Nitrogen Multiple Bonds . . .	339
	5. Miscellaneous Reactions	341
IV.	Dimethylsulfoxide Oxidations	343
	A. Oxidation of Alcohols	345
	B. Oxidation of Halides and Tosylates	352
	C. Other Oxidations	353
V.	Pummerer Rearrangements	356
VI.	Other Reactions Involving DMSO	365
	A. DMSO–DCC and Phenols	365
	B. DMSO and Active Methylene Compounds	370
	C. DMSO and Electron Deficient Species	374
	D. Reduction with Triphenylphosphine	376
VII.	Experimental	376
	A. Preparation of Methylsulfinyl Carbanion · ·	376
	B. Reaction of Methylsulfinyl Carbanion with Benzophenone . .	377

C. Reaction of Esters with Methylsulfinyl Carbanion. Preparation of β-Keto Sulfoxides. General Procedure. 377
D. Reduction of β-Keto Sulfoxides, Preparation of Ketones. General Procedure 378
E. Dimethyloxosulfonium Methylid. General Method of Preparation in Dimethyl Sulfoxide 378
F. Reaction of Dimethyloxosulfonium Methylid with Benzophenone 379
G. Oxidation of Testosterone with DMSO-DCC and Phosphoric Acid 379
H. Oxidation of Yohimbine to Yohimbinone with DMSO–Acetic Anhydride 380
I. Pummerer Rearrangement of β-Keto Sulfoxides 380
   1. To Hemithioacetals 380
   2. To Acetals 381
References 381

I. Introduction

The interest of chemists in dimethylsulfoxide (DMSO) began in the 1950's and was initially due to its properties as a highly polar solvent capable of causing enormous rate increases in a number of reactions, especially in those involving anionic species. Recent reviews on the subject include a consideration of DMSO as a solvent (1), DMSO as an oxidant (2), a bibliography of the chemistry of DMSO for the period 1961–1966 (3), and a more general survey of the chemistry of sulfoxides and sulfur ylids (4). In this review, the author will attempt to present a unifying picture of the chemistry of DMSO. Where useful, extensions of DMSO reactions to other sulfoxides will be commented upon. The literature has been surveyed to the end of 1967.

The physical properties of DMSO have been tabulated and discussed by a number of authors (1,3,5–8). DMSO has pyramidal geometry with the sulfur, oxygen, and carbon atoms at the corners of the pyramid. The carbon–hydrogen and carbon–sulfur bonds appear to be normal, single covalent bonds. Whether the sulfur–oxygen bond is best represented by a semipolar single bond analogous to the nitrogen–oxygen bond in tertiary amine oxides, or by a double bond ($2p$–$3d$ pi bonding) is still open to question (9). In view of the recent trend in usage favoring the double bonded structure, such a designation will also be used here.

The stimulus for regarding the potentials of DMSO as a reagent stems in large part from two publications which illustrate the two main types of reactions which DMSO can undergo. Kornblum and co-workers (10) reported in 1957 that a variety of phenacyl halides were oxidized to phenylglyoxals by simply dissolving these compounds in DMSO at room temperature in the presence of an acid acceptor such as sodium bicarbonate. Later these authors (11) showed that benzyl halides and many primary alkyl tosylates could be converted to aldehydes in relatively good yield (68–85%) by heating in DMSO containing bicarbonate to temperatures of 100–150° for less than 5 min. The oxidations in DMSO offered an obvious advantage over many of the other methods of oxidation since overoxidation to the corresponding acids did not occur even with sensitive aldehydes.

$$ArCOCH_2Br \xrightarrow[25°, 9\,hr]{DMSO} ArCOCHO \quad (70\text{–}95\%)$$

$$ArCH_2Br \xrightarrow[100°, 5\,min]{DMSO} ArCHO$$

$$RCH_2OTs \xrightarrow[150°, 3\,min]{DMSO} RCHO$$

These oxidations demonstrated the nucleophilicity of the oxygen atom of DMSO. They have since been shown to involve displacement of the tosylate or halide function by DMSO to form an intermediate alkoxysulfonium salt which produces a carbonyl compound and dimethylsulfide either by an intra- (12–14) or intermolecular route (14), the pathway depending on the relative acidities of the hydrogens involved. In addition, these reactions suggested that DMSO might react with other electrophilic species to give sulfonium salts of the type **1**. Such expectations have been realized and a wide variety of DMSO reactions have been observed which have involved initial formation of sulfonium salts.

$$RCH_2X + CH_3\overset{O}{\underset{\|}{S}}CH_3 \rightarrow RCH_2O-\overset{+}{S}(CH_3)_2 \quad X^-$$

(**1**)

Intramolecular decomposition

$$\underset{H}{RCH}-O-\overset{+}{S}(CH_3)_2 \xrightarrow{B^-} \underset{H}{RCH}-O-\overset{+}{S}\underset{CH_2^-}{\overset{CH_3}{\diagdown}} \longrightarrow RCHO + CH_3SCH_3$$

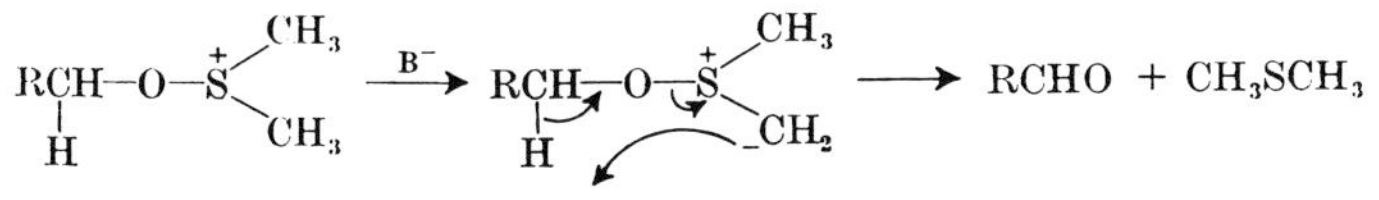

Intermolecular decomposition

$$\underset{H}{RCH}-O-\overset{+}{S}(CH_3)_2 \xrightarrow{B^-} RCHO + CH_3SCH_3$$

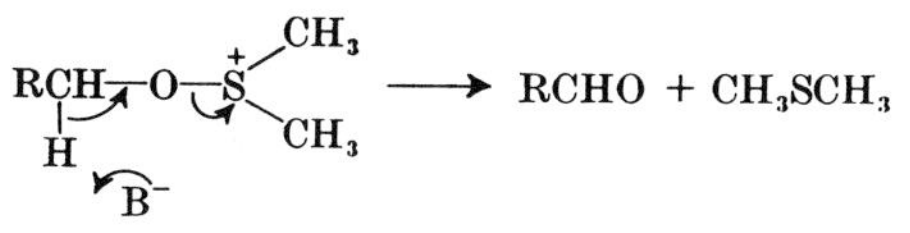

Dimethyloxysulfonium salts, depending on their structure, have been shown to undergo four basic types of transformations: (1) decomposition to a carbonyl compound and dimethylsulfide, (2) nucleophilic displacement on sulphur, (3) rearrangement to an α-substituted sulfide (Pummerer rearrangement), and (4) formation of an oxosulfonium salt.

1. Oxidation

$$(CH_3)_2\overset{+}{S}-OCHRR' \rightarrow RR'CO + CH_3SCH_3$$

2. Nucleophilic displacement

$$(CH_3)_2\overset{+}{S}-OR + N^- \rightarrow N-\overset{+}{S}(CH_3)_2 + \overset{-}{O}R$$

3. Pummerer rearrangement

$$(CH_3)_2\overset{+}{S}-OR \rightarrow CH_3SCH_2OR$$

4. Oxosulfonium salt formation

$$(CH_3)_2\overset{+}{S}-OR \rightarrow (CH_3)_2\underset{+}{\overset{O}{\overset{\|}{S}}}R$$

These transformations, i.e., initial sulfonium salt formation followed by further reaction according to one of the four pathways outlined above, can be used to explain most, if not all, of the chemistry in which DMSO reacts initially as a nucleophile, and can serve as a guideline in the prediction of the feasibility of new reactions. The experimental data which support this overall picture and the more intricate details of the individual steps will be considered at appropriate points in this article.

The other major area of DMSO chemistry, that of the conjugate base of DMSO–methylsulfinyl carbanion 2, was initiated by the work of Corey and Chaykovsky (15,16) who reported that the reaction of DMSO with finely powdered sodium hydride at 70–75° under nitrogen constituted a convenient and efficient synthesis of the sodium salt of the carbanion.* This finding, coupled with a study by these authors of some reactions of methylsulfinyl carbanion, in particular those with sulfonium salts (17), aldehydes (15,16), ketones (15,16), and esters (16,18) has opened a whole new field for the synthetic applicability of

* The trivial names "dimsyl sodium" and "dimsyl potassium" are also used to designate the sodium and potassium salts of methylsulfinyl carbanion. (G. G. Price and M. C. Whiting, *Chem. Ind. (London)*, **1963,** 775.

DMSO. A discussion of these reactions, including useful transformations of the initially formed products, is given in the next section.

II. Methylsulfinyl Carbanion

A. PREPARATION

Because of the relatively low acidity of DMSO, estimated to be 10^4 less than triphenylmethane (19,20), the generation of methylsulfinyl carbanion in stoichiometric yield requires the use of extremely strong bases. The most commonly used reagents are metal hydrides, metal amides, and metal alkyls, with the reagent of choice being closely related to the desired cation.

Sodium methylsulfinyl carbanion, as mentioned in the introduction, is usually and most conveniently prepared by heating finely powdered sodium hydride in DMSO under nitrogen at 70–80° for approximately one hour, or until hydrogen evolution ceases. Longer periods of heating, or higher temperatures, cause significant (16) and at times total decomposition of the carbanion (21). Solutions of methylsulfinyl carbanion are relatively stable at room temperature and lose only approximately 8% of their activity per week (20). The use of an ultrasound generator to promote the reaction of DMSO with sodium hydride at lower temperatures (50°) gives a solution of the carbanion which is even less prone to deterioration (22). This technique of preparation, coupled with freezing of the solution, allows storage of the carbanion solution for considerable periods of time without loss of activity. The extra expense of the ultrasound generator to produce a solution of prolonged stability is generally unnecessary but may be warranted in situations where sodium methylsulfinyl carbanion is used routinely and repeatedly. Anion concentrations may be determined by titration with formanilide using triphenylmethane as indicator (16).

Sodium methylsulfinyl carbanion has also been obtained by reaction of sodium metal with DMSO (20,23). This method, while perhaps intriguing, is not recommended since large amounts of sodium methylsulfenate are also formed which interfere in subsequent reactions (23). Sodium amide in DMSO also readily yields a solution of methylsulfinyl carbanion (15,16,24).

Solutions of the potassium salt in DMSO are usually prepared by reaction with potassium amide. The reaction occurs readily at room temperature and may require cooling if carried out on a large scale. Such solutions are stable for several days if stored under an inert atmosphere (24). The potassium derivative has also been obtained by reaction of DMSO with potassium metal (23). The same objection holds here as in the analogous preparation of sodium methylsulfinyl carbanion. In addition, the reaction of DMSO with potassium metal is very exothermic and dilution with an inert solvent such as benzene is necessary.

The lithium salt is most readily available from reaction of the commercially available alkyllithiums with DMSO (16). Use of alkyllithiums allows preparation of lithium methylsulfinyl carbanion in solvents other than DMSO such as tetrahydrofuran, dimethoxyethane, ether, and benzene (16). The low solubility of the lithium salt in these solvents is, however, potentially a complicating factor in subsequent reactions. DMSO solutions of the lithium methylsulfinyl carbanion have been obtained from reaction with lithium amide (24) and lithium hydride (16). The procedure utilizing hydride is unsatisfactory because the slow rate of reaction at 70–80° is accompanied by significant amounts of decomposition. Lithium metal does not react with DMSO. Other potentially useful metal salts of the carbanion such as the magnesium or zinc derivatives have not been reported.

Equilibrium concentrations of the anion occur in the system potassium t-butoxide–DMSO as is shown, for instance, by the quantitative isolation of an adduct upon reaction with benzophenone (20). In many instances the above system can be substituted for the carbanion solution prepared by the hydride or amide procedures. The exchange of the hydrogen atoms in DMSO via the carbanion occurs readily in aqueous DMSO (25–27) containing sodium hydroxide and, indeed, this reaction has been suggested as a simple and inexpensive synthesis of DMSO-d_6 (25,26).

B. REACTIONS OF METHYLSULFINYL CARBANION

Methylsulfinyl carbanion* undergoes the reactions expected of a strong nucleophilic base. It reacts readily with a variety of electrophilic reagents to give, initially, substituted sulfoxides. The synthetic utility of this reagent lies not so much in the formation of the primary

* Unless stated otherwise, methylsulfinyl carbanion refers to a DMSO solution of the sodium salt of the anion.

products, but in the further transformations which these can undergo. These aspects of DMSO chemistry will be discussed in the following pages.

1. Reaction with Ketones and Aldehydes

The addition of methylsulfinyl carbanion to benzophenone and benzaldehyde to give, after hydrolysis, β-hydroxy sulfoxides in high yield, was first reported by Corey and Chaykovsky (15,16) as proof of the quantitative generation of the anion on reaction of DMSO with sodium hydride.

$$\underset{(2)}{Ph_2CO} + CH_3\overset{O}{\overset{\|}{S}}CH_2^- \rightarrow \underset{(3)}{Ph_2\overset{O^-}{\overset{|}{C}}CH_2\overset{O}{\overset{\|}{S}}CH_3} \xrightarrow{H_2O} \underset{(4)}{Ph_2\overset{OH}{\overset{|}{C}}CH_2\overset{O}{\overset{\|}{S}}CH_3} \quad (86\%)$$

Russell and co-workers (28,29) have described the formation of β-hydroxy sulfoxides from benzophenone, fluorenone, and a number of aromatic aldehydes in DMSO containing potassium t-butoxide (see also ref. 20). Other nonenolizable ketones such as nortricyclanone (5) similarly yield β-hydroxy sulfoxides (30,31). However, when 5 is treated with potassium t-butoxide–H_2O (10:3 ratio) in DMSO at room temperature, only a small amount of the sulfoxide 6 is formed; the major reaction under these conditions involves cleavage to the isomeric bicyclic acids, 7 and 8. Cleavage of nonenolizable ketones in this manner has been shown to be an effective alternative to the Haller-Bauer reaction (sodium amide in benzene).

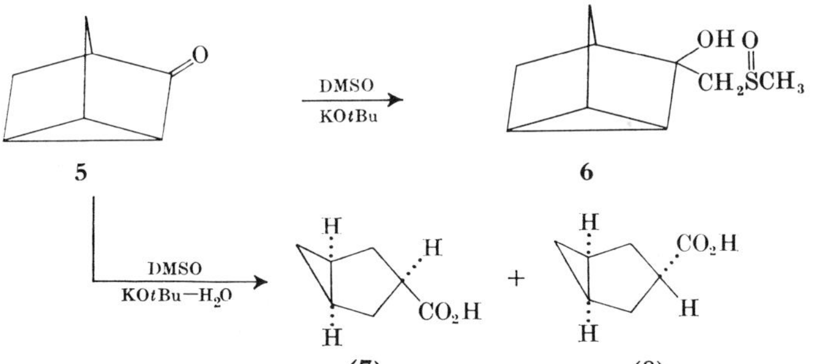

The reaction of sodium methylsulfinyl carbanion with enolizable ketones is accompanied by a significant amount of proton transfer affording enolates which are stable to further attack by the anion, and, on acidification, regenerate the ketone (15,16). Cyclohexanone, for instance, gave only 17% of the adduct **9** together with an 80% recovery of starting material. With cycloheptanone, 64% of the expected β-hydroxy sulfoxide was obtained with only 35% enolization. Part of the problem of enolization can be circumvented by use of the lithium salt of the carbanion in tetrahydrofuran solution; cyclohexanone, under these conditions, gives 45% of **9** and 51% recovered ketone.

A variety of factors such as the nature of the solvent and cation, rates of adduct and enolate formation, and reversibility of the initial adduct may account for the variations. The relative importance of any of these has not been determined.

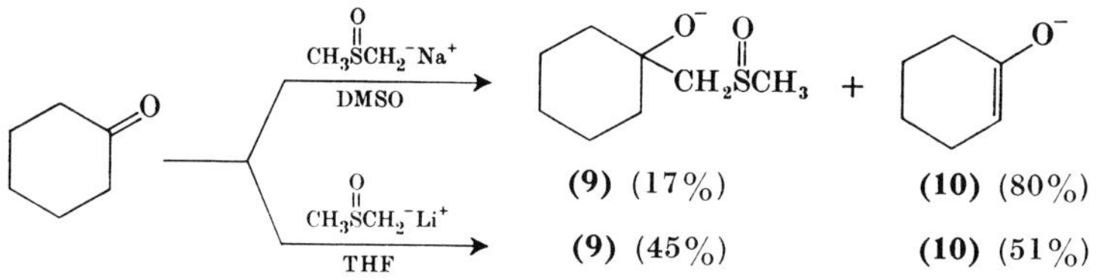

Russell and Becker (29) have described an interesting condensation involving methylsulfinyl carbanion, diphenylmethane, and an aromatic aldehyde which yielded a mixture of **11** and **12**. The amount of **12** formed increased at the expense of **11** as the base concentration, temperature, and time were increased, a 70% yield of **12** being obtained after 2.5 hr at 65°. A mechanistic study by these authors supported the reactions outlined in Scheme 1.

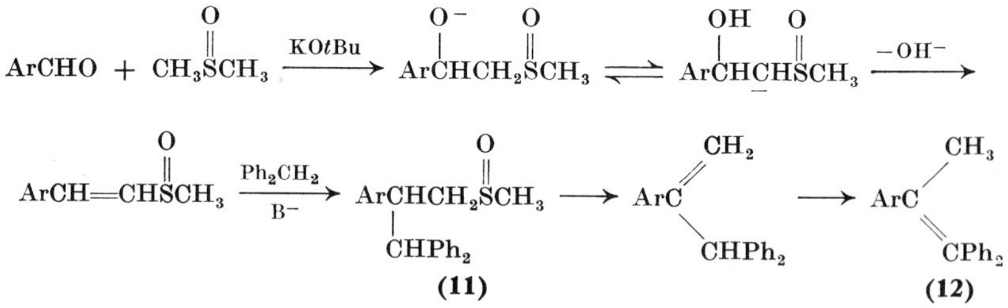

Scheme 1

Attempted replacement of diphenylmethane with other weakly acidic hydrocarbons such as phenyl-*p*-tolylsulfone or fluorene in these reactions was not successful. In the reaction of the sulfone with benzaldehydes, low yields of unsymmetrical stilbenes were isolated. With fluorene and p-methoxybenzaldehyde, a symmetrical tri-carbon condensation occurred to give di-9-fluorenyl-p-methoxyphenylmethane in 70% yield.

$$RC_6H_4CHO + C_6H_5SO_2C_6H_4CH_3 \xrightarrow[KOtBu]{DMSO} RC_6H_4CH{=}CHC_6H_4SO_2C_6H_5$$

R	Yield, %
H	40
p-OCH$_3$	32
p-C$_6$H$_5$SO$_2$	39
p-N(CH$_3$)$_2$	11

As previously mentioned, benzophenone reacts with methylsulfinyl carbanion in DMSO at room temperature to yield the β-alkoxy sulfoxide 3. Under more vigorous conditions, 80–100°, the alkoxide undergoes conversion to diphenylacetaldehyde, probably via 1,1-diphenylethylene oxide (13), and to a mixture of hydrocarbons including 1,1-diphenylethylene, diphenylmethane, and 1,1-diphenylcyclopropane (32, 33). Control experiments showed that the latter two products were derived from reaction of 1,1-diphenylethylene with methylsulfinyl carbanion. (This reaction will be considered in Sec. II-B-6.) The formation of the two primary products, diphenylethylene oxide and 1,1-diphenylethylene, was rationalized in the following manner: Attack of the oxyanion 3 on carbon with concomitant elimination of methanesulfenate gives the epoxide 13. Attack on sulfur produces the 4-membered ring intermediate 14 which could decompose to 1,1-diphenylethylene and methanesulfinate anion, the overall effect being equivalent to the Wittig olefin synthesis. At 65° in DMSO, 3 underwent reversal of formation to benzophenone (80%) and methylsulfinyl carbanion (33), Scheme 2.

Several interesting and potentially useful reactions of β-hydroxy sulfoxides have been reported. Corey and Durst (34) have shown that pyrolysis of the β-hydroxy sulfoxide (4) at 150° for 3 min afforded a 45% yield of 1,1-diphenylethylene. At the present time, this decomposition appears to be restricted to β-hydroxy sulfoxides which cannot undergo the normal sulfoxide pyrolysis (35), and to those which yield highly conjugated olefins.

Epoxide formation

$$\underset{(3)}{Ph_2\overset{O^-}{\underset{|}{C}}-CH_2-\overset{O}{\underset{\|}{S}}CH_3} \xrightarrow{80°} \underset{(13)}{Ph_2C\overset{O}{\diagup\diagdown}CH_2} + CH_3SO^-$$

Olefin formation

$$\underset{(3)}{Ph_2\overset{O^-}{\underset{|}{C}}-CH_2-\overset{O}{\underset{\|}{S}}CH_3} \xrightarrow{80°} \underset{(14)}{Ph_2\overset{\overset{CH_3}{|}}{\underset{|}{C}}-\overset{O-S-O^-}{\underset{|}{CH_2}}} \longrightarrow Ph_2C=CH_2 + CH_3SO_2^-$$

Reversal

$$\underset{(3)}{Ph_2\overset{O^-}{\underset{|}{C}}CH_2\overset{O}{\underset{\|}{S}}CH_3} \xrightarrow{65°} Ph_2C=O + CH_3\overset{O}{\underset{\|}{S}}CH_2^-$$

Scheme 2

The adduct **4**, on exposure to acid (25°, 15 hr) produced 1,1-diphenylethylene in 64% yield (34); again, the generality of this type of reaction has not been demonstrated. The formation of 1,1-diphenylethylene from **4** via pyrolysis or acid-catalyzed reaction may involve

$$\underset{(4)}{Ph_2\overset{OH}{\underset{|}{C}}CH_2\overset{O}{\underset{\|}{S}}CH_3} \begin{array}{c} \xrightarrow[3\ min]{150°} Ph_2C=CH_2 \quad (45\%) \\ \\ \xrightarrow[EtOH,\ 25°]{H^+} Ph_2C=CH_2 \quad (64\%) \end{array}$$

the 4-membered ring intermediate **15** and thus be related to the thermal decomposition of β-hydroxy sulfinamides **16**. The latter compounds have been shown to fragment to olefin, amine, and sulfur dioxide in a stereospecific *cis* manner (34,36).

$$\underset{(15)}{Ph_2\overset{OH}{\underset{|}{C}}-\overset{O-S-CH_3}{\underset{|}{CH_2}}} \rightarrow Ph_2C=CH_2 + CH_3SO_2H$$

$$\underset{(16)}{R\overset{OH}{\underset{|}{C}}-\overset{O}{\underset{\|}{C}}HSNHAr} \rightarrow \underset{(17)}{R\overset{O-SNHAr}{\underset{|}{C}}-\overset{OH}{\underset{|}{CH}}} \rightarrow \overset{R}{\underset{H}{\diagdown}}C=C\overset{H}{\underset{R'}{\diagup}} + ArNH_2 + SO_2$$

TABLE I
Pyrolysis of Aldehyde–Methylsulfinyl Carbanion Adducts (37)

$$\underset{\underset{R'}{|}}{RCHCHSCH_3} \xrightarrow{230°} RCCH_2R' + CH_3SOH$$

(with OH on first C, and S=O on sulfur)

R	R'	Yield, %
Ph	H	77
Ph	CH_3	29
Cyclo-C_6H_{11}	H	26
Cyclo-C_6H_{11}	CH_3	Trace

Russell and co-workers (37) have obtained ketones in pyrolysis of some aldehyde–methylsulfinyl carbanion adducts (Table I). In these examples, normal sulfoxide pyrolysis takes place. These same ketones are available by a two-step sequence involving oxidation of the adducts to β-keto sulfoxides (37) followed by reduction with aluminum amalgam (18,37,38), or, by an alternate two-step process

$$RCCH_2SCH_3 \xleftarrow{MnO_2} RCCH_2SCH_3 \xrightarrow{LiAlH_4} RCCH_2SCH_3$$

(with appropriate O, OH, and H substituents)

Al/Hg ↘   Δ | 230°   ↙ 150°

$$RCCH_3$$

Scheme 3

featuring free-radical decomposition of β-hydroxy sulfides which were obtained from the corresponding sulfoxide on reduction with lithium aluminum hydride (37), Scheme 3 and Table II.

2. Reaction with Imines

Only one example of such a reaction has been reported. Corey and Chaykovsky (16) showed that methylsulfinyl carbanion added to

TABLE II
Free-Radical Decomposition of α-Hydroxy Sulfides (37)

$$\underset{\substack{|\\R'}}{\overset{\substack{OH\\|}}{R\mathrm{CHCHSCH_3}}} \xrightarrow[\text{dicumyl peroxide}]{150°} R\overset{O}{\overset{\|}{\mathrm{C}}}\mathrm{CH_2R'} + \mathrm{CH_3SH}$$

R	R'	Yield, %
Ph	H	93
Ph	CH_3	82
Cyclo-C_6H_{11}	H	67
Cyclo-C_6H_{11}	CH_3	Trace

benzalaniline to give a 92% yield of the β-anilino sulfoxide **18** as a mixture of diastereomers.

$$\mathrm{PhN{=}CHPh} + \mathrm{CH_3\overset{O}{\overset{\|}{S}}CH_2^-} \xrightarrow[25°]{\text{DMSO}} \underset{\substack{|\\ \mathrm{CH_2SOCH_3}\\ \mathbf{(18)}}}{\mathrm{PhNHCHPh}} \quad (92\%)$$

3. Reaction with Esters

The reaction of methylsulfinyl carbanion with esters affords β-keto sulfoxides (16,18,38,41). Because of the great potential of these compounds as intermediates for further transformations, this reaction represents a key use of DMSO. Two equivalents of methylsulfinyl carbanion are required since the β-keto sulfoxide formed by reaction of one equivalent of anion with ester rapidly consumes a second equivalent of base to give a resonance-stabilized carbanion.

$$\mathrm{R\overset{O}{\overset{\|}{C}}OR'} + \mathrm{CH_3\overset{O}{\overset{\|}{S}}CH_2^-} \xrightarrow{\text{DMSO}} \mathrm{R\overset{O}{\overset{\|}{C}}CH_2\overset{O}{\overset{\|}{S}}CH_3} + \mathrm{R'O^-}$$

$$\downarrow \mathrm{CH_3\overset{O}{\overset{\|}{S}}CH_2^-}$$

$$\mathrm{R\overset{O}{\overset{\|}{C}}CH_2\overset{O}{\overset{\|}{S}}CH_3} \xleftarrow{\mathrm{H^+}} \mathrm{R\overset{O}{\overset{\|}{C}}\underset{-}{C}H\overset{O}{\overset{\|}{S}}CH_3}$$

Scheme 4

The formation of β-keto sulfoxides from these reagents is an efficient process with yields generally over 70% and often virtually quantitative (Table III). Because of their high acidity, purification can be accomplished by extraction with base followed by acidification of the aqueous extracts, Scheme 4.

TABLE III
Conversion of Esters to β-Keto Sulfoxides

$$\underset{}{RCOEt} \rightarrow \underset{}{RCCH_2SCH_3}$$
(with C=O groups shown)

R	Yield, %
C_6H_5	79,[a] 88[b], 70[c]
$p\text{-}CH_3C_6H_4$	87[b]
$p\text{-}CH_3OC_6H_4$	98,[a] 95[b]
$p\text{-}BrC_6H_4$	79[a]
$\alpha\text{-}C_{10}H_7$	98[a], 95[b]
$\beta\text{-}C_{10}H_7$	91[b]
α-furyl	71[a]
$Cyclo\text{-}C_6H_{11}$	98[a]
$n\text{-}C_5H_{11}$	70[a]
$n\text{-}C_9H_{19}$	85[b]
$n\text{-}C_{13}H_{27}$	93[c]
$n\text{-}C_{17}H_{35}$	98[a]
$CH_2{=}CH(CH_2)_8$	90[c]
$cis\text{-}C_8H_{17}CH{=}CH(CH_2)_7$	78[c]

[a] Ref. 16.
[b] Ref. 39.
[c] Ref. 41.

Reduction of β-keto sulfoxides with aluminum amalgam in aqueous tetrahydrofuran (18) or with zinc and acetic acid (39) gives methyl ketones in excellent yield (Table IV). β-Keto sulfones and β-keto sulfonamides, which are available by reaction of esters with methylsulfonyl carbanion or dimethylamino sulfonyl carbanion, respectively, are similarly cleaved to methyl ketones (16). The combination of the reaction of an ester with methylsulfinyl carbanion followed by reduction of the product by either of the above methods constitutes an efficient synthesis of methyl ketones.

$$RCOCH_2SOCH_3 \xrightarrow[THF-H_2O]{Al/Hg} RCOCH_3$$

TABLE IV
Reduction of β-Keto Sulfoxides to Methyl Ketones

$$\underset{\text{RCCH}_2\text{SCH}_3}{\overset{\text{O} \quad \text{O}}{\| \quad \|}} \rightarrow \underset{\text{RCCH}_3}{\overset{\text{O}}{\|}}$$

	Yield, %	
R	Al/Hg Reduction (16)	Zinc–Acetic Acid Reduction (39)
C_6H_5	98	88
p-$CH_3C_6H_4$	—	83
p-$CH_3OC_6H_4$	98	87
α-$C_{10}H_7$	89	—
α-furyl	70	—
Cyclo-C_6H_{11}	98	—
n-C_5H_{11}	98	—
n-$C_{17}H_{35}$	98	—

Similarly,

$$RCOCH_2SO_2CH_3 \rightarrow RCOCH_3$$

and,

$$RCOCH_2SO_2N(CH_3)_2 \rightarrow RCOCH_3$$

Gassman and Richmond (38) have described conditions (DMF, NaH, 25°) under which β-keto sulfoxides are mono- and dialkylated at the carbon α to both the carbonyl and sulfoxide function. The alkylated

TABLE V
Alkylation of β-Keto Sulfoxides and Reduction to Ketones

$$\underset{R_1CCH_2SCH_3}{\overset{O \quad O}{\| \quad \|}} \rightarrow \underset{R_1CCR_2R_3SCH_3}{\overset{O \quad O}{\| \quad \|}} \rightarrow \underset{R_1CCHR_2R_3}{\overset{O}{\|}}$$

R_1	R_2	R_3	Yield of ketone, %	Ref.
C_6H_5	CH_3	H	64	38
C_6H_5	CH_3	H	96	37
C_6H_5	CH_2CH_3	H	70	38
C_6H_5	CH_2CH_3	H	35	37
C_6H_5	$CH_2CH_2CH_3$	H	44	38
C_6H_5	$CH_2C_6H_5$	H	76	37
C_6H_5	CH_3	CH_3	54	38
$CH_3(CH_2)_4$	CH_3	H	62	38
$CH_3(CH_2)_4$	CH_2CH_3	H	69	38
$CH_3(CH_2)_4$	CH_3	CH_3	59	38

products were hydrogenolyzed with Al/Hg to give a variety of substituted ketones (Table V). Russell, Sabourin, and Mikol (37) carried out such alkylations in tetrahydrofuran using sodium hydride as base.

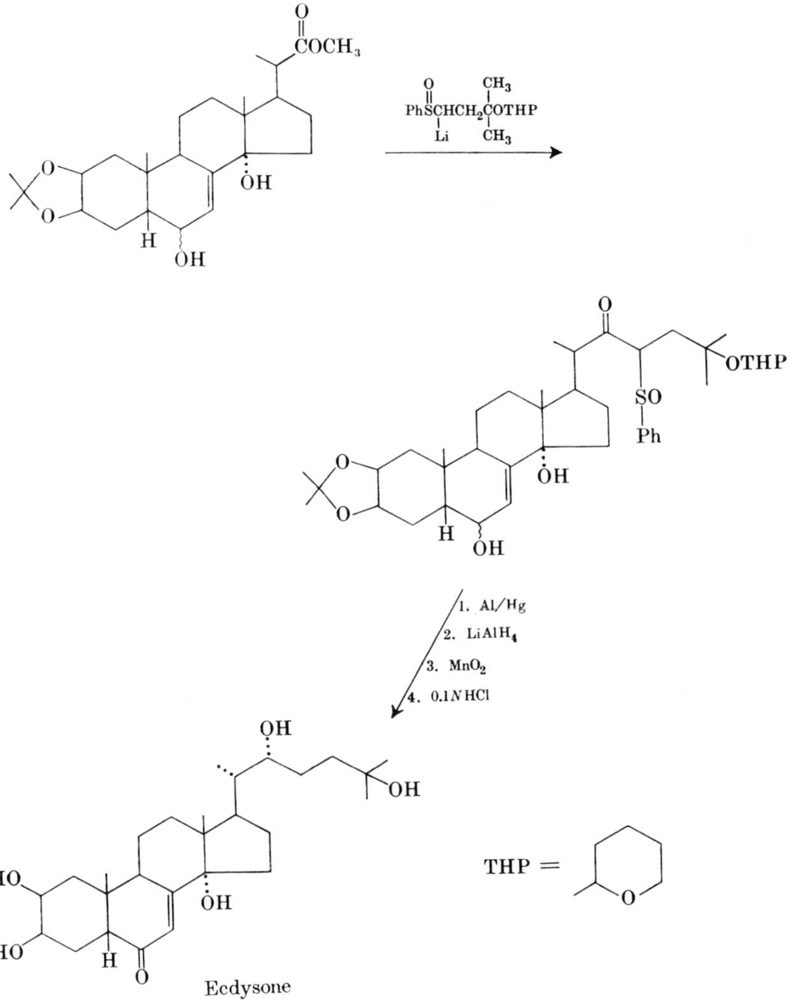

Other sulfoxides, such as phenyl alkyl sulfoxides, are also potentially valuable reagents in the synthesis of ketones from esters. The sulfoxide bearing the desired alkyl group is readily prepared by reaction of sodium thiophenolate with the appropriate halide or tosylate (42) followed by oxidation. The use of the substituted sulfoxides avoids the necessity of alkylating the unsubstituted β-keto sulfoxide which is not an extremely efficient reaction except with simple alkylating agents (37,38). An illustration of the application of such a reagent is provided in the side-chain synthesis of the insect molting hormone ecdysone (43).

On exposure to acid, β-keto sulfoxides undergo the Pummerer rearrangement (39,41) and thereby provide an entry into dicarbonyl systems (the mechanism of the Pummerer reaction will be discussed in Sec. V). Hemithioacetals **19** are readily isolable intermediates in this transformation and are in equilibrium with the α-keto aldehydes **20** under the reaction conditions (39). Iodine in methanol converts β-keto sulfoxides to α-keto acetals in greater than 85% yield by oxidizing the methyl mercaptan to dimethyl disulfide and thereby removing the mercaptan from the equilibrium. Precipitation of methyl mercaptan as cupric mercaptide has been used for the same purpose but is less effective, especially when applied to large-scale reactions (39).

$$\underset{}{\text{RCOCH}_2\text{SOCH}_3} \xrightarrow{\text{H}^+} \underset{\underset{\text{OH}}{|}}{\text{RCOCHSCH}_3} \rightleftharpoons \text{RCOCHO} + \text{CH}_3\text{SH} + \text{H}_2\text{O}$$
$$\quad\quad\quad\quad\quad\quad\quad\quad\quad (19) \quad\quad\quad\quad\quad (20)$$

$$\text{RCOCH}_2\text{SOCH}_3 + \text{I}_2 \xrightarrow{\text{CH}_3\text{OH}} \text{RCOCH(OCH}_3)_2 + \text{CH}_3\text{SSCH}_3$$

Russell and Mikol (39) have reported that in addition to α-keto aldehydes, a number of other products can be obtained from the Pummerer rearrangement of β-keto sulfoxides. For example, reduction of the hemithioacetals **19** with zinc in acetic acid below 25°, or with sodium formaldehyde sulfoxylate at a pH of 7 afforded α-hydroxy

$$\underset{\underset{\text{OH}}{|}}{\text{RCOCHSCH}_3} \begin{cases} \xrightarrow[\text{pH 7}]{\text{NaOSOCH}_2\text{OH}} \text{RCOCH}_2\text{OH} \quad (60\text{–}65\%) \\ \xrightarrow[\text{EtOH}]{\text{NaBH}_4} \underset{\underset{}{}}{\text{RCHCH}_2\text{OH}} \quad (80\text{–}95\%) \\ \quad\quad\quad\quad \overset{\text{OH}}{|} \end{cases}$$

(19)

ketones in 60–65% yield. Reaction of **19** with lithium aluminum hydride in ether, or better, with sodium borohydride in ethanol, resulted in the formation of ethylene glycols. Application to ethyl benzoate, in sequence, of the methylsulfinyl carbanion reaction, Pummerer rearrangement, and sodium borohydride reduction of the hemithioacetal, afforded styrene glycol in 75% overall yield. The formation of α-keto esters, α-hydroxy acids, and pinacols from β-keto sulfoxides was also described.

Becker and Russell employed the methylsulfinyl carbanion–ester reaction in a novel synthesis of ninhydrin (44). Addition of ethyl phthalate to a dry DMSO solution containing sodium methoxide gave an intermediate salt formulated as **21** which upon acidification with $5M$ HCl underwent the Pummerer rearrangement to **22** (80%). Hydrolysis of **22** furnished ninhydrin in 99% yield.

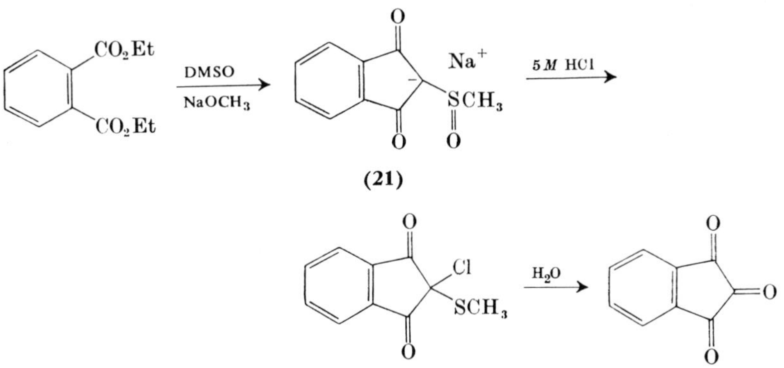

4. *Reaction with Alkyl Halides and Tosylates*

In general, reactions of alkyl halides and tosylates with DMSO solutions of alkali metal alkoxides lead to mixtures of olefins (E_2 elimination) and ethers (S_N2 substitution). The relative amounts of elimination and substitution vary, as expected, with the structure of the alkyl residue, the leaving group, and the alkoxide (45–49). Table VI shows some representative examples. The extraordinary rate increases of these reactions in DMSO compared to alcohols have been of much interest and have been discussed in recent reviews (1,6). Most of these reactions are considered outside the scope of this article since methylsulfinyl carbanion, if it is involved, acts only as a base. A few have, however, shown rather unusual features and will be briefly described in this section.

As indicated in Table VI, substitution products are formed in major amounts in the reaction of primary alkyl halides and tosylates with alkoxides. Efficient substitution in such systems by methylsulfinyl

TABLE VI
Reaction of Alkyl Halides and Tosylates with Alkoxides in DMSO (20–25°)

Substrate	Alkoxide	Product, %		Ref.
		Olefin	Ether	
Octadecyl tosylate	KO*t*Bu	25	71	48
Octadecyl chloride	KO*t*Bu	86	14	48
Octadecyl iodide	KO*t*Bu	90	10	48
24-Cholanyl tosylate	KO*t*Bu	21	78	48
24-Cholanyl chloride	KO*t*Bu	79	21	48
24-Cholanyl iodide	KO*t*Bu	73	17	48
Cyclopentyl benzenesulfonate	KO*t*Bu	76	—	46
Cyclohexyl benzenesulfonate	KO*t*Bu	83	—	46
1-Menthyl benzenesulfonate	KO*t*Bu	50	—	46
2-Octyl benzenesulfonate	KO*t*Bu	19	—	46
Octyl benzenesulfonate	KO*t*Bu	24	67	46
Hexyl benzenesulfonate	KO*t*Bu	20	69	46
Cyclohexyl carbinyl benzenesulfonate	KO*t*Bu	26	60	46
Hexyl benzenesulfonate	NaOMe	—	90	49
2-Octyl benzenesulfonate	NaOMe	27	28	49
Cyclopentyl benzenesulfonate	NaOMe	33	44	49
Cyclohexyl benzenesulfonate	NaOMe	85	5	49

carbanion resulting in the formation of methyl n-alkyl sulfoxides has been reported by Entwistle and Johnstone (50). Pyrolysis of these sulfoxides at 180° afforded terminal olefins in good yield. Pyrolysis of methyl n-alkyl sulfoxides to terminal olefins is synthetically feasible since elimination can occur in only one direction. The formation of sulfenic acids in addition to olefins in these reactions has long been accepted and was finally demonstrated in the pyrolysis of di-t-butyl-sulfoxide by the trapping of t-butylsulfenic acid with electrophilic olefins and acetylenes (51).

$$\text{RCH}_2\text{X} + \text{CH}_3\overset{\overset{\text{O}}{\|}}{\text{S}}\text{CH}_2^- \xrightarrow[25°]{\text{DMSO}} \text{RCH}_2\text{CH}_2\overset{\overset{\text{O}}{\|}}{\text{S}}\text{CH}_3$$

a. $R = n\text{-}C_{11}H_{23}$, $X = Br$ (Yield 73%)

b. $R = n\text{-}C_{15}H_{31}$, $X = OTs$ (Yield 85%)

$$\text{CH}_3(\text{CH}_2)_{10}\text{CH}_2\text{CH}_2\overset{\overset{\text{O}}{\|}}{\text{S}}\text{CH}_3 \xrightarrow[180°, \, 30 \text{ min}]{\text{DMSO}} \text{CH}_3(\text{CH}_2)_{10}\text{CH}=\text{CH}_2 \quad (80\%)$$

A number of sulfonate esters in steroidal (52,53) and carbohydrate (54) systems have been shown to undergo sulfur–oxygen cleavage when exposed to alkoxide or hydroxide ions in DMSO. This type of cleavage appears to be more facile for mesylate than tosylate esters. Chang (52) reported that 3β-cholestanol mesylate (23) and 3α-cholanol mesylate (24) were converted to the corresponding alcohols 25 and 26 in 86 and 87% yield, respectively. Only negligible amounts of the epimeric alcohols were obtained. In contrast, 3β-cholestanol tosylate gave a mixture containing 57% olefinic material, 17% alcohol with retention, and 2% alcohol with inversion.

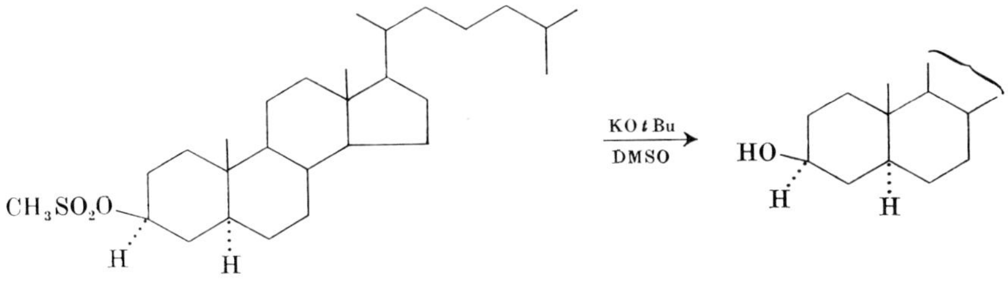

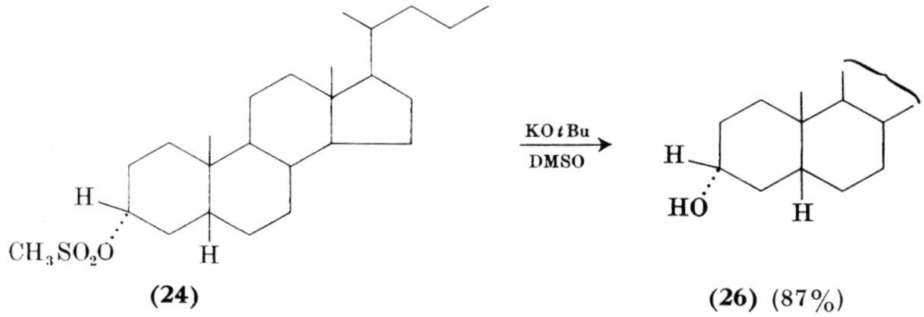

The glucoside mesylate **27** was also cleaved with retention of configuration when heated at 70° in DMSO containing sodium methoxide (54). In this case, in addition to the alcohol **28**, substantial amounts of the ether **29** were also obtained. Oxygen-18 tracer techniques showed that only the methyl group in the ether was derived from methoxide, thereby proving that carbon–oxygen cleavage of the mesylate had not occurred.

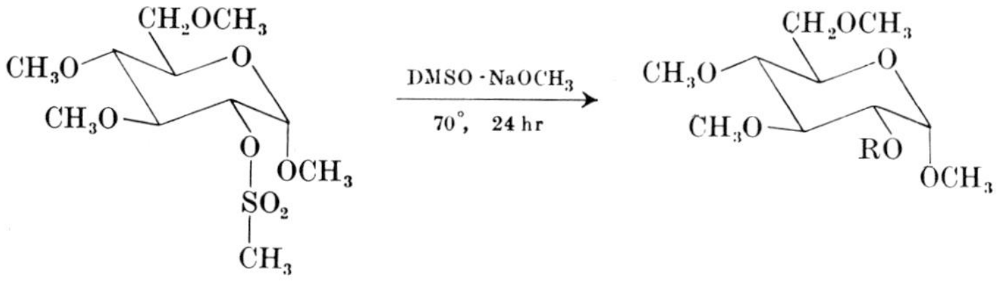

Oxygen–sulfur cleavage in the base-catalyzed hydrolysis of secondary sulfonate esters has been known for some time, especially in carbohydrate chemistry (55), and occurs if S_N2 displacement at carbon is unfavorable because of steric or electronic factors. In **27**, displacement at sulfur leads to the oxyanion **30** and methyl methanesulfonate, the latter substance subsequently serving as the alkylating agent in the conversion **30 → 29**.

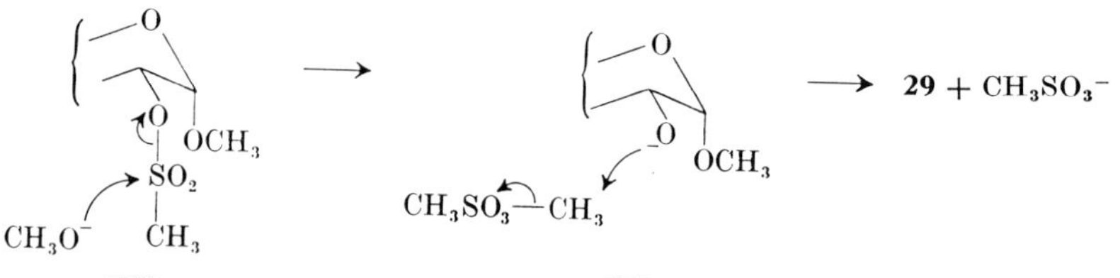

A second possible mechanism which would account for the difference in reactions observed for the mesylate and tosylate esters involves formation of a α-sulfonate ester carbanion **31** followed by elimination of the alkoxide moiety to give the sulfene **32** (56). Methyl methanesulfonate can be formed by the reaction of the sulfene with methanol and again serve to alkylate **30** to **29**. For tosylates such a pathway is not available because of the absence of a hydrogen α to the sulfonyl group, Scheme 5.

$$ROSO_2CH_3 \xrightarrow[CH_3O^-Na^+]{DMSO} ROSO_2CH_2^- \rightarrow RO^- + CH_2=SO_2 + CH_3OH$$
$$\quad\quad\quad\quad\quad\quad\quad (31) \quad\quad\quad (30) \quad\quad (32)$$

$$CH_2=SO_2 + CH_3OH \rightleftharpoons CH_3SO_2OCH_3$$

$$CH_3SO_2OCH_3 + RO^- \rightarrow CH_3SO_3^- + ROCH_3$$

Scheme 5

The occurrence of each of the individual steps of Scheme 5 has been demonstrated, albeit under different circumstances. α-Sulfonate ester carbanions have been obtained by reaction of the esters with *n*-butyllithium in tetrahydrofuran at low temperature and added to carbonyl compounds to produce β-hydroxysulfonate esters **34** (57).

$$CH_3SO_2OCH_3 \xrightarrow[THF,\ -78°]{n\text{-BuLi}} \overset{+}{Li}\overset{-}{CH_2}SO_2OCH_3 \xrightarrow[2.\ H_2O]{1.\ Ph_2CO}$$

$$\quad\quad\quad\quad\quad\quad\quad\quad\quad\quad\quad\quad\quad\quad\quad\quad\quad\quad\quad\quad OH$$
$$\quad\quad\quad\quad\quad\quad\quad\quad\quad\quad\quad\quad\quad\quad\quad\quad\quad\quad Ph_2\overset{|}{C}CH_2SO_2OCH_3 \quad (91\%)$$
$$\quad\quad\quad\quad\quad\quad\quad\quad\quad\quad\quad\quad\quad\quad\quad\quad\quad\quad\quad\quad\quad (34)$$

Decomposition of such a carbanion to yield, after hydrolysis, alcohol with retention of configuration has also been observed (58). *trans*-4-*t*-Butylcyclohexyl mesylate **(35)** was quantitatively metalated to the lithio salt **36** as shown by deuteration. When warmed to room temperature, decomposition of **36** occurred and *trans*-4-*t*-butylcyclohexanol **(37)** was isolated in 88% yield.

Cardenas et al. (59) noted some interesting differences in the reaction of *vic* dibromides in DMSO with potassium *t*-butoxide compared to methylsulfinyl carbanion (generated with sodium or sodium hydride). Treatment of 1,2,5,6-tetrabromocyclooctane (38) with butoxide gave a 49% yield of a mixture of cyclooctatetraene (78%) and styrene (22%). In contrast, reaction of 38 with methylsulfinyl carbanion afforded 1,5-cyclooctadiene (37%). Debromination, rather than dehydrobromination, was also observed for 3β-chloro-5α-bromo-6β-bromocholestane (39) on exposure to methylsulfinyl carbanion.

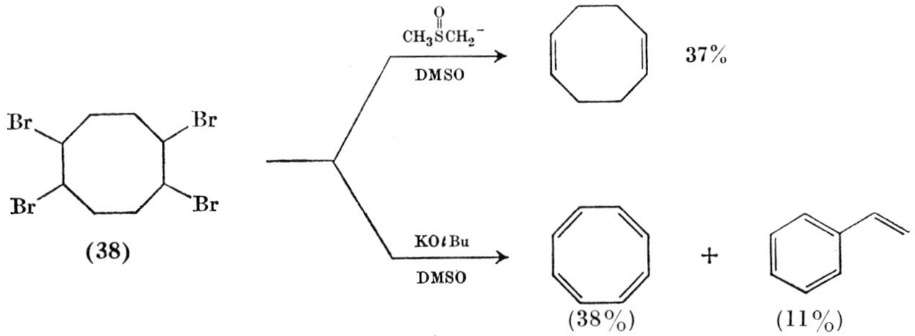

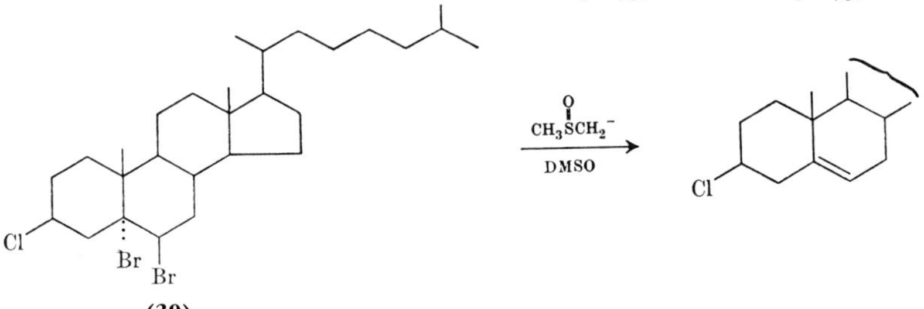

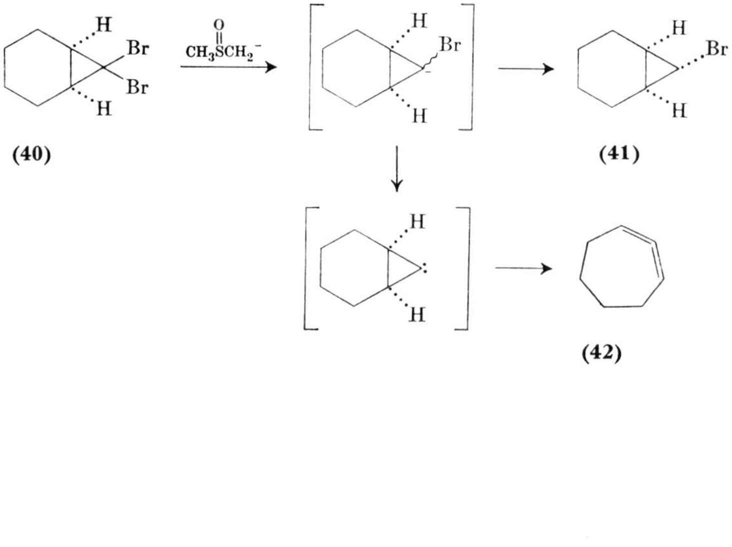

Nucleophilic displacement by methylsulfinyl carbanion on bromine occurs also in *gem*-dibromocyclopropanes (60). Reaction of 7,7-dibromobicyclo[4.1.0]heptane **(40)** with excess sodium methylsulfinyl carbanion at room temperature produced the monobromocyclopropane **41** (mainly *trans*) in 72% yield; **41** has also been obtained from **40** on reduction with tri-*n*-butyltin hydride (61). Prolonged exposure of either the mono- or dibromocyclopropane to the DMSO anion gave 1,2-cycloheptadiene **(42)**, possibly via the cyclopropyl carbene (62).

Carbenoid species may also be involved in the reaction of methylsulfinyl carbanion with benzyl and benzhydryl chlorides (16) which yield *trans*-stilbene (42%) and tetraphenylethylene (98%), respectively.

$$PhCH_2Cl \xrightarrow[DMSO]{CH_3\overset{O}{\underset{\|}{S}}CH_2^-} PhCH=CHPh \quad (42\%)$$

$$Ph_2CHCl \xrightarrow[DMSO]{CH_3\overset{O}{\underset{\|}{S}}CH_2^-} Ph_2C=CPh_2 \quad (98\%)$$

5. Reaction with Aromatic Halides

The reaction of methylsulfinyl carbanion with aromatic halides appears to involve benzyne intermediates. Chlorobenzene reacted exothermically with the DMSO anion to form a mixture of benzyl methyl sulfoxide **(43)** and benzhydryl methyl sulfoxide **(44)** (15,16). When a large excess of anion was employed, only very little of the benzhydryl methyl sulfoxide was obtained.

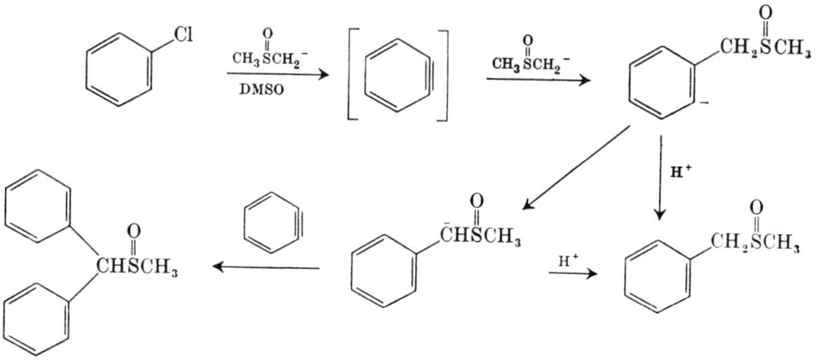

(44)   **(43)**

Cram and Day (63) have reported a rather more complicated example. Treatment of 4-bromo-2,2-paracyclophane **(45)** with potassium *t*-butoxide in DMSO resulted in the formation of the *t*-butyl ether **46** (4%), the phenol **47** (14%), and the thioether phenol **48** (10%). The mechanism leading to **46** and **47** is straightforward, but that proposed

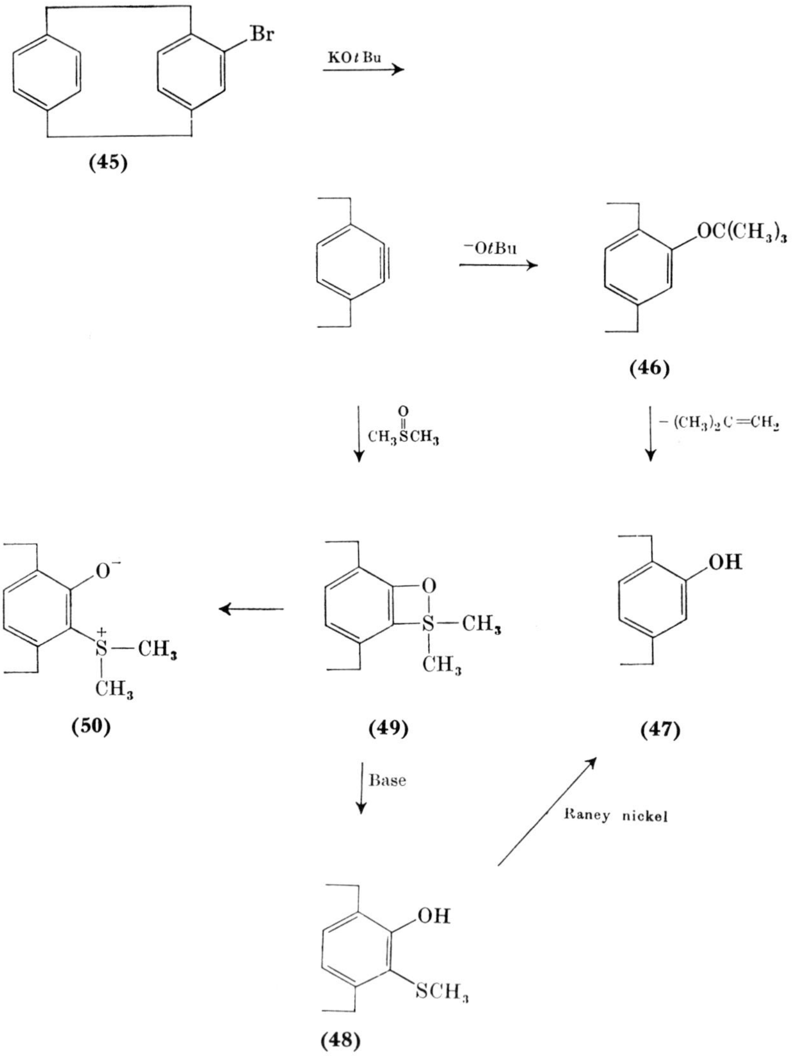

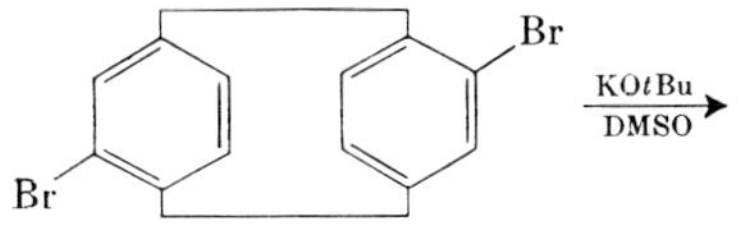

(51) [structure: dibromo paracyclophane] $\xrightarrow{\text{KO}t\text{Bu} \atop \text{DMSO}}$

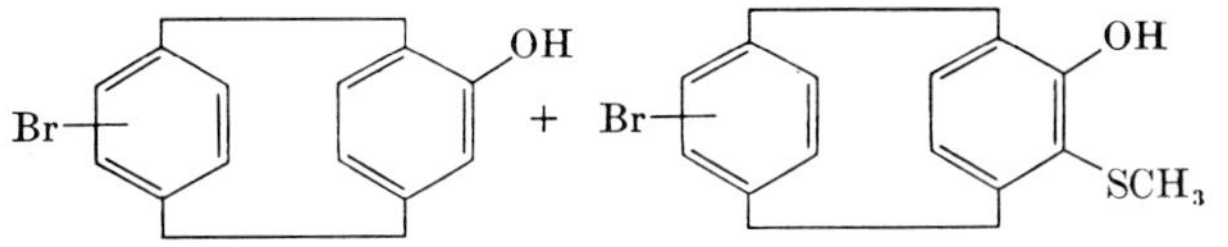

(52) (14%) + (53) (19%)

for the formation of the thiophenol ether contains rather unusual features. It was suggested that DMSO could add to the aryne intermediate to form the tetracovalent sulfur derivative **49**. Demethylation of **49** by a base present in solution with simultaneous ring opening would lead to **48**. A variation in the sequence of the last two steps, i.e., ring opening of **49** to the zwitterionic species **50** followed by demethylation is also a possibility. The structure of **48** was proved by Raney nickel desulfurization to **47**. The isolation of isomeric bromophenols **52** and isomeric bromomethylthiophenols **53** from the reaction of 4,15-dibromo-2,2-paracyclophane **(51)** provides strong evidence for aryne formation in these reactions.

6. Reaction with Aromatic and Olefinic Systems

The addition of methylsulfinyl carbanion to olefinic or aromatic systems occurs if such a reaction leads to a relatively stable carbanion, e.g., benzylic or allylic. Further reaction of this carbanion depends on the nature of R and on reaction conditions.

$$\text{RCH=CH}_2 + \text{CH}_3\overset{\overset{\text{O}}{\|}}{\text{S}}\text{CH}_2^- \rightarrow \text{RCHCH}_2\text{CH}_2\overset{\overset{\text{O}}{\|}}{\text{S}}\text{CH}_3$$

1,1-Diphenylethylene reacts readily with a solution of methylsulfinyl carbanion at 25° to afford, after hydrolysis, a quantitative yield of methyl-3,3-diphenylpropyl sulfoxide **(55)** (64). At higher temperatures (70°) a series of equilibria are set up from which a number of other products are derived, Scheme 6.

The initially formed carbanion **54** can be protonated to the sulfoxide

$$Ph_2C=CH_2 + CH_3\overset{O}{\underset{\|}{S}}CH_2^- \rightleftharpoons Ph_2\overset{-}{C}CH_2CH_2\overset{O}{\underset{\|}{S}}CH_3 \underset{}{\overset{BH}{\rightleftharpoons}} Ph_2CHCH_2CH_2\overset{O}{\underset{\|}{S}}CH_3 + B^-$$
$$(54) \qquad\qquad\qquad (55)$$

γ-elimination ↙   ↗↙ H⁺ / −H⁺   β-elimination ↓

$$Ph_2C{\overset{CH_2}{\underset{CH_2}{\diagup\!\!\diagdown}}} + CH_3SO^- \qquad Ph_2CHCH_2\overset{O}{\underset{\|}{\overset{-}{C}}}\!SCH_3 \qquad Ph_2CHCH=CH_2 + CH_3SOH$$
$$\qquad\qquad\qquad\qquad (56) \qquad\qquad\qquad (57)$$

↓   ↓

$$Ph_2CH_2 + B^- \xleftarrow{BH} Ph_2CH^- + CH_2=CH\overset{O}{\underset{\|}{S}}CH_3 \qquad Ph_2C=CHCH_3$$
$$\qquad\qquad\qquad\qquad\qquad (58)$$

Scheme 6

55 by one of the weak acids present in the reaction mixture. β-Elimination of methanesulfenic acid from **55** affords 3,3-diphenylpropene **(57)** which is readily isomerized to the conjugated olefin **58** under the basic conditions of the reaction. Hofmann et al. (65,66) have shown that such eliminations occur quite readily with a variety of sulfoxides.

$$(CH_3)_2CH\overset{O}{\underset{\|}{S}}CH(CH_3)_2 \xrightarrow[55°, 17\ hr]{DMSO-KOtBu} CH_3CH=CH_2 \quad (95\%)$$

$$(CH_3CH_2CH_2CH_2)_2SO \xrightarrow{DMSO-KOtBu} \text{mixture of butenes} \quad (16\%)$$

The formation of diphenylmethane probably occurs via isomerization of the initially formed carbanion **54** to the α-sulfoxide carbanion **56** which undergoes a reverse Michael addition to methyl vinyl sulfoxide and, after protonation, diphenylmethane.

γ-Elimination of methane sulfenate (E_1cB mechanism) (67) from **54** yields 1,1-diphenylcyclopropane. Baker and Spillet (68) have studied the ratio of β-to γ-elimination of a number of 3-phenyl-2-alkylpropyl sulfoxides in DMSO–DMSO⁻ and triethylamine–KNH_2 mixtures. Cyclopropane formation, which occurs via a carbanionic intermediate, is favored in the more polar solvent, DMSO. The decrease in the ratio of β- to γ-elimination with increasing size of the alkyl group was attributed to the unfavorable inductive effects, and increasing difficulty of the sulfoxide in achieving the conformation required for *trans* 1,2-elimination, Table VII. The sulfoxides were prepared by addition of methylsulfinyl carbanion to β-alkylstyrenes.

TABLE VII

β- and γ-Eliminations from 3-Phenyl-2-Alkylpropyl Sulfoxides

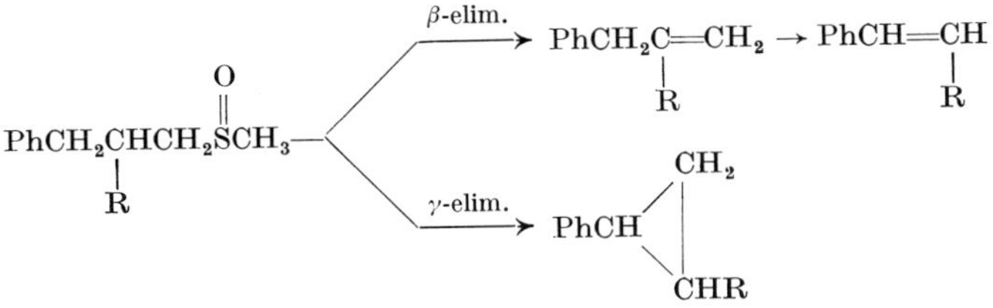

$$PhCH_2CHCH_2SCH_3 \begin{cases} \xrightarrow{\beta\text{-elim.}} PhCH_2C{=}CH_2 \rightarrow PhCH{=}CH \\ \quad\quad\quad\quad\quad\quad | \quad\quad\quad\quad\quad\quad | \\ \quad\quad\quad\quad\quad\quad R \quad\quad\quad\quad\quad\quad R \\ \xrightarrow{\gamma\text{-elim.}} PhCH\overset{CH_2}{\underset{CHR}{\diagdown}} \end{cases}$$

(with R on the starting material)

	$CH_3\overset{O}{\overset{\|}{S}}CH_2^-$ in DMSO[a]		KNH_2 in triethylamine[b]	
	Cyclopropane,[c] %	Olefin, %	Cyclopropane,[c] %	Olefin, %
R = H	0	3	0	32
CH_3	17	5	22	42
C_2H_5	50	19	13	51
i-C_3H_7	67	8	32	50
t-C_4H_9	97	0	38	50

[a] 70°, 48h.
[b] 75°, 24h.
[c] All cyclopropanes had *trans* stereochemistry.

The sequence involving addition of methylsulfinyl carbanion to an olefin, β-elimination of methanesulfenic acid, and finally isomerization, is equivalent to a methylation reaction. A number of examples of such methylations have been reported (69,70). *trans*-Stilbene was converted to α-methylstilbene in 67% yield upon reaction with methylsulfinyl carbanion in DMSO at 25° for 15 min. Stilbazoles, as expected on the basis of the mechanism outlined below, were methylated in the β-position. The yields in a number of examples were 40–80%.

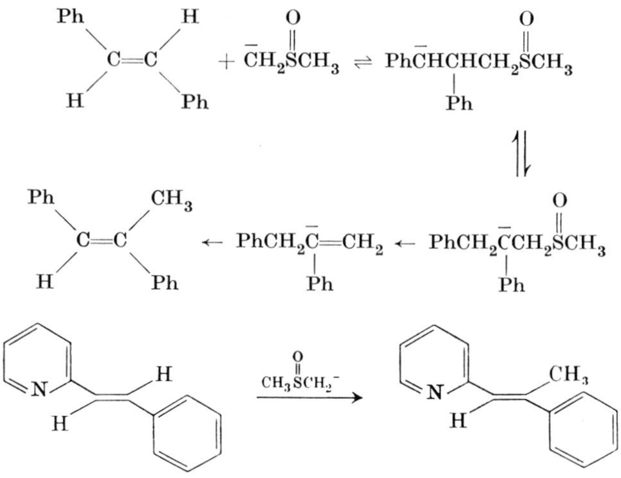

$$\underset{H}{\overset{Ph}{\diagdown}}C=C\underset{Ph}{\overset{H}{\diagup}} + \bar{C}H_2\overset{O}{\overset{\|}{S}}CH_3 \rightleftharpoons Ph\bar{C}HCHCH_2\overset{O}{\overset{\|}{S}}CH_3$$

$$\underset{H}{\overset{Ph}{\diagdown}}C=C\underset{Ph}{\overset{CH_3}{\diagup}} \leftarrow PhCH_2\bar{C}=CH_2 \leftarrow PhCH_2\overset{|}{\underset{Ph}{C}}CH_2\overset{O}{\overset{\|}{S}}CH_3$$

The methylation of some 1,3-dienes has also been performed (70). Butadiene, when added to DMSO containing potassium *t*-butoxide, gave a 50% yield of a mixture of *cis* (20%) and *trans* (80%) 1,3-pentadienes within 1 hr at 55°. Methylation of the pentadiene mixture obtained above afforded a 40% yield of isomeric hexadienes after 17 hr of reaction time. Cyclic dienes such as 1,3-cyclohexadiene and 1,3-cyclooctadiene were found to be less reactive, probably because of the difficulty of achieving a planar allylic system which is necessary for effective stabilization of the carbanion. Norbornadiene was unreactive under these conditions.

Methylation of condensed aromatic systems with methylsulfinyl carbanion has been more successful. A number of workers (70–72) have reported results in this area which underline the synthetic utility of the procedure (see Table VIII). Benzene (70,71), pyridine (71), thianaphthene (71), and phenazine (71), however, failed to yield methylated derivatives even after long reaction times. Anthracene generally gave a mixture of 9-methyl- and 9,10-dimethylanthracene (71).

Mechanistically, aromatic methylations have been suggested to occur in the same manner as olefinic methylations (69–72). The possibility that the negatively charged σ-complex **59**, formed by nucleophilic addition of methylsulfinyl carbanion to the aromatic system, might undergo concerted hydride transfer and elimination of CH_3SO^- to

TABLE VIII
Methylation of Aromatic Systems with Methylsulfinyl Carbanion

Substrate	Base	Mole ratio base/substrate	Time, hr	Temp. °C	Product, %	Ref.
Naphthalene	KOtBu	—	92	55	1-Methylnaphthalene (14) 2-Methylnaphthalene (1)	70
Quinoline	CH$_3$SOCH$_2$Na	5.5	4	70	4-Methylquinoline (98)	71
	CH$_3$SOCH$_2$Na	5	5.5	25	4-Methylquinoline (29)	71
Isoquinoline	CH$_3$SOCH$_2$Na	5.5	4	70	2-Methylisoquinoline (98)	71
	CH$_3$SOCH$_2$Na	3	3	25	2-Methylisoquinoline (51)	72
Benzoxazole	CH$_3$SOCH$_2$Na	5.5	4	65	2-Methylbenzoxazole (50)	71
Anthracene	KOtBu	—	1	55	9-Methylanthracene (45) 9,10-Dimethylanthracene 10	70
	KOtBu	4.5	2	70	9-Methylanthracene (67)	71
	CH$_3$SOCH$_2$Na	4	8	25	9,10-Dimethylanthracene (96)	71
	CH$_3$SOCH$_2$Na	5	5	25	9-Methylanthracene (77) 9,10-Dimethylanthracene (13)	72
Phenanthrene	CH$_3$SOCH$_2$Na	10	4	70	9-Methylphenanthridine (93)	71
	CH$_3$SOCH$_2$Na	10	21	25	9-Methylphenanthridine (86)	72
Acridine	CH$_3$SOCH$_2$Na	5	4	25	9-Methylacridine (74)	72
	CH$_3$SOCH$_2$Na	10	4	70	9-Methylacridine (98)	71

give the methylated hydrocarbon directly has been suggested, but is considered less likely than the stepwise route. The position of methylation is in agreement with the calculated charge densities (73).

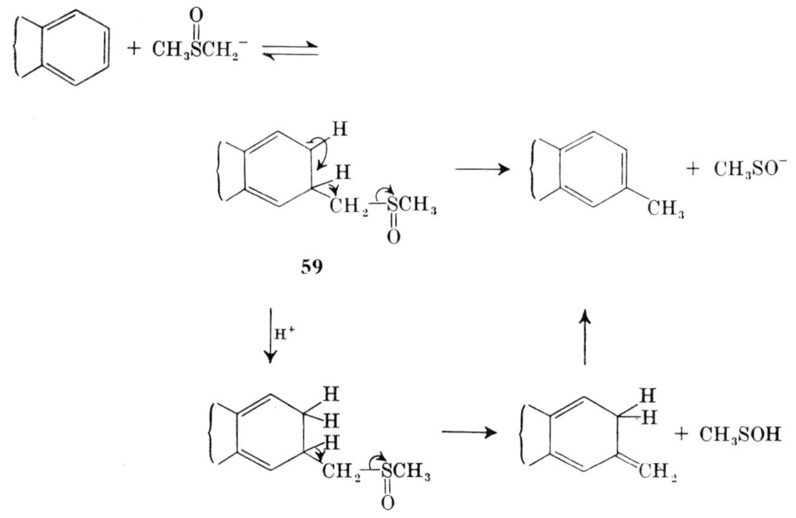

7. *Miscellaneous Reactions of Methylsulfinyl Carbanion*

Methylsulfinyl carbanion in DMSO has been effectively applied to the generation of ylids from the corresponding onium compounds. A modification of the Wittig reaction based on the use of methylsulfinyl carbanion as base and DMSO as solvent has been proposed by Corey (74). The reaction appears to proceed more rapidly in DMSO than in the usual solvents (ether, tetrahydrofuran) and in many instances the yields are significantly better. Highly volatile products can be distilled directly from the reaction mixture. A recent synthesis of a number of deuterium and carbon-14 labeled olefins (75) took particular advantage of such a work-up. The excellent solvent properties of DMSO made possible the generation of the ylid **60** and its use in the synthesis of β,γ-unsaturated acids (76). Other applications of the Corey modification have been reported in the synthesis of a number of natural products (77–80).

A further variation, reported by a group of German workers (81), employs 1,5-diazabicyclo[4.3.0]non-5-ene as base and DMSO as solvent.

This procedure was shown to be especially useful in Wittig reactions involving alkali-sensitive aldehydes.

$$Ph_3\overset{+}{P}CH_2CH_2CO_2H \xrightarrow[DMSO]{2NaH} Ph_3\overset{+}{P}\overset{-}{C}HCH_2CO_2^-$$
(60)

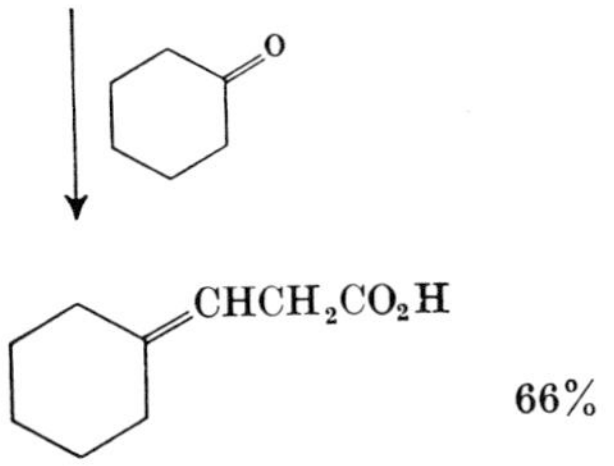

↓ cyclohexanone

cyclohexylidene=CHCH$_2$CO$_2$H   66%

The Sommelet-Hauser rearrangement of the benzyltrimethyl ammonium ion **61 → 62**, usually performed in the liquid ammonia–sodium amide system, is more conveniently carried out at 15–20° in DMSO containing methylsulfinyl carbanion (82). The rearranged amine **62**, formed in 81% yield after 10 min of reaction, was uncontaminated with the isomeric amine **63** which is the main product when the rearrangement is carried out with phenyllithium in hexane (83, 84.)

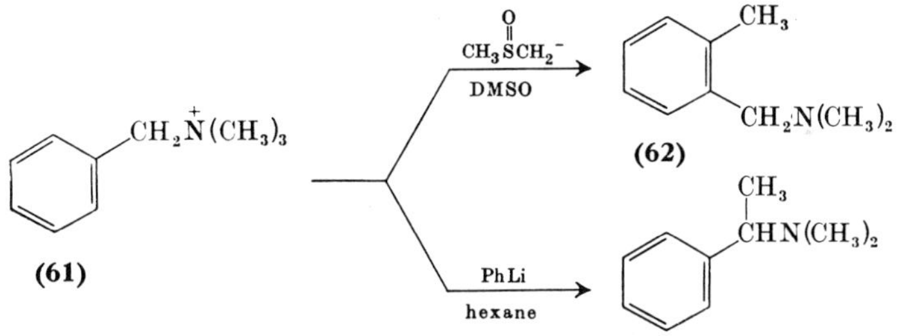

PhCH$_2\overset{+}{N}(CH_3)_3$

(61)

$\xrightarrow[DMSO]{CH_3\overset{O}{\overset{\|}{S}}CH_2^-}$ o-CH$_3$-C$_6$H$_4$-CH$_2$N(CH$_3$)$_2$ (62)

$\xrightarrow[hexane]{PhLi}$ C$_6$H$_5$-CH(CH$_3$)N(CH$_3$)$_2$ (63)

The base-catalyzed autoxidation of sulfoxides was studied by Wallace (85) and Russell and co-workers (86). Among the products identified in various oxidations of DMSO were carbon dioxide, methanesulfonic acid, formic acid, and formaldehyde. The formation of dimethylsulfone was reported by the Russell group but could not be confirmed by Wallace.

In a series of papers, Russell and co-workers have explored the use of

DMSO–KO*t*Bu mixtures containing traces of oxygen for the generation of radical anions in aromatic systems (86) and also for the formation of semidione radical anions from cyclic and acyclic ketones (87). Electron spin resonance studies of the latter compounds have been applied to stereochemical problems.

Iwai and Ide (88) reacted tolan with methylsulfinyl carbanion. At temperatures below 35°, a mixture of the unsaturated sulfoxides **64** and **65** was obtained. When the reaction was carried out without temperature control, the major product was 1,2-diphenylbutadiene **(66)**.

$$PhC{\equiv}CPh + CH_3\overset{O}{\underset{\|}{S}}CH_2^- \xrightarrow[50°]{35°, 4\ hr} \begin{matrix} Ph\\ \diagdown \\ C{=}C \\ \diagup \\ H \end{matrix} \begin{matrix} CH_2\overset{O}{\underset{\|}{S}}CH_3 \\ \diagup \\ \\ \diagdown \\ Ph \end{matrix} + \begin{matrix} Ph \\ \diagdown \\ C{=}C \\ \diagup \\ H \end{matrix} \begin{matrix} Ph \\ \diagup \\ \\ \diagdown \\ CH_2\overset{O}{\underset{\|}{S}}CH_3 \end{matrix}$$

(64)   (65)

$$PhC{-}{-}CPh$$
$$\underset{CH_2}{\|}\ \underset{CH_2}{\|}$$
(66)

All of the reactions of methylsulfinyl carbanion which have been discussed so far have involved reaction with other substrates. A few reports occur in the literature which suggest that lithium methylsulfinyl carbanion can undergo an elimination reaction to yield methyllithium and methylene sulfine **(67)**.

$$CH_3{-}\overset{O}{\underset{\|}{S}}{-}CH_2Li \rightarrow CH_3Li + CH_2{=}\overset{O}{\underset{\|}{S}}:$$
(67)

Franzen (89) has reported that "DMSO reacts with organolithium compounds . . . to a considerable extent according to the following exchange reaction, $(CH_3)_2SO + RLi \rightarrow CH_3SOR + CH_3Li$." Franzen furthermore suggested that such a reaction was common for sulfoxides; however, no experimental results have appeared in support of these comments. The exchange reaction by Franzen can be rationalized in terms of the elimination described above followed by addition of a second equivalent of alkyllithium to the carbon–sulfur bond of the sulfine to produce, after hydrolysis, alkyl methyl sulfoxide (CH_3SOR). Methylene sulfine has also been suggested as a possible intermediate in the formation of n-butyl methyl sulfoxide and t-butyl methyl sulfoxide upon reaction of the respective alkyllithium with N,N-dialkylsulfinamides **68** at $-78°$ (57,90).

$$CH_3SON[CH(CH_3)_2]_2 + RLi \xrightarrow[-78°]{THF} CH_2{=}SO + LiN[CH(CH_3)_2]_2$$
$$(\mathbf{68}) \qquad \qquad \downarrow RLi$$
$$LiCH_2SOR$$

Jacobus and Mislow (91,92) have considered methylene sulfine as a possible intermediate in the base-catalyzed racemization of optically active aryl methyl sulfoxides. Although a number of other mechanisms such as isomerization via a penta-coordinate sulfur species **69** or by inversion of the carbanion **70** could not be definitely ruled out, the sulfine mechanism was considered highly likely since it was able to accommodate all the experimental results.

$$\underset{(\mathbf{69})}{\overset{PhO}{\underset{:CH_3}{\overset{\diagdown\,\|}{S}{-}Ph}}} \qquad \underset{(\mathbf{70})}{\overset{O}{\underset{}{\overset{\|}{Ph\overset{}{S}}{-}\bar{CH}_2}}}$$

$$\underset{}{\overset{O}{\overset{\|}{PhSCH_3}}} \xrightarrow{PhLi} \underset{}{\overset{O}{\overset{\|}{PhSCH_2Li}}} \rightleftharpoons PhLi + CH_2{=}SO \rightleftharpoons \underset{}{\overset{O}{\overset{\|}{LiCH_2SPh}}}$$

The conversion of dibenzylsulfoxide to *trans*-stilbene on exposure to strong base, observed by Wallace et al. (93), can be explained in a similar manner (Scheme 7). Cleavage of the initially formed carbanion **71** to the sulfine **72** and benzyllithium followed by rapid recombination leads to the sulfenate **73**. The conversion of **73** to *trans*-stilbene by

$$\underset{}{\overset{O}{\overset{\|}{PhCH_2SCH_2Ph}}} \underset{}{\overset{KOtBu}{\rightleftharpoons}} \underset{(\mathbf{71})}{\overset{O}{\overset{\|}{Ph\bar{C}HSCH_2Ph}}} \rightleftharpoons \underset{(\mathbf{72})}{[PhCH{=}SO + PhCH_2Li]}$$
$$\downarrow$$
$$PhCH{=}CHPh + [SO^{2-}] \longleftarrow \underset{\underset{(\mathbf{73})}{SO^-}}{\overset{}{PhCH{-}CH_2Ph}}$$

Scheme 7

elimination of [SO^{2-}] has analogy in the base-catalyzed cleavage of tetramethylene sulfoxide to butadiene (66). The rearrangement of dibenzylsulfoxide to **72** is analogous to the Wittig rearrangement of benzyl ethers which has recently been shown to occur either by a carbanion or radical anion elimination–recombination mechanism rather than a concerted 1,2-rearrangement (94–96).

III. Dimethyloxosulfonium Methylid

A. TRIMETHYLOXOSULFONIUM SALTS

The alkylation of DMSO with methyl iodide was initially reported by Kuhn and Trischmann (97) and shown to result in the formation of trimethyloxosulfonium iodide. Major and Hess (98) obtained the corresponding bromide by a less obvious route, i.e., by reaction of phenacyl bromide or ethyl bromoacetate with DMSO. A more systematic examination of the alkylation of DMSO was carried out by Smith and Winstein (99). These authors found that in general both O-alkylated **(74)** and S-alkylated products **(73)** were obtained, the former being products of kinetic and the latter products of thermodynamic control. The rate of isomerization **74 → 73** was found to depend upon the nucleophilicity of the counter ion X$^-$(I$^-$ > NO$_2^-$ > RSO$_3^-$). The suggested route, which is in agreement with the above observation, involves reversibility of the formation of the O-alkyl adduct and competing formation of the S-alkyl derivative.

Nucleophilicity of the sulfur atom in DMSO is only rarely observed. Another clearcut example has been found in the reaction of palladous chloride with DMSO (100). Coordination of sulfur to palladium was suggested for the complex PdCl$_2$[(CH$_3$)$_2$SO]$_2$ on the basis of the S—O stretching frequency which occurred at 1120 cm^{-1}; the S—O frequency of DMSO–metal complexes which coordinate through oxygen occurs below 1010 cm^{-1} (101).

$$\underset{(73)}{\overset{\overset{O}{\|}}{\underset{\underset{R}{|+}}{CH_3SCH_3}}} \xleftarrow{RX} \underset{}{\overset{\overset{O}{\|}}{CH_3SCH_3}} \rightleftharpoons \underset{(74)}{\overset{\overset{OR}{|}}{\underset{+}{CH_3SCH_3}}}$$

In addition to the above results, Smith and Winstein reported the important observation that trimethyloxosulfonium salts undergo proton exchange more rapidly in neutral solution than trimethylsulfonium salts in basic media (102,103). The remarkable ease of proton exchange prompted the investigations of Corey and Chaykovsky (17,104) regarding the generation of dimethyloxosulfonium methylid (75) and its application to synthesis.

$$(CH_3)_2\overset{O}{\overset{\|}{S}}CH_3 + (CH_3)_2\overset{O}{\overset{\|}{\underset{+}{S}}}-\overset{}{\underset{-}{CH_2}} \xrightarrow{D_2O} (CH_3)_2\overset{O}{\overset{\|}{\underset{+}{S}}}CH_2D$$
$$(75)$$

Alkoxysulfonium salts, e.g., 74, are available by a number of routes. Their importance both synthetically and mechanistically stems from the fact that they have been shown to be intermediates in the Moffatt-Pfitzner oxidation (see Sec. IV for a more complete discussion regarding the formation and chemistry of these compounds). In contrast, only a few oxosulfonium salts have been described. In all instances except one, these salts had no hydrogen atoms β to the sulfur function. The lone exception to this is the zwitterionic compound 76 formed by heating 1,3-propane sultone in DMSO at 85°. Here again, the O-alkylated salt 77 was formed initially and was readily isolated when the reaction was carried out at room temperature. Isomerization to 76 occurred on heating at 85° in DMSO (105).

<pre>
                                    (CH₃)₂S⁺—O(CH₂)₃SO₃⁻
                              25°   (77)
         O   O   │ 85°
         │   +   CH₃SCH₃   ↓
         SO₂   ‖   O
                                          ‖
                              85°   (CH₃)₂S(CH₂)₃SO₃⁻
                                          +
                                         (76)
</pre>

Attempts at preparing some other oxosulfonium salts such as dimethylethyloxosulfonium iodide (78) by alkylation of dimethyloxosulfonium methylid (75) with methyl iodide have not been successful and only dimethylsulfoxide has been isolated from such a reaction (106). This result was explained in terms of the instability of 78 to β-elimination.

$$(CH_3)_2\overset{O}{\overset{\|}{\underset{+}{S}}}-\underset{-}{CH_2} + CH_3I \rightarrow (CH_3)_2\overset{O}{\overset{\|}{\underset{+}{S}}}CH_2CH_3\ I^- \rightarrow CH_3\overset{O}{\overset{\|}{S}}CH_3 + CH_2=CH_2$$
$$(75) \qquad\qquad\qquad (78)$$

Trimethyloxosulfonium ions can be demethylated by such bases as pyridine and quinoline (97), the methylated bases being formed in 97 and 94% yield, respectively, eq. a. Addition of the ylid **75** to phenols, carboxylic acids, or oximes also resulted in methylation of these compounds presumably via trimethyloxosulfonium salts formed *in situ* (107,108). These reactions are generalized in eq. b. The formation of thioanisole from thiophenol and **73a** has been observed by Wallace and Mahon (109) who suggested the species **79**, formed by addition of thiophenolate to **73a**, as a possible intermediate in the reaction. At the present time, the latter pathway should be considered less likely than the straightforward mechanism represented by eqs. a and b.

a. $(CH_3)_2\overset{+}{S}(O)-\overset{-}{CH_2}$ (**75**) + pyridine $\longrightarrow$ N-methylpyridinium + $CH_3S(O)CH_3$

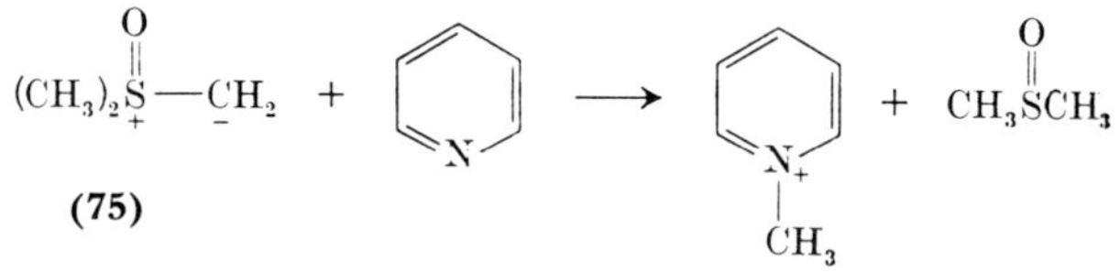

b. $AH + (CH_3)_2\overset{+}{S}(O)-\overset{-}{CH_2}$ (**75**) $\rightleftharpoons$ $A^- + (CH_3)_2\overset{+}{S}(O)-CH_3 \longrightarrow ACH_3 + CH_3S(O)CH_3$

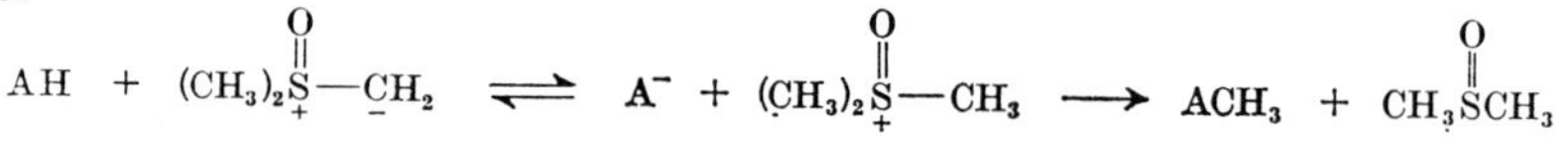

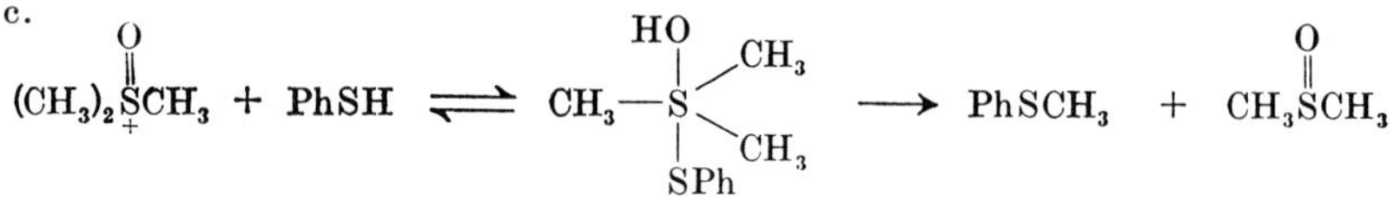

c. $(CH_3)_2\overset{+}{S}(O)CH_3$ (**73a**) $+ PhSH \rightleftharpoons CH_3-\underset{SPh}{\overset{HO}{S}}(CH_3)(CH_3)$ (**79**) $\longrightarrow PhSCH_3 + CH_3S(O)CH_3$

B. PREPARATION OF DIMETHYLOXOSULFONIUM METHYLID

A particularly convenient and inexpensive preparation of solutions of dimethyloxosulfonium methylid (**75**) in DMSO, tetrahydrofuran, or dioxane involves interaction of trimethyloxosulfonium salts with sodium hydride (17,104). In DMSO, the formation of the ylid is complete within 15–20 min at room temperature; in the ether solvents it is necessary to heat for 3–4 hr at 65° in order to complete the reaction. Tetrahydrofuran solutions of **75**, prepared in this manner, are stable for several months if kept at 0° and under an inert atmosphere. The concentration of ylid in such solutions is readily determined by titration with standard acid in water.

Dimethyloxosulfonium methylid (**75**) may be represented by the hybrid structures **75** ↔ **75a** ↔ **75b** ↔ **75c**. The factors responsible for stabilization and bonding in carbanions α to sulfur functions have recently been reviewed in considerable depth (9,110,111) and will not be repeated here. The structure **75** will be used to represent dimethyloxosulfonium methylid throughout this article because the author feels that it best conveys its nucleophilic character. At the present time, dimethyloxosulfonium methylid is the only known representative of this type of ylid (no stablizing group other than the sulfur function). This may be partly due to the unavailability of other trialkyloxosulfonium salts, but even should such salts become available the generation of ylids from these salts would likely be complicated by competing β-elimination to form olefins and sulfoxides (106).

$$(CH_3)_2\overset{O}{\underset{+}{\overset{\|}{S}}}-\overset{-}{CH_2} \leftrightarrow (CH_3)_2\overset{O}{\overset{\|}{S}}=CH_2 \leftrightarrow (CH_3)_2\overset{O^-}{\underset{+}{\overset{|}{S}}}=CH_2 \leftrightarrow (CH_3)_2\overset{O^-}{\underset{2+}{\overset{|}{S}}}-\overset{-}{CH_2}$$

(**75**)   (**75a**)   (**75b**)   (**75c**)

C. REACTIONS OF DIMETHYLOXOSULFONIUM METHYLID

The initial investigations of Corey and Chaykovsky indicated considerable synthetic utility of dimethyloxosulfonium methylid, especially as a methylene transfer reagent in reactions with polar double bonds. In addition, useful differences in the reactivity between **75** and the closely related dimethylsulfonium methylid (**80**) were uncovered; these will be referred to at appropriate places in the discussion. Recent reviews on sulfonium ylids are by Johnson (111) and Bloch (4).

$$(CH_3)_2\overset{+}{S}-\overset{-}{CH_2} \leftrightarrow (CH_3)_2S=CH_2$$
(**80**)

1. Reaction with Ketones and Aldehydes

The reactivity of the ylid **75** toward ketones and aldehydes can be expressed in terms of eq. a and as such is comparable to the diazomethane–carbonyl reaction. The process involving this ylid is, however, not complicated by the formation of insertion products which accompany the diazomethane reaction (112). The formation of epoxides from ketones and aldehydes by reaction with the ylid is restricted to those which are not excessively prone to enolate formation.

In these instances preferential proton transfer occurs between the carbonyl compound and **75**, thereby precluding further reaction, eq. b.

a. $R_2C=O + (CH_3)_2\overset{+}{\underset{-}{S}}-CH_2 \overset{O}{\|} \rightarrow R_2C\overset{O}{\triangle}CH_2 + CH_3\overset{O}{\overset{\|}{S}}CH_3$

(**75**)

b. $Ph\overset{O}{\overset{\|}{C}}CH_2Ph + \mathbf{75} \rightarrow Ph\overset{O^-}{\overset{|}{C}}=CHPh + (CH_3)_2\overset{+}{\overset{O}{\overset{\|}{S}}}CH_3$

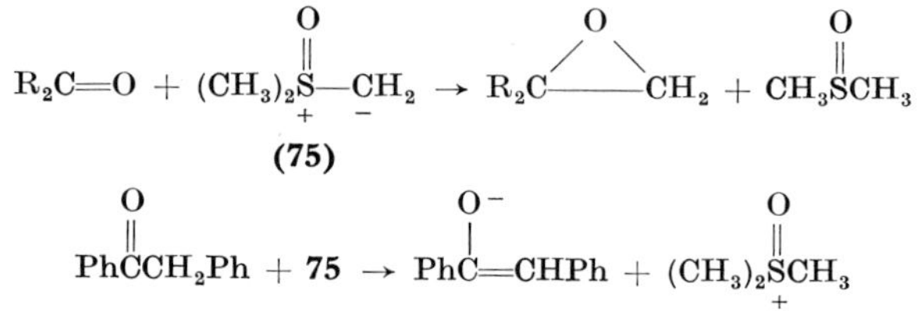

The formation of epoxides probably occurs via initial and reversible attack of **75** on the carbonyl compound to form the betaine **81** which can cyclize with concomitant expulsion of dimethylsulfoxide (16). The possibility existed that **81** might decompose via the cyclic intermediate **82**, in analogy with the decomposition of the corresponding phosphorus betaine **83**, and thus produce an olefin and dimethylsulfone (111,113). This type of decomposition has not been observed for betaines such as **81**, or for the corresponding sulfonium derivatives **84** which also give only epoxides.

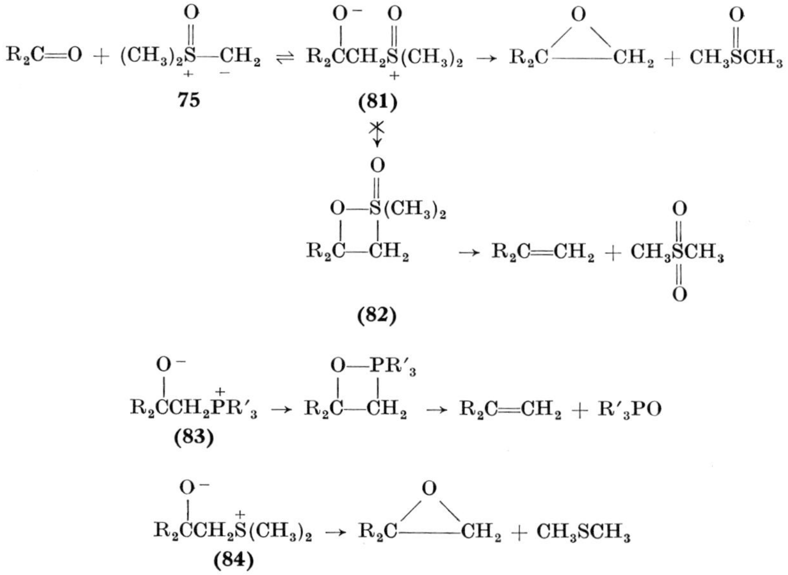

$R_2C=O + (CH_3)_2\overset{+}{\underset{-}{S}}-CH_2 \rightleftharpoons R_2\overset{O^-}{\underset{|}{C}}CH_2\overset{+}{\overset{O}{\overset{\|}{S}}}(CH_3)_2 \rightarrow R_2C\overset{O}{\triangle}CH_2 + CH_3\overset{O}{\overset{\|}{S}}CH_3$

75   (**81**)

$\downarrow\!\!\!\!\!\times$

$\begin{matrix} & O \\ & \| \\ O-\!\!\!&S(CH_3)_2 \\ | & | \\ R_2C-\!\!\!&CH_2 \end{matrix} \rightarrow R_2C=CH_2 + CH_3\overset{O}{\underset{O}{\overset{\|}{\underset{\|}{S}}}}CH_3$

(**82**)

$R_2\overset{O^-}{\underset{|}{C}}CH_2\overset{+}{P}R'_3 \rightarrow R_2\overset{O-PR'_3}{\underset{|}{C}}\!\!-\!\!\overset{|}{C}H_2 \rightarrow R_2C=CH_2 + R'_3PO$

(**83**)

$R_2\overset{O^-}{\underset{|}{C}}CH_2\overset{+}{S}(CH_3)_2 \rightarrow R_2C\overset{O}{\triangle}CH_2 + CH_3SCH_3$

(**84**)

The reaction between carbonyl compounds and **75** when carried out in DMSO or tetrahydrofuran generally gives excellent yields of the desired product which is easily isolated and purified. Typical yields are shown in Table IX; for comparison, data obtained using dimethylsulfonium methylid **(80)** are also included. Because of the greater stability of **75** compared to **80**, reactions in which both ylids lead to the same product are more conveniently carried out using the former reagent.

Holt and Lowe (114) have reported a simple benzofuran synthesis by interaction of **75** with salicylaldehydes. Intermediates in the benzofuran formation are 3-hydroxy-2,3-dihydrobenzofurans **(85)** which can be isolated in good yield if exposure to acids is avoided on work-up. o-Hydroxyacetophenone and o-hydroxybenzalaniline underwent analogous reactions. The mechanism of the formation of these products is of interest since it may involve formation of the furan ring without the intermediacy of the epoxide **86** and thus provides concrete evidence as to the initial formation of a zwitterionic species such as **87** in the transfer of the methylene group from dimethyloxosulfonium methylid to a carbonyl compound.

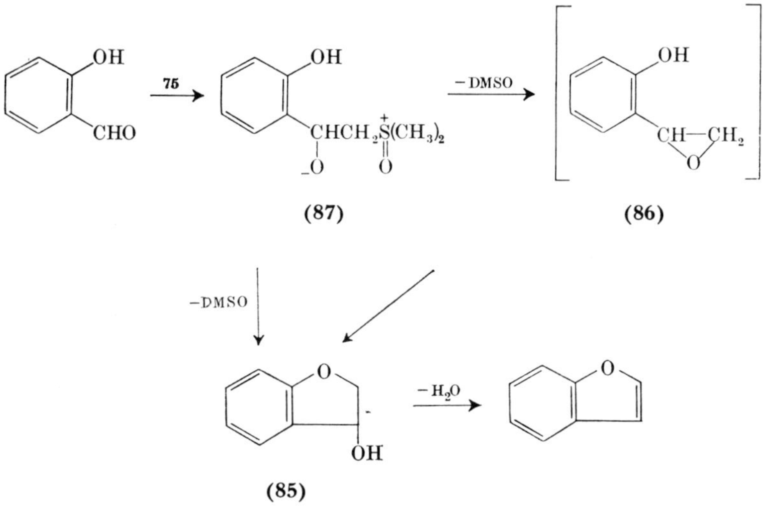

Methylene transfer from **75** to cyclohexanones occurs selectively and in such a way that the newly formed carbon–carbon linkage is equatorial (17,115). This selectivity is exemplified by the formation

TABLE IX
Reaction of Dimethyloxosulfonium Methylid (**75**) and Dimethylsulfonium Methylid (**80**) with Ketones and Aldehydes

Substrate	Reagent	Product	Yield, %	Ref.
Ph_2CO	75	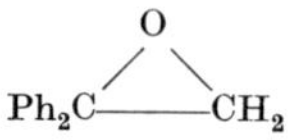 $Ph_2C\text{—}CH_2$ epoxide	90	17
	80	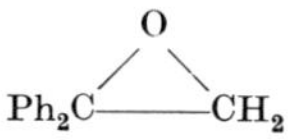 $Ph_2C\text{—}CH_2$ epoxide	84	17
	80	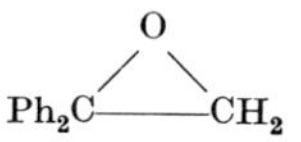 $Ph_2C\text{—}CH_2$ epoxide	82	126
PhCHO	75	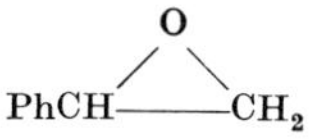 $PhCH\text{—}CH_2$ epoxide	56	17
	80	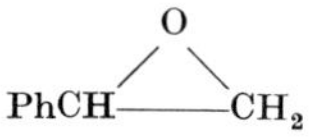 $PhCH\text{—}CH_2$ epoxide	75	17
	80	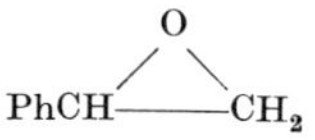 $PhCH\text{—}CH_2$ epoxide	65	126
Cycloheptanone	75	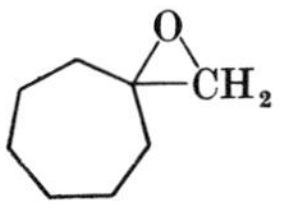 cycloheptanone spiro epoxide with CH_2	71	17
	80	,,	75	126
	80	,,	97	17
Cyclohexanone	80	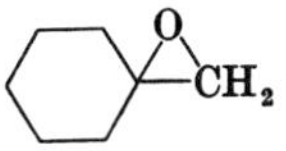 cyclohexanone spiro epoxide with CH_2	74	126
4-t-Butylcyclohexanone	75	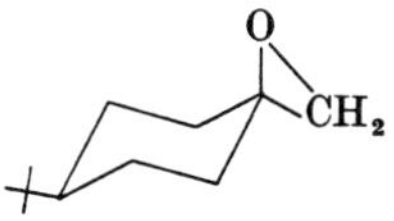 (axial O, equatorial CH_2)	89	17
4-t-Butylcyclohexanone	80	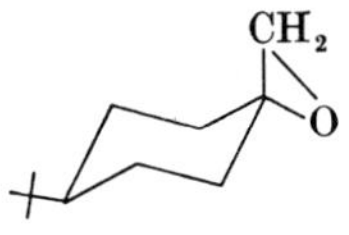 (axial CH_2, equatorial O)	77[a]	17
3,3,5-Trimethylcyclohexanone	75	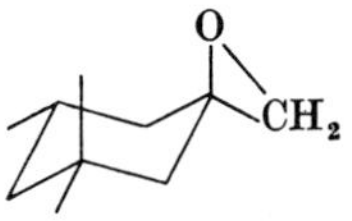 trimethylcyclohexanone spiro epoxide with CH_2	78	17

(*continued*)

TABLE IX (*continued*)

3,3,5-Trimethylcyclohexanone	**80**	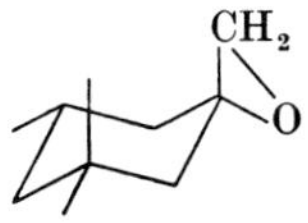	88[b]	17
4-Phenylcyclohexanone	**75**	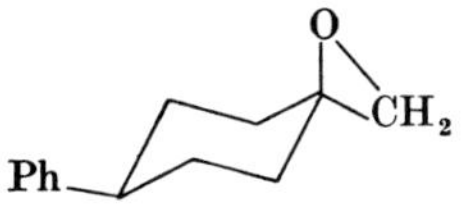	72	17
1-Acetylcyclohexene	**75**	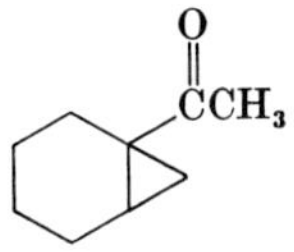	54	17
Carvone	**75**	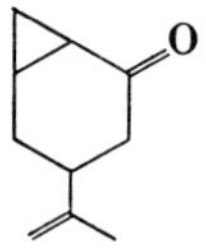	81	17
Eucarvone	**75**	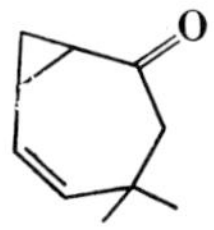	88	17
Eucarvone	**80**	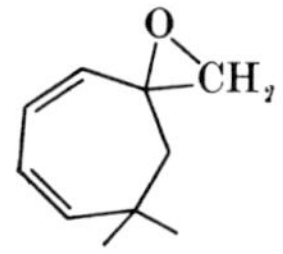	93	17
Pulegone	**80**	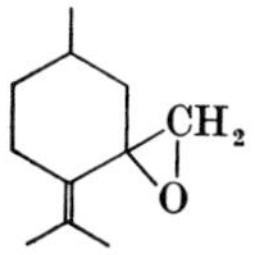	90	17
Bicyclo [2,2,1] hept-2-en-7-one	**75**	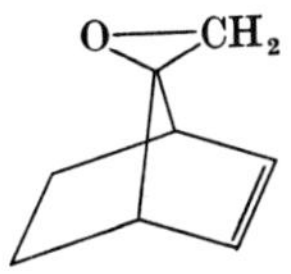	72	120
Benzalacetophenone	**75**	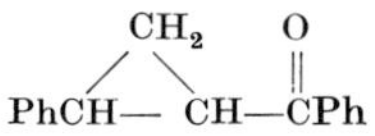	95	17

(*continued*)

TABLE IX (continued)

Substrate	Ylid	Product	Yield (%)	Ref.
Benzalacetophenone	80	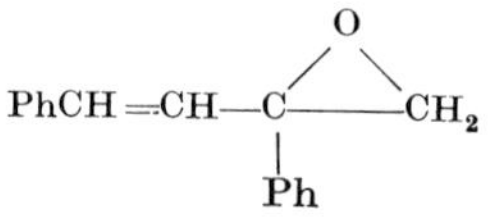 PhCH=CH−C(Ph)(O−CH2) epoxide	87	17
Salicylaldehyde	75	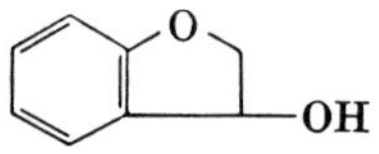 2,3-dihydrobenzofuran-2-yl−OH	68	114
5-Bromosalicylaldehyde	75	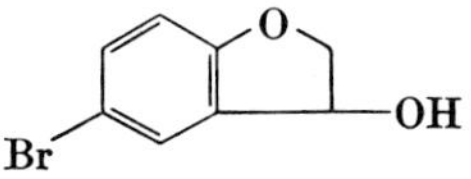 5-Br-2,3-dihydrobenzofuran-2-yl−OH	79	114
5-Chlorosalicylaldehyde	75	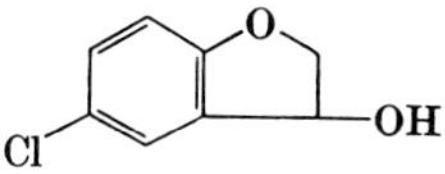 5-Cl-2,3-dihydrobenzofuran-2-yl−OH	78	114
3-Methoxysalicylaldehyde	75	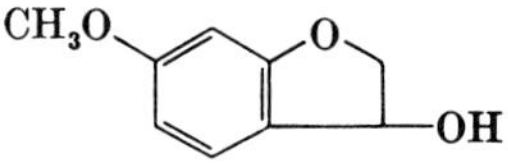 7-CH3O-2,3-dihydrobenzofuran-2-yl−OH	38	114
2-Hydroxy-1-naphthaldehyde	75	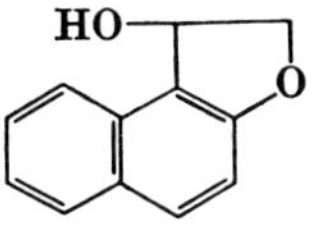 1-HO-naphtho[2,1-b]furan	86	114
o-Hydroxyacetophenone	75	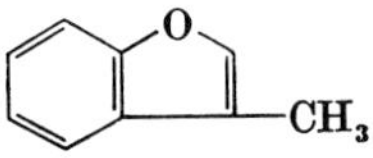 2-methylbenzofuran	80	114
Δ-4-Cholesten-3-one	75	Enolization	0	17
Δ-4-Cholesten-3-one	80	Isomeric mixture	90	17
Deoxybenzoin	75	Enolization	0	17
Deoxybenzoin	80	Enolization	0	17

[a] 83% isomer as shown.
[b] 55% isomer as shown.

of the epoxides **88** and **89** in 78 and 89% yield from the corresponding ketones. The stereochemistry of **89** was shown by lithium aluminum hydride reduction to **90** (94%). Overend and co-workers have observed similar stereochemical results using carbohydrate substrates (116). Dimethylsulfonium methylid **(80)**, on the other hand, underwent mainly, but not exclusively, axial addition to 4-t-butylcyclohexanone to afford after reduction with lithium aluminum hydride an 83/17 ratio of *cis/trans* 4-*t*-butyl-1-methylcyclohexanol (the stereochemistry refers to the *t*-butyl and methyl groups).

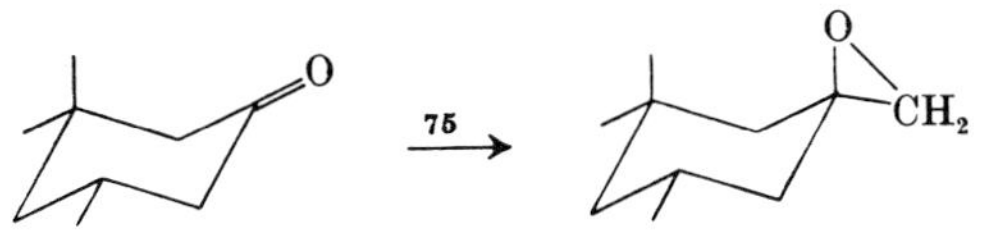

(88)

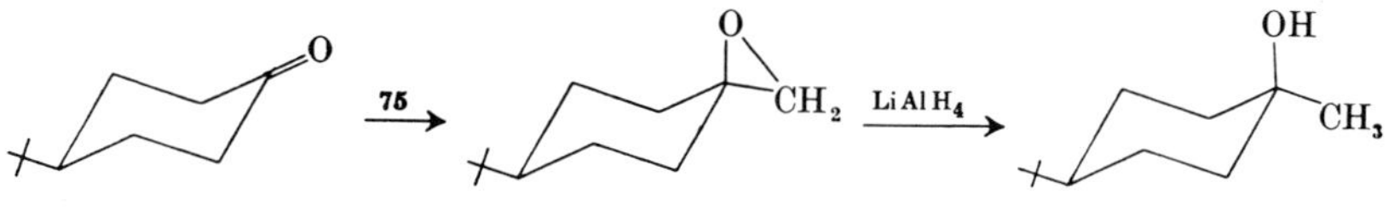

(89)   (90)

Complementary selectivity of the two ylids has also been reported by Cook et al. (115). Reaction of dihydrotestosterone (91) with 75 and 80 afforded stereospecifically the epoxides 92 (methylene group equatorial, 78%) and 93 (methylene group axial, 90%), respectively. The stereochemistry of the epoxides was proved by conversion to the tertiary alcohols 94 and 95, followed by dehydration with phosphorus oxychloride. Since the latter requires a *trans* and coplanar arrangement of a hydrogen and the hydroxyl group (117), dehydration of the equatorial alcohol 95 can and does lead only to the exocyclic olefin 96.

The observed equatorial addition by dimethyloxosulfonium methylid can be rationally explained. Addition of a bulky reagent to a six-membered ring ketone is generally considered to be sterically more favorable from the equatorial direction. Such addition of 75 leads to the betaine intermediate 97 which can cyclize to the observed product. Addition from the axial direction results in the formation of the intermediate 98. The stereoelectronic requirements for ring closure are such that the oxygen and sulfur functions take up a *trans* coplanar arrangement (118). In such an arrangement, the sulfur function in the intermediate 98 encounters very strong steric interactions with the *syn* axial protons on carbons 3 and 5, thereby probably making cyclization to the epoxide a higher energy process than the reversal to the starting materials. Qualitatively, the same situation should exist for the reaction of dimethylsulfonium methylid if the methylene transfer occurs by this mechanism. It has been argued (115) that the

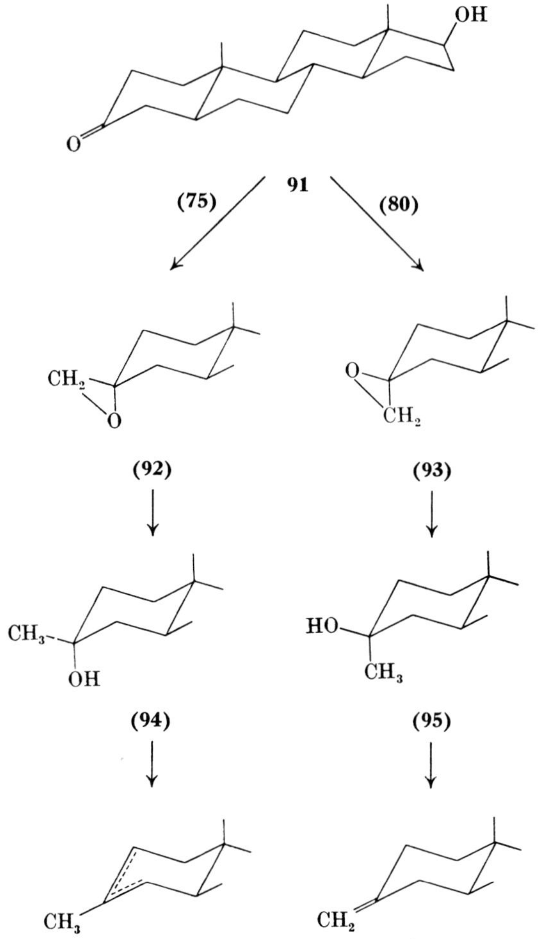

328 T. DURST

(75) 91 (80)

(92) (93)

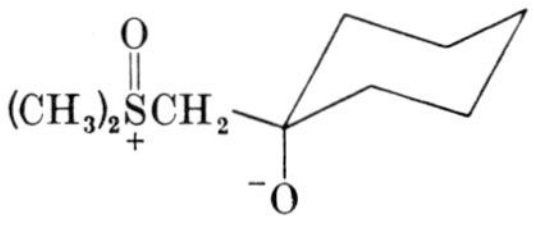

(94) (95)

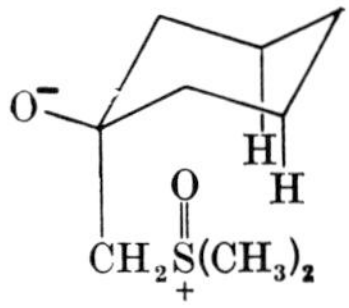

(96)

(97) (98) (99)

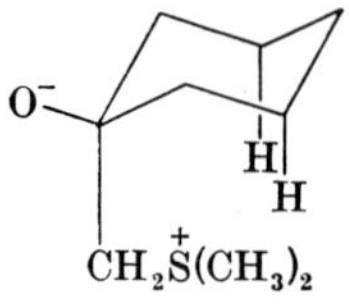

latter reagent is smaller than the oxosulfonium ylid and that steric compression in the cyclization of **99** would not be as prohibitive as in **98**. Admitting for the moment that cyclization from **99** may be possible, it is difficult to justify the very high proportion of initial axial attack by the sulfonium ylid.

The tendency for axial carbon–carbon bond formation in the reactions of **80** with cyclohexanones persists even with 3,3,5-trimethylcyclohexanone [ratio of axial to equatorial CH_2, 55:45 (17)] despite the strong adverse effects of the axial 3-methyl group which should affect not only the axial approach of the reagent but also introduce prohibitive steric interactions in the transition state leading to epoxide formation.

It seems reasonable that the detailed mechanism for methylene transfer differs for the two reagents. More experimental data are, however, needed to support proposals which might be made at this time. The complexity of the situation here may be similar to that found in the reduction of ketones with metal hydrides. Despite the fact that hydride reductions have been studied quite thoroughly, especially in the steroid field (19,119), there remains a lack of understanding and agreement as to the relative importance of the various factors which can influence the stereochemical results of such reductions.

The stereospecific methylene transfer from dimethyloxosulfonium methylid to bicyclo[2.2.1]hept-2-en-7-one to yield the epoxide **101** has been explained in the following manner. Attack of the ylid on the side *syn* to the double bond is sterically favored by the absence of two *exo* hydrogens. In addition, **102** may be stabilized by attractive interactions between the positively charged sulfur atom and the pi orbitals of the double bond. The involvement of the pi orbitals may also account for the stereospecific acid-catalyzed rearrangement of **101** to the aldehyde **103** (120).

Control of the stereochemistry of metal hydride reduction and Grignard addition to carbonyl compounds by the presence of neighboring oxygen or amine functions is well documented (121,122). Similar control ought to be possible as well for the methylene transfer from sulfur ylids such as **75** and **80**, thereby enhancing the synthetic utility of these reagents.

A further difference between **75** and **80** is observed in their reaction with α,β-unsaturated ketones. The former reagent produces cyclopropyl ketones while the latter affords exclusively α,β-unsaturated

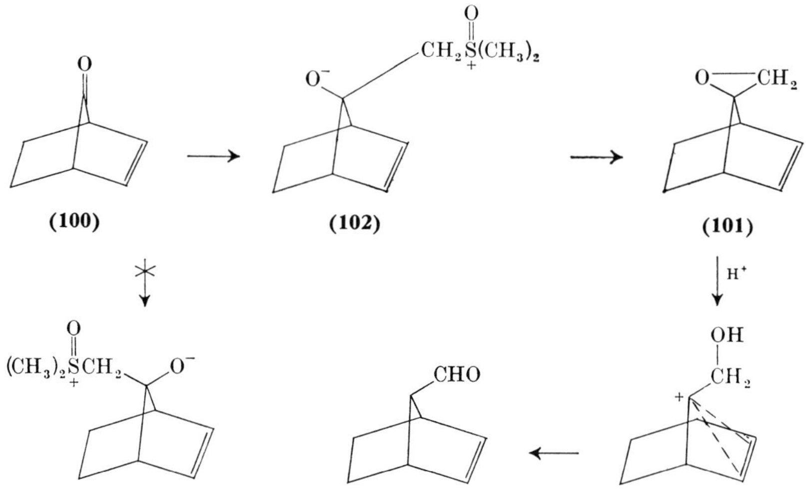

[Scheme showing structures 100, 102, 101, 103 with reaction arrows]

epoxides (17,123–126) (Table IX). This difference may be related to the lower nucleophilicity and larger size of dimethyloxosulfonium methylid.

$$\text{RCH=CHCR'} \xrightarrow{\text{O}} \begin{array}{l} \xrightarrow{75} \text{RCH—CHCR'} \text{ (with CH}_2\text{ epoxide and C=O)} \\ \xrightarrow{80} \text{RCH=CHC(R')—CH}_2 \text{ (with epoxide O)} \end{array}$$

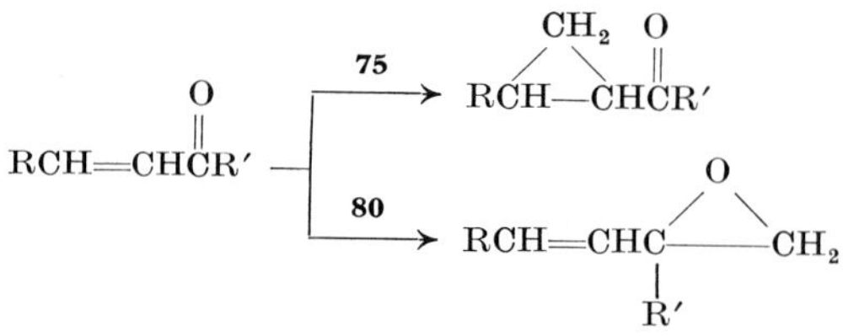

Thus, in their reactions with ketones, dimethyloxosulfonium methylid and dimethylsulfonium methylid would seem to complement rather than simply duplicate each other. The availability of reagents such as these which show stereospecific complementary reactivity can often be of decisive importance in the planning and execution of a synthetic scheme. Application of dimethyloxosulfonium methylid has been reported in the synthesis of the natural product d,l-rimuene (127).

2. Reaction with Carboxylic Acid Derivatives

A number of different processes have been observed in reactions involving dimethyloxosulfonium methylid and carboxylic acid derivatives. Carboxylic acids, as was mentioned in Section III-A, are converted by **75** to the corresponding methyl esters. Acid chlorides (128–131), anhydrides (129,131), or phenyl esters (128) react with two equivalents of **75** to form the highly stabilized acylated oxosulfonium ylids, e.g., **104**. Such ylids, which are also produced by the interaction of **75** with ketenes (129), are readily isolable substances of high thermal stability. They exhibit greatly reduced nucleophilicity and react further only with very strong electrophiles such as acid chlorides, carbamoyl chlorides or isocyanates (131) affording diacylated or acylcarbamoyl ylids **105** and **106**.

$$\overset{O}{\underset{\|}{R\overset{}{C}X}} + 2(CH_3)_2\overset{O}{\underset{\underset{-}{\|}}{\overset{+}{S}}}-CH_2 \rightarrow R\overset{O}{\underset{\|}{\overset{}{C}}}CH_2-\overset{O}{\underset{\underset{+}{\|}}{S}}(CH_3)_2 \xrightarrow{-H^+} R\overset{O}{\underset{\|}{\overset{}{C}}}\overset{-}{\underset{}{C}}H-\overset{O}{\underset{\underset{+}{\|}}{S}}(CH_3)_2$$

(104)

$$104 + R'\overset{O}{\underset{\|}{\overset{}{C}}}Cl \rightarrow R\overset{O}{\underset{\|}{\overset{}{C}}}-\overset{-}{\underset{\underset{+}{(CH_3)_2SO}}{C}}-\overset{O}{\underset{\|}{\overset{}{C}}}R'$$

(105)

$$104 + R'N\!=\!C\!=\!O \rightarrow R\overset{O}{\underset{\|}{\overset{}{C}}}-\overset{-}{\underset{\underset{+}{(CH_3)_2SO}}{C}}-\overset{O}{\underset{\|}{\overset{}{C}}}NHR'$$

(106)

The carbamoyl substituted oxosulfonium ylids such as **107**, derived from **75** and phenyl isocyanate, are considerably more reactive than the acylated derivatives (131). Reaction of **107** with isobutyraldehyde in the presence of a small amount of isobutyric acid afforded the unsaturated amide **108** in 40% yield. The epoxide **109** was suggested as a probable intermediate.

$$PhN\!=\!C\!=\!O + 75 \rightarrow PhNH\overset{O}{\underset{\|}{\overset{}{C}}}\overset{-}{\underset{}{C}}H-\overset{O}{\underset{\underset{+}{\|}}{S}}(CH_3)_2$$

(107)

$$\downarrow (CH_3)_2CHCHO$$

$$\underset{(108)}{PhNH\overset{O}{\underset{\|}{\overset{}{C}}}CH\!=\!CH\overset{OH}{\underset{|}{\overset{}{C}}}(CH_3)_2} \leftarrow \underset{(109)}{PhNH\overset{O}{\underset{\|}{\overset{}{C}}}CH\overset{O}{\overset{\diagup\diagdown}{-}}CHCH(CH_3)_2}$$

In the presence of toluenesulfonic acid, **107** is converted to the corresponding oxosulfonium salt from which dimethylsulfoxide is readily displaced by nucleophilic reagents such as thiophenol or aniline. The formation of α-iodopropionanilide (39%) on attempted methylation of **107** with methyl iodide probably involves a similar displacement (131).

$$\mathbf{107} + H^+ \rightarrow PhNH\overset{O}{\overset{\|}{C}}CH_2\overset{O}{\overset{\|}{\underset{+}{S}}}(CH_3)_2 \xrightarrow{PhSH} PhNH\overset{O}{\overset{\|}{C}}CH_2SPh + CH_3\overset{O}{\overset{\|}{S}}CH_3$$
$$(81\%)$$

$$\mathbf{107} + CH_3I \rightarrow PhNH\overset{O}{\overset{\|}{C}}\underset{I}{CH}CH_3 + CH_3\overset{O}{\overset{\|}{S}}CH_3$$
$$(39\%)$$

van Leusen and Taylor (132) have employed dimethyloxosulfonium methylid in a novel synthesis of some nitrogen heterocyclic compounds. Treatment of *N*-methylisatoic anhydride **(110)** with **75** led to the formation of the stable ylid **112** in 70% yield presumably via loss of

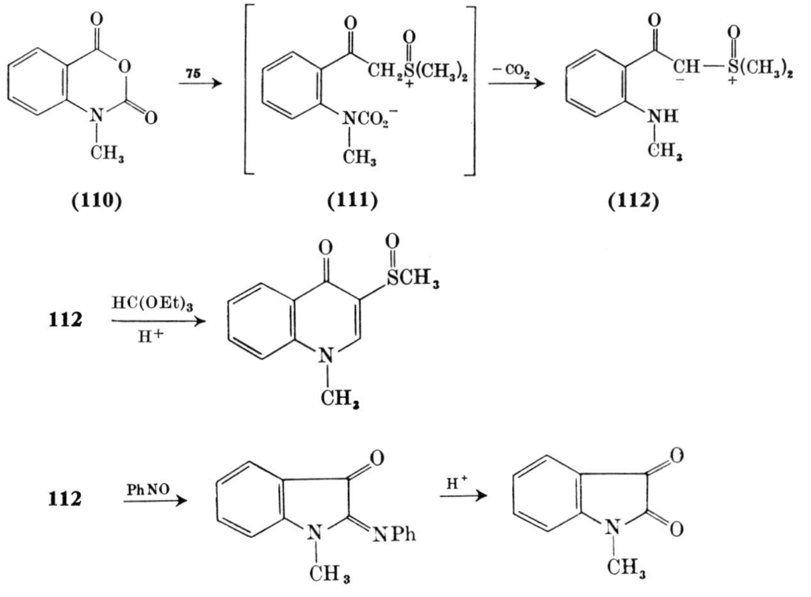

Scheme 8

carbon dioxide from the intermediate **111**. The conversion of **112** to quinolin-4-one and indoxyl derivatives is shown in Scheme 8.

Saturated aliphatic esters do not react with **75** under the usual reaction conditions (128). Modification of other functional groups in the presence of such esters is therefore possible. House and co-workers (133) were thus able to obtain the ester epoxide **114** from the keto ester **113**; again methylene transfer appeared to have occurred with formation of an equatorial carbon–carbon bond.

cyclohexanone with CH$_2$CO$_2$Et substituent → (via **75**) → epoxide with CH$_2$ and CH$_2$CO$_2$Et substituents

(113)   (114)

α,β-Unsaturated esters undergo conjugate addition with dimethyloxosulfonium methylid to afford cyclopropyl esters (124,134–136). Trost and co-workers (135) found that ethyl *trans*-cinnamate was converted by **75** to ethyl 2-phenylcyclopropane carboxylate in about 30% yield (99% *trans* isomer). Nozaki et al. (136) observed a small amount (3–4%) of asymmetric induction in accordance with the Prelog rule (137) upon reaction of **75** with (+)-menthyl esters of *trans*-cinnamic acids. In agreement with the Trost group (135), these workers obtained almost exclusively *trans*-2-arylcyclopropane carboxylic acid derivatives.

$$\text{ArCH}=\text{CHCO}_2\text{R} \xrightarrow{75} \text{Ar}-\underset{\text{H}}{\overset{}{\text{C}}}\overset{\text{CH}_2}{\underset{}{\diagup\!\!\diagdown}}\underset{\text{CO}_2\text{R}}{\overset{}{\text{C}}}-\text{H} \quad (20\text{--}60\%)$$

In the reaction of ethyl *trans*-cinnamate with **75**, Corey and Chaykovsky (124) obtained, in addition to the cyclopropyl ester, a crystalline sulfur-containing product which, on the basis of analytical and spectroscopic data, was assigned the cyclic ylid structure **115a**. In a second report (128), these authors found the formation of such cyclic ylids to be a general process if the reaction was carried out at room temperature in tetrahydrofuran solution. The cyclopropyl esters and the cyclic ylids are presumably both formed from the same intermediate **115**.

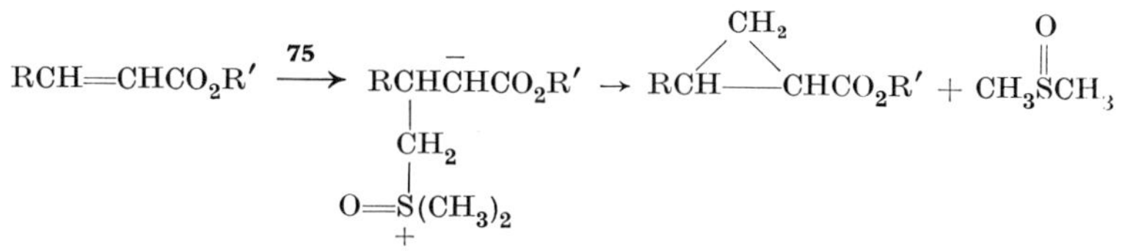

$$RCH{=}CHCO_2R' \xrightarrow{75} RCH\bar{C}HCO_2R' \rightarrow RCH\overset{CH_2}{\underset{}{\triangle}}CHCO_2R' + CH_3\overset{O}{\underset{\|}{S}}CH_3$$

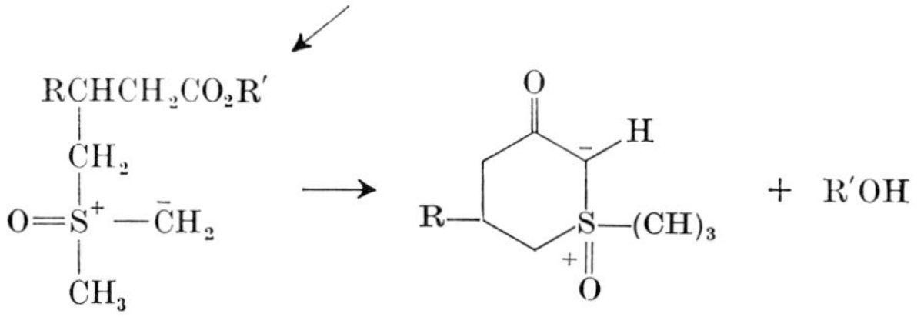

$$\begin{array}{c} RCHCH_2CO_2R' \\ | \\ CH_2 \\ | \\ O{=}\overset{+}{S}{-}\bar{C}H_2 \\ | \\ CH_3 \end{array}$$

(115)

(115a) — gives cyclic β-keto sulfoxonium ylid with R, S(CH₃), + R'OH

One of the most interesting properties of β-keto oxosulfonium ylids is the susceptibility to photochemical cleavage of the dipolar carbon–sulfur bond. The ylids **116** (R = Ph or cyclo-C_6H_{11}), when irradiated at 253 mμ in alcoholic solvent, are converted to esters **117**, presumably via keto carbene and ketene intermediates. Trost (134) has reported similar photochemical behavior for dimethylsulfonium phenacylid and was able to trap the keto-carbene with cyclohexene. A similarity thus exists in the photochemical behavior of α-diazoketones and β-keto sulfur ylids.

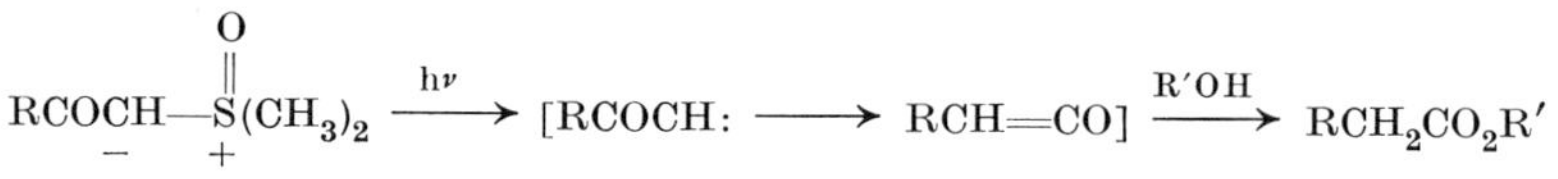

$$RCOCH{-}\overset{+}{S}(CH_3)_2 \xrightarrow{h\nu} [RCOCH{:} \longrightarrow RCH{=}CO] \xrightarrow{R'OH} RCH_2CO_2R'$$

(116)   R = Ph, cyclo-C_6H_{11} **(117)**

$$PhCOCH{-}\overset{+}{S}(CH_3)_2 + \text{cyclohexene} \xrightarrow{h\nu} \text{bicyclic-COPh} + \text{other products}$$

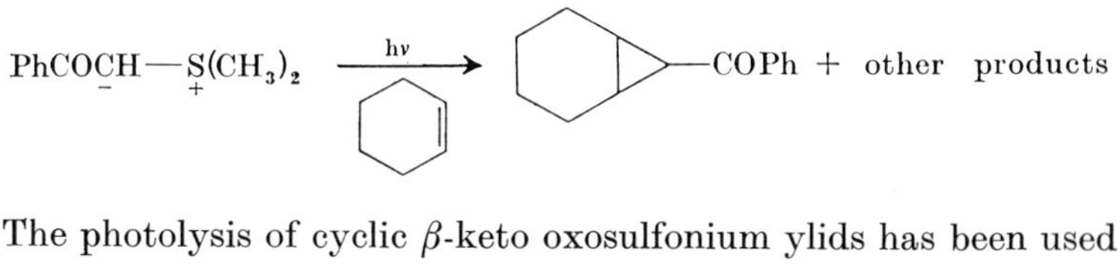

The photolysis of cyclic β-keto oxosulfonium ylids has been used as part of a novel synthesis of cyclopentanones (128). Irradiation of **118**, derived from ethyl Δ¹-cyclohexenyl carboxylate and **75**, at 253 mμ in methanol produced the sulfoxide **119** in 80% yield. Oxidation of **119** to the corresponding sulfone, followed by cyclization with *t*-butoxide, gave the ketosulfone **120** which was hydrogenolized with aluminum amalgam (16) to *trans*-hydrindan-2-one; the overall yield from **118** was 60%. In a similar sequence, 3-phenylcyclopentanone was produced from ethyl cinnamate in 30% yield.

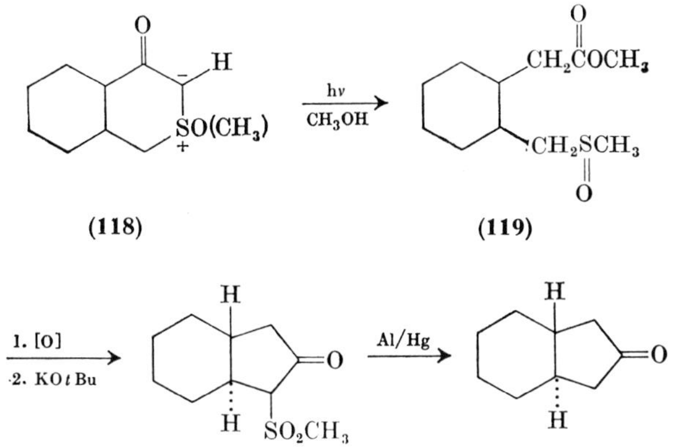

Trost and co-workers (135) investigated the reaction of dimethyloxosulfonium methylid **(75)** with ethyl phenylpropiolate in an attempt to prepare ethyl 2-phenylcyclopropene carboxylate. They obtained, however, a product which, on the basis of analysis and spectroscopic data [infrared C=O at 6.0 μ; ultraviolet λ_{max}^{EtOH} 346 mμ (ε = 16100); NMR singlets at ppm = 2.96 (6H), 4.78 (1H), and 6.28 (1H)], was assigned the resonance-stabilized ylid structure **121**. Ide and Kishida (138) reported similar results. The yields of ylids of the type **121**, obtained with a variety of aromatic substituents, were of the order of 60–100%. Other acetylenic derivatives such as ethyl acetylenedicarboxylate, benzoyl acetylene, phenyl *p*-tolylsulfonyl acetylene and 1,4-diphenyl-1,3-butadiyne were also reported to react with **75** to yield stabilized ylids (138); these products, however, were not described. Tolan was unreactive toward dimethyloxosulfonium methylid.

Ide and Kishida also described some interesting transformations of the ylid **121**. Reduction with zinc in acetic acid afforded a 1:9 mixture of ethyl 3-phenyl-2-butenoate **(122)** and ethyl 3-phenyl-3-butenoate **(123)**, the latter being readily isomerized to **122** on exposure to base. This reduction is reminiscent of the zinc-acetic acid (39) and aluminum amalgam reductions (16) of various β-keto sulfur compounds.

Upon treatment with triethylamine **121** was converted in good yield to the butadiene **124**. A possible mechanistic sequence is shown in Scheme 9.

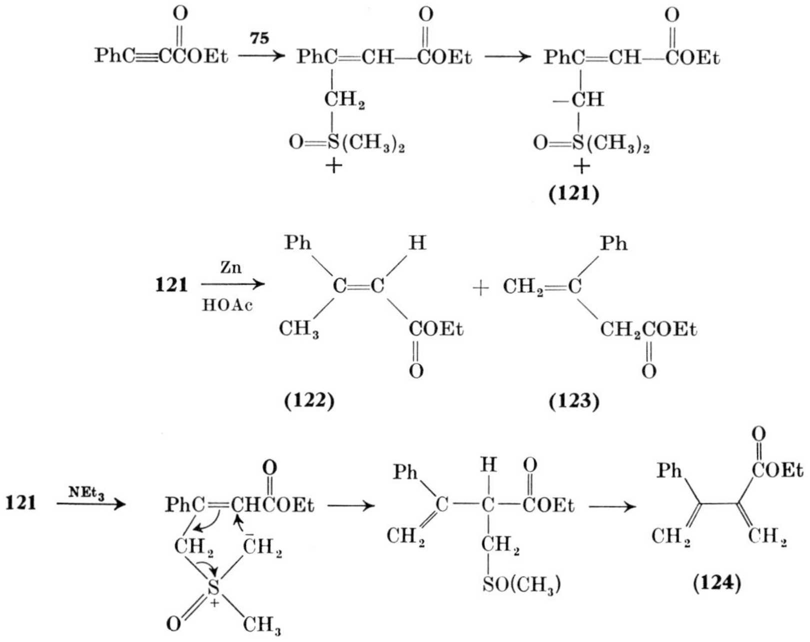

Scheme 9

In common with cinnamate esters, *trans*-*N*,*N*-dimethylcinnamamide reacted stereoselectively with the ylid **75** to yield only *trans*-*N*,*N*-dimethyl-2-phenylcyclopropane carboxamide (30%) (134). König, Metzger, and Seelert (139,140) reported in a detailed study that reaction of **75** with α,β-unsaturated primary or secondary amides took a different course and gave as the major product pyrrolidinones **127** in yields of 45–95%; cyclopropyl amides and several other substances (see below) were generally formed as minor products. The betaine **125** formed by addition of **75** to the unsaturated amide can further react along a number of routes: (*1*) ring closure to cyclopropyl derivatives with simultaneous expulsion of dimethylsulfoxide, (*2*) proton shift from nitrogen to carbon to form **126** which cyclizes to the pyrrolidinone **127**, again expelling DMSO, and (*3*) proton shift to give the ylid **128** which adds a second equivalent of amide resulting in yet another betaine which again partitions itself among the various possible pathways.

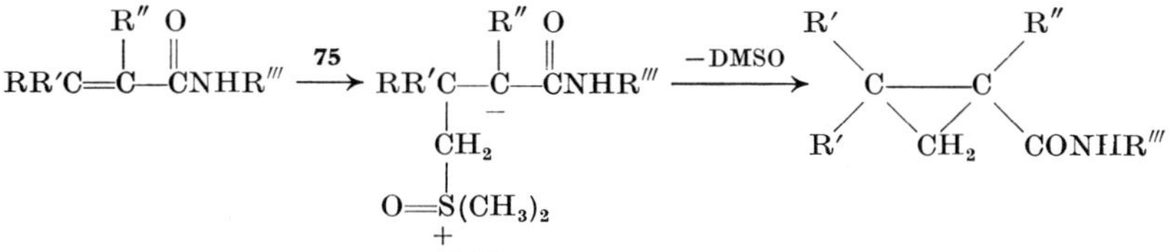

$$RR'C=\underset{\underset{}{R''}}{C}-\underset{}{\overset{O}{\overset{\|}{C}}}NHR''' \xrightarrow{75} RR'C-\underset{\underset{\underset{+}{O=S(CH_3)_2}}{\underset{}{CH_2}}}{\overset{\underset{}{R''}}{\overset{|}{C}}}-\overset{O}{\overset{\|}{C}}NHR''' \xrightarrow{-DMSO} \underset{R'}{\overset{R'}{\diagdown}}C\underset{CH_2}{\text{——}}C\underset{CONHR'''}{\overset{R''}{\diagup}}$$

(125)

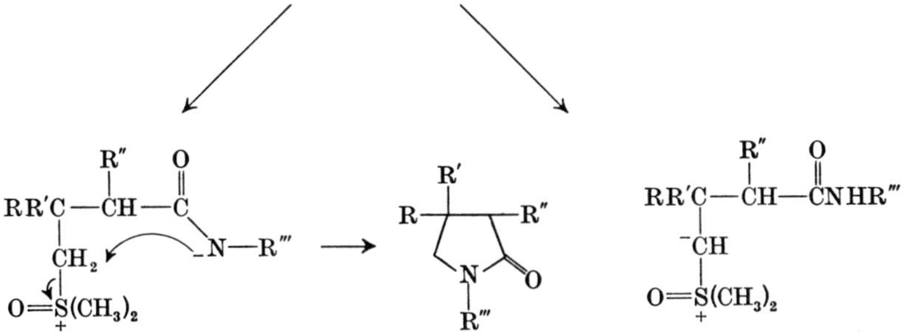

(126)   (127)   (128)

Interestingly, the doubly unsaturated amide **129** which could conceivably have yielded the 7-membered ring compound **130** gave a mixture of the dicyclopropyl amide **131** and the cyclopropyl pyrrolidinone **132**.

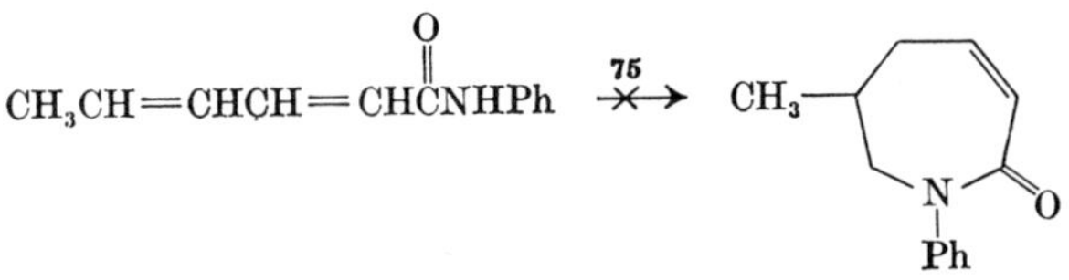

$$CH_3CH=CHCH=CH\overset{O}{\overset{\|}{C}}NHPh \xrightarrow{75} \not\rightarrow CH_3\diagdown\text{...}\diagup\underset{Ph}{N}\diagdown O$$

(129)   (130)

↓ 75

$$CH_3CH\underset{CH_2}{-}CH-CH-CH\overset{O}{\overset{\|}{C}}NHPh \;+\; CH_3CH\underset{CH_2}{-}CH\text{...}\underset{Ph}{N}\diagdown O$$

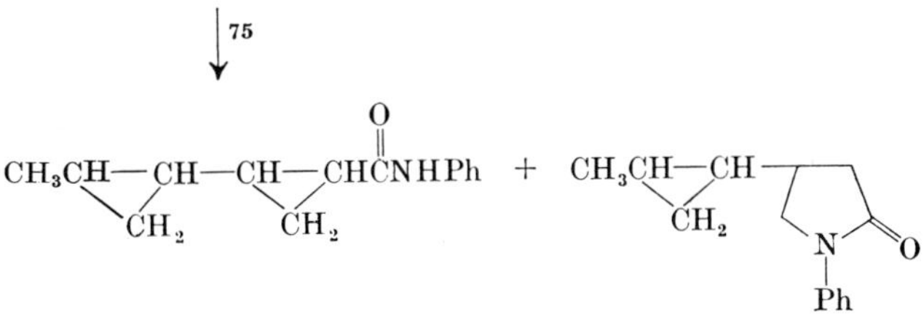

(131)   (132)

3. Additions to Conjugated Olefinic Systems

Michael addition of dimethyloxosulfonium methylid to conjugated ketonic systems resulting in the formation of cyclopropyl ketones was initially observed by Corey and Chaykovsky (17) and has been discussed in an earlier part of this section. Since then, cyclopropyl formation has been reported for a number of other Michael receptors such as

TABLE X
Cyclopropane Formation on Reaction of Dimethyloxosulfonium Methylid with Some Unsaturated Systems

$$R_1R_2C=CR_3R_4 \xrightarrow{75} R_1R_2C\overset{CH_2}{\underset{}{\diagup\!\diagdown}}CR_3R_4$$

Substituents					
R_1	R_2	R_3	R_4	Yield	Ref.
Ph	Ph	H	H	35	17
Ph	H	H	COPh	95	17
Ph	H	H	CO_2Et	31	135
				54	126
Ph	H	H	CO_2tBu	65	135
Ph	H	CO_2Et	CO_2Et	60	135
Ph	H	H	$CO_2(-)$ menthyl	42	136
Ph	H	H	$CO_2(+)$ bornyl	49	136
Ph	H	H	CN	48	135
Ph	H	H	$CON(CH_3)_2$	39	135
Ph	H	H	SO_2Ph	87	142
CH_3	H	CH_3	SO_2Ph	40	142
CH_3	H	C_2H_5	SO_2Ph	40	142

α,β-unsaturated esters (124,135,136), amides (106,141), nitriles (106,135), and sulfones (142). The yields of cyclopropyl derivatives vary considerably for the different systems since in some cases, e.g., esters and amides, alternate reactions are possible. A number of representative examples are presented in Table X.

The ylid **75** does not transfer a methylene group to dienes or aryl conjugated ethylenes (17,108). In contrast, a 35% yield of 1,1-diphenylcyclopropane was obtained on reaction of the more reactive dimethylsulfonium methylid (**80**) with 1,1-diphenylethylene (17).

Reaction of aromatic nitro compounds with **75** resulted in the formation of a mixture of methylated derivatives in rather low yield

(108,143,144). Anthracene afforded 45% of 9-methylanthracene but other aromatic compounds such as diphenylsulfone, methyl benzoate, benzonitrile, pyridine, or quinoline did not react even under forcing conditions (108,144). Methylations have also been reported for the reaction of **80** with some condensed hydrocarbons (145). These reactions, while presently of little synthetic applicability, are of some mechanistic interest.

Traynelis and McSweeney (143) made the observation that methylation of aromatic nitro compounds occurred mainly *ortho* to the nitro group (*o/p* ratio > 10:1) and, furthermore, in *meta* substituted nitrobenzenes, methylation occurred at the more highly hindered *ortho* group. These authors suggested that a "complex" between the ylid and the nitro group may direct the ylid to the *ortho* position. Decomposition of the intermediate **133** formed from such an attack has been suggested to occur by concerted hydride shift and elimination of dimethylsulfoxide (see **133**). Alternate mechanisms are (1) intramolecular hydrogen abstraction with elimination of DMSO, followed by aromatization (**134**), and, (2) in analogy with the proposed mechanism for aromatic methylations with methylsulfinyl carbanion (see page 314), protonation to the cyclohexadiene **135**, elimination of DMSO, and again aromatization.

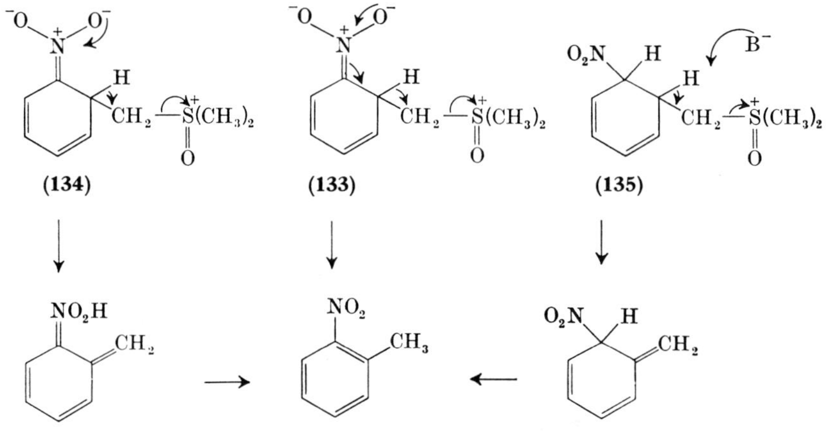

(134)   (133)   (135)

4. Reaction with Carbon–Nitrogen Multiple Bonds

Relatively few investigations have been made regarding the addition of dimethyloxosulfonium methylid to carbon–nitrogen double bonds.

Corey and Chaykovsky (17) reported that benzalaniline and **75** led to the formation of three products: 1,2-diphenylaziridine (**136**) (44%), acetophenone anil (**137**) (22%), and the aminosulfoxide **138** (19%). Similar results were obtained by the Metzger group (108,146,147). The formation of these products can be rationalized on the basis of the intermediate **139** formed by attachment of **75** to the electrophilic carbon of benzalaniline. The cyclization of **139** to the aziridine requires no further comment. Acetophenone anil could arise via a concerted hydride shift and elimination (structure **140**) or, more likely, by a prototropic shift to **141**, elimination of DMSO, and isomerization. The aminosulfoxide may be due to reaction of a small amount of methylsulfinyl carbanion with benzalaniline (16) (DMSO being present either as solvent or generated during the reaction), or as suggested by Metzger et al. (108), by demethylation of the protonated **139**. Other Schiff bases such as cyclohexylidenecyclohexylamine, or *p*-methoxybenzylidene cyclohexylamine did not react under conditions which sufficed for benzalaniline.

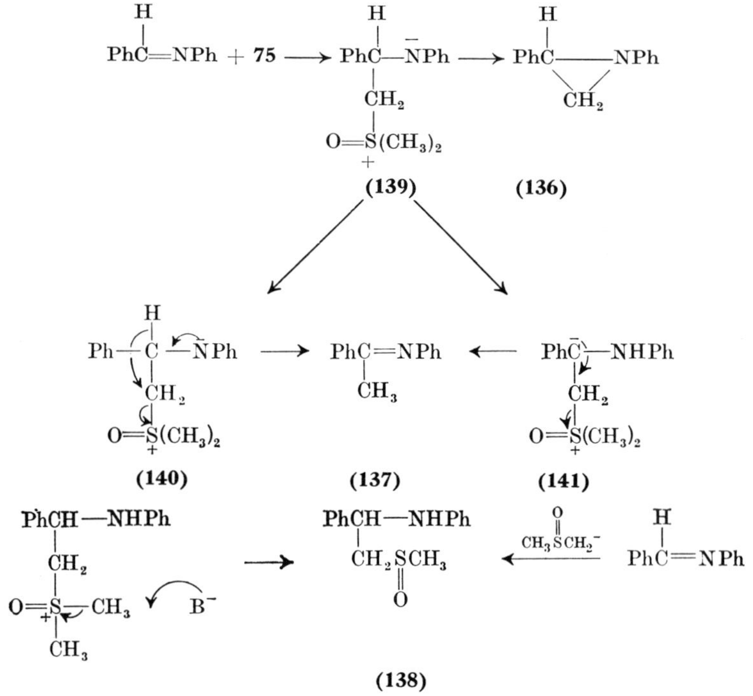

In contrast, the addition of dimethylsulfonium methylid **(80)** to C=N bonds occurs much more cleanly. Benzalaniline was converted to the aziridine **136** in high yield (17,148). In a novel application of **80**, Hortman and Robertson (149) were able to obtain a 60% yield of the azabicyclobutane **142** by reaction with 3-phenyl-2H-azirine. Clearly, the sulfonium ylid **80** is a better reagent for methylene transfer to a C=N bond than the oxosulfonium ylid **75**.

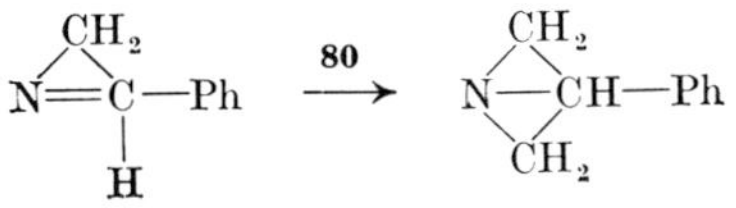

$$\underset{H}{\overset{CH_2}{N=C-Ph}} \xrightarrow{80} \underset{CH_2}{\overset{CH_2}{N-CH-Ph}}$$

(142)

The reaction of dimethyloxosulfonium methylid with aromatic nitriles proceeds by nucleophilic addition followed by prototropic rearrangement (104,108,150), thereby forming salts of the type **143**. When **75** was generated in benzonitrile as solvent, a second crystalline material, assigned structure **144**, was isolated in low yield (108). This compound, which was obtained by addition of a second molecule of benzonitrile to **143** and subsequent cyclization, is of theoretical interest since it may possibly exhibit some aromatic character. The NMR data of the compound, which show in addition to the aromatic and methyl protons a two-hydrogen singlet at 6.30 ppm downfield from TMS, do not require such an interpretation.

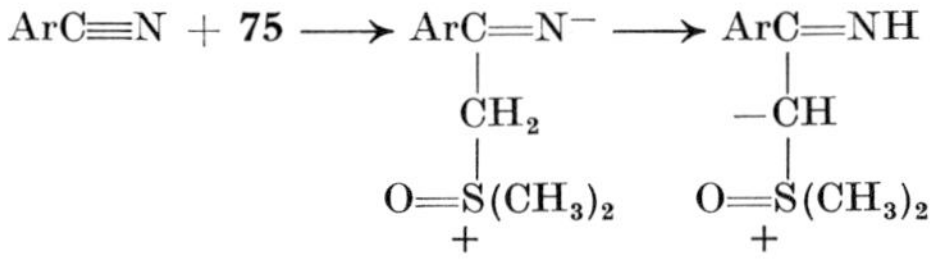

$$ArC\equiv N + 75 \longrightarrow \underset{\underset{+}{O=S(CH_3)_2}}{\underset{CH_2}{ArC=N^-}} \longrightarrow \underset{\underset{+}{O=S(CH_3)_2}}{\underset{-CH}{ArC=NH}}$$

(143)

143 + PhC≡N ⟶

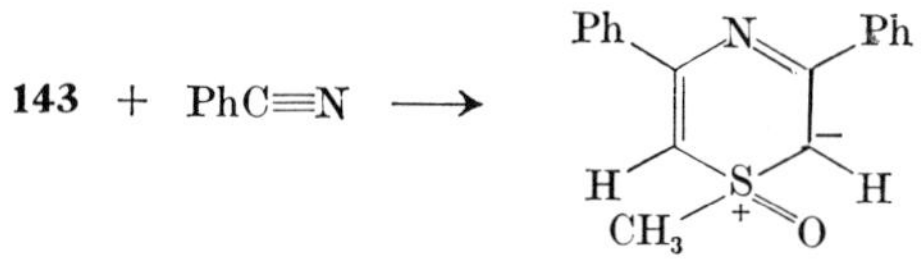

(144)

5. Miscellaneous Reactions

Sulfonyl halides, as might be expected in analogy with the behavior of carboxylic acid halides, are converted to stable α-sulfonyloxosulfonium ylids, e.g., **145** on reaction with **75** (151). The conversion is most general for sulfonyl fluorides where yields of expected ylids are usually in the 40–90% range. Aromatic sulfonyl chlorides failed to react in this manner, undergoing instead displacement on chlorine and elimination of sulfinic acids (152). Methanesulfonyl chloride, in contrast, afforded an oxosulfonium ylid in 72% yield. A sulfene (56) is a possible intermediate in the latter reaction. Unlike the β-keto oxosulfonium ylids, these derivatives did not undergo photolytic cleavage to α-sulfonyl carbenes.

$$RSO_2F + 2CH_2^-\overset{O}{\underset{+}{\overset{\|}{S}}}(CH_3)_2 \longrightarrow RSO_2CH^-\overset{O}{\underset{+}{\overset{\|}{S}}}(CH_3)_2$$

(145)

$$CH_3SO_2Cl + 75 \longrightarrow [CH_2=SO_2] \overset{75}{\longrightarrow} CH_3SO_2CH\overset{O}{\underset{+}{\overset{\|}{S}}}(CH_3)_2$$

The 1,3 dipoles benzonitrile oxide and phenyl azide undergo two successive methylene transfers with **75** to afford 3-phenyl-Δ^2-isoxazoline **(146)** (10%) and 1-phenyl-Δ^2-1,2,3-triazoline **(147)** (80%),

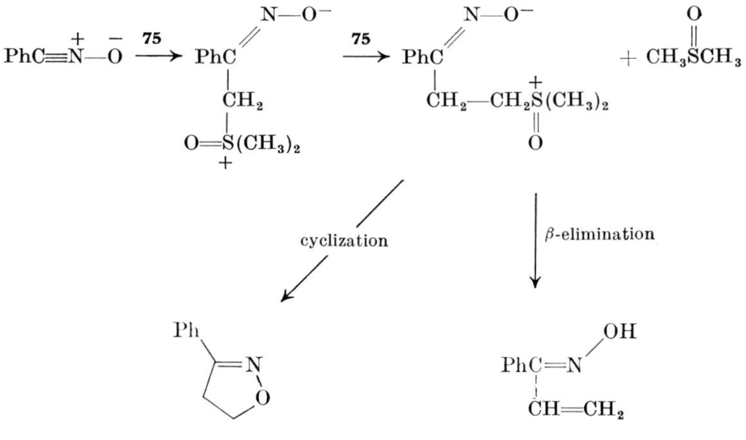

(146)

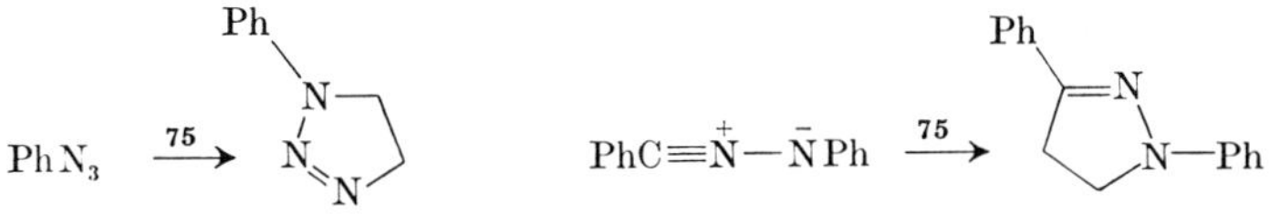

(147) **(148)**

respectively; C,N-diphenyl nitrile imine similarly gives a 45% yield of **148** (153,154). Mechanistically, these reactions were formulated as shown for benzonitrile oxide. Other dipolar reagents such as azoxybenzene, quinoline N-oxide, and diphenyl diazomethane failed to form 5-membered ring heterocyclic compounds with **75**. Diphenyl diazomethane underwent oxidation to benzophenone, a reaction which may involve initial decomposition of the azo compound to a carbene (see following Section).

Quite recently Turfariello and Lee (155) reported methylene insertion on reaction of dimethyloxosulfonium methylid with trialkyl and triaryl boranes. The reactions were pictured as occurring via initial addition of the ylid to the borane to form the betaine **149**, followed by alkyl migration with expulsion of dimethyl sulfoxide. Since the product **150** is susceptible to further reaction, mixture of various homologs were generally obtained.

$$R_3B + 75 \xrightarrow[0°]{THF} R_2\bar{B}-CH_2-\overset{O}{\underset{+}{\overset{\|}{S}}}(CH_3)_2 \longrightarrow R_2BCH_2R + CH_3\overset{O}{\overset{\|}{S}}CH_3$$

(149)   (150)

IV. Dimethylsulfoxide Oxidations

The oxidation of alcohols to the corresponding carbonyl compounds has always been an important synthetic procedure. Even though many preparative methods are now available for such conversions, the restrictions which accompany some of them make new procedures highly desirable. The recent development of a number of mild and efficient procedures in which DMSO plays the role of oxidant has been an important addition to the tools available to the synthetic chemist for such conversions. Successful applications of the various procedures have been reported in a variety of fields including alkaloids, carbohydrates, steroids, nucleosides, and nucleotides. Important advantages of oxidation by these methods, as compared to many of the old procedures, become obvious upon consideration of the mechanism of the reactions. For instance, oxidation of primary alcohols can proceed only to the aldehyde stage, a factor of considerable importance when compounds highly susceptible to further oxidation are involved. The reactions, in most cases, occur reasonably rapidly under mild, and in some cases almost neutral conditions, thus minimizing the chances of isomerization or occurrence of other changes in the molecule. Particular examples of the effectiveness of the dimethyl sulfoxide–dicyclohexylcarbodiimide (DMSO–DCC) procedure are the oxidation of cholesterol to Δ^5-3-cholestenone in 66% yield (156), the conversion of 3-methylenecyclobutanol to 3-methylenecyclobutanone (157), and the oxidation of the α-silyl alcohol **151** to the corresponding ketone **152** (158). The pyridine–chromic acid method gives mainly conjugated ketone in the first two examples and cleavage of the silicon–carbon bond in the last.

The recent comprehensive review by Epstein and Sweat (159) covers the literature through the early part of 1966. In view of this, emphasis in this section will be on very recent work and on mechanistic aspects which correlate the various oxidation procedures among themselves and to other DMSO reactions.

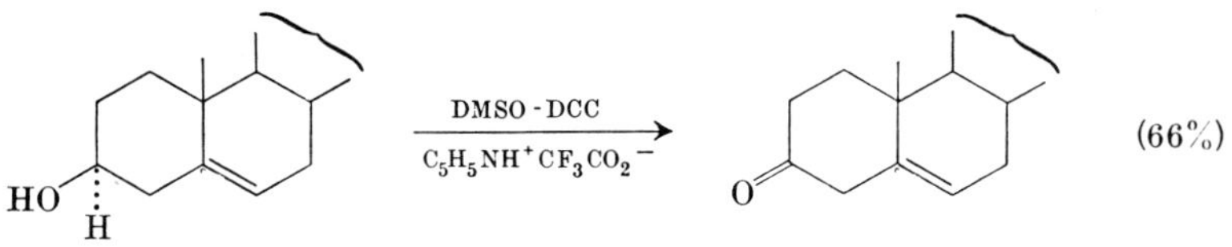

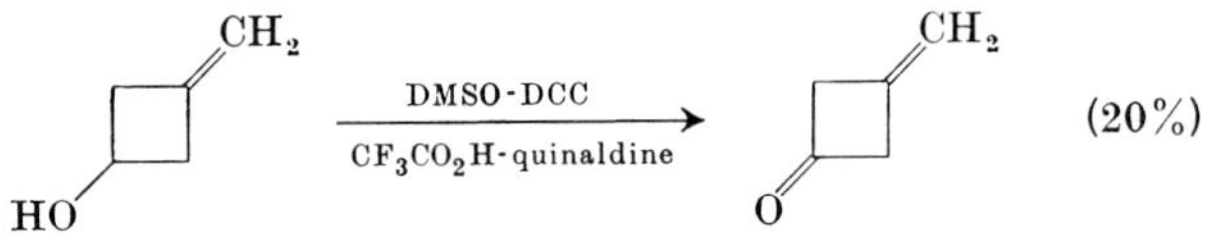

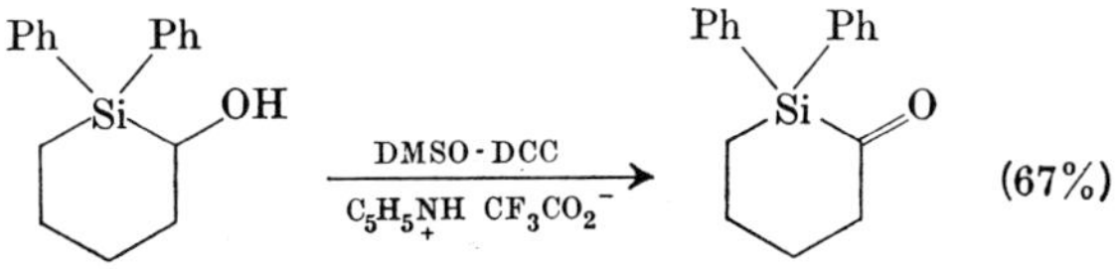

Very strong evidence has been presented by a number of workers that most oxidations involving DMSO occur via intermediate dimethylalkoxysulfonium salts **(153)** which subsequently react with a base to give the oxidized derivative and dimethylsulfide. Of special importance in this connection are the studies of Johnson (160,161) and Torssell (162,163) who isolated alkoxysulfonium salts and showed that they were indeed converted to carbonyl compounds on treatment with base.

DMSO oxidations can be divided into two broad classes depending on how the alkoxysulfonium salt **153** is generated. The first group of DMSO oxidations concerns itself almost exclusively with the oxidation of alcohols to carbonyl compounds. Here the required alkoxysulfonium salt is formed by reaction of an alcohol with oxysulfonium salts of the type **154** which are produced by the interaction of DMSO with an electrophilic species E present in solution. A variety of substances have served to "activate DMSO" to nucleophilic attack on sulfur. The requirements are that the electrophilic species E react much more rapidly with DMSO than with alcohols, and that the group OE formed from such a reaction be a good leaving group.

In the second group of DMSO oxidations of which the Kornblum oxidation is a representative, the alkoxysulfonium salt **153** is obtained by nucleophilic displacement of a tosyl or halide function by the oxygen atom of dimethylsulfoxide. The acid-catalyzed opening of epoxides (164,165) and aziridines (205) in DMSO also leads to alkoxysulfonium salts. The distinguishing feature of this group is that the oxygen atom in DMSO is transferred to the substrate being oxidized.

$$\text{E} + \text{CH}_3\overset{\text{O}}{\underset{\|}{\text{S}}}\text{CH}_3 \longrightarrow (\text{CH}_3)_2\overset{+}{\text{S}}\text{—OE}$$
$$(\mathbf{154})$$

$$\downarrow \text{RR'CHOH}$$

$$\text{RR'CHX} + \text{CH}_3\overset{\text{O}}{\underset{\|}{\text{S}}}\text{CH}_3 \longrightarrow \text{RR'CHO—}\overset{+}{\text{S}}(\text{CH}_3)_2 \quad \text{X}^-$$
$$(\mathbf{153})$$

A. OXIDATION OF ALCOHOLS

The most detailed mechanistic study has been carried out on a technique discovered and developed by Pfitzner and Moffatt (156,166, 167) in which a combination of dicyclohexylcarbodiimide **155** and a proton source—usually polyphosphoric acid or pyridinium trifluoroacetate—serves as a source of the electrophile E. The observations and conclusions obtained from these studies are generally applicable to other systems with only minor variations. The mechanism proposed by Fenselau and Moffatt (167) for this oxidation is presented in Scheme 10. Evidence obtained for these steps is discussed below.

Oxygen-18 labeling experiments (167) have shown that the oxygen

1. $C_6H_{11}N=C=NC_6H_{11}$ + $CH_3\overset{O}{\underset{\|}{S}}CH_3$ $\xrightarrow{H^+}$ $C_6H_{11}N=CNHC_6H_{11}$
   (155) $\qquad\qquad\qquad\qquad\qquad\qquad\qquad\qquad\;\;\; |$
   $\qquad\qquad\qquad\qquad\qquad\qquad\qquad\qquad\;\;\; O$
   $\qquad\qquad\qquad\qquad\qquad\qquad\qquad\qquad\;\;\; |$
   $\qquad\qquad\qquad\qquad\qquad\qquad\qquad\qquad +\overset{}{S}(CH_3)_2$
   $\qquad\qquad\qquad\qquad\qquad\qquad\qquad\qquad\quad$ (156)

2. $C_6H_{11}\overset{H^+}{\underset{\curvearrowleft}{N}}=CNHC_6H_{11}$ $\longrightarrow$ $C_6H_{11}NH\overset{O}{\underset{\|}{C}}NHC_6H_{11}$ + $RR'CHO\overset{+}{-}\overset{}{S}(CH_3)_2$
   $\qquad\quad |$ $\qquad\qquad\qquad\qquad\qquad\qquad$ (157) $\qquad\qquad\qquad$ (158)
   $\qquad\quad O$
   $\qquad\quad |$
   $\qquad +\overset{}{S}(CH_3)_2$
   $\qquad\quad\;\nwarrow$
   $\qquad\qquad\;\; RR'CH\overset{\cdot\cdot}{O}H$

3. $RR'\underset{H}{\overset{O\,\diagdown\,}{\underset{|}{C}}}\underset{\;\;CH_2}{\overset{+}{\underset{|}{S}}CH_3}$ $\longrightarrow$ $RR'C=O$ + CH_3SCH_3
   $\quad$ (159)

Scheme 10.

atom of DMSO is transferred to the dicyclohexylcarbodiimide. This result is compatible with the initial formation of the sulfonium isourea **156** by addition of DMSO to protonated DCC, followed by displacement of N,N'-dicyclohexylurea **(157)** by the alcohol, thereby yielding the alkoxysulfonium salt **158**. It eliminates the alternate sequence to the alkoxysulfonium salt, i.e., reaction of the alcohol with DCC to form the isourea **156a** and subsequent conversion to the alkoxysulfonium salt and N,N'-dicyclohexylurea on reaction with DMSO. This conclusion is further corroborated by the report that oxidation of ^{18}O-labeled

$C_6H_{11}N=C=NC_6H_{11}$ + $RR'CHOH$ $\xrightarrow{H^+}$ $C_6H_{11}N=CNHC_6H_{11}$
$\qquad\qquad\qquad\qquad\qquad\qquad\qquad\qquad\qquad\qquad\qquad |$
$\qquad\qquad\qquad\qquad\qquad\qquad\qquad\qquad\qquad\qquad\qquad O$
$\qquad\qquad\qquad\qquad\qquad\qquad\qquad\qquad\qquad\qquad\qquad |$
$\qquad\qquad\qquad\qquad\qquad\qquad\qquad\qquad\qquad\qquad\qquad CHRR'$
$\qquad\qquad\qquad\qquad\qquad\qquad\qquad\qquad\qquad\qquad\quad$ (156a)

156a + $CH_3\overset{O}{\underset{\|}{S}}CH_3$ $\xcancel{\longrightarrow}$ $RR'CHO\overset{+}{-}S(CH_3)_2$ + $C_6H_{11}NH\overset{O}{\underset{\|}{C}}NHC_6H_{11}$
$\qquad\qquad\qquad\qquad\qquad\qquad\quad$ (158) $\qquad\qquad\qquad\quad$ (157)

$R = H,\; R' = p\text{-}NO_2C_6H_4$

alcohols by the DMSO–DCC method led to aldehydes with retention of the isotope (168,169) and by a control experiment which showed that the isourea **156a** (R = H, R' = p-nitrophenyl) was inert under the conditions of the oxidation reaction (167).

The second step of the mechanism (step 2 in Scheme 10) involves nucleophilic attack by an alcohol upon the sulfonium isourea **156** with formation of the alkoxysulfonium compound **158** and the insoluble dicyclohexylurea. Such a step is amply supported by data obtained by other workers which illustrate the ease with which alkoxysulfonium salts undergo nucleophilic attack on sulfur. Alkoxysulfonium salts are readily hydrolyzed to sulfoxides (160–163). Exchange of the alkoxy function with other alcohols or alkoxides has also been observed. These reactions have been shown to occur with inversion of configuration at sulfur (170–172).

$$\underset{+}{\overset{\overset{\displaystyle OR''}{|}}{R\overset{}{S}R'}} + R'''OH \rightleftharpoons \underset{\overset{|}{OR'''}}{\overset{+}{R\overset{}{S}R'}} + R''OH$$

$$\downarrow H_2O \qquad\qquad \downarrow H_2O$$

$$\underset{\overset{\|}{O}}{RSR'} \qquad\qquad \underset{RSR'}{\overset{O}{\|}}$$

The final step in this mechanism, the conversion of the alkoxysulfonium salt to a carbonyl compound and dimethylsulfide, can occur either via formation of the ylid **159** and subsequent collapse by a cyclic mechanism (step 3 in Scheme 10) or by E_2-type elimination as shown in **160**. The following evidence has been presented (160,162, 167,173) to show that the former pathway is the preferred route unless the hydrogen α to the oxygen is labilized by the presence of an electron-withdrawing group. Oxidation of 1,1-dideuteriobutanol-1 in the presence of unlabeled DMSO, DCC, and anhydrous phosphoric acid gave 1-deuteriobutyraldehyde and dimethylsulfide-d_1 as determined by NMR and mass spectrometry. Under the same conditions, oxidation of unlabeled butanol-1 by hexadeuteriodimethylsulfoxide yielded completely unlabeled butyraldehyde and dimethylsulfide-d_5. The formation of these products can be reasonably explained only in terms of ylid formation and cyclic decomposition. Since only one of the six deuterium atoms is lost in the reaction involving DMSO-d_6, it appears that the ylid **159** is very efficient as an internal base and is not reprotonated to the alkoxysulfonium salt **158**.

The mechanism outlined in Scheme 10 requires both acid and base catalysis, in agreement with the observations that strong mineral acids do not promote oxidation (166). In view of the ease of α-hydrogen exchange in sulfonium (100,101) and oxosulfonium salts (99), ylid formation from the alkoxysulfonium salt **158** should be possible with such bases as $H_2PO_4^-$, HPO_4^{2-}, or pyridine.

Results which are essentially identical to those of the labeling experiments described above have been obtained by Johnson and Phillips (160,161) and Torssell (162,163). The important additional feature was that these authors performed the labeling experiments on pure alkoxysulfonium salts which had been prepared by different routes. Their results are summarized in eqs. a and b.

a. $\text{PhSCH}_3\overset{\text{OCD}_3}{\underset{+}{|}} \xrightarrow[\text{THF}]{\text{NaH}} \text{PhSCH}_2\text{D} + \text{CD}_2\text{O}$

b. $(CH_3)_2CHCH_2O-\overset{+}{S}(CD_3)_2 \xrightarrow[\text{DMSO}]{\text{NEt}_3} (CH_3)_2CHCHO + CH_3SCD_2H$

Sweat and Epstein (173) studied the DMSO–DCC oxidation mechanism by using tritiated cholestanol and measuring the tritium

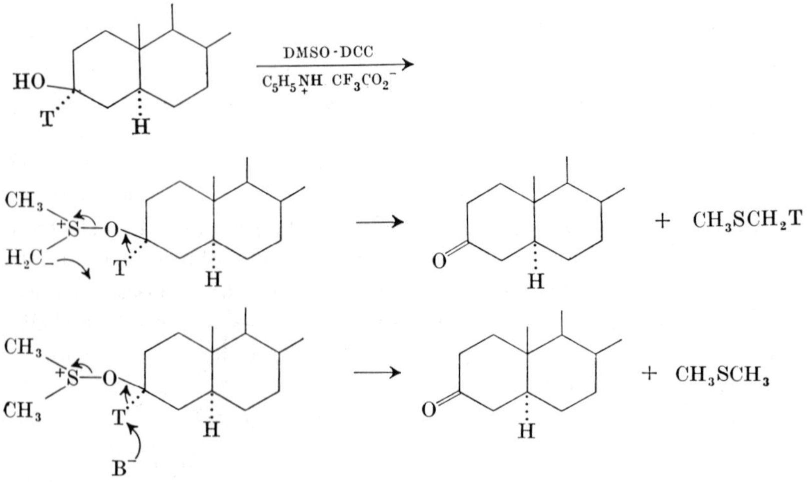

(160)

label appearing in the dimethyl sulfide formed in the reaction. These authors agree that the primary pathway in this oxidation involves the intermediate **158a**, but also suggest that a small portion of the reaction proceeds via an elimination reaction involving an external base, as depicted in **160**. The latter proposal was based on the fact that a small, but real amount of tritium label escaped into the medium and was exchanged into dicyclohexyl urea.

In addition to the labeling experiments, Johnson and Phillips (160) found that diphenylmethoxysulfonium fluoroborate **(161)** yielded no formaldehyde on treatment with sodium methoxide in methanol, but was instead converted to diphenylsulfoxide and, presumably, dimethyl ether. Thus if oxidation is to occur, the alkoxysulfonium salt should possess a hydrogen α to the positively charged sulfur atom.

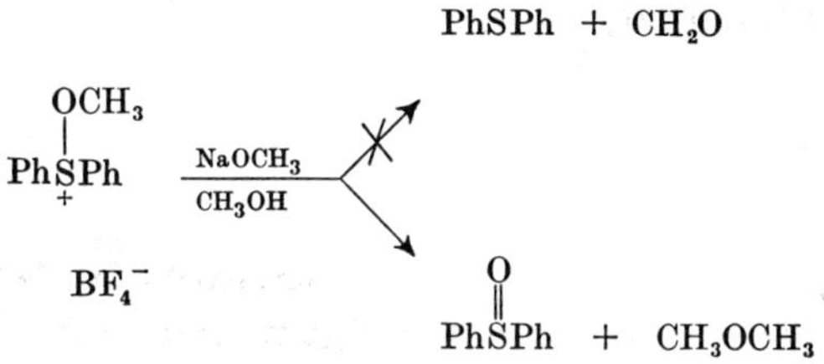

$$\underset{(161)}{\underset{BF_4^-}{\overset{OCH_3}{PhSPh}}} \xrightarrow[CH_3OH]{NaOCH_3} \begin{array}{c} PhSPh + CH_2O \\ \\ \overset{O}{\underset{\parallel}{PhSPh}} + CH_3OCH_3 \end{array}$$

The oxidation reactions are usually accompanied by formation of a small amount of by-product which has been identified as the thiomethoxymethyl ethers of the general formula **162**. The formation of these compounds, which bear a strong resemblance to the products obtained in the Pummerer reaction, will be discussed in detail in the next section.

$$RR'CHOH \xrightarrow{DMSO-DCC} RR'CO + RR'CHOCH_2SCH_3$$
$$(162)$$

The oxidation of alcohols by an acetic anhydride–DMSO mixture was initially reported by Albright and Goldman (174). Here, reaction of DMSO with acetic anhydride leads to the acylated sulfonium salt **163**. S_N2 displacement of the acetate function by an alcohol furnishes the same alkoxysulfonium salt **158** obtained in the DMSO–DCC procedure. Acetate ion, which is produced in the initial reaction, can serve as the base required for the ylid formation (169). Benzoic anhydride or phosphorus pentoxide (169,175,176) have successfully replaced acetic anhydride.

The acetic anhydride–DMSO procedure appears to suffer from a number of disadvantages when compared to the DMSO–DCC technique such as a greater tendency to produce side products such as acetates and thiomethoxymethyl ethers. The procedure does offer the advantage of oxidizing highly hindered alcohols which are inert to the DMSO–DCC conditions, and as such has found considerable use in the carbohydrate field (177) and in the oxidation of sterically hindered steroidal alcohols (178). This difference in the reactivity of the two reagents may reflect the difference in size between the sulfonium isourea **156** (from DCC and DMSO) and the acetoxy sulfonium salt **163**.

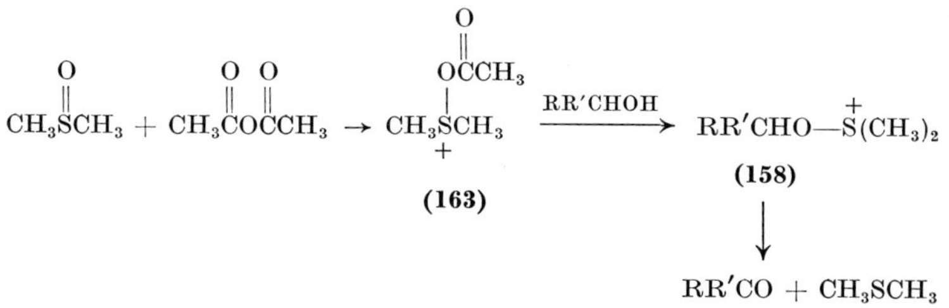

$$CH_3\overset{O}{\overset{\|}{S}}CH_3 + CH_3\overset{O}{\overset{\|}{C}}O\overset{O}{\overset{\|}{C}}CH_3 \rightarrow CH_3\overset{+}{\underset{|}{S}}CH_3 \xrightarrow{RR'CHOH} RR'CHO\text{---}\overset{+}{S}(CH_3)_2$$
$$\overset{\overset{O}{\overset{\|}{O}CCH_3}}{}$$
(163)   (158)

$$\downarrow$$

$$RR'CO + CH_3SCH_3$$

Efficient oxidation of alcohols in DMSO–sulfur trioxide–pyridine–triethylamine mixtures has recently been reported by Parikh and Doering (179). A number of advantages of this system over the DMSO–DCC and DMSO–acetic anhydride methods were pointed out. These include rapid reaction, an uncomplicated isolation procedure, and the absence of significant amounts of by-product. However, as in the DMSO–DCC method, highly hindered alcohols remain inert.

Torssell (162,163) has questioned the existence of a free alkoxysulfonium salt during the oxidation of alcohols by the DMSO–DCC reagent, since addition of either the sulfonium salt **164** or **165** to the

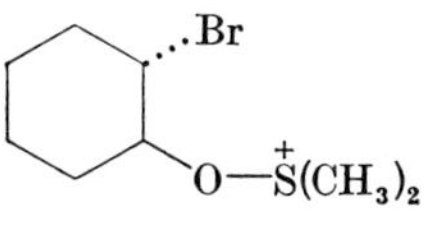

(164)

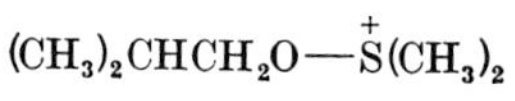

(165) $(CH_3)_2CHCH_2O\text{---}\overset{+}{S}(CH_3)_2$

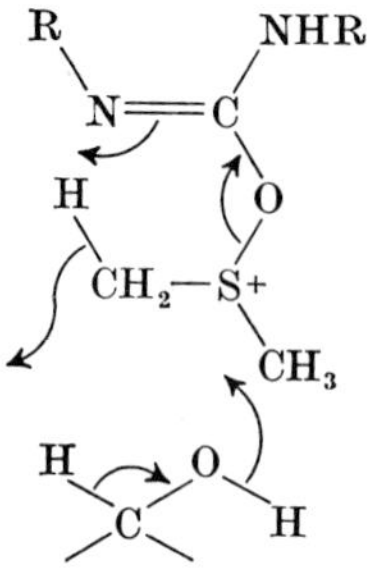

(166)

usual DMSO–DCC–phosphoric acid mixture failed to yield significant quantities of carbonyl compounds. He suggested instead the termolecular mechanism shown in **166**, reasoning that "at the very moment the alcohol displaces the urea a strong base is formed which abstracts a proton from the S-methyl group and thus creates the cyclic intermediate."

Although it is difficult to be certain, it appears that the conditions which Torssell employed are in fact not identical to those which exist in the actual DMSO–DCC reaction. In the DMSO–DCC–anhydrous phosphoric acid oxidation of an alcohol, an equivalent of base is generated in the initial reaction of DMSO with DCC (Reaction 1 in Scheme 10) which can later serve to deprotonate the alkoxysulfonium salt. Under the Torssell conditions, the alkoxysulfonium salt is added to the initial reaction mixture, no base is present, and none is generated other than possibly a small amount due to autoprotolysis of the phosphoric acid. Thus, in the absence of base only a small amount of carbonyl formation is observed.

A similar situation occurs in the DMSO–acetic anhydride reaction. Again a base (in this case acetate ion) required for ylid formation is formed in the first step of the reaction sequence. Addition of the preformed alkoxysulfonium salt to a DMSO–acetic anhydride mixture would not be expected to yield any oxidation because of the absence of base (169).

In view of the questionable nature of the experiments, the very high entropy requirements of a transition state such as **166**, and the fact that "free" alkoxysulfonium salts are oxidized to carbonyl compounds by base, the author feels that the original proposal by Fenselau and Moffatt (167) remains the more likely.

An interesting variation in the route to alkoxysulfonium salts was reported in 1964 by Barton and co-workers (180). Alcohols were initially converted to chloroformates **167** by reaction with phosgene.

$$RR'CHOH \xrightarrow{COCl_2} \underset{(167)}{RR'CHOCCl} \xrightarrow{DMSO} [RR'CHOCOS(CH_3)_2]$$

$$\downarrow DMSO \qquad \swarrow -CO_2$$

$$\underset{(158)}{RR'CHO-\overset{+}{S}(CH_3)_2} \xrightarrow{B(Ph)_4^-} \text{tetraphenyl borate salt}$$

Sequential addition of dimethylsulfoxide and triethylamine gave reasonable yields (~60%) of the corresponding carbonyl compounds. The intermediacy of an alkoxysulfonium salt in this sequence was suggested by Barton and later confirmed by Torssell (163) who was able to precipitate such salts from the reaction mixture as tetraphenyl borates.

B. OXIDATION OF HALIDES AND TOSYLATES

These oxidations differ from those of the alcohols in that the alkoxysulfonium salt is formed by direct nucleophilic displacement of a leaving group by DMSO and that the oxygen atom of DMSO becomes the carbonyl oxygen of the newly formed ketone or aldehyde. The reactions are generally carried out by heating the substrate in DMSO containing bases such as sodium bicarbonate or collidine which are capable of decomposing the intermediate alkoxysulfonium salts to carbonyl compounds and dimethyl sulfide and also neutralizing the acid which is liberated in the displacement reaction. In most cases, the main route of decomposition is the cyclic pathway discussed in the previous section (169,173). Torssell (163) has shown by deuterium-labeling experiments that phenacyl sulfonium salts, e.g., **168**, in which the acidity of the hydrogen α to the oxygen is greatly increased by the presence of a carbonyl group, are decomposed by direct abstraction of that proton. A similarity exists between this reaction of DMSO and those of t-amine oxides, since the salts derived in both cases are capable of forming aldehydes and ketones when exposed to base.

$$\text{PhC(=O)}-\overset{\curvearrowleft}{\text{CH}}-\text{O}-\overset{+}{\text{S}}(\text{CH}_3)_2 \xrightarrow{\text{base}} \text{PhCCHO} + \text{CH}_3\text{SCH}_3$$
$$\underset{\text{H}}{|}$$
(168)

DMSO oxidations of this type are synthetically useful for α-haloesters and acids (181), phenacyl halides (10,182), benzyl halides (11,183), primary sulfonates (11,183), and primary iodides (11,184). Primary alkyl chlorides and bromides do not react, but can be oxidized by initial conversion to the corresponding tosylates on treatment with silver toluenesulfonate (11). Oxidation of secondary halides and tosylates is not generally synthetically feasible since elimination to olefin becomes a competing and at times the major reaction (185-189).

Exceptions to the above generalization are secondary α-keto derivatives which have been oxidized in satisfactory yield to α-diketones (188).

The order of reactivity described in the preceding paragraph is most consistent with an S_N2 mechanism for the formation of the dimethylalkoxysulfonium salts, although in some instances, such as in the oxidation of benzhydryl derivatives, an S_N1 route is more probable (184). The suggestion has been made (185) that the dimethylalkoxysulfonium salts are intermediates in both the oxidation and elimination reactions. Iacona and co-workers (187) rejected this proposal on the basis of some studies in steroidal systems.

In steroidal systems, axial tosylates and halides gave a higher ratio of elimination to substitution than the corresponding equatorial isomers. Such would not be expected if an alkoxysulfonium salt formed by an S_N2 substitution were the intermediate in the elimination reaction. Displacement of an axial group results in the formation of an equatorial alkoxysulfonium salt which cannot fulfill the *trans* stereoelectronic requirements of an E_2 elimination.

C. OTHER OXIDATIONS

DMSO has also been employed in the oxidation of a variety of other functional groups. Among the conversions which have been reported are the following: thiols to disulfides (189–194), sulfides to sulfoxides (195), amines to carbonyl compounds via diazonium salt intermediates (196), carbenes to carbonyl compounds (197), epoxides to α-hydroxy aldehydes or ketones (198–200), and ketones to α-hydroxy acids (201).

The oxidation of thiols to disulfides can be carried out using either the DMSO–DCC procedure, or simply by heating the thiol in DMSO. In the latter procedure, the acidity of the thiol greatly affects the ease of oxidation. Whereas aromatic thiols are oxidized at room temperature within 24 hr, aliphatic derivatives require heating at 160°. Wallace and Mahon (192) suggested on the basis of kinetic studies that the initial reaction between thiol and sulfoxide leads to formation of a "thiol-sulfoxide" **169** which on further reaction with thiol forms the disulfide, dimethylsulfide, and water.

$$CH_3\overset{O}{\overset{\|}{S}}CH_3 + RSH \rightarrow CH_3\underset{SR}{\overset{OH}{\overset{|}{S}}}CH_3 \xrightarrow{RSH} RSSR + CH_3SCH_3 + H_2O$$

(169)

An intermediate analogous to **169** may also be involved in the DMSO oxidation of HBr and HI to Br_2 and I_2 (202). Since bromine is generated *in situ*, solutions of DMSO containing HBr can be used as a medium for brominations (203). In the Kornblum oxidation of α-bromo ketones, such brominations can be a nuisance unless the HBr is effectively removed. Reaction of 2-bromocyclohexanone with dimethylsulfoxide in the absence of base led to 1-bromo-2-hydroxy-cyclohex-1-en-3-one **(170)** in 70% yield rather than cyclohexane-1,2-dione **(171)**; under similar conditions, the bromocyclopentanone **172** also gave the brominated product **173** rather than the desired dione (204).

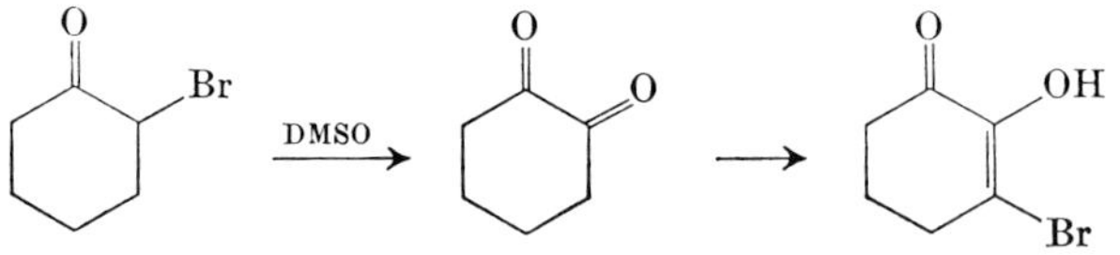

The nucleophilic opening of 3-membered heterocyclic compounds by DMSO leads to alkoxysulfonium salts which decompose to carbonyl compounds and dimethylsulfide in the usual manner. Monosubstituted epoxides are thus converted by DMSO–boron trifluoride–etherate via alkoxysulfonium salts, e.g., **174**, to α-hydroxy aldehydes (199). Ring opening followed by oxidation of the intermediate sulfonium salt by DMSO has also been reported for the *N*-acyl aziridine **175** (205) which afforded *N*-desyl-*p*-nitrobenzamide **(176)** in 80% yield after 17 hr at 115–120°.

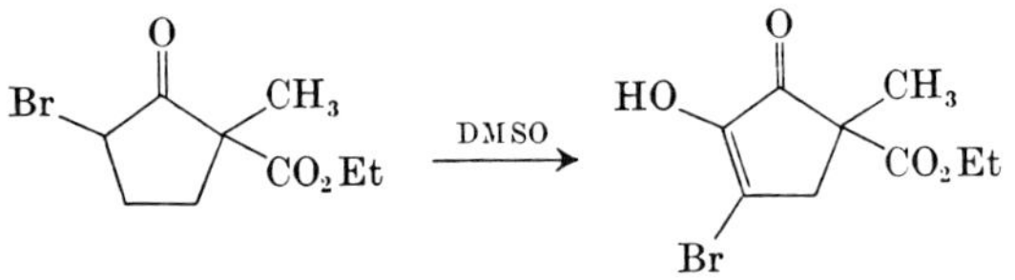

The interception of bromonium ions by DMSO, which may be classified as the opening of a 3-membered ring species, has recently been described (163,206,207) and is potentially of synthetic value. Dalton and Jones (206) have shown that reaction of *trans*-stilbene with *N*-bromo-succinimide in DMSO containing small quantities of water afforded *erythro*-1-bromo-1,2-diphenylethanol **(178)**. Reaction in ^{18}O-labeled

DMSO yielded bromohydrin which had incorporated greater than 95% of the labeled oxygen; no label was incorporated from ^{18}O-enriched water. These results are consonant with the formation of an intermediate bromonium ion which is efficiently trapped by DMSO affording

$$\underset{RCH-CH_2}{\overset{O}{\diagup\diagdown}} + \underset{CH_3SCH_3}{\overset{O}{\overset{\|}{}}} \xrightarrow{BF_3 \cdot Et_2O}$$

$$\underset{(174)}{\overset{O^-}{\underset{|}{RCHCH_2O}} - \overset{+}{S}(CH_3)_2} \longrightarrow \underset{|}{\overset{OH}{\underset{|}{RCHCHO}}} + CH_3SCH_3$$

$$\underset{(175)}{p\text{-}NO_2C_6H_4\overset{O}{\overset{\|}{C}}\underset{\diagdown CH_2}{\overset{\diagup CHPh}{N}}} + CH_3\overset{O}{\overset{\|}{S}}CH_3 \rightarrow p\text{-}NO_2C_6H_4\overset{O^-}{\underset{|}{C}}=NCH_2\overset{Ph}{\underset{|}{CH}}O-\overset{+}{S}(CH_3)_2$$

$$\downarrow$$

$$\underset{(176)}{p\text{-}NO_2C_6H_4\overset{O}{\overset{\|}{C}}NHCH_2\overset{O}{\overset{\|}{C}}Ph} + CH_3SCH_3$$

the *erythro*-sulfonium salt **177** and eventually the *erythro*-bromohydrin **178**. Torssell (163) has found that treatment of cyclohexene with bromotrinitromethane in DMSO gives the brominated sulfonium salt **179**—isolated as the tetraphenyl borate. Bromination of cyclohexene in DMSO–dimethoxyethane at $-10°$ affords *trans*-2-bromocyclohexanol on work-up (163). Conceivably, conditions may be found where the intermediate **179** could, prior to isolation, be oxidized to 2-bromocyclohexanone, thereby providing for a simple conversion of an olefin to an α-bromo carbonyl compound.

$$\underset{H}{\overset{Ph}{\diagdown}}C=C\underset{Ph}{\overset{H}{\diagup}} \xrightarrow{NBS} \underset{H}{\overset{Ph}{\diagdown}}\overset{Br_+\cdots}{\underset{Ph}{C-C}}H \xrightarrow{DMSO}$$

$$\underset{(177)}{\underset{H}{\overset{Ph}{\diagdown}}\overset{H}{\underset{Br}{C}}\diagup\overset{+}{O-S(CH_3)_2}\diagdown\underset{Ph}{}} \xrightarrow{H_2O} \underset{(178)}{\underset{H}{\overset{Ph}{\diagdown}}\overset{H}{\underset{Br}{C}}\diagup\overset{}{OH}\diagdown\underset{Ph}{}}$$

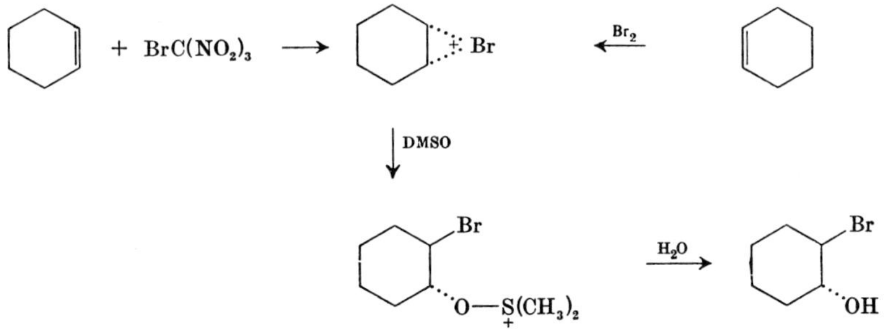

$$\text{cyclohexene} + \text{BrC(NO}_2)_3 \longrightarrow \text{[bromonium intermediate]} \xleftarrow{Br_2} \text{cyclohexene}$$

$$\downarrow \text{DMSO}$$

$$\text{trans-2-bromocyclohexyl-O-}\overset{+}{S}(CH_3)_2 \xrightarrow{H_2O} \text{trans-2-bromocyclohexanol}$$

(179)

The oxidation of carboxylic, sulfenic, sulfinic, and sulfonic acid chlorides and the reactions of inorganic halides with DMSO will be discussed in connection with the Pummerer rearrangement.

V. Pummerer Rearrangements

During the last 60 years there have been reported a number of reactions, generally referred to as Pummerer rearrangements, in which a sulfoxide bearing at least one α-hydrogen is reduced to a sulfide and concomitantly oxidized at the α-position. An early example was provided in 1909 by Smythe (208) who showed that dibenzylsulfoxide was cleaved in aqueous acid to give benzaldehyde and benzylmercaptan. Shortly thereafter, Pummerer (209) reported the acid-catalyzed cleavage of α-(phenylsulfinyl) propionic acid **(180)** to thiophenol and pyruvic acid, and the acetic anhydride-induced rearrangement of ethyl phenylsulfinylacetate **(181)** to ethyl α-phenylthio-α-acetoxy-acetate **(182)**.

Sulfoxides, such as β-disulfoxides (210), β-keto sulfoxides (40,41), and the β-sulfinyl acids and esters (210) mentioned above, appear to be particularly susceptible to acid-catalyzed rearrangement. In fact, Russell et al. (40) found that some of the β-keto sulfoxides formed in the methyl sulfinyl carbanion–ester reaction rearranged to hemithio-acetals on the acid work-up of the reaction. Most alkyl sulfoxides, including DMSO, are considerably more stable to acids at room temperature, but are decomposed on prolonged exposure. Such sulfoxides do undergo Pummerer-type rearrangements in the presence of other electrophilic reagents. A large number of compounds have been used to initiate such rearrangements. Among them are: carboxylic

$$\text{PhCH}_2\overset{\underset{\|}{O}}{\text{S}}\text{CH}_2\text{Ph} \xrightarrow[\text{H}_2\text{O}]{\text{H}^+} \text{PhCHO} + \text{PhCH}_2\text{SH}$$

$$\underset{\underset{\text{CH}_3}{|}}{\text{Ph}\overset{\underset{\|}{O}}{\text{S}}\text{CHCO}_2\text{H}} \xrightarrow[\text{H}_2\text{O}]{\text{H}^+} \text{CH}_3\overset{\underset{\|}{O}}{\text{C}}\text{CO}_2\text{H} + \text{PhSH}$$

(180)

$$\text{Ph}\overset{\underset{\|}{O}}{\text{S}}\text{CH}_2\overset{\underset{\|}{O}}{\text{C}}\text{OEt} \xrightarrow{\text{Ac}_2\text{O}} \underset{\underset{\underset{O}{\|}}{\underset{\text{OCCH}_3}{|}}}{\text{Ph}\overset{\underset{\|}{O}}{\text{S}}\text{CHCOEt}}$$

(181)   **(182)**

acid chlorides (211–213); anhydrides (208,209,214–220); isocyanates (221); organic sulfur acid chlorides (RSCl, RSOCl, RSO$_2$Cl) (222–224); a host of inorganic halides including thionyl chloride (211), boron trichloride (225), and silicon tetrachloride (225); various phosphorus chlorides and oxychlorides (213,226); phosphorus pentoxide (175,176); and dicyclohexylcarbodiimide, the reagent in the Pfitzner-Moffatt oxidation. Many other initiators could be suggested.

The mechanism of the Pummerer rearrangement has been the subject of a number of recent investigations. The acetic anhydride reaction has been studied in greatest detail, and a discussion of its mechanism will, for the most part, suffice for the other processes.

Little doubt exists that the first step in the reaction of a sulfoxide, for example DMSO, with acetic anhydride results in the formation of the acetoxysulfonium salt **163**. The details of the rearrangement from **163** to acetoxymethyl methyl sulfide **183** have, however, been subjected to much speculation (211,214–220). Various possible pathways which have been suggested are shown in eqs. a–d.

It would seem to the author that the only mechanisms which can seriously be considered are mechanisms a and b. The question which remains is whether the ylid **184**, formed by proton abstraction from **163**, rearranges by an intramolecular process (in a solvent cage) or by an intermolecular route. The other suggestions can be considered highly unlikely since nucleophiles attack nucleophilic centers.

The recent work of Johnson and co-workers (214) provides strong support for the intermolecular process. A number of alkoxysulfonium

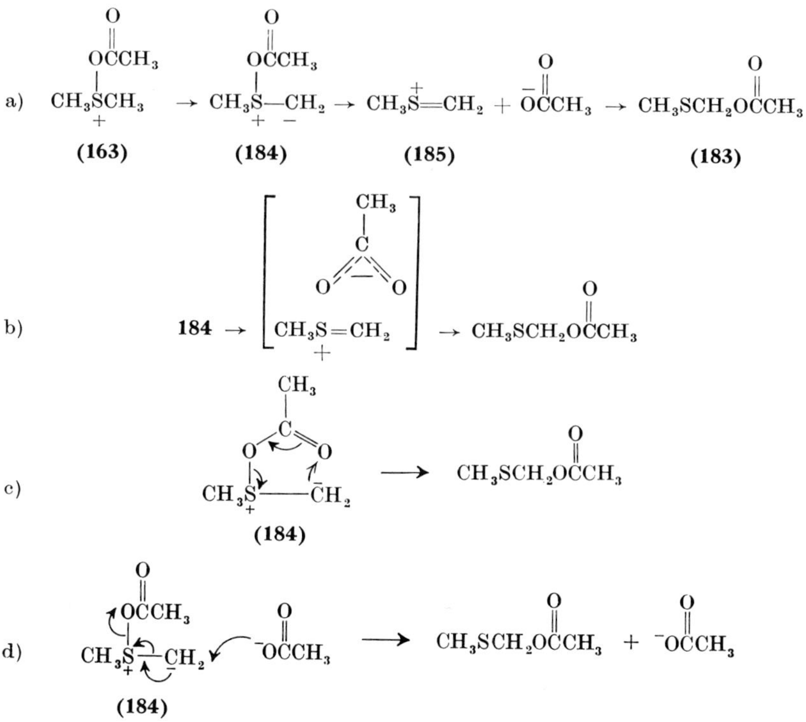

a) [reaction scheme: (163) → (184) → (185) + ⁻OCCH₃ → (183)]

b) [reaction scheme: 184 → cyclic intermediate → CH₃SCH₂OCCH₃]

c) [reaction scheme showing (184) rearrangement → CH₃SCH₂OCCH₃]

d) [reaction scheme showing (184) → CH₃SCH₂OCCH₃ + ⁻OCCH₃]

salts such as **186** were found to undergo both (*1*) oxidation to formaldehyde and (*2*) rearrangement to hemithioacetals. Simultaneous rearrangement of **186** and the ^{14}C-labeled salt **188** yielded products which showed that considerable crossover had occurred and thus provided conclusive evidence that the alkoxy group exchanged into

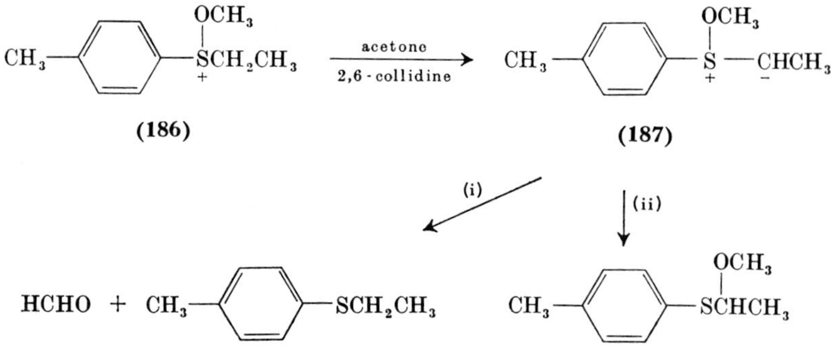

[reaction scheme: (186) $\xrightarrow[\text{2,6-collidine}]{\text{acetone}}$ (187), with (i) giving HCHO + CH₃-C₆H₄-SCH₂CH₃ and (ii) giving CH₃-C₆H₄-SCHCH₃ with OCH₃]

the medium during the α-rearrangement. Sulfur-stabilized ions such as carbonium ion **185** are therefore established as intermediates in the Pummerer rearrangements. This ion is reasonably stable and has been isolated by Meerwein (227) as the hexachloroantimonate. It is amusing to note that loss of the acetate from the ylid **184** converts a carbon with carbanion character to one with carbonium ion character.

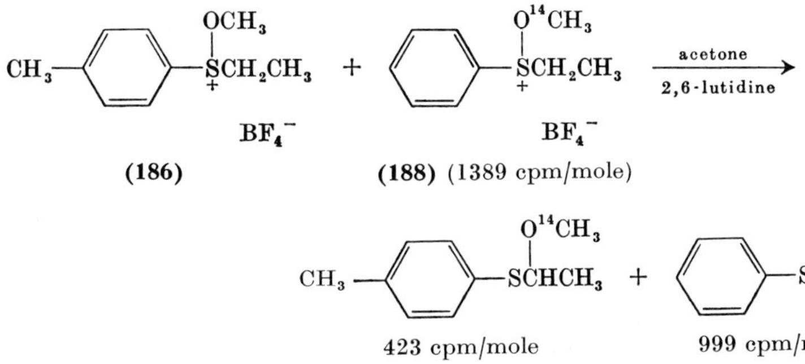

$$CH_3-\langle C_6H_4\rangle-\overset{OCH_3}{\underset{+}{S}}CH_2CH_3 \quad BF_4^- \quad + \quad \langle C_6H_5\rangle-\overset{O^{14}CH_3}{\underset{+}{S}}CH_2CH_3 \quad BF_4^- \xrightarrow[2,6\text{-lutidine}]{\text{acetone}}$$

(**186**)   (**188**) (1389 cpm/mole)

$$CH_3-\langle C_6H_4\rangle-\overset{O^{14}CH_3}{S}CHCH_3 \quad + \quad \langle C_6H_5\rangle-\overset{O^{14}CH_3}{S}CHCH_3$$

423 cpm/mole   999 cpm/mole

Evidence which indicates that the conclusions derived above for the alkoxysulfonium salt rearrangement are indeed applicable to the acetic anhydride reaction was also provided by the Johnson group (214). In the reaction of acetic anhydride with unsymmetrical sulfoxides, such as methyl isopropyl sulfoxide (**189**), migration of the acetoxy group proceeded to the least substituted α-carbon to give α-acetoxymethyl isopropyl sulfide (**190**) in 69% yield. Similar migrations were observed in reactions involving methyl n-propyl and methyl n-butyl sulfoxide. The direction of migration was ascribed to the difference in acidities of the α-protons in the intermediate sulfonium salt **191**. The ylid **191a** once formed is immediately converted to product, and thus its formation is the product-determining step.

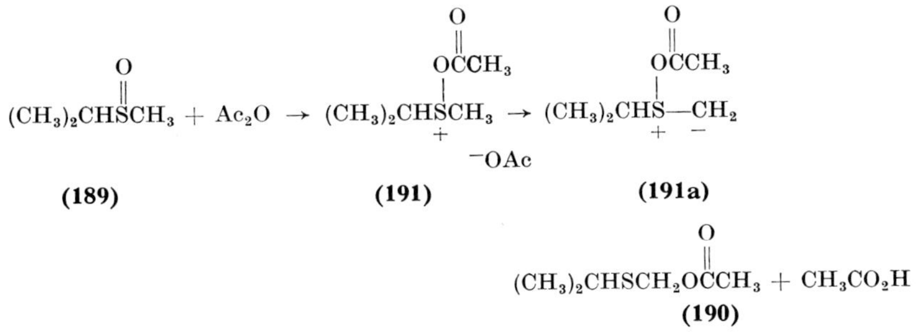

$$(CH_3)_2CH\overset{O}{\overset{\|}{S}}CH_3 + Ac_2O \rightarrow (CH_3)_2CH\underset{+}{\overset{OCCH_3}{\underset{|}{S}}}CH_3 \rightarrow (CH_3)_2CH\underset{+}{\overset{OCCH_3}{\underset{|}{S}}}-\overset{-}{CH_2}$$

(**189**)   (**191**) ^-OAc (**191a**)

$$(CH_3)_2CHSCH_2O\overset{O}{\overset{\|}{C}}CH_3 + CH_3CO_2H$$

(**190**)

This assumption is based on the analogy that ylids such as **187** are not reprotonated to a significant extent, but are converted rapidly to product (160).

Reaction of the alkoxysulfonium salt **192** with sodium acetate in DMSO (214) afforded α-acetoxymethyl isopropyl sulfide **(190)** in 69% yield, together with methoxymethyl isopropyl sulfide **(193)** (20%) and methyl isopropyl sulfide **(194)** (6%). Again, acetate migration had occurred to the least substituted carbon. The formation of these products was rationalized in the following way. Methyl isopropyl sulfide **(194)** is formed by cyclic decomposition of the ylid, **195**. The acetoxymethyl and methoxymethyl isopropyl sulfides result from an initial displacement of methoxide by acetate ion affording the acetoxysulfonium salt **191** which collapses via an ylid to the sulfur-stabilized carbonium ion **196** and acetate ion. Competition for the ion **196** by both methoxide and acetate accounts for the products **190** and **193**. The formation of **193** via the ylid **195** was ruled out since such ylids generally undergo exclusively the cyclic decomposition to a carbonyl compound and a sulfide (160).

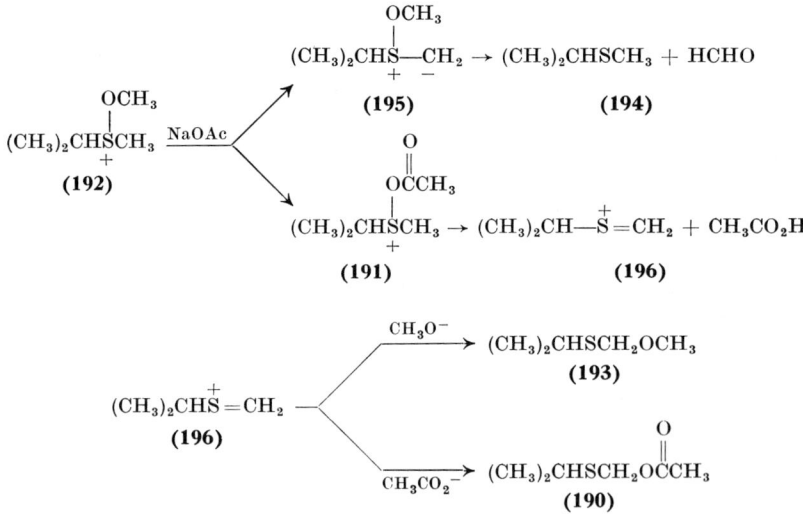

The other Pummerer rearrangements in all likelihood occur by very similar mechanisms. For example, the reaction of sulfoxides with thionyl chloride (211), which leads to α-chlorosulfides **197**, sulfur dioxide, and HCl, probably has the ions **198, 199,** and **200** as intermediates. The chlorosulfonium salt **199** is also an intermediate in the chlorinolysis of sulfides to α-chlorosulfides (211). A more direct route from **198** to **200** is also possible which involves ylid formation and fragmentation thereof to **200**, sulfur dioxide, and chloride ion. The rearrangement of the chlorosulfonium chloride **199** to the chloromethyl sulfide **197** has been suggested to occur intramolecularly along a rather picturesque route in which a chloronium ion "rides downhill from sulfur to carbon on an electron cloud" (211).

$$\underset{\text{}}{\text{RSCH}_3} + \text{SOCl}_2 \rightarrow \underset{\underset{\text{Cl}^-}{+}}{\overset{\overset{\text{O}}{\|}}{\underset{\text{}}{\text{RSCH}_3}}} \rightarrow \underset{\underset{\text{Cl}}{|}}{\overset{\overset{\text{O}}{\|}}{\underset{\text{}}{\text{RSCH}_3}}} \overset{\text{Cl}^-}{\underset{+}{}} \leftarrow \text{Cl}_2 + \text{RSCH}_3$$

(198)   (199)

$$\text{RSCH}_2\text{Cl} \leftarrow \overset{+}{\text{RS}}=\text{CH}_2 \leftarrow \underset{\underset{\text{Cl}}{|}}{\overset{+}{\text{RS}}-\overset{-}{\text{CH}_2}}$$

(197)   (200)

The rationalization of the thiomethoxymethyl ether formation in the DMSO oxidation can be made in terms of the above discussion. Sweat and Epstein (173) have pointed out that these products are not formed when the intermediate alkoxysulfonium salt is generated by direct nucleophilic displacement of a tosylate or halide function by DMSO.

This observation is in agreement with the work of Johnson and Phillips (160,214), who showed that the Pummerer-type rearrangement occurs to a negligible extent in salts of the type **201**.

$$\underset{\substack{+ \\ \text{BF}_4^-}}{\overset{\overset{\text{OCH}_3}{|}}{\text{PhSCH}_3}} \xrightarrow{\text{base}} \underset{+}{\overset{\overset{\text{OCH}_3}{|}}{\text{PhS}-\overset{-}{\text{CH}_2}}} \begin{cases} \xrightarrow{\text{oxidation}} \text{PhSCH}_3 + \text{HCHO} & (>99\%) \\ \xrightarrow{\text{rearrangement}} \text{PhSCH}_2\text{OCH}_3 & (<1\%) \end{cases}$$

(201)   (202)

In the initial sulfonium salt **203**, X = CH₃CO or C₆H₁₁N = CNHC₆H₁₁, generated in the DMSO–Ac₂O or in the DMSO–DCC oxidation procedures respectively, ylid formation can lead only to elimination of $CH_2\overset{+}{=}SCH_3$, which consumes some of the alcohol to produce the thioethers. The amount of oxidation versus thiomethoxy methyl ether formation will thus depend on the relative rates of hydrogen abstraction (ylid formation) and nucleophilic displacement on sulfur by alcohol (alkoxysulfonium salt formation).

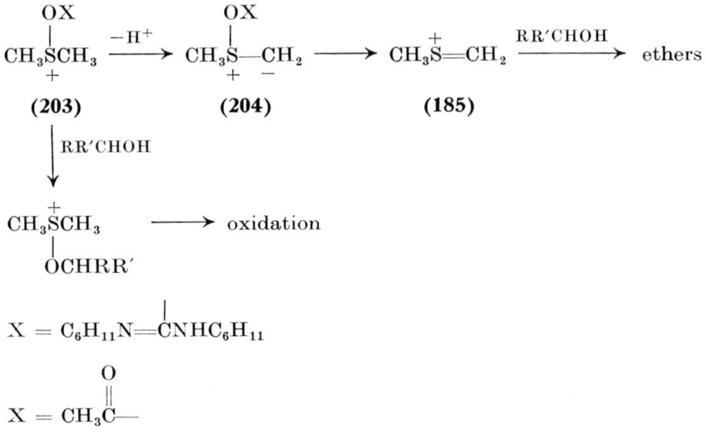

$$\underset{(203)}{\underset{+}{CH_3\overset{\overset{OX}{|}}{S}CH_3}} \xrightarrow{-H^+} \underset{(204)}{\underset{+\quad -}{CH_3\overset{\overset{OX}{|}}{S}-CH_2}} \longrightarrow \underset{(185)}{CH_3\overset{+}{S}=CH_2} \xrightarrow{RR'CHOH} \text{ethers}$$

$$\Big\downarrow RR'CHOH$$

$$\underset{}{CH_3\overset{+}{S}CH_3} \longrightarrow \text{oxidation}$$
$$\underset{}{|}$$
$$OCHRR'$$

$$X = C_6H_{11}N=\overset{|}{C}NHC_6H_{11}$$

$$X = CH_3\overset{\overset{O}{\|}}{C}-$$

Generally, significantly more thioether formation is observed in the acetic anhydride reaction than in the DCC reaction. This probably reflects the efficiency of the bases present in the two reaction mixtures in promoting ylid formation; acetate, the base present in the acetic anhydride reaction, is more efficient than the conjugate base of phosphoric acid.

Every one of the ions **185** formed in the decomposition of the ylid **204** need not, however, consume alcohol. Other nucleophilic species in the solution will also react with **185** as is shown by the isolation of the by-products, acetoxymethyl methyl sulfide **(183)** in the acetic anhydride reaction and the pyridinium salt **205** in the pyridine–pyridinium trifluoroacetate-catalyzed DMSO–DCC reaction (166).

The nucleophilicity of the alcohol should affect its rate of reaction with **203** and, as a result, affect the ratio of the products formed from the two possible routes. This is illustrated in the reaction of phenols with both the DMSO–DCC and DMSO–Ac$_2$O reagents which will be discussed in the next section. Acidic phenols such as the *o*- and *p*-nitrophenol give, as expected, higher yields of thiomethoxy methylethers than do the less acidic derivatives.

The reaction of Grignard reagents with sulfoxides is formally similar to a Pummerer rearrangement. Potter (228) reported in 1960

$$\underset{\underset{\text{SCH}_3}{|}}{\underset{\underset{\text{CH}_2}{|}}{\overset{\bigcirc}{\text{N}^+}}} \quad \text{X}^-$$

(205)

that *p*-tolyl methyl sulfoxide **(206)** and *p*-tolyl benzyl sulfoxide **(207)** reacted with phenylmagnesium bromide to furnish, among other products, *p*-tolyl benzyl sulfide **(208)** (50%) and *p*-tolyl benzhydryl sulfide **(209)** (90%), respectively. Oda and Yamamoto (229) treated dimethylsulfoxide with various Grignard reagents and obtained the expected substituted sulfides in 20–35% yield.

$$p\text{-CH}_3\text{C}_6\text{H}_4\overset{\overset{\text{O}}{\|}}{\text{S}}\text{CH}_3 \xrightarrow{\text{PhMgBr}} p\text{-CH}_3\text{C}_6\text{H}_4\text{SCH}_2\text{Ph} \quad (50\%)$$
$$\quad\quad\quad\text{(206)} \quad\quad\quad\quad\quad\quad\quad\quad\quad \text{(208)}$$

$$p\text{-CH}_3\text{C}_6\text{H}_4\overset{\overset{\text{O}}{\|}}{\text{S}}\text{CH}_2\text{Ph} \xrightarrow{\text{PhMgBr}} p\text{-CH}_3\text{C}_6\text{H}_4\text{SCHPh}_2 \quad (90\%)$$
$$\quad\quad\quad\text{(207)} \quad\quad\quad\quad\quad\quad\quad\quad\quad \text{(209)}$$

$$\text{CH}_3\overset{\overset{\text{O}}{\|}}{\text{S}}\text{CH}_3 \xrightarrow{\text{RMgX}} \text{CH}_3\text{SCH}_2\text{R} \quad (20\text{--}35\%)$$

A group of French workers (230) investigated the DMSO–phenyl magnesium bromide reaction in more detail and identified a variety of products by comparison of VPC retention times. Mechanistically, the more important products were methyl phenyl sulfide **(210)**, benzyl methyl sulfide **(211)**, ethyl phenyl sulfide **(212)** (minor component), and phenol (minor product). Two simultaneous reactions were suggested to occur. Both involved addition of the Grignard reagent to the sulfoxide to give the tetracovalent sulfur derivative **213**, disproportionation of which (231) gives rise to the pairs methyl phenyl sulfide–methanol and dimethylsulfide–phenol. To account for the sulfides **211** and **212**, the formation of the carbanion **214** was invoked, which could undergo a Stevens-like 1,2-rearrangement to either **211** or **212**.

$$\text{CH}_3\overset{\overset{\text{O}}{\|}}{\text{S}}\text{CH}_3 + \text{PhMgBr} \rightarrow \underset{\underset{\text{Ph}}{|}}{\text{CH}_3\overset{\overset{\text{OMgBr}}{|}}{\text{S}}\text{CH}_3} \rightarrow (\text{CH}_3\text{SCH}_3 + \text{PhOH})$$

$$\textbf{(213)} \qquad + (\text{CH}_3\text{SPh} + \text{CH}_3\text{OH})$$
$$\textbf{(210)}$$

$$-\text{H}^+ \downarrow$$

$$\text{CH}_3\text{CH}_2\text{SPh} + \text{CH}_3\text{SCH}_2\text{Ph} \leftarrow \underset{\underset{\text{Ph}}{|}}{\text{CH}_3\overset{\overset{\text{OMgBr}}{|}}{\text{S}}\text{—CH}_2^-}$$

(212) **(211)** **(214)**

Another possible route to **211** might be via the complexed sulfonium salt **215** undergoing successively ylid formation, elimination to the ion **185**, and finally addition of the Grignard reagent. Such a mechanism would account for the high yield of product obtained by Potter in the reaction of benzyl phenyl sulfoxide with phenylmagnesium bromide but could not readily explain the formation of the ethyl phenyl sulfide obtained by the French workers in the DMSO reaction.

$$\text{CH}_3\overset{\overset{\text{O}}{\|}}{\text{S}}\text{CH}_3 + \text{PhMgBr} \longrightarrow \underset{+}{\text{CH}_3\overset{\overset{\text{OMgPh}}{|}}{\text{S}}\text{CH}_3}$$

$$\textbf{(215)}$$

$$\downarrow$$

$$\text{CH}_3\text{SCH}_2\text{Ph} \xleftarrow{\text{PhMgBr}} \overset{+}{\text{CH}_3\text{S}}=\text{CH}_2$$
$$\textbf{(185)}$$

Ratts and Yao (232,233) have recently described a rearrangement of some phenacylsulfonium ylids which bears a close analogy to the Pummerer reaction. Reflux of an aqueous solution of dimethylphenacylsulfonium ylid **216** for 5 hr afforded α-thiomethoxymethylstyrene **(217)** in 66% yield. A number of other alkyl- and arylmethylphenacylsulfonium ylids underwent the same rearrangement. The authors suggested that the ylid **216** in a hydroxylic solvent could give rise to the isomeric ylid **218** which rearranges to **217** by an intramolecular pathway. An intermolecular rearrangement, analogous to that demonstrated for the alkoxysulfonium salts (214), does not appear reasonable in this case since the ion **(185)**, when free from the enolate **219**, would rapidly be destroyed by reaction with water.

$$\underset{(216)}{\text{PhCCH}-\overset{+}{\underset{\text{CH}_3}{\overset{\text{CH}_3}{\text{S}}}}} \longrightarrow \underset{(218)}{\text{PhC}\overset{\text{O}}{\underset{\text{CH}_2}{\diagdown}}\overset{+}{\underset{\text{CH}_3}{\overset{\text{CH}_2}{\text{S}}}}}$$

$$\underset{(217)}{\overset{\text{OCH}_2\text{SCH}_3}{\underset{|}{\text{PhC}=\text{CH}_2}}} \longleftarrow \left[\underset{(219)}{\overset{\text{O}^-}{\underset{|}{\text{PhC}=\text{CH}_2}}} + \underset{(185)}{\text{CH}_2=\overset{+}{\text{SCH}_3}} \right]$$

VI. Other Reactions Involving DMSO

A. DMSO–DCC AND PHENOLS

A natural extension of the DCC–DMSO oxidation of alcohols was the application of these reaction conditions to phenols. Such an investigation was simultaneously communicated by two groups (234,235) who found that these reactions were considerably more complicated and gave rise to a variety of interesting products. The full papers by Burdon and Moffatt (236,237) discuss the formation of the various products in considerable detail.

The predominant reaction with most simple phenols is the introduction of thiomethoxymethyl groups in the available *ortho* positions. Thus phenol itself gives a mixture of 27% 2-(thiomethoxymethyl)-phenol **(220)** and 16% 2,6-(dithiomethoxymethyl)phenol **(221)**; in addition, a minor product, 1,3-benzoxathiane **(222)** was obtained in 4% yield. Other phenols which had free *ortho* positions produced the corresponding products in similar yields. The more acidic phenols such as *p*-nitrophenol gave, in addition to these products, significant amounts of thiomethoxymethyl ethers **223**. A possible mechanistic significance of the formation of the latter products which appear to be unique for the acidic phenols was discussed in the last section.

Thiomethoxymethylations have also been performed using DMSO–acetic anhydride mixtures (237,238). The results of these reactions are qualitatively similar to those of the DMSO–DCC procedure. The formation of acetates is an important side reaction, especially for the more acidic phenols in the acetic anhydride modification, thereby seriously limiting its usefulness.

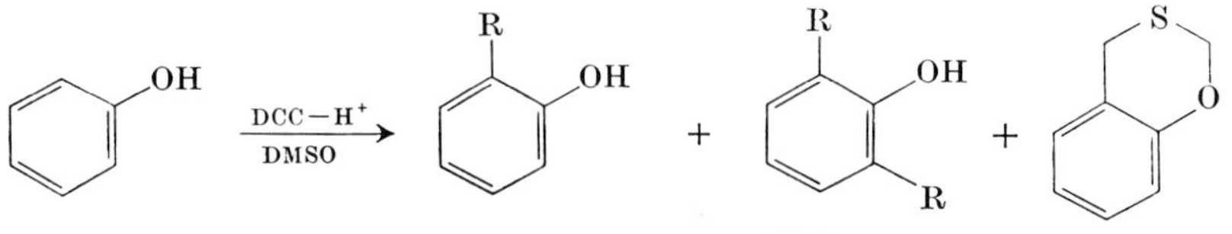

(220) (27%) **(221)** (16%) **(222)** (4%)

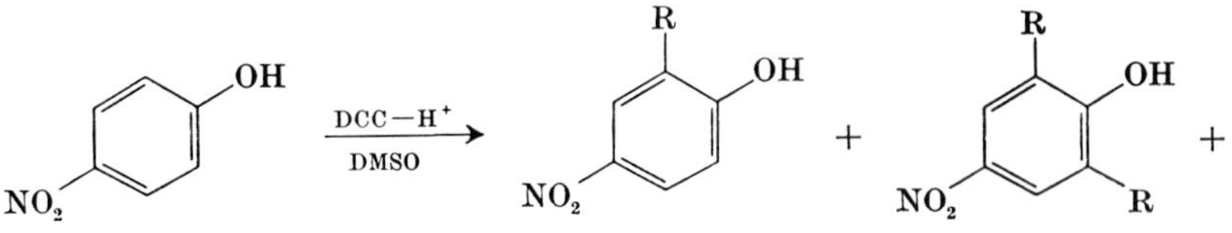

(25%) (11%)

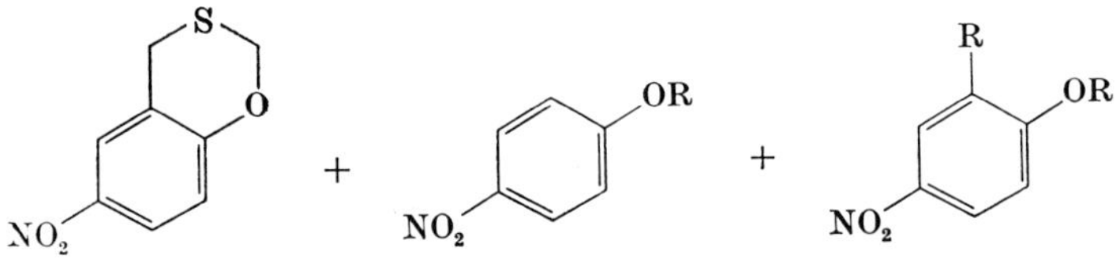

(3%) **(223)** (3%) **(233a)** (14%)

R=CH$_2$SCH$_3$

Sulfoxides other than DMSO have been used in these reactions. Thus, dibenzyl sulfoxide and tetramethylene sulfoxide reacted with o-cresol under the usual conditions to give the monoalkylated derivatives **224** and **225** in 26 and 45% yield, respectively.

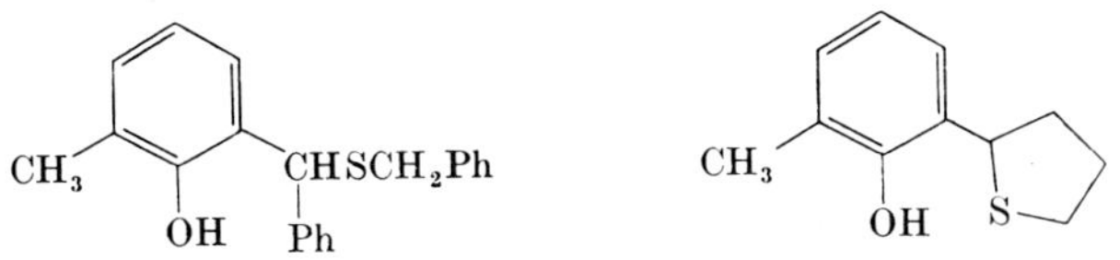

(224) **(225)**

The mechanism proposed for the formation of the *ortho*-alkylated products involves initial attack of the phenolic oxygen on the DMSO–DCC adduct (Section IV) to form an aryloxysulfonium salt **226**. Proton abstraction yields the ylid **227** which alkylates the available *ortho* position, eventually forming thiomethoxymethylphenols, Scheme 11. This mechanism is closely related to the Sommelet rearrangement of benzyldimethylsulfonium salts **228** to 2-(thiomethoxymethyl)toluene **(229)** with sodium amide in liquid ammonia (239).

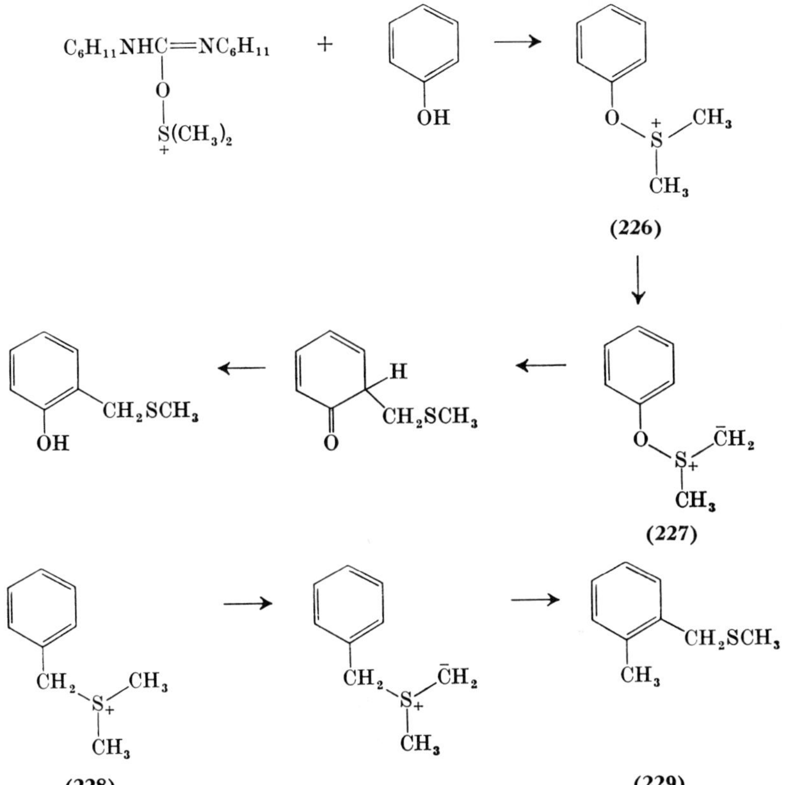

Scheme 11

The formation of the 1,3-benzoxathianes is more difficult to rationalize. It has been suggested (235,237) that in view of the low yield of these products, the mechanism possibly involves an initial bimolecular reaction between the sulfonium salt **226** and the ylid **227**, Scheme 12. Benzoxathianes become the major product with phenols containing suitable leaving groups, such as chlorine, in the *ortho* position, e.g., 2,6-dichlorophenol. Here intramolecular displacement of a chloride

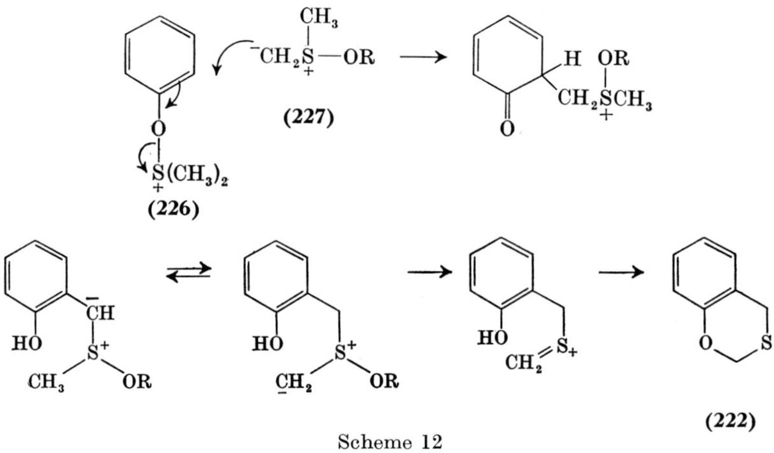

Scheme 12

in the ylid **230** produces the 5-membered ring sulfonium salt **231** which is converted in a relatively straightforward manner to 8-chloro-1,3-benzoxathiane **(232)**, Scheme 13.

The reactions of 2,6-disubstituted phenols can be interrupted at the cyclohexadienone stage (237). Upon careful work-up, these compounds could usually be isolated in high yield. Treatment of the dienones

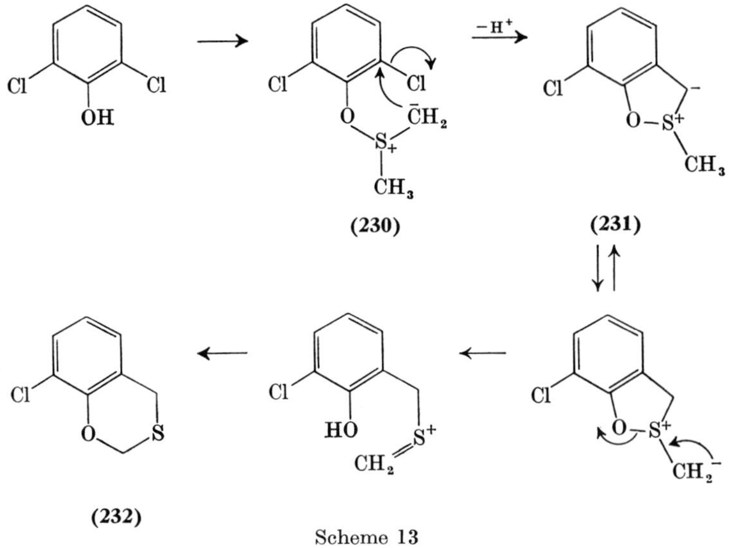

Scheme 13

with acids led to migration of the thiomethoxymethyl group to an open *meta* or *para* position in the ring. The acid-catalyzed rearrangement involves generation of the sulfur-stabilized carbonium ion **185** which is usually recaptured intramolecularly but can, with high concentrations of a suitable acceptor molecule such as another phenol, give some intermolecular alkylation. These transformations are depicted for 2,6-dimethylphenol in Scheme 14.

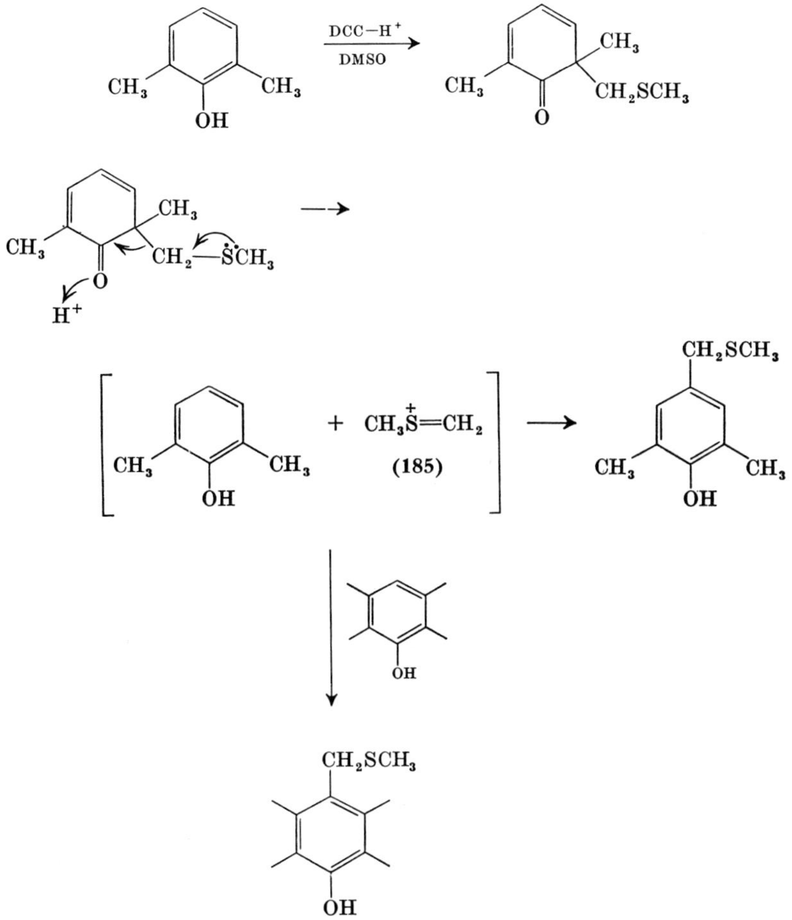

Scheme 14

In contrast to the above reactions, phenol and phenols bearing substituents having negative Hammett σ-constants react with DMSO to produce p-dimethylsulfonio phenols **233** in yields which were for the most part greater than 50% (240). Anisole and toluene failed to yield

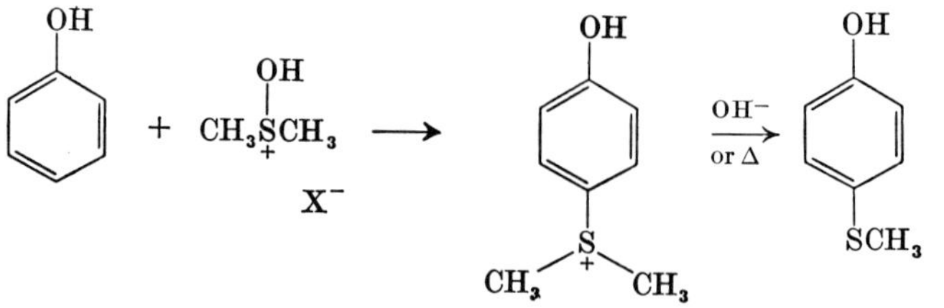

sulfonium salts under these conditions. These results are in agreement with a nucleophilic aromatic substitution by protonated dimethyl sulfoxide. Pyrolysis or base treatment of the sulfonium salts afforded p-hydroxythioanisoles.

B. DMSO AND ACTIVE METHYLENE COMPOUNDS

A number of authors have described the formation of stabilized sulfonium ylids by "condensing" sulfoxides with active methylene compounds in the presence of protonic acids (241,242); DCC–polyphosphoric acid (243,244), acetic anhydride (244–248), thionyl chloride (241), or phosphorus pentoxide (248).

These reactions can be mechanistically interpreted along the lines discussed for the DMSO oxidation of alcohols and the DCC–H⁺ or acetic anhydride-catalyzed reaction of DMSO with phenols. 2,4-Pentanedione will be used as the active methylene compound in the following discussion. Nucleophilic attack by the enolate ion of the active methylene compound on the sulfonium salt **234** would give the enol sulfonium salt **235** which could undergo oxygen-to-carbon migration to the diketo sulfonium salt **236**. Alternately, **236** could be formed directly by attack of the carbanion of the active methylene compound on **234**. Loss of a proton from **236** would be expected to occur spontaneously in the polar reaction medium to give the resonance-stabilized ylid **237**.

Other sulfoxides may replace DMSO in these reactions. Thus these methods, especially the DMSO–DCC–polyphosphoric acid modification

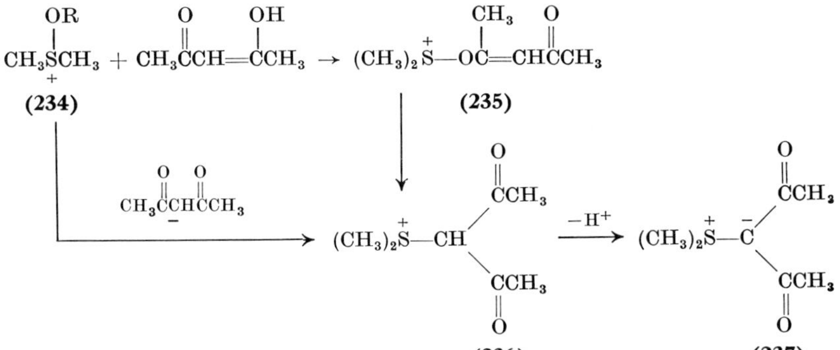

$$\underset{(234)}{\overset{OR}{\underset{+}{CH_3\overset{|}{S}CH_3}}} + \underset{}{CH_3\overset{O}{\overset{\|}{C}}CH=\overset{OH}{\overset{|}{C}}CH_3} \rightarrow \underset{(235)}{(CH_3)_2\overset{+}{S}-O\overset{CH_3}{\overset{|}{C}}=CH\overset{O}{\overset{\|}{C}}CH_3}$$

$$\underset{}{CH_3\overset{O}{\overset{\|}{C}}\overset{-}{CH}\overset{O}{\overset{\|}{C}}CH_3} \longrightarrow \underset{(236)}{(CH_3)_2\overset{+}{S}-CH\overset{\overset{O}{\overset{\|}{C}CH_3}}{\diagdown\overset{\|}{C}CH_3\atop\overset{\|}{O}}} \xrightarrow{-H^+} \underset{(237)}{(CH_3)_2\overset{+}{S}-\overset{-}{C}\overset{\overset{O}{\overset{\|}{C}CH_3}}{\diagdown\overset{\|}{C}CH_3\atop\overset{\|}{O}}}$$

(243), constitute a rather general approach to resonance-stabilized ylids. Some examples are given in Table XI. Ylids derived from β-diketones generally show two infrared maxima in the carbonyl region separated by about 30–50 cm^{-1}, with the lower wavelength band occurring in the 1540–1560 cm^{-1} range. Those from the β-ketoesters and β-ketoamides also show a low wavelength band below 1600 cm^{-1} and a higher band between 1680 and 1630 cm^{-1}.

Most of the ylids containing dialkylsulfonium groups larger than those of the parent dimethylsulfonium compounds show a magnetic nonequivalence of the α-methylene group which is dependent on the rest of the molecule and the solvent (243,249,250). See structures 238 and 239.

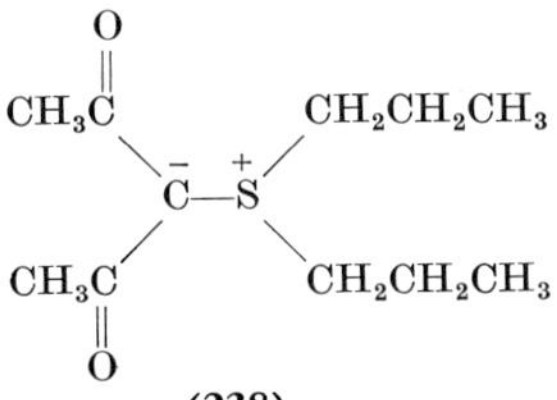

$$\underset{(238)}{\overset{CH_3\overset{O}{\overset{\|}{C}}}{\diagdown}\overset{-}{C}-\overset{+}{S}\overset{CH_2CH_2CH_3}{\diagup}\atop\overset{CH_3\overset{\|}{C}}{\diagup}\overset{}{\overset{\|}{O}}\overset{CH_2CH_2CH_3}{\diagdown}} \qquad \delta H_A = 2.89, \delta H_B = 3.91, \text{ and } J_{AB} = 12 \text{ cps}$$

$$\underset{(239)}{\overset{\overset{N}{\overset{\|\|\|}{C}}}{\diagdown}\overset{-}{C}-\overset{+}{S}\overset{CH_2CH_3}{\diagup}\atop\overset{C}{\diagup}\overset{}{\overset{\|\|\|}{N}}\overset{CH_2CH_3}{\diagdown}} \qquad \delta H_A = \delta H_B = 3.01$$

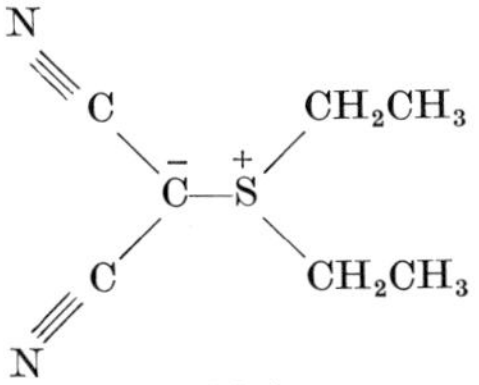

TABLE XI
Resonance-Stabilized Sulfur Ylids from Sulfoxides and Active Methylene Compounds

$$R_1R_2CH_2 + R_3R_4SO \rightarrow R_1R_2\overset{-}{C}\text{—}\overset{+}{S}R_3R_4$$

Sulfoxide	Active methylene compound	Method	Yield, %	Ref.
DMSO	$(NC)_2CH_2$	$SOCl_2$	40	241
DMSO	$(NC)_2CH_2$	DCC	57	243
DMSO	$(NC)_2CH_2$	Ac_2O	40	244
DMSO	$(NO_2)_2CH_2$	Ac_2O	36	245
DMSO	$(CH_3CO)_2CH_2$	DCC	57	243
DMSO	$(CH_3CO)_2CH_2$	Ac_2O	5	248
DMSO	$(CH_3OCO)_2CH_2$	DCC	40	243
DMSO	CH_3COCH_2COEt	DCC	35	243
DMSO	$NCCH_2COEt$	DCC	62	243
DMSO	CH_3COCH_2CNHPh	DCC	49	243
DMSO	$NCCH_2P(OEt)_2$	DCC	46	243
DMSO	$(PhSO_2)_2CH_2$	Ac_2O	67	247
DMSO	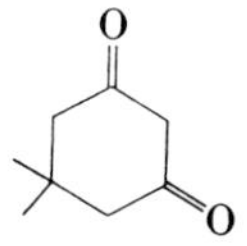 5,5-dimethylcyclohexane-1,3-dione	DCC	59	243
DMSO	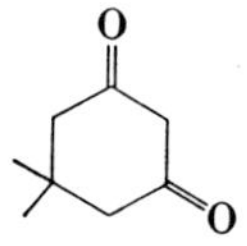 5,5-dimethylcyclohexane-1,3-dione	Ac_2O	24	248
DMSO	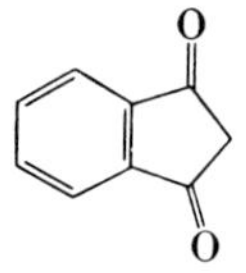 indane-1,3-dione	DCC	80	243

(*continued*)

TABLE XI (*continued*)

Sulfoxide	Active methylene compound	Method	Yield, %	Ref.
DMSO	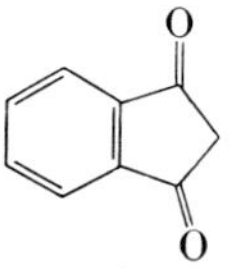 1,3-indandione	Ac$_2$O	63	244
DMSO	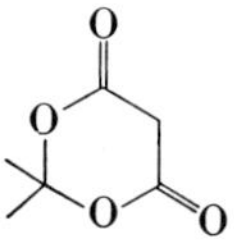 2,2-dimethyl-1,3-dioxane-4,6-dione	DCC	40	244
DMSO	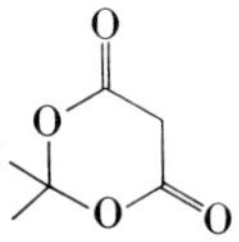 2,2-dimethyl-1,3-dioxane-4,6-dione	Ac$_2$O	80	244
(CH$_3$CH$_2$)$_2$SO	(NC)$_2$CH$_2$	DCC	71	244
(CH$_3$CH$_2$CH$_2$)$_2$SO	NCCH$_2$COEt	DCC	41	244
PhS(O)CH$_3$	(CH$_3$CO)$_2$CH$_2$	Ac$_2$O	44	248
PhS(O)CH$_3$	5,5-dimethyl-1,3-cyclohexanedione	Ac$_2$O	27	248
(PhCH$_2$)$_2$SO	(NC)$_2$CH$_2$	Ac$_2$O	40	248
(CH$_2$)$_4$SO	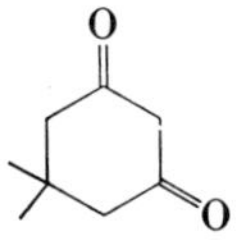 5,5-dimethyl-1,3-cyclohexanedione	DCC	58	248
(CH$_2$)$_4$SO	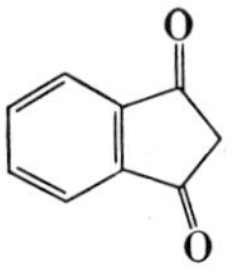 1,3-indandione	DCC	45	248

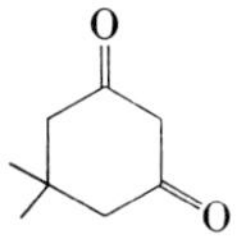

Related to these reactions is the formation of sulfonyl sulfilimines **240** from DMSO and primary sulfonamides by refluxing the reagents in toluene in the presence of P_2O_5 (230). A number of primary amides, such as di- and trichloroacetamide, also react with DMSO under these conditions to afford acylsulfilimines (251).

$$RSO_2NH_2 + CH_3\overset{O}{\overset{\|}{S}}CH_3 \xrightarrow{P_2O_5} (CH_3)_2\overset{+}{S}-NHSO_2R \xrightarrow{-H^+} (CH_3)_2\overset{+}{S}-\overset{-}{N}SO_2R$$
(240)

The reaction of DMSO with phosphoric anhydride and mono-N-alkylsulfonamides in refluxing xylene takes a different course, yielding methylene bis-sulfonamides **241** (230,252). Formally, the latter reaction is similar to the formation of methylene bis-acetamide **(242)** when DMSO is refluxed for an extended period with acetamide (253).

$$RSO_2NHR' + CH_3\overset{O}{\overset{\|}{S}}CH_3 \xrightarrow[\text{xylene}]{P_2O_5} RSO_2\overset{R'}{\underset{}{N}}-\overset{+}{S}\diagdown^{CH_3}_{CH_3} \longrightarrow$$

$$RSO_2\overset{R'}{\underset{}{N}}CH_2SCH_3 \xrightarrow[-CH_3SH]{+H^+} RSO_2\overset{R'}{\underset{}{N}}-CH_2{}^- \xrightarrow{RSO_2NHR'} RSO_2\overset{R'}{\underset{}{N}}CH_2\overset{R'}{\underset{}{N}}SO_2R$$
(241)

$$CH_3\overset{O}{\overset{\|}{S}}CH_3 \xrightarrow{180°} [HCHO] \xrightarrow{CH_3\overset{O}{\overset{\|}{C}}NH_2} CH_3\overset{O}{\overset{\|}{C}}NHCH_2NH\overset{O}{\overset{\|}{C}}CH_3$$
(242)

Scheme 15

Formaldehyde, formed on decomposition of DMSO, was suggested (253) and proved as intermediate (252) in the latter reaction. However, since formaldehyde does not react with sulfonamides when heated in xylene (252), its intermediacy in the sulfonamide–DMSO reaction was ruled out and the alternate route shown in Scheme 15 was suggested.

C. REACTION WITH ELECTRON-DEFICIENT SPECIES

A number of interesting preliminary results have been reported regarding the reaction of carbenes and nitrenes with DMSO. These will be presented here without mechanistic speculations since such would be highly premature.

Oda and co-workers (197) have shown that carbenes are oxidized by DMSO to carbonyl compounds. Dichlorocarbene, generated in DMSO from ethyl trichloroacetate and sodium methoxide, was converted to phosgene (17%) which was identified as dimethylcarbonate; dimethyl sulfide was also produced and isolated as the mercuric chloride complex (20%). Alkaline cleavage to tosylhydrazones in DMSO at 100–160° was also investigated by these authors and found to give carbonyl compounds. The products based on tosylhydrazone were benzophenone (64%), acetophenone (46%), benzaldehyde (40%), and cyclohexanone (12%). In contrast to these results, Dieckmann (254) reported that photolysis of bis(phenylsulfonyl)diazomethane (243) in DMSO afforded the oxosulfonium ylid 244 (10%), presumably via a carbene intermediate.

$$RR'C=NNHSO_2C_6H_4pCH_3 \xrightarrow[DMSO]{NaOCH_3} RR'CO$$

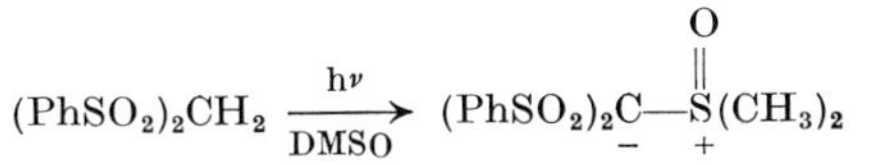

$$(PhSO_2)_2CH_2 \xrightarrow[DMSO]{h\nu} (PhSO_2)_2\overset{-}{C}\!-\!\overset{+}{\underset{\underset{\|}{O}}{S}}(CH_3)_2$$
$$\quad\quad(243) \quad\quad\quad\quad\quad\quad\quad (244)$$

Horner and Christmann (255) observed an analogous reaction for nitrenes. Photolysis of benzoyl azide or benzenesulfonyl azide in DMSO gave the sulfoximines 245 and 246, respectively, in approximately 30% yield. Very recently, Kwart and Kahn (256,257) reported that benzenesulfonyl azide reacted with DMSO in the absence

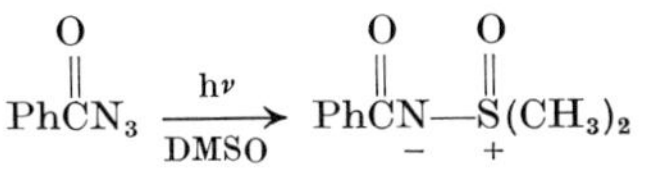

$$Ph\overset{\overset{O}{\|}}{C}N_3 \xrightarrow[DMSO]{h\nu} Ph\overset{\overset{O}{\|}}{C}\overset{-}{N}\!-\!\overset{+}{\underset{\underset{\|}{O}}{S}}(CH_3)_2$$
$$(245)$$

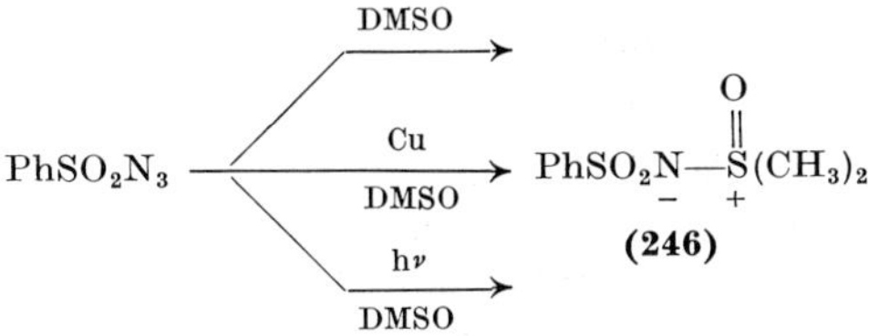

$$PhSO_2N_3 \begin{matrix} \xrightarrow{DMSO} \\ \xrightarrow[DMSO]{Cu} \\ \xrightarrow[DMSO]{h\nu} \end{matrix} PhSO_2\overset{-}{N}\!-\!\overset{+}{\underset{\underset{\|}{O}}{S}}(CH_3)_2$$
$$\quad\quad\quad\quad\quad\quad (246)$$

of irradiation also to give 246. The rate of formation of 246 was increased 25-fold on addition of copper to the reaction mixture.

Whether all of the sulfonyl azide reactions proceed through a common intermediate, possibly a nitrene or a heterocyclic species formed by a 1,3-dipolar addition of the azide to DMSO, has not been established.

D. REDUCTION WITH TRIPHENYLPHOSPHINE

Castrillón and Szmant (258) found that sulfoxides are reduced to sulfides upon heating with triphenylphosphine in carbon tetrachloride. Thus, dimethyl sulfoxide and triphenylphosphine gave dimethyl sulfide (82%) and triphenylphosphine oxide. The procedure is of synthetic interest since it allows the reduction of sulfoxides, generally in excellent yield, in the presence of other functional groups, such as nitro groups, which are sensitive to the more common reducing agents. The solvent, carbon tetrachloride, appears to be involved in the reaction since no reduction took place in benzene.

Reduction of sulfoxides by triphenylphosphine also takes place in the presence of acids (213,259). Kinetic studies indicated that the rate-determining step was nucleophilic attack by the phosphine on the protonated sulfoxide.

$$\underset{\text{RSR}}{\overset{\text{O}}{\|}} + \text{Ph}_3\text{P} \xrightarrow[\text{H}_2\text{O}]{\text{H}^+} \left[\underset{+\overset{|}{\text{PPh}_3}}{\overset{\overset{\text{OH}}{|}}{\text{RSR}}} \right] \rightarrow \text{RSR} + \text{Ph}_3\text{PO} + \text{H}_2\text{O}$$

VII. Experimental*

A. PREPARATION OF METHYLSULFINYL CARBANION (16)

A weighed amount of sodium hydride (50% mineral oil dispersion; Metal Hydrides, Inc.) is placed in a three-necked, round-bottomed flask and washed three times with light petroleum ether by swirling, allowing the hydride to settle, and decanting the liquid portion in order to remove the mineral oil. The flask is immediately fitted with a mechanical stirrer, a reflux condenser, and a rubber cap through which reagents can be introduced via hypodermic syringe (a pressure-compensated dropping funnel may also be used). A three-way stopcock, connected to the top of the reflux condenser, is connected to a water aspirator and a source of dry nitrogen. The system is

* Reprinted with permission of the authors and the American Chemical Society.

evacuated until the last traces of petroleum ether are removed from the sodium hydride and is then placed under nitrogen by evacuating and filling with nitrogen several times. The aspirator hose is removed and this arm of the stopcock is connected to a mercury-sealed U tube, to which the system is opened. Dimethyl sulfoxide (distilled from calcium hydride, bp 64° at 4 mm) is introduced via hypodermic syringe or dropping funnel and the mixture is heated with stirring to 70–75° until the evolution of hydrogen ceases. A mixture of 0.05 mole of sodium hydride and 20–30 ml of dimethyl sulfoxide requires about 45 min for complete reaction and yields a somewhat cloudy, pale yellow-gray solution of the sodium salt.

B. REACTION OF METHYLSULFINYL CARBANION WITH BENZOPHENONE (16)

A solution of sodium methylsulfinyl carbanion was prepared under nitrogen from 0.05 mole of sodium hydride and 20 ml of dimethyl sulfoxide. To this solution, with stirring at room temperature, was added 4.55 g (0.025 mole) of benzophenone in 10 ml of dimethyl sulfoxide over a 3-min period. The reaction mixture became warm and was then allowed to stir at room temperature for 2 hours. This was followed by the addition of 50 ml of cold water and extraction of the precipitated solid with chloroform. The combined extracts were washed three times with water, dried over anhydrous sodium sulfate, and evaporated to yield a white solid which was recrystallized from 45 ml of ethyl acetate to give 5.6 g (86.2%) of the hydroxy sulfoxide adduct as colorless prisms, mp 144–146°. Recrystallization twice again gave the analytical sample, mp 148–148.5°.

C. REACTION OF ESTERS WITH METHYLSULFINYL CARBANION. PREPARATION OF β-KETO SULFOXIDES. GENERAL PROCEDURE (16)

A 1.5–2M solution of methylsulfinyl carbanion in dimethyl sulfoxide is prepared under nitrogen in the usual manner from sodium hydride and dry dimethyl sulfoxide. An equal volume of dry tetrahydrofuran is added and the solution is cooled in an ice bath during the addition, with stirring, of the ester (0.5 equiv. based on 1 equiv. of carbanion; neat if liquid or dissolved in dry tetrahydrofuran if solid) over a period of several minutes. The ice bath is removed, stirring is continued for 30 min and the reaction mixture is then poured into three times its volume of water, acidified with aqueous hydrochloric acid to a pH of about 3–4 (pH paper), and thoroughly extracted with chloroform. The combined extracts are washed three times with water, dried over anhydrous sodium sulfate, and evaporated to yield the β-keto sulfoxide as a white or pale yellow crystalline solid. The crude product is triturated with cold ether or isopropyl ether and filtered to give the product in a good state of purity.

D. REDUCTION OF β-KETO SULFOXIDES. PREPARATION OF KETONES. GENERAL PROCEDURE. (16)

The compound to be reduced, dissolved in 10% aqueous tetrahydrofuran (60 ml/g of compound), is placed in a reaction vessel equipped with a stirrer. Aluminum amalgam (10 g-atoms of aluminum/mole of compound) is then freshly prepared as follows. Aluminum foil is cut into strips approximately 10 cm × 1 cm and immersed, all at once, into a 2% aqueous solution of mercuric chloride for 15 sec. The strips are rinsed with absolute alcohol and then with ether and cut immediately with scissors into pieces approximately 1 cm square which are dropped directly into the reaction vessel. For the reduction of the conjugated aromatic compounds, the reaction vessel should be cooled to 0° prior to the addition of the amalgam and stirring then continued for 10 min. at this temperature for completion of the reduction. Longer reaction times and/or higher temperatures lead to pinacol formation by further reduction of the ketone formed. With the nonconjugated compounds, the reaction mixture is heated at 65° for 60–90 min after addition of the amalgam. The reaction mixture is then filtered and the filtered solids are washed with tetrahydrofuran. The filtrate is concentrated to remove most of the tetrahydrofuran, ether is added, and the ether phase is separated from the water, dried over anhydrous sodium sulfate, and evaporated to leave the ketone, usually in a high state of purity.

E. DIMETHYLOXOSULFONIUM METHYLID. GENERAL METHOD OF PREPARATION IN DIMETHYL SULFOXIDE (17)

A weighed amount of sodium hydride (50% mineral oil dispension) was placed in a three-necked, round-bottomed flask and washed three times with light petroleum ether by swirling and decanting the liquid portion in order to remove the mineral oil. The flask was immediately fitted with a mechanical stirrer, a reflux condenser, and a rubber stopper through which reagents were introduced via hypodermic syringe (a pressure-compensated dropping funnel may also be used). A three-way stopcock, connected to the top of the reflux condenser, was connected to a water aspirator and a source of dry nitrogen. The system was evacuated until the last traces of petroleum ether were removed from the sodium hydride, the vacuum broken, and 1 equiv. of powdered trimethyloxosulfonium iodide or chloride introduced through one of the side arms of the flask. The system was placed under nitrogen by evacuating and filling with nitrogen several times. The aspirator hose was removed and this arm of the stopcock was connected to a mercury-sealed U tube to which the system was opened. Dimethyl sulfoxide [distilled from calcium hydride, bp 64° (4 mm)] was introduced slowly via hypodermic syringe or dropping funnel, the stirrer was started, and a vigorous evolution of hydrogen ensued, which ceased after 15–20 min to give a milky white reaction mixture.

F. REACTION OF DIMETHYLOXOSULFONIUM METHYLID WITH BENZOPHENONE (17)

A solution of the ylid was prepared under nitrogen from 0.03 mole of sodium hydride, 6.6 g (0.03 mole) of trimethyloxosulfonium iodide, and 30 ml of dimethyl sulfoxide. A solution of 4.55 g (0.025 mole) of benzophenone in 10 ml of dimethyl sulfoxide was added with stirring and the reaction mixture heated to 50° for 1 hr. After cooling and adding 60 ml of water, the mixture was extracted with ether, and the combined extracts were washed twice with water, dried over anhydrous sodium sulfate, and evaporated to yield 4.4 g (89.9%) of 1,1-diphenylethylene oxide as a white crystalline solid, mp 52–56°.

G. OXIDATION OF TESTOSTERONE WITH DMSO–DCC AND PHOSPHORIC ACID (156)

Testosterone (5.7 g, 20 mmoles) was dissolved in DMSO (20 ml) and benzene (10 ml) containing DCC (12.4 g, 60 mmoles). Anhydrous orthophosphoric acid (0.4 ml of a $5M$ solution in DMSO, 2 mmoles) was then added, and the mixture was kept at room temperature for 2 hr. Thin layer chromatography (chloroform–ethyl acetate, 4:1) then showed the presence of very little testosterone. Ethyl acetate (50 ml) was added followed by a solution of oxalic acid (5 g) in methanol. After 30 min, the dicyclohexylurea (12.7 g) was removed by filtration and washed with ethyl acetate. The solution was then extracted with aqueous sodium bicarbonate and water, dried over sodium sulfate, and evaporated to dryness leaving 5.7 g of an oil which rapidly crystallized. Crystallization from 20 ml of methanol gave androst-4-ene-3,17-dione (5.0 g, 87.5%), mp 169–170°.

H. OXIDATION OF YOHIMBINE TO YOHIMBINONE WITH DMSO–ACETIC ANHYDRIDE (169)

To a mixture of 886 g of yohimbine and 7.55 liters of dry dimethyl sulfoxide was added 5.05 liters of acetic anhydride. The mixture was stirred at room temperature for 18 hr. The mixture was diluted with 16.8 liters of ethanol, stirred for 1 hr, and diluted with 4.2 liters of water. Concentrated ammonium hydroxide (11 liters) was added while maintaining the temperature at 15–30° by cooling and the mixture was then diluted with 16.8 liters of water. Filtration gave a solid which was washed with water and dried to give 818 g (93%) of tan crystals, mp 248–250° decomp. This was slurried twice with 4 liters of ethanol and filtered to give 742 g (84%) of yohimbinone, mp 253–254° decomp.

I. PUMMERER REARRANGEMENT OF β-KETO SULFOXIDES

1. To Hemithioacetals (39)

A solution of 50 g of ω-(methylsulfinyl)-acetophenone in 100 ml of DMSO was diluted with 150 ml of water and acidified with 100 ml of concentrated hydrochloric acid. After standing at room temperature for 24 hr, the white precipitate was removed by filtration, pulverized, and dried for 24–36 hr at room temperature. Recrystallization of the product from Skelly B gave a 93–95% yield of the methyl hemimercaptal of phenylglyoxal as colorless needles, mp 106–107°.

For β-keto sulfoxides which were not appreciably soluble in aqueous DMSO, the rearrangement was effected by dissolving the β-keto sulfoxide in DMSO (about 5 ml DMSO per gram of sulfoxide), adding concentrated hydrochloric acid (2 ml per gram of sulfoxide), and allowing the solution to stand at room temperature for 12–24 hr. Water was then added until an oil began to precipitate. Cooling of the solution with stirring caused a solid to form. Further dilution with water to four or five times the original volume and cooling in an ice bath for 1 hr followed by filtration yielded the product as a pale yellow solid which was generally purified by crystallization from Skelly B or benzene.

2. To Acetals (41)

1,1-Dimethoxyundecan-2-one. 1-Methylsulfinylundecan-2-one (11.6 g, 0.05 mole) was dissolved in 100 ml of methanol containing 8.0 g (0.031 mole) of iodine. The solution was refluxed for 90 min and then allowed to cool. Most of the methanol was removed at room temperature on a rotary evaporator under aspirator vacuum. The dark residual oil was taken up in 50 ml of chloroform and extracted twice with 50-ml portions of saturated sodium thiosulfate solution. The very light yellow chloroform solution was dried with anhydrous magnesium sulfate and solvent removed under vacuum. The residual oil (11.8 g) was subjected to simple distillation through a Vigreux head giving 9.8 g (85% yield) of a colorless liquid boiling at 85° (0.2 mm). Gas chromatography on a 5-ft, ⅜in. Ucon Polar column showed >95% purity for the keto acetal.

ACKNOWLEDGMENT

The author would like to express his appreciation to Prof. R. R. Fraser for helpful comments and discussions.

REFERENCES

1. D. Martin, A. Weise, and H. J. Niclas, *Angew Chem.*, **79,** 340 (1967); *Angew. Chem. Intern. Ed. Engl.*, **6,** 318 (1967).
2. W. W. Epstein and F. W. Sweat, *Chem. Rev.*, **67,** 247 (1967).
3. N. Kharasch and B. S. Thyagarajan, *Quart. Rev. Sulfur Chem.*, **1,** 1 (1967).
4. J. C. Bloch, *Ann. Chim.*, **1965,** 419.
5. O. Ranky and D. C. Nelson, *Organic Sulfur Compounds*, Vol. I, N. Kharasch, Ed., Pergamon, London, 1961, pp. 170–182.
6. A. J. Parker, in *Advances in Organic Chemistry*, Vol. 5, R. A. Raphael, E. C. Taylor, and H. Wynberg, Eds., Interscience, New York, 1965; pp. 1–46.
7. C. Agami, *Bull. Soc. Chim. France*, **1965,** 1021.
8. Crown Zellerbach Corporation, Camas, Washington; Dimethylsulfoxide Technical Bulletin.
9. C. C. Price and S. Oae, *Sulfur Bonding*, Ronald Press, New York, 1962, pp. 129–148.
10. N. Kornblum, J. W. Powers, G. J. Anderson, W. J. Jones, H. O. Larson, O. Levand, and W. M. Weaver, *J. Am. Chem. Soc.*, **79,** 6562 (1957).
11. N. Kornblum, W. J. Jones, and G. J. Anderson, *J. Am. Chem. Soc.*, **81,** 4113 (1959).
12. K. E. Pfitzner and J. G. Moffatt, *J. Am. Chem. Soc.*, **87,** 5661 (1965).
13. C. R. Johnson and W. G. Phillips, *J. Org. Chem.*, **32,** 1926 (1967).
14. Torssell, K., *Acta Chem. Scand.*, **21,** 1 (1967).
15. E. J. Corey and M. Chaykovsky, *J. Am. Chem. Soc.*, **84,** 866 (1962).

16. E. J. Corey and M. Chaykovsky, *J. Am. Chem. Soc.*, **87,** 1345 (1965).
17. E. J. Corey and M. Chaykovsky, *J. Am. Chem. Soc.*, **87,** 1353 (1965).
18. E. J. Corey and M. Chaykovsky, *J. Am. Chem. Soc.*, **86,** 1639 (1964).
19. E. C. Steiner and J. M. Gilbert, *J. Am. Chem. Soc.*, **85,** 3054 (1963).
20. A. Ledwith and N. McFarlane, *Proc. Chem. Soc.*, **1964,** 108.
21. W. S. MacGregor, 153rd American Chemical Society Meeting, Miami Beach, Florida, April 12, 1967.
22. S. Sjöberg, *Tetrahedron Letters*, **1966,** 6383.
23. D. E. O'Connor and W. I. Lyness, *J. Org. Chem.*, **30,** 1620 (1965).
24. A. Ratajczak, F. A. L. Anet, and D. J. Cram, *J. Am. Chem. Soc.*, **89,** 2072 (1967).
25. E. Buncel, E. A. Symons, and A. W. Zabel, *Chem. Commun.*, **1965,** 173.
26. W. Frühstorfer and B. Hampel, German Pat., 1,171,422; *Chem. Abstr.*, **61** 6921e (1964).
27. J. I. Brauman and N. J. Nelson, *J. Am. Chem. Soc.*, **88,** 2332 (1966).
28. G. A. Russell, E. G. Janzen, H. D. Becker, and F. J. Smentowski, *J. Am. Chem. Soc.*, **84,** 2652 (1962).
29. G. A. Russell and H. D. Becker, *J. Am. Chem. Soc.*, **85,** 3406 (1963).
30. P. G. Gassman, J. L. Lumb, and F. V. Zalar, *J. Am. Chem. Soc.*, **89,** 946 (1967).
31. P. G. Gassman and F. V. Zalar, *Tetrahedron Letters*, **1964,** 3031, 3251.
32. E. J. Corey and M. Chaykovsky, *J. Org. Chem.*, **28,** 254 (1963).
33. C. Walling and L. Bollyky, *J. Org. Chem.*, **28,** 256 (1963).
34. E. J. Corey and T. Durst, *J. Am. Chem. Soc.*, **88,** 5656 (1966).
35. C. A. Kingsbury and D. J. Cram, *J. Am. Chem. Soc.*, **82,** 1810 (1960).
36. E. J. Corey and T. Durst, *J. Am. Chem. Soc.*, **90,** 5553 (1968).
37. G. A. Russell, E. Sabourin, and G. J. Mikol, *J. Org. Chem.*, **31,** 2854 (1966).
38. P. G. Gassman and G. D. Richmond, *J. Org. Chem.*, **31,** 2355 (1966).
39. G. A. Russell and G. J. Mikol, *J. Am. Chem. Soc.*, **88,** 5498 (1966).
40. H. D. Becker, G. J. Mikol, and G. A. Russell, *J. Am. Chem. Soc.*, **85,** 3410 (1963).
41. T. L. Moore, *J. Org. Chem.*, **32,** 2786 (1967).
42. V. N. Ipatieff, H. Pines, and B. S. Friedman, *J. Am. Chem. Soc.*, **60,** 2731 (1938).
43. J. B. Siddal, A. D. Cross, and J. H. Fried, *J. Am. Chem. Soc.*, **88,** 862 (1966).
44. H. D. Becker and G. A. Russell, *J. Org. Chem.*, **28,** 1896 (1963).
45. P. Veeravagu, R. T. Arnold, and E. W. Eigenmann, *J. Am. Chem. Soc.*, **86,** 3072 (1964), and references therein.
46. C. H. Snyder and A. R. Sato, *J. Org. Chem.*, **29,** 742 (1964).
47. C. H. Snyder, *Chem. and Ind. (London)*, **1963,** 121.
48. N. F. Wood and F. C. Chang, *J. Org. Chem.*, **30,** 2054 (1965).
49. C. H. Snyder and A. R. Sato, *J. Org. Chem.*, **30,** 673 (1965).
50. I. D. Entwistle and R. A. Johnstone, *Chem. Commun.*, **1965,** 29.
51. R. J. Shelton and K. E. Davis, *J. Am. Chem. Soc.*, **89,** 719 (1967).
52. F. C. Chang, *Tetrahedron Letters*, 305 (1964).
53. F. C. Chang and N. F. Wood, *Steroids*, **4,** 55 (1964).

54. D. H. Ball, E. D. M. Eades, and L. Long, Jr., *J. Am. Chem. Soc.*, **86,** 3579 (1964).
55. R. S. Tipson, *Advan. Carbohydrate Chem.*, **8,** 107 (1953).
56. G. Opitz, *Angew. Chem.*, **79,** 161 (1967); See *Angew. Chem. Intern. Ed. Engl.*, **6,** 107 (1967), for a review of sulfene chemistry.
57. E. J. Corey and T. Durst, *J. Am. Chem. Soc.*, **88,** 5656 (1966).
58. E. J. Corey and T. Durst, unpublished observations.
59. C. G. Cardenas, A. N. Khafaji, C. L. Osborn, and P. D. Gardner, *Chem. Ind. (London)*, **1965,** 345.
60. C. L. Osborn, T. C. Shields, B. A. Shoulders, C. G. Cardenas, and P. D. Gardner, *Chem. Ind. (London)*, **1965,** 766.
61. D. Seyferth, H. Yamazaki, and D. L. Alleston, *J. Org. Chem.*, **28,** 703 (1963).
62. L. Skattebøl, *Tetrahedron Letters*, **1961,** 167.
63. D. J. Cram and A. C. Day, *J. Org. Chem.*, **31,** 1227 (1966).
64. C. Walling and L. B. Bollyky, *J. Org. Chem.*, **29,** 2699 (1964).
65. J. E. Hofmann, T. J. Wallace, and A. Schriesheim, *J. Am. Chem. Soc.*, **86,** 1561 (1964).
66. J. E. Hofmann, T. J. Wallace, P. A. Argabright, and A. Schriesheim, *Chem. Ind. (London)*, **1963,** 1243.
67. C. L. Bumgardner, *J. Am. Chem. Soc.*, **83,** 4423 (1961).
68. R. Baker and M. J. Spillet, *Chem. Commun.*, **1966,** 757.
69. M. Feldman, S. Danishefsky, and R. Levine, *J. Org. Chem.*, **31,** 4322 (1966).
70. P. A. Argabright, J. E. Hofmann, and A. Schriesheim, *J. Org. Chem.*, **30,** 3233 (1965).
71. G. A. Russell and S. A. Weiner, *J. Org. Chem.*, **31,** 248 (1966).
72. H. Nozaki, Y. Yamamoto, and R. Nayori, *Tetrahedron Letters*, **1966,** 1123.
73. A. Streitweiser, Jr., *Molecular Orbital Theory for Organic Chemists*, Wiley, New York, 1962, pp. 307–356 and 392–412.
74. R. Greenwald, M. Chaykovsky, and E. J. Corey, *J. Org. Chem.*, **28,** 1128 (1963).
75. J. G. Atkinson, M. H. Fisher, D. Horley, A. T. Morse, R. S. Stuart, and S. Syness, *Can. J. Chem.*, **43,** 1614 (1965).
76. H. S. Corey, Jr., J. R. D. McCormick, and W. E. Swensen, *J. Am. Chem. Soc.*, **86,** 1884 (1964).
77. G. Drehfahl, K. Ponsold, and H. Schick, *Ber.*, **98,** 604 (1965).
78. E. J. Corey, R. B. Mitra, and H. Uda, *J. Am. Chem. Soc.*, **86,** 485 (1964).
79. E. J. Corey and S. Nozoe, *J. Am. Chem. Soc.*, **85,** 3527 (1963).
80. A. M. Krubiner and E. P. Oliveto, *J. Org. Chem.*, **31,** 24 (1966).
81. H. Oedinger, H. J. Kabbe, F. Möller, and K. Eiter, *Ber.*, **99,** 2012 (1966).
82. K. P. Klein and C. R. Hauser, *J. Org. Chem.*, **31,** 4276 (1966).
83. A. R. Lepley and R. H. Becker, *Tetrahedron*, **21,** 2365 (1965); *J. Org. Chem.*, **30,** 3888 (1965).
84. G. Wittig, R. Mangold, and G. Fellestchin, *Ann.*, **560,** 116 (1948).
85. T. J. Wallace, *J. Org. Chem.*, **30,** 4017 (1965).
86. G. A. Russell, E. G. Janzen, H. D. Becker, and F. S. Smentowski, *J. Am. Chem. Soc.*, **84,** 2652 (1962); G. A. Russell, E. G. Janzen, and E. J. Strom *J. Am. Chem. Soc.*, **84,** 4155 (1962).

87. G. A. Russell, P. R. Whittle, and J. McDonnell, *J. Am. Chem. Soc.*, **89**, 5515 (1967), and previous papers.
88. I. Iwai and J. Ide, *Chem. Pharm. Bull. (Tokyo)*, **13**, 663 (1965).
89. V. Franzen, *Special Publication, No. 19*, The Chemical Society, London, 1965, p. 172.
90. E. J. Corey and T. Durst, unpublished observations.
91. J. Jacobus and K. Mislow, *J. Am. Chem. Soc.*, **89**, 5228 (1967).
92. K. Mislow, *Record of Chemical Progress*, **28**, 217 (1967).
93. T. J. Wallace, H. Pobiner, J. E. Hofmann, and A. Schriesheim, *Proc. Chem. Soc. (London)*, **1963**, 137.
94. P. T. Lansbury, V. A. Pattison, J. D. Sidler, and J. B. Bieber, *J. Am. Chem. Soc.*, **88**, 78 (1966).
95. P. T. Lansbury and V. A. Pattison, *J. Am. Chem. Soc.*, **84**, 4295 (1962); *J. Org. Chem.*, **27**, 1933 (1962).
96. V. Schollköpf and W. Fabian, *Ann.*, **642**, 1 (1961).
97. R. Kuhn and H. Trischmann, *Ann*, **611**, 117 (1958).
98. R. T. Major and H. J. Hess, *J. Org. Chem.*, **23**, 1563 (1958).
99. S. G. Smith and S. Winstein, *Tetrahedron*, **3**, 317 (1958).
100. F. A. Cotton and R. Francis, *J. Am. Chem. Soc.*, **82**, 2986 (1960).
101. R. S. Drago and D. Meek, *J. Phys. Chem.*, **65**, 1446, (1961).
102. W. E. von Doering and A. H. Hoffmann, *J. Am. Chem. Soc.*, **77**, 521 (1955).
103. F. A. Cotton, J. H. Fassnacht, W. D. Horrocks, Jr., and N. A. Nelson, *J. Chem. Soc.*, **1959**, 4138.
104. E. J. Corey and M. Chaykovsky, *J. Am. Chem. Soc.*, **84**, 867 (1962).
105. G. Natus and E. J. Goethals, *Bull. Soc. Chim. Belg.*, **74**, 450 (1965).
106. H. König, H. Metzger, and K. Seelert, *Ber.*, **98**, 3712 (1965).
107. H. Metzger, H. König, and K. Seelert, *Tetrahedron Letters*, **1964**, 867.
108. H. König, H. Metzger, and K. Seelert, *Ber.* **98**, 3724 (1965).
109. T. J. Wallace, and J. J. Mahon, *Chem. Ind. (London)*, **1965**, 765.
110. A. B. Burg, in *Organic Sulfur Compounds*, Vol. 1., N. Kharasch, Ed., Pergamon Press, New York, 1961, pp. 30–40.
111. A. W. Johnson, *Ylid Chemistry*, Academic Press, New York and London, 1962, pp. 304–310.
112. E. S. Gould, *Mechanism and Structure in Organic Chemistry*, Holt, Rinehart, and Winston, New York, 1960, pp. 628–629.
113. A. W. Johnson and R. B. LaCount, *J. Am. Chem. Soc.*, **83**, 417 (1961).
114. B. Holt and P. A. Lowe, *Tetrahedron Letters*, **1966**, 683.
115. C. E. Cook, R. C. Corley, and M. E. Wall, *Tetrahedron Letters*, **1965**, 891.
116. R. D. King, W. G. Overend, J. Wells, and N. R. Williams, *Chem. Commun.*, **1967**, 726.
117. D. H. R. Barton, A. S. Campos-Neves, and R. C. Cookson, *J. Chem. Soc.*, **1956**, 3500.
118. A. W. Johnson, V. J. Hubry, and J. L. Williams, *J. Am. Chem. Soc.*, **86**, 918 (1964).
119. M. Hanack, *Conformation Theory*, Academic Press, New York and London, 1965, pp. 270–273.
120. R. K. Bly and R. S. Bly, *J. Org. Chem.*, **28**, 3165 (1963).

121. D. J. Cram and D. R. Wilson, *J. Am. Chem. Soc.*, **85**, 1245 (1963).
122. H. B. Henbest and J. McEntee, *J. Chem. Soc.*, **1961**, 4478.
123. E. J. Corey and M. Chaykovsky, *J. Am. Chem. Soc.*, **84**, 3782 (1962).
124. E. J. Corey and M. Chaykovsky, *Tetrahedron Letters*, **1963**, 169.
125. V. Franzen and H. E. Driessen, *Tetrahedron Letters*, **1962**, 661.
126. V. Franzen and H. E. Driessen, *Ber.*, **96**, 1881 (1963).
127. R. E. Ireland and L. N. Mander, *Tetrahedron Letters*, **1964**, 3453.
128. E. J. Corey and M. Chaykovsky, *J. Am. Chem. Soc.*, **86**, 1640 (1964).
129. H. Metzger and H. König, *Tetrahedron Letters*, **1964**, 3003.
130. H. Metzger and H. König, *Z. Naturforsch.*, **18b**, 987 (1963).
131. H. König and H. Metzger, *Ber.*, **98**, 3733 (1965).
132. A. M. van Leusen and E. C. Taylor, *J. Org. Chem.*, **33**, 66 (1968).
133. H. O. House, S. G. Boots, and V. K. Jones, *J. Org. Chem.*, **30**, 2519 (1965).
134. B. M. Trost, *J. Am. Chem. Soc.*, **89**, 138 (1967); **88**, 1587 (1966).
135. C. Kasier, B. M. Trost, J. Beeson, and J. Weinstock, *J. Org. Chem.*, **30**, 3972 (1965).
136. J. Nozaki, H. Ito, D. Tunemento, and K. Kondo, *Tetrahedron*, **22**, 441 (1966).
137. V. Prelog, *Helv. Chem. Acta*, **36**, 308 (1953).
138. J. Ide and Y. Kishida, *Tetrahedron Letters*, **1966**, 1787.
139. H. König, H. Metzger, and K. Seelert, *Ber.*, **98**, 3712 (1965).
140. H. Metzger and K. Seelert, *Angew. Chem.*, **75**, 919 (1963); *Angew. Chem. Intern. Ed. Engl.*, **2**, 624 (1963).
141. P. T. Izzo, *J. Org. Chem.*, **28**, 1713 (1963).
142. W. E. Truce and V. V. Badiger, *J. Org. Chem.*, **29**, 3277 (1964).
143. V. J. Traynelis and J. V. McSweeney, *J. Org. Chem.*, **31**, 243 (1966).
144. H. Metzger, H. König, and K. Seelert, *Tetrahedron Letters*, **1964**, 867.
145. B. M. Trost, *Tetrahedron Letters*, **1966**, 5761.
146. H. Metzger and K. Seelert, *Z. Naturforsch.*, **18b**, 336 (1963).
147. H. Metzger and K. Seelert, *Z. Naturforsch.*, **18b**, 335 (1963).
148. V. Franzen and H. E. Driessen, *Ber.*, **96**, 1881 (1963).
149. A. G. Hortman and D. A. Robertson, *J. Am. Chem. Soc.*, **89**, 5944 (1966).
150. H. König, H. Metzger, and K. Seelert, *Ber.*, **98**, 3724 (1965).
151. W. E. Truce and G. D. Madding, *Tetrahedron Letters*, **1966**, 3681.
152. C. M. Suter, *Organic Chemistry of Sulfur Compounds*, Wiley, New York, 1944, p. 504.
153. G. Gaudino, A. Umani-Ronchi, P. Brava, and M. Acampora, *Tetrahedron Letters*, **1967**, 107.
154. A. Umani-Ronchi, P. Brava, and G. Gaudino, *Tetrahedron Letters*, **1966**, 3477.
155. J. J. Turfariello and L. T. C. Lee, *J. Am. Chem. Soc.*, **88**, 4757 (1966).
156. K. E. Pfitzner and J. G. Moffatt, *J. Am. Chem. Soc.*, **87**, 5670 (1965).
157. P. Dowd and K. Sachdev, *J. Am. Chem. Soc.*, **89**, 715 (1967).
158. A. G. Brook and J. B. Pierce, *J. Org. Chem.*, **30**, 2566 (1965).
159. W. W. Epstein and F. W. Sweat, *Chem. Rev.*, **67**, 247 (1967).
160. C. R. Johnson and W. G. Phillips, *J. Org. Chem.*, **32**, 1926 (1967).
161. C. R. Johnson and W. G. Phillips, *Tetrahedron Letters*, **1965**, 2101.
162. K. Torssell, *Tetrahedron Letters*, **1966**, 4445.

163. K. Torssell, *Acta Chem. Scand.*, **21,** 1 (1967).
164. E. Brouse and M. D. LeFort, *Compt. Rend.*, **261,** 1990 (1965).
165. T. Cohen and T. Tsuji, *J. Org. Chem.*, **26,** 1681 (1961).
166. K. E. Pfitzner and J. G. Moffatt, *J. Am. Chem. Soc.*, **87,** 5661 (1965).
167. A. H. Fenselau and J. G. Moffatt, *J. Am. Chem. Soc.*, **88,** 1762 (1966).
168. J. D. Albright and L. Goldman, *J. Am. Chem. Soc.*, **87,** 4214 (1965).
169. J. D. Albright and L. Goldman, *J. Am. Chem. Soc.*, **89,** 2416 (1967).
170. N. J. Leonard and C. R. Johnson, *J. Am. Chem. Soc.*, **84,** 3701 (1962).
171. C. R. Johnson, *J. Am. Chem. Soc.*, **85,** 1020 (1963).
172. C. R. Johnson and D. McCants, Jr., *J. Am. Chem. Soc.*, **87,** 5404 (1965).
173. F. W. Sweat and W. W. Epstein, *J. Org. Chem.*, **32,** 835 (1967).
174. J. D. Albright and L. Goldman, *J. Org. Chem.* **30,** 1107 (1965).
175. K. Onodera, S. Hirano, and N. Kashimura, *J. Am. Chem. Soc.*, **87,** 4651 (1965).
176. J. Onodera, S. Hirano, N. Kashimura, F. Masuda, T. Yajima, and N. Miyazaki, *J. Org. Chem.*, **31,** 1291 (1966).
177. H. Sowa and G. H. S. Thomas, *Can. J. Chem.*, **44,** 836 (1966).
178. M. F. Lappert and J. K. Smith, *J. Chem. Soc.*, **1961,** 3224.
179. R. J. Parikh and W. E. von Doering, *J. Am. Chem. Soc.*, **89,** 5506 (1967).
180. D. H. R. Barton, and B. J. Gardner, and R. H. Wightman, *J. Chem. Soc.*, **1964,** 1855.
181. I. M. Hunsberger and J. M. Tien, *Chem. Ind. (London)*, **1959,** 88.
182. R. T. Major and H. J. Hess, *J. Org. Chem.*, **23,** 1563 (1958).
183. H. R. Nace and J. J. Mongale, *J. Org. Chem.*, **24,** 1792 (1959).
184. A. P. Johnson and A. J. Pelter, *J. Chem. Soc.*, **1964,** 520.
185. F. X. Jarreau, M. B. Tchoubar, and R. Goutarel, *Bull. Soc. Chim. France,* **1962,** 887.
186. D. N. Jones and M. A. Saeed, *J. Chem. Soc.*, **1963,** 4657.
187. R. N. Iacona, A. T. Rowland, and H. R. Nace, *J. Org. Chem.*, **29,** 3495 (1964).
188. H. R. Nace and R. N. Iacona, *J. Org. Chem.*, **29,** 3498 (1964).
189. H. R. Nace, *J. Am. Chem. Soc.*, **81** 5428 (1959).
190. J. B. Jones and D. C. Wigfield, *Can. J. Chem.*, **44,** 2517 (1966).
191. T. J. Wallace and J. J. Mahon, *J. Org. Chem.* **30,** 1502 (1965).
192. T. J. Wallace and J. J. Mahon, *J. Am. Chem. Soc.*, **86,** 4099 (1964).
193. T. J. Wallace, *J. Am. Chem. Soc.*, **86,** 2018 (1964).
194. C. N. Yiannos and V. J. Karabinos, *J. Org. Chem.*, **29,** 3246 (1963).
195. H. Searles and H. R. Hays, *J. Org. Chem.*, **23,** 2028 (1958).
196. K. H. Scheit and W. Kampe, *Angew. Chem.*, **77,** 811 (1965); *Angew Chem. Intern. Ed. Engl.*, **4,** 787 (1965).
197. R. Oda, M. Mieno, and Y. Hayashi, *Tetrahedron Letters,* **1967,** 2363.
198. E. Brousse and M. D. Lefort, *Compt. Rend.*, **261,** 1990 (1965).
199. T. Cohen and T. Tsuji, *J. Org. Chem.*, **26,** 1681 (1961).
200. T. Tsuji, *Tetrahedron Letters,* **1966,** 2413.
201. I. Lilien, *J. Org. Chem.*, **29,** 1631 (1964).
202. D. Landini and F. Montanian, *Tetrahedron Letters,* **1964,** 2691.
203. T. L. Fletcher and H. L. Pan, *J. Org. Chem.*, **24,** 141 (1959).

204. K. Sato, S. Suzuki, and Y. Kojima, *J. Org. Chem.* **32**, 399 (1967).
205. H. W. Heine and T. Newton, *Tetrahedron Letters*, **1967**, 1859.
206. D. R. Dalton and D. G. Jones, *Tetrahedron Letters*, **1967**, 2875.
207. D. R. Dalton, J. B. Hendrickson, and D. G. Jones, *Chem. Commun.*, **1966**, 591.
208. J. A. Smythe, *J. Chem. Soc.*, **95**, 349 (1909).
209. R. Pummerer, *Ber.*, **43**, 1401 (1910).
210. W. J. McKenny, J. A. Walsh, and D. A. Davenport, *J. Am. Chem. Soc.*, **83**, 4019 (1961).
211. F. G. Bordwell and B. M. Pitt, *J. Am. Chem., Soc.*, **77**, 572 (1955).
212. E. H. Amonoo-Neizer, S. K. Ray, R. A. Shaw, and B. C. Smith, *J. Chem. Soc.*, **1965**, 6250.
213. S. K. Ray, R. A. Shaw, and B. C. Smith, *Nature*, **196**, 372 (1962).
214. C. R. Johnson, J. C. Sharp, and W. G. Phillips, *Tetrahedron Letters*, **1967**, 5299.
215. W. E. Parham and M. D. Bhasvar, *J. Org. Chem.*, **28**, 2686 (1963).
216. L. P. Horner and P. Kaiser, *Ann.*, **626**, 19 (1959).
217. W. E. Parham and R. Koncos, *J. Am. Chem., Soc.*, **83**, 4034 (1961).
218. S. Oae and M. Kise, *Tetrahedron Letters*, **1967**, 1409.
219. S. Oae, T. Kitao, and S. Kawamura, *Tetrahedron*, **19**, 1783 (1963).
220. S. Oae, T. Kitao, S. Kawamura, and Y. Kitaoka, *Tetrahedron*, **19**, 817 (1963).
221. W. R. Sorenson, *J. Org. Chem.*, **24**, 978 (1959).
222. A. Senning, *Chem. Commun.*, **1967**, 64.
223. R. E. Boyle, *J. Org. Chem.*, **31**, 3880 (1966).
224. N. J. Leonard and C. R. Johnson, *J. Am. Chem. Soc.*, **84**, 3701 (1962).
225. F. W. Lappert and J. K. Smith, *J. Chem. Soc.*, **1965**, 7102.
226. R. Rätz and O. J. Sweeting, *Tetrahedron Letters*, **1963**, 529.
227. H. Meerwein, K. E. Zenner, and R. Gipps, *Ann.*, **688**, 67 (1965).
228. H. Potter, 137th Meeting, American Chemical Society, Cleveland, Ohio, April 30, 1960, p. 30.
229. R. Oda and Y. Yammamota, *J. Org. Chem.*, **26**, 4679 (1961).
230. A. Sekera, J. E. Fauvet, and P. Rumpf, *Ann. Chim.*, **1965**, 413.
231. V. Grignard, *Traite de Chimie Organique*, **1937**, 364.
232. K. W. Ratts and A. N. Yao, *J. Org. Chem.*, **33**, 70 (1968).
233. K. W. Ratts and A. N. Yao, *J. Org. Chem.*, **31**, 1869 (1966); **31**, 1185 (1966).
234. M. G. Burdon and J. G. Moffatt, *J. Am. Chem. Soc.*, **87**, 4656 (1965).
235. K. E. Pfitzner, J. P. Marino, and R. A. Olofson, *J. Am. Chem. Soc.*, **87**, 4658 (1965).
236. M. G. Burdon and J. G. Moffatt, *J. Am. Chem. Soc.*, **88**, 5855 (1966).
237. M. G. Burdon and J. G. Moffatt, *J. Am. Chem. Soc.*, **89**, 4725 (1967).
238. Y. Hayashi and R. Oda, *J. Org. Chem.*, **32**, 457 (1967).
239. C. R. Hauser, S. W. Kantor, and W. R. Brasen, *J. Am. Chem. Soc.*, **75**, 2660 (1953).
240. E. Goethals and P. de Radzitzky, *Bull. Soc. Chim. Belg.*, **73**, 546 (1964).
241. W. J. Middleton, E. L. Buhle, J. G. McNally, Jr., and M. Zanger, *J. Org. Chem.*, **30**, 2384 (1965).
242. E. Goethals and P. Radzitzky, *Bull. Soc. Chim. Belg.*, **73**, 579 (1964).

243. A. F. Cook and J. G. Moffatt, *J. Am. Chem. Soc.*, **90,** 740 (1968).
244. A. Hochreiner and F. Wessely, *Monatsh. Chem.*, **97,** 1 (1966).
245. A. Hochreiner, *Monatsh. Chem.*, **97,** 823 (1966).
246. A. Hochreiner and F. Wessely, *Tetrahedron Letters,* **1965,** 721.
247. R. Gompper and H. Euchner, *Ber.*, **99,** 527 (1966).
248. H. Nozaki, Z. Morita and K. Kondo, *Tetrahedron Letters,* **1966,** 2913.
249. A. Hochreiner and W. Silhan, *Monatsh. Chem.*, **97,** 1477 (1966).
250. R. K. Ratts, *Tetrahedron Letters,* **1966,** 4707.
251. D. S. Tarbell and C. Weaver., *J. Am. Chem. Soc.*, **63,** 2939 (1941).
252. A. Sekera and P. Rumpf, *Compt. Rend.*, **260,** 2252 (1965).
253. V. J. Traynelis and W. L. Hergenrother, *J. Org. Chem.*, **29,** 221 (1964).
254. J. Diekmann, *J. Org. Chem.*, **30,** 2272 (1965).
255. L. Horner and A. Christmann, *Ber*, **96,** 388 (1963).
256. H. Kwart and A. A. Kahn, *J. Am. Chem. Soc.*, **89,** 1950 (1967).
257. H. Kwart and A. A. Kahn, *J. Am. Chem. Soc.*, **89,** 1951 (1967).
258. S. P. Castrillón and H. H. Szmant, *J. Org. Chem.*, **30,** 1338 (1965).
259. H. H. Szmant and O. Cox., *J. Org. Chem.*, **31,** 1595 (1966).

AUTHOR INDEX

Numbers in parentheses are reference numbers and indicate that the author's work is referred to although his name is not mentioned in the text. Numbers in *italics* show the pages on which the complete references are listed.

A

Abegg, V. D., *251*
Abel, E. W., 115(36), *236*
Acampora, M., 343(153), *385*
Acton, N., *255*
Adam, W., 20, *98*
Adams, D. M., 153(117), *239*
Agahigian, H., 70(279), *104*
Agami, C., 286(7), *381*
Agnes, G., 164, *240*
Agranat, I., 55(242,244), 56(242), 81(308), *103*, *105*
Aguilo, A., *249*
Akhmedov, I. M., 209(263), *244*
Akiyama, S., 41(196), *101*
Albright, J. D., 349, 351(169), 352(169), 380(169), *386*
Alden, R., 80(303), *105*
Alderson, T., 213, 214(288), 235(288), *245*
Ali, M. A., 64(267), 70(267), *104*
Allegra, G., *253*
Allen, A. D., 116(40), *236*, *248*
Allen, M. J., 278, *283*
Allendoerfer, R. D., 30(142), *99*
Alleston, D. L., 307(61), *383*
Altman, L. J., 4(22), 5(33), 6(33,35), 81(33), *95*, *96*
American Petroleum Institute, 5(26), *95*
Amiel, Y., 38(178), 43(203), 50(221, 222), 53(222), 54(222), *101*, *102*
Amonoo-Neizer, E. H., 357(212), *387*
Anastassiou, A. G., 93(366), *108*
Anderson, C. B., 139(88), *238*, *255*
Anderson, G. J., 286(10), 287(11), 352(10,11), *381*
Anderson, J. D., 264(39–41), 269(39–41), 278(39,60), 279(39), 280(40), *282*
Anderson, T., 119, 154(118), *237*, *239*
Andreas, S., 5(33), 6(33), 8(33b), 81(33), *96*, 264(42), 269(42), *264*
Anet, F. A. L., 289(24), 290(24), *382*
Arai, S., 28(129), *99*
Argabright, P. A., 310(66), 311–313(70), 318(66), *383*
Armit, J. W., 1, 62, *94*
Armstrong, R. K., 230(336), *246*
Arnold, R. T., 301(45), *382*
Asahi Kasei Co., *249*
Asamiya, K., 168(164), *241*
Asano, T., 74(289), *105*
Ashida, T., 84(321), *106*
Atherton, N. M., 88(342), *107*
Atkinson, J. G., 314(75), *383*
vanAuken, T. V., 220(310), *246*
Avram, M., 15(74), 16(75,77), 58(250), 59(250,253), 60(253), 86(332), *97*, *103*, *104*, *106*
Azatyan, V. D., 30(149), *100*

B

Babaeva, R. B., *253*
Backes, L., 92(362), *107*
Badger, G. M., 50, 51(227,228,230), *102*, *103*
Badiger, V. V., 338(142), *385*
Badische Anilin Soda Fabrik A.G., 154(121–123), *239*

Baer, F., 89(351), *107*
Baezner, C., 264(34), *282*
Bahary, W., 4(21), *95*
Baikie, P. E., 87(339), *107*
Bailar, J. C., *252*
Bailey, A. S., 87(340), *107*
Bailey, D. L., 209(254), *243*
Bailey, N. A., 42(199–201), 44(199), *101*, 153(116), *239*
Bailor, J. C., Jr., 202(224), *242*
Baird, M. C., 116(43), *236, 247, 251*
Baird, W. C., 139, 233(90), *238, 249*
Baizer, M. M., 264(39–41), 269(39–41), 278(39,60), 279(39,63), 280(40), *282, 283*
Baker, R., *105*, 310, *383*
Baker, W., 2(10), *95*
Ball, D. H., 303(54), 304(54), *383*
Bangert, K. F., 91(357), *107*
Bank, H. M., 208, *243*
Banks, D., 61, *104*
Barnes, G. H., 206(235), *243*
Barth, W. E., 92(361,362), *107*
Barton, D. H. R., 327(117), 351, *384, 386*
Basolo, F., 161(142), *240*
Bastiansen, O., 30(138), *99*
Bath, S. S., 116(45), 195, *237*
Battiste, M., 8(40), 12(60), *96*
Bauld, N. L., 29(136), 61, 93(364), *99, 104, 107*, 259(10), 261(10), *281*
Bayer, O., 164(156), *240*
Bazant, V., 207(238), *243*
Bechter, M., 114(27), 130(27,70), *236, 237*
Becker, A., 230(341), *247*
Becker, H. D., 291(28,29), 292, 301, 315(86), 316(86), 356(40), *382, 383*
Becker, R. H., 315(83), *383*
Beeson, J., 333(135), 335(135), 338(135), *385*
Behr, O. M., 40(192a,192b), *101*
Belinskii, L. I., 258(2), *281*
Belov, A. D., 135(84,85), *238*
Belov, A. P., *249*
Belyakova, Z. V., 210(273), *244*

Ben, V. R., 92(358),*107*
Ben-Efraim, D. A., 43(203), 50(225), 52(231), *102, 103*
Benitez, A., 209(253), *243*
Benkeser, R. A., 209, 210(265,266), *244, 253*, 276, *282*
Bennett, M. A., 189(197), *242*
Bennett, R. F., *250*
Benson, R. E., 31–33(156), *100*, 187(191), 198(213), *241, 242*
Bergmann, E. D., 25, 47(218), 55(242, 244), 56(242), 63(262), 81(308), *98, 102–105, 248, 251*
Berkowitz, L. M., 230(333), *246*
Berlin, A. J., *254*
Bertelli, D. J., 26, 77, *98, 105*
Berthier, G., 24(106), 54(236), 62(236), 71(236), 77(236), *98, 103*
Beynon, P. J., *255*
Bhasvar, M. D., 357(215), *387*
Bibler, J. P., 194(206,207), *242*
Bieber, J. B., 318(94), *384*
Biellmann, J. F., *252*
Binnig, F., 76(294), 94(370), *105, 108*
Birch, A. J., 205, *243, 252*
Bird, C. W., 150(109), *239*
Birnbaum, K., 113, *235*
Biskup, M., 45(212), *102*
Blank, B., 230(334), *246*
Blattman, H. R., 45(210), 88(346), *102, 107*
Bloch, J. C., 286(4), 321, *381*
Blomquist, A. T., 11, 15(70), 16,17(81), 90, *96, 97, 107*, 219(298), 220, *245*
Bloomfield, J. J., 37, *101*
Blum, J., 193, 195(205), 234(205), *242, 248, 251*
Bly, R. K., 325(120), 329(120), *384*
Bly, R. S., 325(120), 329(120), *384*
Boche, G., 84(323,324), *106*
Bock, H., *253*
Boecke, R., *255*
Boehm, T., 164(157), *240*
Boekelheide, V., 44, 45(210,211), 70, 87(340), 88(342–346), *102, 104, 107*

AUTHOR INDEX 391

Böll, W. A., 35(164), 36(166,169,171–173), *100*
Boer, D. H. W. den, 54(237,238), 63(237,238), 77(237,238), *103*
Boer, P. C. den, 54(237,238), 63(237,238), 77(237,238), *103*
Boer-Veenendaal, P. C. den, 54(238), 77(238), *103*
Bohrer, J. C., 220, *245*
Bollyky, L. B., 293(33), 309(64), *382, 383*
Bonati, F., *247*
Bonner, W. A., 259, 279(12), *281*
Booth, B. L., *247*
Boots, S. G., 333(133), *385*
Bordence, C., *250*
Bordwell, F. G., 357(211), 360(211), 361(211), *387*
Borisov, S. N., *253*
Bothner-By, A. A., 43(203), *102*
Bott, R. W., 208(250), *243*
Bottomley, F., *248*
Boyd, G. V., 90, *107*
Boyle, R. E., 357(223), *387*
Bräunling, H., 94(370), 108
Brasen, W. R., 367(239), *387*
Brastow, W. C., 119(50), *237*
Brauman, J. I., 26(118), 55(240), *99, 103*, 290(27), *382*
Brava, P., 343(153,154), *385*
Braye, E. H., 14, *97*
Bredt, J., 264, *281*
Bregman, J., 44(205), 50(223), *102*
Bremser, W., 87(337), *106*
Breslow, R., 2, 3(15,16,18,19), 4(21,22), 5, 6(33,35), 12(60), 19, 21(94,95), 22(96), 29, 70, 77(297), 79(297), 80(305,306), 81(33), *94–96, 98, 99, 104, 105*
Brewis, S., 155(125,127), 156(125), 175, *239, 241*
Bright, G. M., 92(359), *107*
Britelli, D. R., 92(360), *107*
Brook, A. G., 344(158), *385*
Brookhart, M., 84(322), *106*
Brouse, E., 345(164), 353(198), *386*

Brown, E. A., 263, *281*
Brown, J. M., 83, *106*
Brown, J. W., *251*
Brown, M., *252*
Brown, M. S., 29(136), *99*
Brown, R. D., 54(236), 62(236), 71(236), 77(236), *103*
Bruckner, G., 213(283), *245*
Brunner, H., 41(195), *101*
Bryan, R. F., 10(46), *96*
Bryant, D. R., 134, 135(82), 136, *238*
Bryce-Smith, D., 26, *98*, 177(171), 178, 218(171), *241*
Buhle, E. L., 370(241), 372(241), *387*
Bumgardner, C. L., 310(67), *383*
Buncel, E., 290(25), *382*
Bunyan, P. J., 262, *281*
Burdon, M. G., 365, 367(237), 368(237), *387*
Burg, A. B., 321(110), *384*
Burger, G., 168, *241*
Burkoth, T. L., 84(329), *106*
Burr, M., 3(17), *95*
Burreson, B. J., *255*
Burrous, M. L., 210(266), *244*
Burt, G. D., 18(86), *97*
Burwell, R. L., 201, *242*

C

Cahn, R. S., 223(316), *246*
Calder, I. C., 38(183), 39(187), 40(183,187), 44(183), 45(214), 47(183,214), 50(224), 52(183), 53(183), 54(234), 87(341), 89(349), *101–103, 107*
Calundann, G. W., 230(337), 231, *246*
Calvin, G., 161(143), *240*
Cambell, I. D., 41(194), 47(194), *101*
Campos-Neves, A. S., 327(117), *384*
Canale, A. J., 213(282,286), *245*
Cantrell, T. S., 31(153,154), *100*
Capri, E., 190(199), *242*
Caputo, J. A., *255*
Cardenas, C. G., 305, 307(60), *383*

Caress, E. A., 226, *246*
Carnaban, J. C., *255*
Carrington, A., 30(144,147), 84(326), *99, 106*
Carty, D., *247*
Carwood, R. F., 262, *281*
Casanova, J., 230(339), *247*, 259(10), 261(10), *281*
Caserio, M. C., 11(50), 17(83), *96, 97*
Cassidy, J. P., 269(49), *282*
Castrillón, S. P., 376, *388*
Catone, D. L., 116(41a), *236*
Cava, M. P., 58(251), 59–61, 80 (300), 89(300), *103–105*
Ceasar, G. P., 83(314), *106*
Cenini, S., *247*
Chalk, A. J., 134, 212, *238, 245*
Chalvet, O., 72(282), 77(282,) *105*
Chang, F. C., 301(48), 302(48), 303, *382*
Chang, H. W., 3(15,16,18,19), 4(22), 21(94,95), 22(96), 29, *95, 98, 99*
Charman, H. B., *252*
Charman, H. F., *249*
Chatt, J., 113, 115(35,38), 149, 153 (117), 192(202), 197, 198, *235, 236, 239, 242*
Chaykovsky, M., 288, 289(15,16), 290 (16), 291, 292(15,16), 293(32), 295, 296(16,18), 297(16,18), 298(16), 307(15,16), 314(74), 319, 320(17, 104), 322(16), 323–326(17), 329(17), 330(17,123,124), 331(128), 333, 334 (128), 335(16), 338, 340, 341(17, 104), 376(16), 377(16), 378(16,17), 379(17), *381–385*
Chemical Society Special Publication, 80(299), *105*
Cherkasova, E. M., 277, *282*
Chernyshev, E. A., 208(247,249), *243*
Chernysheva, T. I., *253*
Chesnut, D. B., 32(157), *100*
Chevallier, Y., *252*
Chickos, J., 7(39), *96*
Chin, C. G., 85(330a), *106*
Chiusoli, G. P., 164, *240*

Christ, H., 114(26,28,29,31), 128(28), 130(28), *236*
Christmann, A., 375, *388*
Chvalovsky, V., 207(238), *243*
Ciabattoni, J., 82(311), *106*
Ciampelli, E., 213(283), *245*
Citron, J. D., *253*
Clar, E., 75, *105*
Clark, D., 132(75), *238*
Clauss, K., 40(191), *101*
Clement, W. H., 121, 132, 233(57), *237, 238*
Closs, G. L., 83(317), *95, 106*
Closson, R. D., 161(141), *240*
Coates, G. E., 112(5), 114(32), 161 (143), *235, 236, 240*
Coffey, R. S., *252*
Coffield, T. H., 161(141), *240*
Cohen, L. A., 260(13), *281*
Cohen, S., 12(54,56), *96*
Cohen, S. G., 12(56), *96*
Cohen, T., 345(165), 353(199), 354 (199), *386*
Collins, D. M., *255*
Collman, J. P., 112(7), 116(39,46), 165 (158), 194(46), *235–237, 240, 247, 248, 250*
Colombo, A., *253*
Conia, J. M., 162(151), *240*
Conti, F., 113(15), 171(165), *235, 241, 247, 248*
Cook, A. F., 370–372(243), *388*
Cook, C. D., *248*
Cook, C. E., 323(115), 327, *384*
Cook, N. C., 211, 212(280), *244*
Cookson, R. C., 86(333), *106*, 219 (304), *245*, 327(117), *384*
Cope, A. C., 183(179), 220, 221(311), 226, *241, 245, 246, 248, 254*
Corey, E. J., 5(27), 17, *95*, 146(99), 230(339), *239, 247*, 259(10), 261, *281*, 288, 289(15,16), 290(16), 291, 292(15,16), 293, 294(34,36), 295, 296 (16,18), 297(16,18), 298(16), 305 (57,58), 307(15,16), 314, 317(57, 90), 319, 320(17,104), 322(16), 323–

326(17), 329(17), 330(17,123,124), 331(128), 333, 334(128), 335(16), 338, 340, 341(17,104), 376(16), 377 (16), 378(16,17), 379(17), *381–385*
Corey, H. S., Jr., 314(76), *383*
Corley, R. C., 323(115), 327(115), *384*
Corradini, P., 223(317), 224(319), 225(320), *246*
Cossee, P., 115(34), *236*
Cotton, F. A., 318(100), 319(103), 348(100), *384*
Coulson, C. A., 13(61), 51(229), 54 (237), 63(237), 64(267), 70(267), 77 (237), *97*, *102–104*
Covitz, F. H., 264(38), 268(38), 269, *282*
Cox, O., 376(259), *388*
Craig, D. P., 54, 63(235), 77(235), *103*
Cram, D. J., 289(24), 290(24), 293 (35), 294(35), 308, 329(121), *382*, *383*, *385*
Cramer, R., 134(80), 216(290), *238*, *245*, *254*
Cramer, R. D., 187(189), 202, *241*
Criegee, R., 14, *97*
Cross, A. D., 300(43), *382*
Crown Zellerbach Corp., 286(8), *381*
Cruse, R., 72(288), 74(288), *105*
Cunico, R. F., 209, *244*, *253*

D

Dailey, B. P., 83(314), *106*
Dall'asta, G., 213(287), 217, *245*
Dalton, D. R., 354, *387*
Danielisz, M., 26(114), *98*
Danishefsky, S., 311(69), 312(69), *383*
Dauben, H. J., 28(125,126,132), 29, 77, 92(358), *99*, *105*, *107*
Dauby, R., 213(284), *245*
Daudel, R., 72(282), 77(282), *105*
Davenport, D. A., 356(210), *387*
Davidson, J. M., 146, *239*, *249*
Davidson, N., 72(281), *104*
Davis, J. E., 230(343), *247*

Davis, K. E., 302(51), *382*
Davison, A., 27(120), *99*
Dawallu, A., 199(217), *242*
Day, A. C., 308, *383*
Dean, F. M., 230(338), *246*
Dehmlow, E. V., 6, 20(89), *96*, *98*
Dehn, J. S., 261, *281*
Denham, J. M., 8(41), *96*
Dent, W. T., 114(18), 166(160), 233 (18), *236*, *240*
De Renzi, A., 222, 226(312), *246*, *249*
Dessy, R. E., 264(35), 266, 267(35), *282*
Dettmeier, U., 33(159), *100*
Dewar, M. J. S., 2, 13(62), 38, 51, 78 (180), 80, 89(300), *94*, *97*, *101*, *105*
Dewhirst, K. C., *253*
Diekmann, J., 375, *388*
Dietl, H., 114(30,31), *236*, *247*
DiLuzio, J. W., 161(140), *240*
Di Maio, G., 38(183), 40(183), 44 (183), 47(183), 52(183), 53(183), *101*
Dinu, D., 58(250), 59(250), *103*
Dinulescu, I., 16(77), 58(250), 59(250, 253), 60(253), *97*, *103*, *104*
Distillers Company Ltd., 143(95), *238*
Dixon, J. A., 230(346), *247*
Djerassi, C., 205, 230, *243*, *246*, *252*
Dobler, M., 35(167), *100*
Dodge, R. P., 14(67), *97*
Dodson, P. A., 260(14), *281*
Doering, W. v. E., 2, 24, 25(110), 29, 54(104), 71, 78, *94*, *98*, *99*, 319 (102), 350, *384*, *386*
Doganges, P. T., *255*
Dolejs, L., 275(53), *282*
Dolf Bass, J., 34(162), *100*
Dolgaya, M. E., 208(247, 249), *243*
Donati, M., 113(15), 171(165), *235*, *241*, *247*, *248*
Doran, M. A., 61(258), *104*
Douglas, B. E., 47(219), *102*
Dovoretzky, I., 116(47), *237*
Dowd, P., 4(22), *95*, 344(157), *385*
Doyle, J. R., 222(313), *246*
Drago, R. S., 318(101), 348(101), *384*

Drehfal, G., 314(77), *383*
Dreyer, D. L., 26, *98*
Driessen, H. E., 324(126), 330(125, 126), 338(126), 341(148), *385*
Drydon, H. L., Jr., 272(51), *282*
Drysdale, J. J., 25(111), *98*
Dunathan, H. C., 17, *97*
Duncanson, L. A., 113, *235*
Dunitz, J. D., 14(68), 35(167), *97*, *100*
Dunny, S., *253*
Du Pont de Nemours, E. I., & Co., 199(215), *242*, *249*
Durst, T., 293, 294(34,36), 305 (57, 58), 317(57,90), *382–384*
Duty, R., 276, *282*
Dvorakian, G. A., 20(92), *98*

E

Eaborn, C., 207(237), 208(250), *243*
Eades, E. D. M., 303(54), 304(54), *383*
Eberhardt, G. C., *252*
Eberson, L., 84(325), *106*
Efraty, A., 83(315), *106*, 219(307), *245*
Eglinton, G., 38, 40, 41(194), 47(194), *101*
Egorov, Yu. P., 208(249), *243*
Eicher, T., 5(32), 81(310), *95*, *105*
Eigenmann, E. W., 301(45), *382*
Eimer, J., 37(175), *101*
Eischens, R. P., 202(227), *243*
Eiter, K., 314(81), *383*
Elbs, K., 265, *282*
Elian, M., 16(77), *97*
Elix, J. A., 38(183), 40(183), 44(183), 47(183), 50(226–228), 51(227,228), 52(183), 53(183), 62(260), 76(293), 94(375), *101*, *102*, *104*, *105*, *108*
Ellis, A. F., *250*
Ellis, L. E., 55(240), *103*
Emerson, G. F., 16(76,78), 59(76), *97*
Emken, E. A., *252*
Engelhardt, V. A., 154(118), *239*
Engle, R. R., 230, *246*

Englert, G., 93(367), *108*
Ennis, C. L., 94(374), *108*
Entwistle, I. D., 302, *382*
Epstein, W. W., 286(2), 344, 347(173), 348, 352(173), 361, *381*, *385*, *386*
Errede, L. A., 269(46,48,49), *282*
Eschinazi, H. E., 162(147–149), *240*
Euchner, H., 370(247), 372(247), *388*
Evans, D., 198(212), 201(212), *242*, *251*
Evans, M. V., 12(55), *96*

F

Fabian, W., 19(88), *98*, 318(96), *384*
Faget, C., 162(151), *240*
Faisst, W., 93(367), *108*
Falmar, W., 55(247), 57(247), *103*
Farbwerke Hoechst, 143(94,96), *238*
Farcasiu, M., 16(77), *97*
Farnum, D. G., 3(17), 7, 10, *95*, *96*
Fassnacht, J. H., 319(103), *384*
Fauvet, J. E., 363(230), 374(230), *387*
Fehlhaber, H. W., 230(342), *247*
Feldman, M., 311(69), 312(69), *383*
Fellestchin, G., 315(84), *383*
Fenselau, A. H., 345, 347(167), 351, *386*
Fessenden, R. W., 28(130), *99*
Field, A. E., 197, *242*
Figueras, J., 264(29), 272(29), *281*
Filatova, E. I., 209(252), *243*
Finkelstein, M., 84(325), *106*
Finley, K. T., 258(5), *281*
Firnhaber, B., 199(217), *242*
Fischer, E. O., 112(8), 113(8), 150(110), 168, *235*, *239*, *241*
Fischer, L. P., *254*
Fischer, U., 55(241,245), 72(288), 74(288), *103*, *105*
Fisher, M. H., 314(75), *383*
Fitzpatrick, J. D., 16(78), 18(85), 19(87), *97*
Fleicher, R., 64(268), *104*
Fletcher, T. L., 354(203), *386*

Foote, C. S., 156, *239*
Fordice, M. W., *254*
Fraenkel, G. K., 30(141,143), *99*
Francis, R., 318(100), 348(100), *384*
Franken, E. N., *252*
Frantz, A. M., 10, *96*
Franzen, V., 316, 324(126), 330(125, 126), 338(126), 341(148), *384*, *385*
Freedman, H. H., 10, 15, 20, *96–98*
Freidrich, E. C., 27(122), *99*, *105*
Freiesleben, W., 120(53), *237*
Freudenberger, V., 93(368), *108*
Fried, J., *251*
Fried, J. H., 300(43), *382*
Friedman, B. S., 300(42), *382*
Friedrich, E. C., *248*
Fritz, H. P., 15(74), 16(75,79b), *97*
Fritz, K., 64(268), *104*
Frühstorfera, W., 290(26), *382*
Frye, H., 157(129), 227, *240*, *246*
Fuchs, R., *255*
Fuest, R. W., 229, *246*
Fujimoto, H., *253*
Fujiwara, Y., 144(97), *238*, *249*

G

Gaitlis, J. M., 80(302), *105*
Gal, P., 4(22), *95*
Galantay, E., 70(279), *104*
Galazzi, M. C., *253*
Galbraith, A. R., 38(185), 40(192a), *101*
Games, M. L., 15(73), 83(73), *97*, 219 (303,305–307), *245*
Ganellin, C. R., 220(309,310), *245*
Gaoni, Y., 38(183), 40(183), 42(198, 199), 43(198,203), 44(183,199,204, 206, 207), 45(213,214), 47(183,214), 50(221), 52(183,232,233), 53(183, 232,233), 54(233), *101–103*
Gardiol, H., 264(34), *282*
Gardner, B. J., 351(180), *386*
Gardner, P. D., 305(59), 307(60), *383*
Garnett, J. L., 146(101,103), *239*, *250*

Garratt, P. J., 31(150,151), 32(150), 33(150), 38(183), 39(187), 40(183, 187), 44(183), 45(214), 47(183,214), 50(224), 52(183), 53(183), 87(341), 89(349), *100–102*, *107*
Garst, J. F., 84(328), *106*
Gaspar, P. P., 29, *99*
Gassman, P. G., 291(30,31), 295(38), 296(38), 298, 300(38), *382*
Gaudino, G., 343(153,154), *385*
Gault, F. G., 162(144), *240*
Gemert, J. T. van, 214(289), *245*
Genas, M., 158(134), *239*
Gendell, J., 92(362), *107*
Georgian, V., 230(334), *246*
Gerloch, M., 42(201), *101*
Gerlock, J. L., 93(363), *107*
German, E. H., *254*
Gerson, F., 36(173), 45(211), *100*, *102*
Giannini, U., 213(283), *245*
Giddings, S. A., 113(14), *235*
Gilbert, J. M., 289(19), 329(19), *382*
Gill, N., *251*
Gillard, R. D., 153(116), *239*
Ginsberg, A. P., 115(37), *236*
Ginsburg, D., 2(9), 24(9), 34(9), 38 (9), *94*
Gipps, R., 359(227), *387*
Glaser, C., 38, *101*
Glass, G. P., 5(25b), *95*
Gleicher, G. J., 13(62), 38, 51, 78 (180), *97*, *101*
Gleu, K., 264(31), 265, *282*
Glocking, F., 114(32), *236*
Godwin, T. H., 54(237), 63(237), 77 (237), *103*
Goethals, E. J., 319(105), 370(240, 242), *384*, *387*
Gold, E. H., 9(43), *96*
Goldman, L., 349, 351(169), 352(169), 380(169), *386*
Golino, C., 26, *98*
Golubstov, S. A., 210(273), *244*
Gomper, R., 370(247), 372(247), *388*
Goodman, L., 209(253), *243*
Gould, E. S., 321(112), *384*

Goutarel, R., 352(185), 353(185), *386*
Graf, F., 41(193,197), *101*
Greaves, E. O., 178(172), *241*
Green, M., *249*
Green, M. L. H., 114(16), 115(37), *236*
Green, N., 139, *238*
Greenwald, R., 314(74), *383*
Gregorian, R. S., 269(48), *282*
Griffin, C. E., 47(219), *102*
Griffin, G. W., 93(366), *108*, 260, 278 (15), *281*
Grigg, R., 5(26), *95*
Grignard, V., 363(231), *387*
Grimme, W., 33(159), 36(168), 37 (177), 86(331), 87(338), *100, 101, 106, 107*
Grishko, A. N., 208(246), 210(270), *243, 244*
Grob, C. A., 228(326), *246*
Grohmann, K., 38(183), 40(183), 44 (183), 47(183), 52(183), 53(183), 85 (330), 87(336), *101, 106*
Gross, D. E., 137, *238*
Groves, J. T., 80(305), *105*
Grunder, H. T., 87(337), *106*
Günther, G., 35(165), *100*
Günther, H., 45(212), 87, *102, 107*
Gunji, N., 113(13), *235*
Gunning, H. E., 83(316), *106*
Guseinov, M. M., 209(263), *244*
Guseinzade, B. M., *253*
Gutzwiller, J., 205, *243*
Guy, R. G., 153(117), *239*
Guyer, A., 199(216), *242*
Guyer, P., 199, *242*

H

Haddad, Y. M. Y., 206(234), *243*
Häfner, K. H., 67(274), *104*
Hafner, K., 2(10), 26, 64, 67, 68(10d), 69, 70, 91, *95, 98, 104, 107*
Hafner, W., 114(19), 119(51,52), 121 (51,55), 122(52), 123(51), 140(52), 141(52), 228, *236, 237, 246*

Hagihara, N., 15(71), *97*, 116, *236, 248, 251, 254*
Hall, J. R., 9(42), *96*
Hallman, P. S., *251*
Halpern, J., 112, 200(4,219–221), *235, 242*
Hammer, H., 199, *242*
Hammond, W. B., 5(28), *95*
Hampel, B., 290(26), *382*
Hanack, M., 329(119), *384*
Hancock, R. I., *249*
Hardy, W. B., *250*
Harris, R. O., *248*
Harrison, A. G., 28(126), *99*
Harrison, D. E., *248*
Harrod, J. F., 134, 200(220,221), 200, *238, 242, 245*
Hasegawa, N., *254*
Hashimoto, H., *249*
Haszeldine, R. N., 139, *238, 247*
Hauser, C. R., 315, 367(239), *383, 387*
Hausser, K. H., 41(195), *101*
Hawthone, J. O., 162(150), *240*
Hayashi, Y., 353(197), 365(238), 375 (197), *386, 387*
Hayden, P., 132(75), *238*
Haynie, R., 5(30), *95*
Hays, H. R., 353(195), *386*
Hecht, J. K., 221(311), *246*
Hechte, W., 84(323), *106*
Heck, R. F., 114(33), 192, *236, 242, 248, 251*
Hedberg, K., 30(138), *99*
Hedberg, L., 30(138), *99*
Hegenberg, P., 82(312), *106*
Heidelberger, M., 1(4), 30(4), *94*
Heilbronner, E., 36(173), 45(210,211), 87(337), 88(346), *100, 102, 106, 107*
Heimbach, P., 228(327), *246, 248*
Heine, H. W., 345(205), 354(205), *387*
Helden, R. van, 145, *239, 249*
Hemidy, J. F., 162(144), *240*
Henbest, H. B., 206(234), *243, 252*, 329(122), *385*
Henderson, W., 41(194), 47(194), *101*
Hendrickson, J. B., 354(207), *387*

Henry, P. M., 125(65–67), 133, *237*, *249*
Hergenrother, W. L., 374(253), *388*
Heront, V., 275(53), *282*
Herzog, K., 114(29), *236*
Hess, B. A., 87(340), *107*
Hess, H. J., 318, 352(182), *384*, *386*
Hewett, W. A., 213(282,286), *245*
Hey, D. H., 262, *281*
Hickner, R. A., 210(265), *244*
Hill, M., *247*
Hill, R., 22(96), *98*
Hinchcliffe, A., 88(348), *107*
Hirai, H., 142(91), *238*, *254*
Hirano, S., 349(175,176), 357(175, 176), *386*
Hirata, Y., *96*
Hirschfeld, F. L., 50(223), *102*
Hobey, W., 28(124), *99*
Hochmann, P., 94(371), *108*
Hochreiner, A., 370(244–246), 371(249), 372(244, 245), 373(244), *388*
Hodges, R. J., *250*
Hodgins, T., 230(337), 231, *246*
Hönig, C., 67(274), *104*
Höver, H., 3(15,16), *95*
Hof, L. P. van't, *252*
Hoffman, E. G., 64, *104*
Hoffman, H., 37(177), *101*
Hoffman, N. E., 162(145,146), *240*
Hoffmann, A. H., 319(102), *384*
Hofmann, J. E., 310, 311–313(70), 317(93), 318(66), *383*, *384*
Hogeveen, H., *254*
Hojo, K., 85(330a), *106*
Holmes, J. D., 27(119), *99*
Holt, B., 323, 326(114), *384*
Hong, P., *251*
Honnen, L. R., 28(126), *99*
Horley, D., 314(75), *383*
Horner, L. P., 357(216), 375, *387*, *388*
Horrocks, W. D., Jr., 319(103), *384*
Horspool, W., 77(297), 79(297), *105*
Hortman, A. G., 341, *385*
Hosaka, S., 155(124), 156(124), 159(136), 172(166,167), 175(124,166), *239*, *241*

Hosking, J. W., *248*
Hoskyns, W. F., 209(255), *244*
House, H. O., 333, *385*
Hoyt, J. M., 269(46,48), *282*
Hruby, V. J., 90, *107*, 327(118), *384*
Huber, H., 84(323,324), *106*
Hudec, J., 86(333), *106*
Hübel, W., 14, *97*
Hückel, E., 2, *94*
Hünig, S., 204(203), *243*
Hüttel, R., 114(17,26–31), 128, 130(27,28,70), *236*, *237*, *248*
Hughes, P. R., 155(125,127), 156(125), 175(168), *239*, *241*
Huisgen, R., 84(323,324), *106*
Hunsberger, I. M., 352(181), *386*
Hunter, F. R., 28(125), *99*
Huntsman, W. D., 17(82), *97*
Hurwitz, M. D., 146(102), *239*
Husband, J., 206(234), *243*
Hush, N. S., 61(256), *104*
Hwang, B., 59(252), 60, *104*

I

Iacona, R. N., 352(187,188), 353, *386*
Ibers, J. A., 116(44), *236*
Ichikawa, K., *249*, *250*
Ide, J., 316, 335, *384*, *385*
Igoshin, V. A., *249*
Ikan, R., 25, *98*
Ikeda, S., *248*
Imamura, S., 114(24), 166(161), 168, 170(163), 234(161), *236*, *241*
Imperial Chemical Industries, Ltd., 131(72), 132(76), 154(120), *237–239*
Ingold, C. K., 223(316), *246*
Inoue, T., 186, *241*
Ipatieff, V. N., 300(42), *382*
Ireland, R. E., 330(127), *385*
Isayama, K., *250*
Ishii, K., *254*
Ishii, Y., *250*, *255*
Itatani, H., 202(224), *242*, *252*
Ito, H., 333(136), 338(136), *385*

Ito, M., 12(58), *96*, 122(60), *237*
Iwai, I., 316, *384*
Iwamoto, N., 159(137), 178(174), 184, 185, *240*, *241*
Iwashi, H., 260(13), *281*
Izumi, T., *248*, *255*
Izzo, P. T., 55(241,246,247), 57(246, 247), *103*, 338(141), *385*

J

Jackman, L. M., 42(199), 43(203), 44(199), *101*, *102*
Jacobsen, G., 178(173), *241*
Jacobus, J., 317, *384*
James, B. R., 200(220,221), *242*, *252*
Janata, J., 92(362), *107*
Janzen, E. G., 93(363), *107*, 291(28), 315(86), 316(86), *382*, *383*
Jardine, F. H., 189(195,229), 198(212), 201(212,223), 202, 203(195), *242*, *243*, *251*, *252*
Jarolím, V., 275(53), *282*
Jarreau, F. X., 352(185), 353(185), *386*
Jauhnal, G. S., *248*
Jenner, E. L., 187(189,190), 202(189), 213, 214(288), 235(288), *241*, *245*
Jensen, L. H., 3(14), *95*
Jiang, S. H. K., 92(358), *107*
Jira, R., 119(51,52), 120(53), 121(51, 55), 122(52), 123(51), 126, 140(52), 141(52), *237*
Jo, T., *251*
Johnson, A. P., 352(184), 353(184), *386*
Johnson, A. W., 29(134), *99*, 321, 322(111,113), 327(118), *384*
Johnson, C. R., 287(13), 344, 347(160, 161, 170–172), 348, 349, 357, 359(214), 360(160,214), 361, 365(214), *381*, *385–387*
Johnson, H. W., 220(309,310), 221(311), *245*, *246*
Johnson, W. S., 34, *100*

Johnstone, R. A., 302, *382*
Jonassen, H. B., 227, *246*
Jones, D. G., 354, *387*
Jones, D. J., 115(37), *236*
Jones, D. N., 352(186), *386*
Jones, D. W., 219(304), *245*
Jones, E. N., *254*
Jones, E. R. H., 178, *241*
Jones, J. B., 353(190), *386*
Jones, J. K. N., 230(340), *247*
Jones, P. R., *253*
Jones, V. K., 333(133), *385*
Jones, W. J., 286(10), 287(11), 352(10,11), *381*
Jones, W. M., 8(41), 55(241), 94(374), *96*, *103*, *108*
Julg, A., 24(108), *98*
Julia, M., 258(3), *281*
Junge, B., 41(197), *101*
Jutz, C., 26, *98*

K

Kabasakalian, P., 263, *281*
Kabbe, H. J., 314(81), *383*
Kaeriyama, R., 54(238), 63(238), 77(238), *103*
Kaesz, H. D., 27(122), *99*
Kagan, E. G., *253*
Kagan, G. I., 208(246), 210(270), *243*, *244*
Kahn, A. A., 375, *388*
Kaiser, C., 333(135), 335(135), 338(135), *385*
Kaiser, E. M., 276(57), *282*
Kaiser, E. T., 259(10), 261(10), *281*
Kaiser, P., 357(216), *387*
Kajimoto, T., 160(138), 163(138), 164(138), *240*
Kakudo, M., 84(321), *106*, *248*
Kampe, W., 353(196), *386*
Kanakkanatt, A. T., 162(146), *240*
Kandil, S. A., 264(35), 266, 267(35), *282*
Kang, J. W., 116(39), *236*, *247*

Kantor, S. W., 367(239), *387*
Karabinos, V. J., 353(194), *386*
Karasawa, S., 89(353), *107*
Kasahara, A., 168(164), *241*, *248*, *255*
Kasai, N., *248*
Kashimura, N., 349(175,176), 357 (175,176), *386*
Kashiwagi, T., *248*
Katagiri, S., 24(107), 72(282), 77 (282), *98*, *105*
Kato, M., 83(316), *106*
Katsuno, R., *254*
Katz, T. J., 9, 30, 31(150–152,155), 32(150), 33(150), 66,68, *96*, *99*, *100*, *104*, 218, *245*, *255*
Kaufman, J. J., 72(282), 77(282), *105*
Kaufmann, M., 266(44), *282*
Kaufold, M., 33(159), *100*
Kawamura, S., 357(219,220), *387*
Kawashima, Y., *255*
Kealy, T. J., 198(213), *242*
Keaveney, W. P., 217(294), *245*
Kebarle, P., 83(316), *106*
Keeton, M., 153(116), *239*
Keller, C. E., 26(118), *99*
Keller, H., 15(74), 16(75), *97*, 221 (311), *246*
Kemp, W., 75(291), *105*
Kende, A. S., 7(38), 55(241,246,247), 57(246,247), *96*, *103*
Kerwin, J. F., 230(334), *246*
Ketley, A. D., *254*
Khafaji, A. N., 305(59), *383*
Khalilova, E. M., 210(274,275), *244*
Khan, A. M., 94(372), *108*
Kharasch, M. S., 113, 232(12), *235*
Kharasch, N., 286(3), *381*
Kiji, J., 114(24), 151(112,113), 153 (115),154, 155(124), 156(124), 166 (159,161), 168, 172(166), 175(124, 166), 234(161), *236*, *239–241*
Kikuchi, S., 122(60), *237*
King, R. D., 326(116), *384*
Kingsbury, C. A., 293(35), 294(35), *382*
Kintner, R. R., 162(152), *240*

Kioussis, D., 199(217), *242*
Kise, M., 357(218), *387*
Kishida, Y., 335, *385*
Kiskup, M., 36(171), *100*
Kistiakowsky, G. B., 4(25a), 5(25b), *95*
Kitahara, Y., 55(243), 74(289), 84 (321), *103*, *105*, *106*
Kitao, T., 357(219,220), *387*
Kitaoka, Y., 357(220), *387*
Kitazume, S., *248*
Kitching, W., 134(83), 135(83), *238*
Kivelevich, D., 19(88), *98*
Klager, K., 30(137), *99*
Klein, K. P., 315(82), *383*
Kline, G. B., 20(90), *98*
Knight, J. A., 5(26), *95*
Knight, J. C., 230(338), *246*
Knothe, L., 93(367,369), *108*
Knox, L. J., 2, 24, 25(110), 78(110), *94*, *98*
Kochs, P., *248*
Koehl, W. J., Jr., 259, 263, *281*
Kölbel, H., 199, *242*
Koenig, G., 40(191), *101*
König, H., 319(106), 320(107,108), 321(106), 331(129–131), 322(131), 336(106,108), 339(108,144), 340 (108,146,147), 341(108,150), *384*, *385*
Kohda, S., 89(353), *107*
Kohll, C. F., *249*
Kojer, H., 119(51), 121(51), 123(51), *237*
Kojima, Y., 354(204), *387*
Komarov, N. V., *253*
Koncos, R., 357(217), *387*
Kondo, K., 333(136), 338(136), 370 (248), *385*, *388*
Kopp, E., 121(56), *237*
Kopp, O., 265, *282*
Kornblum, N., 286, 287(11), 352(10, 11), *381*
Korte, S., 36(168), *100*
Kovenshkov, Yu. D., 5(29), *95*
Kozikowski, J., 161(141), *240*

Kratzer, J., 114(17,27), 128(69), 130(27), *236*, *237*
Kraut, J., 80(303), *105*
Krebs, A., 5(31,32), 6(35), 81(307), *95*, *96*, *105*
Kreienbuhl, P., *251*
Kreiter, C. G., 16(75), 26(118), 27(122), *97*, *99*
Kreuder, M., 67(274), *104*
Krubiner, A. M., 314(80), *383*
Kruger, C. R., 209(257), *244*
Krupica, J., 280, *283*
Kubo, M., 25(112), *98*
Kubota, M., *248*
Kuhn, H., 89(351), *107*
Kuhn, R., 318, *384*
Kukina, G. A., *248*
Kuli-Zade, T. S., *248*
Kuljian, E., 157(129), 227, *240*, *246*
Kumada, M., 207(239), *243*
Kurashiki Rayon Co., *249*
Kurematsu, S., *254*
Kuri, Z., 28(129), *99*
Kurita, K., *96*
Kursanov, D. N., 5(29), *95*
Kusunoki, Y., *254*
Kwart, H., 375, *388*
Kwiatkowski, S. J., 264, *281*
Kwitowski, P. T., 93(365), *108*

L

Lacher, J. R., 12(54), *96*
La Count, R. B., 67, 68(275), *104*, 322(113), *384*
Laitinen, H. A., 264, *281*
LaLancette, E. A., 11, 31(156), 32(156,157), 33(156), *96*, *100*
LaLonde, R. T., 259(10), 261(10), *281*
Lambert, R. F., 276(57), *282*
LaMonica, G., *247*
Landini, D., 354(202), *386*
Lansbury, P. T., 318(94,95), *384*
La Placa, S. J., 116(44), *236*
Lappert, F. W., 357(225), *387*
Lappert, M. F., 350(178), *386*
Lardy, I. A., 40(192b), *101*
Larson, H. O., 286(10), 352(10), *381*
Lavrova, K. F., 208(246), 210(270), *243*, *244*
Lawson, D. N., 116(43), *236*
Lawton, R. G., 92(361,362), *107*
Ledwith, A., 289–291(20), *382*
Lee, L. T. C., 343, *385*
LeFort, M. D., 345(164), 353(198), *386*
Leftin, H. P., 142, *232*
Le Goff, E., 63, 67, 68(275), *104*
Leites, L. A., 208(249), *243*
Lennard Jones, J. E., 13(61), *97*
Leonard, N. J., 264(29,30), 272, *281*, *282*, 347(170), 357(224), *386*, *387*
Lepley, A. R., 315(83), *383*
Leusen, A. M. van, 332, *385*
Levand, O., 286(10), 352(10), *381*
Levine, R., 311(69), 312(69), *383*
Lewis, B. B., 230(334), *246*
Lewis, G. E., 50(226–228), 51(227, 228,230), *102*, *103*
Leyshon, K., 208(250), *243*
Leznoff, C. C., 89(352), *107*
Liehr, A. D., 13(61), *97*
Liesenfelt, H., *252*
Lilien, I., 353(201), *386*
Lin, Y., *105*
Lindley, J., 139, *238*
Lindsey, R. V., Jr., 134(80), 187(189, 190), 202(189), 213, 214(288), 235(288), *238*, *241*, *245*
Ling, C.-Y., 92(362), *107*
Link, H., 228(326), *246*
Linsen, B. G., *252*
Liu, L. H., 220, *245*
Lloyd, D. M. G., 2(11), 33(158), *95*, *100*
Lloyd, W. G., *249*
Lockhart, J., 3(18), *95*
Long, L., Jr., 303(54), 304(54), *383*
Long, R., 114(18), 166(160), 233(18), *236*, *240*
Longstaff, P. A., 189(197), *242*

Longuet-Higgins, H. C., 13, 30(147), 38, 47(217), 51, 75(292), 89(217, 349), *97*, *99*, *101*, *102*, *105*, *107*
Loshner, A., 81(310), *105*
Lossing, F. P., 23, 28(126), *98*, *99*
Lowe, P. A., 323, 326(114), *384*
Lu, C.-S., 61(255), *104*
Lubuzh, E. D., 208(247), *243*
Ludwig, P., 14(65), *97*
Lumb, J. L., 291(30), *382*
Lund, H., 266, *282*
Lunde, P., 266(44), *282*
Lupin, M. S., 114(23), 176(23), *236*, *247*
Lyashenko, L. N., *253*
Lydon, J. E., 216(293), *245*
Lyness, W. I., 289(23), 290(23), *382*
Lyons, J. E., 211, 212(280), *244*, *253*

M

Maahs, S., 82(312), *106*
McBee, E. T., 230(337), 231, *246*
McCants, D., Jr., 347(172), *386*
McCapra, F., 260(14), *281*
McClung, R., 31(155), *100*
McConnell, H. M., 28(127), *99*
McCorkingdale, N. J., 6(37), *96*
McCormick, R. D., 314(76), *383*
McDonagh, P. M., 209(256,259), *244*
McDonnell, J., 316(87), *384*
McEntee, J., 329(122), *385*
McFarlane, N., 289–291(20), *382*
McFarlane, W., 27(120), *99*
MacGregor, P. T., 55(246), 57(246), *103*
MacGregor, W. S., 289(21), *382*
McKenny, W. J., 356(210), *387*
McKeon, J. E., 134, 135(82), 136, *238*
McLachlan, A. D., 28(124), *99*
McNally, J. G., Jr., 370(241), 372(241), *387*
MacNevin, W. M., 113(14), *235*
McOmie, J. F. W., 15(74), 16(75), *97*
McQuillin, F. J., 201(223), 202, *242*

McSweeney, J. V., 339, *385*
McVey, S., 189(196), *242*
Madding, G. D., 341(151), *385*
Maglio, G., 224(319), *246*
Magnani, A., 230(334), *246*
Mague, J. T., 116(43), *236*, *251*
Mahler, J. E., 26(118), *99*
Mahon, J. J., 320, 353, *384*, *386*
Maier, W., 37(175), *101*
Maitlis, P. M., 15(70,73), 16(79a,81) 17(81), 83(73,315), *97*, *106*, 177 (170), 178(172), 189(196), 219, *241*, *242*, *245*, *247*
Major, R. T., 318, 352(182), *384*, *386*
Mak, T. C. W., 61(255), *104*
Makishima, S., 142(91), *238*
Maksimova, N. G., 210(271), *244*
Malatesta, L., 14, *97*, 219, *245*
Malera, A., 44(206), *102*
Mamedov, M. A., 209(263), *244*
Manatt, S. L., 3(20), *95*
Mander, L. N., 330(127), *385*
Mangham, J. R., 162(153), *240*
Mango, F. D., 116(47), *237*, 259, 279 (12), *281*
Mangold, R., 315(84), *383*
Marica, E., 16(77), 86(332), *97*, *106*
Marino, J. P., 365(235), 367(235), *387*
Mark, H. B., 92(362), *107*
Mark, V., 72(283), *105*
Markushina, I. A., 275, *282*
Marrice, W. E., *250*
Marsden, J., 86(333), *106*
Martin, D., 286(1), 301(1), *381*
Martin, D. J., 39(189), *101*
Martin, K. R., 47(219), *102*
Masada, H., *251*
Masamune, S., 83(316), 85, *106*
Mason, R., 42(199–201), 44(199), 88 (342), *101*, *107*, 153(116), *239*
Mason, S. F., 225(320), *246*
Masuda, F., 349(176), 357(176), *386*
Mateescu, G., 15(74), 16(75,77), 58 (250), 59(250,253), 60(253), 86 (332), *97*, *103*, *104*, *106*
Matsuda, M., *249*

Matsumura, Y., *248*
Matteson, D. S., 25(111), *98*
Mawby, R. J., 161(142), *240*
Mayer, J., 38(183), 40(183), 43(202), 44(183), 47(183), 52(183), 53(183), 71, *101*
Mayer, J. R., 25(110), 78, *98*
Mayo, C., 113(12), 232(12), *235*
Mayo, F. R., 146(102), *239*
Meador, W. R., 25(110), 78(110), *98*
Meals, R. N., *253*
Mechoulam, R., 230(344), *247*
Meckel, W., 86(331), *106*
Meek, D., 318(101), 348(101), *384*
Meerwein, H., 359, *387*
Meinwald, Y. C., 16(80), *97*
Meisels, A., 230(343), *247*
Melnikov, N. N., 277, *282*
Memon, N. A., *252*
Menzie, G. K., 209(260), *244*
Merk, U., 90(356a), *107*
Meter, J. P. van, 59(252), *104*
Metzger, H., 319(106), 320(107,108), 321(106), 331(129–131), 332(131), 336, 338(106,108), 339(108,144), 340, 341(108,150), *384, 385*
Meuche, D., 45(210), *102*
Meyers, M. B., 260(14), *281*
Mez, H. C., 14(68), *97*
Michael, J. V., 4(25a), *95*
Michael, K. W., *253*
Michelotti, F. W., 217(294), *245*
Michl, J., 90(354), *107*
Middleton, W. J., 370(241), 372(241), *387*
Mieno, M., 353(197), 375(197), *386*
Mikol, G. J., 295(37), 296(37), 297(39), 298(37,39), 299, 300, 335(39), 356(40), 380(39), *382*
Milgram, J., 228(329), *246*
Mills, O. S., 14(68), 87(339), *97, 107*
Minachev, K. M., 209(261,262), *244*
Mironov, V. F., 210(268,271), *244*
Mirra, J., 5(30), *95*
Mislow, K., 34(160), 38, *100*, 317, *384*
Misono, A., *254*

Misumi, S., 41(196), *101*
Mitchell, M. J., 19(88), 80(300), 89(300), *98, 105*
Mitchell, R. H., 86(334), *106*
Mitchell, T. R. B., 206(234), *243*
Mitra, R. B., 314(78), *383*
Mitsuhashi, H., 190(199), *242*
Miyasaka, T., 88(345), *107*
Miyazaki, N., 349(176), 357(176), *386*
Mizuno, N., *96*
Möller, F., 314(81), *383*
Moffatt, J. G., 287(12), 344(156), 345, 347(167), 348(166), 351, 362(166), 365, 367(237), 368(237), 370–372 (243), 379(156), *381, 385–388*
Moffitt, W. E., 13(61), *97*
Mohacsi, E., 6(35), *96*
Moiseev, I. I., 120, 122, 125, 131–133, 135(84,85), 136, 141, 162, *237, 238, 248, 249*
Moller, K. E., 158(133), *240*
Molyneux, R. J., 45(210), 88(344), *102, 107*
Mongale, J. J. 352(183), *386*
Montanian, F., 354(202), *386*
Moore, T. L., 296(41), 297(41), 356(41), 381(41), *382*
deMore, W. B., 72(281), *104*
Morelli, D., *247*
Morgan, C. R., *254*
Morgan, R. A., 222(313,314), *246*
Morikawa, M., 147, 151(112,113), 153(115), 154, 159(137), 166(159,161), 178(174), 234(161), *239–241*
Morimoto, M., 41, *101*
Morita, Z., 370(248), 372(248), 373(248), *388*
Moritani, I., 81(309), *105*, 144(97), *238, 249*
Morrell, M. L., 28(125), *99*
Morse, A. T., 314(75), *383*
Mosettig, E., 164(155), *240*
Moss, R. E., 84(326,327), *106*
Motroni, G., 213(287), *245*
Mottus, E. H., 264(30), 272(30), *282*
Mozingo, R., 164(155), *240*

Mrowca, J. T., 66(272), *104*, 218, *245*
Müller, H. R., 204(230), *243*
Müller, W. H., 199, *242*
Mukai, T., 25(112), *98*
Mulligan, P. J., 86(335), *106*
Murahashi, S., *251*
Murata, I., 6(35), 55(243), 74(289), 84(321), *96, 103, 105, 106*
Murrell, J. N., 88(348), *107*
Musco, A., 157(130), 224(319), *240, 246*
Musher, J. I., 80, *105*
Musolf, M. C., 208(248), *243*

N

Nace, H. R., 352(183,187–189), 353(187–189), *386*
Nagarajan, K., 17(83), *97*
Nagy, P. L. I., 114(16), *236*
Nakagawa, M., 41(196), *101*
Nakajima, T., 24(107), 54(238), 63(238), 72(282), 77(238,282), 89(353), *98, 103, 105, 107*
Nakamura, A., 15(71), *97*, 113(13), *235*
Nakata, H., 230(335), *246*
Nametkin, N. S., *253*
Napier, D. R., 58(251), 61, *103, 104*
Nathan, E. C., 82(311), *106*
National Distillers & Chemical Corp., *250*
Natta, G., 213(287), 217, *245*
Natus, G., 319(105), *384*
Nayori, R., 312(72), 313(72), *383*
Nealy, D. L., 9(44), *96*
Neikam, W. C., 9(42), *96*
Nelson, D. C., 286(5), *381*
Nelson, L. E., 210(266), *244*
Nelson, N. A., 319(103), *384*
Nelson, N. J., 290(27), *382*
Nemoto, Y., 54(238), 63(238), 77(238), *103*
Nenitzescu, C. D., 15(74), 16(75,77), 58(250), 59, 60, 86(332), *97, 103, 104, 106*

Nerlekar, P. G., *253*
Netto, N., 157(130), *240*
Newman, M. S., 162(153), *240, 251*
Newton, T., 345(205), 354(205), *387*
Nicholson, C., 31(152), *100*
Nicholson, J. K., 184, 216, 229(330), *241, 245, 246*
Nicholson, J. M., 83(320), *106*
Niclas, H. J., 286(1), 301(1), *381*
Nikiforova, A. V., 131, *237*
Nishida, S., 81(309), *105*
Nishijama, K., *250*
Nitta, I., 23(101), *98*
Niu, H. Y., 12(55,58), *96*
Nogi, T., 157(131), 158(131), 179(176), 180(176,177), 181(177,178), *240, 241*
Nonaka, T., 277(59), *282*
Novotný, L., 275(53), *282*
Nozaki, H., 312(72), 313(72), 370(248), 372(248), 373(248), *383, 388*
Nozaki, J., 333, 338(136), *385*
Nozoe, S., 314(79), *383*
Nozoe, T., 24(105), 25, *98*
Nyberg, K., 84(325), *106*
Nyholm, R. S., 112(6), 115(6), *235*

O

Oae, S., 286(9), 321(9), 357(218–220), *381, 387*
Oberender, F. G., 230(346), *247*
O'Brien, D. H., *253*
Occolowitz, J. L., 83, *106*
O'Connor, D. E., 289(23), 290(23), *382*
Oda, R., *248*, 353(197), 363, 365(238), 375, *386, 387*
Odabashyan, G. V., 207(240), 209(261,262), *243, 244*
Odaira, Y., 143(93), 144(93), *238*
Oedinger, H., 314(81), *383*
Oga, T., 122(60), *237*
Ogawa, S., 28(130), *99*

Ogburn, S. C., 119(50), *237*
Ogliaruso, M., 83(320), *106*
O'Hara, R. K., 66(269), *104*
Ohnishi, S., 23(101), *98*
Ohno, K., 160(138), 163(138), 164(138), 189, 190(198), 191(200), 192, 195(203), 234(203), *240, 242, 250, 251*
Oishi, T., 143(93), 144(93), *238*
Okada, H., *249*
Okamura, W. H., 66(270), 89(350), *104, 107*
Okawara, R., 207(239), *243*
Okita, H., 209(258), *244*
Olah, G., *251*
Olechowski, J. R., 227, *246*
Oligaruso, M., 31(155), 84(322), *100, 106*
Oliveto, E. P., 314(80), *383*
Olofson, R. A., 365(235), 367(235), *387*
Onodera, K., 349(175,176), 357(175,176), *386*
Opitz, G., 304(56), 342(56), *383*
Opitz, K., 5(34), *96*
Oppenheimer, E., *251*
Orchin, M., 111(1), *235*
Orfanos, V., 91(357), *107*
Orgel, L. E., 13, *97*
Ort, M. R., 278(60), *282*
Osborn, C. L., 305(59), 307(60), *383*
Osborn, J. A., 116(43), 188(194), 189(195,229), 198(212), 201(212), 203(195,228,229), *236, 241–243, 251, 252*
Oshima, A., *255*
Oth, J. F. M., 47, *102*
Overberger, C. G., 263, *281*
Overend, W. G., *255*, 326(116), *384*
Ownings, F. F., 230(334), *246*

P

Pacifici, J. G., 93(363), *107*
Paiaro, G., 157(130), 222, 223, 224(319), 225(320–322), 226(312), *240, 246, 249*
Palchik, R. I., 210(269,272), *244*

Palumbo, R., 157(130), 223(317), *240, 249*
Pan, H. L., 354(203), *386*
Panunzi, A., 222, 223, 225(320–322), 226(312), *246*
Paolella, N., 70(279), *104*
Pappas, B., 34, *100*
Pappo, R., 230(341), *247*
Parham, W. E., 357(215,217), *387*
Parikh, R. J., 350, *386*
Parikh, V. M., 230(340), *247*
Park, J. D., 12(54), *96*
Parker, A. J., 286(6), 301(6), *381*
Parshall, G. W., 114(25), 187(188), 224(25), *236, 241*
Partington, J. R., 1(1,2), *94*
Pasquinelli, E. A., 263, *281*
Pattison, V. A., 318(94,95), *384*
Pauson, P. L., 115(35), *236*
Pawson, B. A., *254*
Pearson, R. G., 161(142), *240*
Pek, G. Yu., 135(84), *238, 248*
Pelchowicz, Z., 47(218), *102*
Pelter, A. J., 352(184), 353(184), *386*
Perkins, N. A., 26, *98*
Perlmutter, H. D., 30(146), *99*
Pestunovich, V. A., *253*
Peters, D., 63, *104*
Petersen, R. C., 84(325), *106*
Peterson, R. A., 5(32), 6(35), *95, 96*
Petrov, A. A., 211(277), *244*
Petrov, A. D., 207(240), 208(249), 209(251,252), 210(272), 211(276), *243, 244*
Petrovich, J. P., 264(40,41), 269(40,41), 278(60), 280(40), *282*
Pettit, R., 16, 18, 19(87), 26, 27(119), 59, 90(356a), *97, 99, 107*
Pfannstiel, K., 264(31), 265, *282*
Pfitzner, K. E., 287(12), 344(156), 345, 348(166), 362(166), 365(235), 367(235), 379(156), *381, 385–387*
Phillips, F. C., 119(49), *237*
Phillips, J. B., 44, 88(342,343), *102, 107*

Phillips, W. G., 287(13), 344(160,161), 347(160,161), 348, 349, 357(214), 359(214), 360(160,214), 361, 365 (214), *381, 385, 387*
Pichler, H., 199(217), *242*
Pierce, J. B., 344(158), *385*
Pike, R. M., 209(256,259), *243*
Pines, A. N., 209(254), *243*
Pines, H., 162(148), *240*
Pino, P., 199, *242*
Pirkle, W. H., 5(26), *95*
Piszkiewicz, L. W., *252*
Pitt, B. M., 357(211), 360(211), 361 (211), *387*
Plattner, P. A., 111(3), *235*
Pliskin, W. A., 202(227), *243*
Ploss, G., 67(274), *104*
Pobiner, H., 317(93), *384*
Pollock, D., 219(303), *245*
Pomerantseva, M. G., 210(273), *244*
Ponomarenko, V. A., 209(261,262), *244*
Ponomarev, A. A., 275, *282*
Ponsold, K., 314(77), *383*
Poole, M. D., 51(229), *102*
Pople, J. A., 47(216), 89(216), *102*
Popp, F. D., 264(25), *281*
Porai-Koshits, M. A., *248*
Porri, L., 217, *245, 253*
Posner, J., 5(32), 6(35), *95, 96*
Post, H. W., 209(255), *244*
Potter, H., 363, *387*
Pottie, R. F., 23, *98*
Powell, D. L., 12(55,59), 82(59), *96*
Powell, H. M., 222(315), *246*
Powell, J., 184, *241, 247*
Powers, J. W., 286(10), 352(10), *381*
Pratt, L., 27(120), *99*
Pregaglia, G. F., 113(15), *235, 248*
Prelog, V., 223(316), *246*, 333, *385*
Preston, N. W., 33(158), *100*
Pretzer, W., 36(171,172), *100*
Price, C. C., 286(9), 321(9), *381*
Price, G. G., 382
Prigge, H., 228, *246*
Prince, R. H., 198, *242*

Prinzbach, H., 55(241,244), 72, 73 (286,287), 74(288), 93, *103, 105, 108*
Pritchard, H. O., 72(281), *104*
Proctor, G. R., 94(372,373), *108*
Pryde, W. J., 219(303), *245*
Pryon, R. S., 55(241), *103*
Pullman, B., 24(106), 54(236), 62 (236), 71(236), 77(236), *98, 103*
Pummerer, R., 356, 357, *387*
Puthenpurackal, T., 162(145), *240*

Q

Quinkert, G., 5(34), *96*
Quinlin, W. J., 37, *101*

R

Rabinovich, D., 50(223), *102*
Radlick, P., 33(159), *100*
Radzitzky, P. de, 370(240,242), *387*
Rätz, R., 357(226), *387*
Ranky, O., 286(5), *381*
Rao, V. N. M., 83(317), *94, 106*
Raphael, R. A., 6(37), 40, 41(194), 47(194), *96, 101*
Rappoport, Z., 134(83), 135(83), *238*
Raspin, K. A., 198, *242*
Ratajczak, A., 289(24), 290(23), *382*
Rathousky, J., 207(238), *243*
Ratts, K. W., 364, 371(250), *387, 388*
Rawitscher, M., 41(195), *101*
Ray, S. K., 357(212,213), 376(213), *387*
Rees, L., 94(372), *108*
Regal, W., 89(351), *107*
Regan, C. M., 2(12), 55(12), 57(12), 61(12), *95*
Reid, D. H., 75(290), 94(371), *105, 108*
Reilly, C. A., 31(152), *100*
Reinmuth, W. H., 4(21), 30(145), *95, 99*
Reinsalu, V. P., *248*

Reitz, D. C., 23(103), *98*
Renfrew, A. H., 94(373), *108*
Reppe, W., 30, *99*
Rhodes, R. E., 202, *242*
Rhone-Poulenc, S. A., 216(291), *245*
Richmond, G. D., 295(38), 296(36), 298, 300(38), *382*
Riedel, H. W., 26(114), *98*
Rieger, P. H., 30(142), *99*
Rieke, R., 31(155), *100*
Rifi, M. R., 28(132), 29, *99*, 264(37), 267, 268, 279(37), *282*
Rinehart, R. E., 213(285), 217(295), 229, *245, 246*
Roberts, J. D., 2(12), 3(20), 11, 17, 20,55(12), 57(12), 61(12), *95–98*
Robertson, D. A., 341, *385*
Robinson, R., 1, 62, *94*
Robinson, S. D., 114(21), 171(21), *236*
Rodd, E. H., 258(1), *281*
Roman, V. K., *253*
Romeyn, H., 213(285), *245*
Roper, W. R., 116(46), 165(158), 194(46), *237, 240*
Rosen, W., 33(159), *100*
Rosenberg, J. L. v., 26(118), *99*
Rosenberger, M., 66(269,271), *104*
Rosenman, H., *248*
Ross, S. D., 84(325), *106*
Roth, H. D., 35(163), *100*
Rowland, A. T., 352(187), 353(187), *386*
Rowland, J. R., 61(256), *104*
Rull, T., 158(132,134), *240*
Rumpf, P., 363(230), 374(230,252), *387, 388*
Rusina, A., 197, *242*
Russel, D. R., 153(116), *239*
Russell, G. A., 291, 292, 295, 296(37), 297(39), 298(37,39), 299–301, 312(71), 313(71), 315, 316(86,87), 335(39), 356, 380(39), *382–384*
Ruttinger, R., 119(51), 121(51), 123(51), *237*
Ryan, G., 80(305,306), *105*
Ryan, J. W., 206, 208(245), 209(260), 210(267), *243, 244, 253*
Rylander, P. N., 230(333), *246*

S

Saam, J. C., 207(243), 208, *243*
Sabel, A., 119(52), 122(52), 140(52), 141(52), *237*
Sabourin, E., 295(37), 296(37), 298(37), 299, 300(37), *382*
Sacco, A., 161(139), *240*
Sachdev, K., 344(157), *385*
Sado, A., 4(23), *95*
Sadykh-Zade, S. I., 209(251,252,263), 210(274,275), 211(276), *243, 244, 253*
Saeed, M. A., 352(186), *386*
Saegusa, T., *250*
Sajus, L., *252*
Sakai, M., 83(320), *106*
Sakai, S., *250, 255*
Sakurai, B., 264(27), *281*
Salem, L., 38, 51, *101*
Salimov, A., *253*
Sandel, V. R., 20(92), *98*
Santarella, G., 14(69), *97*, 219(300–302), *245*
Sarel, S., 230(345), *247*
Sargent, M. V., 5(26), 38(183), 40(183), 44(183), 47(183), 52(183), 53(183), 62(260), 76(293), 94(375), *95, 101, 104, 105, 108*
Sasada, Y., 84(321), *106*
Sato, A. R., 301(46,49), 302(46,49), *382*
Sato, K., 354(204), *387*
Sawai, H., 142(91), *238*
Schaefgen, J. R., 269(47), *282*
Schaum, H., 69, *104*
Schechter, H., 31(153,154), *100*
Scheidegger, U., 93(368), *108*
Scheiss, P. W., 228(326), *246*
Scheit, K. H., 353(196), *386*
Schick, H., 314(77), *383*
Schlichting, O., 30(137), *99*

Schmid, H., *248*
Schmidt, G. M. J., 50(223), *102*
Schneider, G., 70, *104*
Schneider, R. F., 162(146), *240*
Schnell, B., 21, *98*
Schollköpf, V., 318(96), *384*
Schomaker, V., 14(67), *97*
Schott, H., *248*
Schrader, B., 81(307), *105*
Schrauzer, G. N., 27(121), *99*
Schriesheim, A., 310(65,66), 311–313 (70), 317(93), 318(66), *383*, *384*
Schröch, W., 36(169), *100*
Schröder, G., 14, 30(139), 47, *97*, *99*, *102*
Schubert, W. M., 162(152), *240*
Schulman, J., 28(123), 68, *99*, *104*
Schultz, H. P., 264(25), *281*
Schultz, R. G., 114(22), 137, 176(22), *236*, *238*
Schulz, G., 67(274), *104*
Schuman, G., 164(157), *240*
Scott, A. I., 260(14), *281*
Scott, C. J., 262, *281*
Scott, W. T., 6(37), *96*
Searle, G. H., 225(320), *246*
Searles, H., 353(195), *386*
Sedlmeier, J., 119(51,52), 121(51,55), 122(52), 123(51), 126, 140(52), 141(52), *237*
Seelert, K., 319(106), 320(107,108), 321(106), 336, 338(106,108), 339(108,144), 340(108,146,147), 341(108,150), *384*, *385*
Seidel, H., *253*
Seider, R. T., 85(330a), *106*
Seip, D., 72(286), 73(286), 93(367), *105*, *108*
Sekera, A., 363(230), 374(230,252), *387*, *388*
Selin, T. G., 207(242), *243*
Selwitz, C. M., 121, 132, 233(57), *237*, *238*
Semmelhack, M. F., 146(99), *239*
Senning, A., 357(222), *387*
Senoff, C. V., 116(40), *236*, *248*
Serge, A., *247*

Setliff, F. L., 93(366), *108*
Seyferth, D., 307(61), *383*
Seyler, R. C., 113(12), 232(12), *235*
Shani, A., 36(170), *100*
Sharkey, W. H., 25(111), *98*
Sharp, J. C., 357(214), 359(214), 365(214), *387*
Sharts, C. M., 11(51), *96*
Shaw, B. L., 114(20,21,23), 115(38), 171(20,21), 175(23), 184, 194(202), 197, 198, 216, 229(330), *236*, *241*, *242*, *245–247*
Shaw, R. A., 357(212,213), 376(213), *387*
Shchukovskaya, L. L., 210(269,272), *244*
Shearer, H. M. M., 14(68), *97*
Shelton, R. J., 302(51), *382*
Shen, T. Y., 178, *241*
Sheppard, N., 15(74), 16(75), *97*, 153(117), *239*
Shibano, T., *254*
Shida, J., 28(129), *99*
Shields, T. C., 307(60), *383*
Shiihara, I., 209(255,258), *244*
Shikhiev, I. A., 210(275), *244*, *253*
Shimanouchi, H., 84(321), *106*
Shimizu, Y., 190(199), *242*
Shinohara, H., *254*
Shono, T., *248*
Shostakovskii, M. F., 208(246), *243*
Shoulders, B. A., 307(60), *383*
Shryne, T. M., 213(286), *245*
Sicher, J., 280, *283*
Siddal, J. B., 300(43), *382*
Sidler, J. D., 318(94), *384*
Sieber, R., 119(51,52), 121(51,58), 122(52,58), 123(51,58), 140(52), 141(52), *237*
Siekman, R. W., 183(179), *241*
Siep, D., 55(241), *103*
Siew, L. C., 30(148), *100*
Silhan, W., 371(249), *388*
Silverstein, R. M., 209(253), *243*
Silvestri, A. J., 66(273), *104*
Simmons, H. E., 20(90), 32(157), *98*, *100*

Singh, U. P., 50(228), 51(228,230), *102*, *103*
Sjöberg, S., 289(22), *382*
Skattebøl, L., 307(62), *383*
Smentowski, F. J., 291(28), 315(86), 316(86), *382*, *383*
Smidt, H. P., 213(285), *245*
Smidt, J., 114(19), 119, 121, 122, 126, 140(52), 141, 228, *236*, *237*, *246*
Smiley Irelan, J. R., 37(176), *101*
Smith, B. C., 357(212,213), 376(213), *387*
Smith, C. D., 70, *104*
Smith, D. E., 30(145), *99*
Smith, H. P., 217(295), *245*
Smith, I. C. P., 28(128), *99*
Smith, J. K., 350(178), 357(225), *386*, *387*
Smith, S. G., 318, 348(99), *384*
Smutny, E. J., 11, *96*, *254*
Smythe, J. A., 356, 357(208), *387*
Snatke, G., 230(342), *247*
Snyder, C. H., 301(46,47,49), 302(46, 49), *382*
Snyder, L. C., 13(61), 22, 28, 54(97), 77(97), *97–99*
Sokolov, B. A., 207(240), 208(246), 209(261,262), 210(270), *243*, *244*
Sollich, W. A., 146(101,103), *239*
Sommer, L. H., *253*
Sondheimer, F., 36(170), 38, 39, 40 (183,187), 41(186), 42(181,182,198, 199), 43(198,202,203), 44(181,183, 199,204,206,207), 45(213,214), 47 (181–183,214), 48(181,182), 49(220), 50(220-222, 224,225), 52(183,231– 233), 53(183,220,222,232,233), 54 (220,222,233,234), 62(260), 71, 76 (293), 85(330), 86(334,335), 87 (336), 89(349,350,352), 94(375), *100–108*, 230(344), *247*
Sonogashira, K., 116, *236*, *251*
Sorenson, W. R., 357(221), *387*
Sorm, F., 275, *282*
Sowa, H., 350(177), *386*
Spathe, H., 178(173), *241*

Spector, M. L., 132, 134, 135(79), 141 (74), 142, 184, *238*, *241*
Speier, J. L., 206, 207(241,243), 208, 209(260), 210(267), *243*, *244*, *253*
Spialter, L., *253*
Spillet, M. J., 310, *383*
Spotswood, T. M., 50(228), 51(228), *102*
Sprecher, M., 230(344), *247*
Sprenger, H. E., 82(313), *106*
Staab, H. A., 41, 76, 93, *101*, *105*, *107*
Stackelberg, M. v., 264(36), *282*
Stadnichuk, M. D., 211(277–278), *244*
Ställberg-Stenhagen, S., 274, *282*
Starcher, P. S., 134–136(82), *238*
Steadman, T. R., *254*
Steiner, E. C., 289(19), 329(19), *382*
Stern, E. W., 132, 134, 135(79), 141 (74), 142, 184, *238*, *241*
Stern, R., *252*
Stewart, D. G., 75(291), *105*
Stichnoth, B., 264(32), 265, *282*
Stille, J. K., 222, *246*
Stolberg, U. G., 187(189), 202(189), *241*
Stork, G., 230(343), *247*
Stracke, W., 264(36), *282*
Strauss, H. L., 30(141,143), *99*
Strausz, O. P., 83(316), *106*
Streibl, M., 275(53), *282*
Streith, J., 5(27), 17, *95*
Streitwieser, A., 2(10,12), 4(10a), 23, 34(10a), 54(10a), 55(12), 57(12), 61 (12), 78(10a), *95*, *98*, 314(73), *383*
Strom, E. J., 315(86), 316(86), *383*
Stuart, R. S., 314(75), *383*
Sturm, E., 67(274), 88(344), *104*, *107*
Sugino, K., 277(59), *282*
Sugiyana, H., 77(297), 79(297), *105*
Sultanov, R., 210(274), *244*
Sundaralingam, M., 3(14), *95*
Susuki, T., 155(124), 156(124), 175 (124), 176(169), *239*, *241*
Suter, C. M., 342(152), *385*
Suzuki, S., 354(204), *387*
Svadkovskaya, G. E., 259(9), *281*

Weinberg, N. L., 263, *281*
Weiner, S. A., 312(71), 313(71), *383*
Weinlich, J., 5(34), *96*
Weinstock, J., 333(135), 335(135), 338(135), *385*
Weise, A., 286(1), 301(1), *381*
Wells, J., 326(116), *384*
Wendel, K., 19(88), 70, *98*, *104*
Werner, H., 112(8), 113(8), *235*
Wessely, F., 370(244,246), 372(244), 373(244), *388*
West, P., 61(258), *104*
West, R., 4(23), 12(55,58,59), 80(302), 82(59), 93(365), *95*, *96*, *105*, *108*, 207(242), *243*
Wheatley, P. J., 72(284), *105*
Wheland, G. W., 13(61), *97*
White, E. H., 17, *97*
White, W. A., 222(315), *246*
Whitehurst, D. D., 222(313), *246*
Whitfield, G. H., 166(160), *240*
Whiting, M. C., 178, *241*, 382
Whittle, P. R., 316(87), *384*
Wiersdorff, W. W., 5(34), *96*
Wigfield, D. C., 353(190), *386*
Wightman, R. H., 351(180), *386*
Wilcox, C. F., 9(44), *96*
Wiley, D. W., 24, 25(110), 78(110), *98*
Wilke, G., *248*
Wilkinson, A. J., 114(18), 233(18), *236*
Wilkinson, G., 27(120), *99*, 114(25), 188(194), 189(195,229), 198, 201 (212), 203, 224(24), *236*, *241–243*, *247*, *251*, *252*
Wilkinson, G. W., 116(43), *236*
Wilkinson, P. R., 214(289), *245*
Williams, D. H., 5(26), *95*
Williams, J. L., 327(118), *384*
Williams, N. R., 326(115), *384*
Williamson, K. L., 34(162), *100*
Willstätter, R., 1, 30, *94*
Wilson, D. R., 329(121), *385*
Wilt, J. W., *251*
Wilt, M. H., 162(150), *240*
Winkler, H. J. S., 220(310), 221(311), *246*

Winstein, S., 26(118), 27(122), 31 (155), 83(320), 84(322), *99*, *100*, *105*, *106*, 134(83), 135(83), 139(88), *238*, 318, 348(99), *384*
Winter, R., 230(339), *247*
Witkop, B., 260(13), *281*
Witt, H. S., 213(285), *245*
Wittig, G., 40, *101*, 264(32), 265, *282*, 315(84), *383*
Wohlfahrt, T., 264(33), 265, *282*
Wojcicki, A., 194(206,207), *242*
Wolff, M. E., 230(334), *246*
Wolovsky, R., 38(178,183), 39, 40 (183,187), 41(186), 43(203), 44 (183,206), 47(183), 49(220), 50(220, 222,224), 52(183,231), 53(183,220, 222), 54(220,222), 89(349), *101– 103*, *107*
Wood, D. E., 28(127), *99*
Wood, J. K., 258(8), *281*
Wood, N. F., 301(48), 302(48), 303 (53), *382*
Woodward, R. B., 156, *239*
Wratten, R. J., 88(342), *107*
Wristers, H. J., 17(82), *97*
Wysocki, D. C., 39, 40(188), *101*

Y

Yager, W. A., 21(95), *98*
Yaguchi, Y., 54(238), 63(238), 77 (238), *103*
Yajima, T., 349(176), 357(176), *386*
Yamada, K., *96*
Yamaguchi, K., 28(129), *99*
Yamaguchi, M., 209(258), *244*, *252*
Yamakawa, M., 25(112), *98*
Yamamoto, A., *248*
Yamamoto, Y., 312(72), 313(72), 363, *383*, *387*
Yamazaki, H., *248*, *254*, 307(61), *383*
Yannoni, C. S., 83(314), *106*
Yanuka, Y., 230(345), *247*
Yao, A. N., 364, *387*
Yasuoka, N., *248*

Yiannos, C. N., 353(194), *386*
Yoshida, M., 30(148), *100*
Yoshimiura, T., *248*
Young, A. E., 10(47), *96*
Young, J. F., 188(194), 189(195,229), 203(195,228,229), *241–243*
Young, W. C., 134(83), 135(83), *238*
Youngman, E. A., 213(286), *245*
Yuan, C., 2(13), *95*
Yukawa, T., 143(93), 144(93), *238*

Z

Zabel, A. W., 290(25), *382*
Zahnow, E. W., 264(42), 269(42), *282*
Zahradnik, R., 54(239), 65(239), 77(239), 90, 94(371), *103, 107, 108*
Zakharkin, L. I., 155(126), *239*
Zakharova, I. A., *248*
Zalar, F. V., 291(30,31), *382*
Zandastra, P. J., 23(102), *98*
Zanger, M., 370(241), 372(241), *387*
Závada, J., 280, *283*
Zeise, W. C., 113(9), *235*
Zenner, K. E., 359(227), *387*
Ziegenbein, W., 82(313), *106, 255*
Ziegler, K., 21, *98*
Zimmerman, R., 207(241), *243*
Zingales, F., 14(69), *97*, 219(299–301), *245*
Zoeller, J. H., 93(364), *107*
Zwanenburg, B., 6(37), *96*

SUBJECT INDEX

A

Acetaldehyde, 128, 134, 140, 205
Acetamide, 150
Acetic anhydride, 140
Aceton, reductive coupling of, 277
Acetone, 128, 129
Acetophenone, 138
Acetophenone anil, 340
β-Acetoxyethylmercuric chloride, 141
α-Acetoxymethyl isopropylsulfide, 359
Acetylene, carbonylation of, 186
Acetylenecarboxylates, carbonylation of, 186
Acetylenedicarboxylate, 226
Acetylenic compounds, carbonylation of, 185, 197
Acrylonitrile, 130, 151, 224
  reductive coupling of, 277, 278
Acyl halides, decarbonylation of, 171, 199, 200
Acyloin cyclization, 275
Acyloxy radical, 259
Acylsulfilimines, 374
Acyltriapentafulvalenes, double bond character of, 57
  electrophilic substitution reactions of, 57
  NMR spectrum of, 57
Addition, of ethylene to butadiene, 222
  of ethylene to methyl acrylate, 223
Addition reactions, 221
  of ethylene, 224
  of norbornadiene, 226
Alcohols, oxidation of, 139, 345
Aldehyde formation, 167
Aldehyde–methylsulfinyl carbanion adducts, pyrolysis of, 295
Aldehydes, decarbonylation of, 170, 197, 200

Alkoxide anion, nucleophilic attack of, 149
Alkoxysulfonium salts, 319, 345
  decomposition of, 347
Alkyl halides, carbonylation of, 203
Alkyl iodides, oxidation of, 352
Alkyl sulfonates, oxidation of, 352
Alkyl tosylates, oxidation of, 287
Allene, 184, 195
Allene complexes, carbonylation of, 184
Allyl acetate, 142, 144
Allyl alcohol, carbonylation of, 195
Allyl chloride, carbonylation of, 242
π-Allyl complexes, 122
π-Allylic complex, 122, 134, 136, 137, 138, 144, 154, 155, 156, 176, 178, 184, 237
Allylic compounds, carbonylation of, 174
π-Allylpalladium chloride, 155, 174, 192, 193, 238, 239
  synthesis of, 241
t-Amine oxides, reaction with dimethylsulfoxide, 352
Amines, carbonylation of, 192
  oxidation of, 353
2-Amino-6-ethoxybenzothiazole, 277
2-Amino-5-ethoxyphenyl thiocyanate, 277
2-Amino-1,6-methano[10]annulene, 36
Annelated fulvalenes, 72
Annelated pentalenes, 63
[10]Annulene, 84
  dipole moments of bridged derivatives of, 87
  substituted derivatives, 86
[10]Annulene hydroquinone, 86
[12]Annulene, 38, 41
[14]Annulene, 38, 43
  conformational isomers of, 43

413

NMR spectrum of, 43
  temperature dependency of, 44
[16]Annulene, 47, 54
  antiaromaticity of, 54
  NMR spectrum of, 47
  paramagnetic ring current of, 54
[18]Annulene, 38, 48
  bond lengths in, 88
  chemical reactivity of, 50
  conformational effects in, 88
  from dehydroannulenes, 50
  electronic spectrum of, 50
  NMR spectrum of, 50
  x-ray analysis of, 50
[18]Annulene dioxide monosulfide, 51
[18]Annulene monoxide disulfide, 51
[18]Annulene trioxide, 51
  electronic spectrum of, 51
  NMR spectrum of, 51
[18]Annulene trisulfide, 51
  NMR spectrum of, 51
[20]Annulene, 52
[22]Annulene, 51
[22]- and [26]Annulene, bond alternation between, 38
[24]Annulene, 53
  NMR spectrum of, 53
  properties of, 54
  stability of, 53
[26]Annulene, 51
[30]Annulene, 38, 54, 89
  aromaticity of, 54
  bond alternation of, 54
Anodic cyclizations, by Kelbe reactions, 259
  by methoxylation, 262
Aromatic sextet, 1
trans-2-Arylcyclopropane carboxylic acid, derivatives of, 333
Aryl methyl sulfoxides, base-catalyzed racemization of, 317
Asymmetric induction, 233, 234
Asymmetric olefins, resolution of, 121
Azabicyclobutane, derivatives of, 341
Azirines, 345

Azobenzene complex, carbonylation of, 191
Azobenzene, reductive coupling of, 278

B

Benzalaniline, reductive coupling of, 278
2H-Benz[c,d]azulene, 70
  Diels-Alder adduct of, 70
  electrophilic substitution of, 70
Benz[c,d]azulenyl ions, 70
Benzisoazoline-4-carboxylic acid, 265
Benzo-[c]-cinnoline, 265
Benzocyclobutadiene, 58
  reactions of, 58
Benzocyclobutadienequinone, 61
  IR spectrum of, 61
Benzocyclobutadienyl iron, carbonyl complex, 59
  reactions of, 59
Benzocyclopropene, 36
Benzofuran, 323
Benzonitrile oxide, reaction with dimethyloxosulfonium methylid, 342
Benzo-octalene, 78
  NMR spectrum of, 78
  synthesis of, 78
  UV spectrum of, 78
Benzopentalene, 63
Benzophenone, 138, 291
Benzosesquifulvalenes, NMR spectra of, 74
  synthesis of, 73
2,3-Benzosesquifulvalene-1, 4-quinone, 74
Benzothiazoles, 277
1,3-Benzoxathians, 365, 367
O-Benzoylbenzoic acids, electrolysis of, 262
  electrolytic reduction of, 264
Benzvalenes, 57
Benzyl halides, oxidation of, 287, 352

SUBJECT INDEX

Benzyl hydrogen, β,β-dimethylglutarate, electrolysis of, 275
7-Benzylidine-8,9-benzo-7 H-cyclohepta[a]naphthalene, 25
11-Benzylidene-9,10-benzo-11H-cyclohepta[a]naphthalene, 25
N-Benzyl-N-methylethanolamine, 263
3-Benzyloxazolidine, 263
Benzyne, 276
Benzyne intermediates, 307
Bicyclobutane, 260
  derivatives of, 267
Bicyclo[6.2.0]deca-1,3,5,7-tetraene, 62
Bicyclo[6.2.0]deca-2,4,6,9-tetraene, 85
Bicyclo[5.4.1.]dodecapentaenylium fluoroborate, 37
  NMR spectrum of, 37
Bicyclo[2,2,1]heptene-2, 225
Bicyclo[2.2.0]hexa-1,3-diene, 57
Bicylo[2.2.0]hexadiene, 18
Bicyclo[2.2.0]hexatriene, 57
Bicyclo[3.1.0]hexatriene, 55
Bicyclo[6.1.0]-nonene, 158
Bicyclo(3,3,1)nonen-2-one-9, 163
Bicyclo[5.1.0]octadienyl cation, 27
  homoaromatic ion of, 27
Bicyclo[3.3.0]octane, 158, 261
Bicyclo[5.1.0]octane, 261
Bicyclo[2.1.0]pent-2-ene, 55
  NMR spectrum of, 55
Bicyclo[9.3.0]tetradeca-1,5,7,11,13-pentaene-3,9-diyne, 71
  basicity of, 71
  IR spectrum of, 71
  NMR spectrum of, 71
Bipehnyl, 153, 154
Biphenylene, dianion of, 61
  monoanion of, 61
  monocation of, 61
  x-ray study of, 61
Biphenyl formation, mechanism of,153
1,4-Biscyanomethyl-2,3,5,6-tetraphenylbenzene, 272
1,11-Bisdehydro[12]annulene, 39
  IR spectrum of, 39
  NMR spectrum of, 39

1,8-Bisdehydro[14]annulene, 42
  electrophilic substitution of, 44
  NMR spectrum of, 42
  radical anion, ESR spectrum of, 88
  x-ray crystallographic analysis of, 42
1,3-Bisdehydro[16]annulene, 47
1,9-Bisdehydro[16]annulene, 45
  NMR spectrum of, 47
Bisdehydro[20]annulene, 52, 53
  NMR spectrum of, 52
2,3-Bis(dicarbethoxymethyl)-1,2,3,4-tetrahydroquinoxaline, 269
  synthesis of, 279
O-Bis(α-dicarbethoxyvinylamino)benzene, 269
2,3-Bis(ethoxycarboxylmethyl)-1,4-dioxane, 269
1,2-Bis(2-ethoxycarboxylvinyloxy)ethane, electrohydrocyclization of, 269
1,3-Bis(dimethylamino)pentalene, spectral properties of, 91
  stability of, 91
  synthesis of, 91
Bishomocyclopentadienide anion, 83
  NMR spectrum of, 83
  UV spectrum of, 83
$anti$-1,6:8,13-Bismethano[14]annulene, 45
1,2-Bis(triphenylphosphoranyl)benzocyclobutene, 90
Bond alternation, 38
Bond alternation effect, 51
$trans$-2-Bromocyclohexanol, 355
1-Bromo-2-hydroxycyclohex-1-en-3-one, 354
2-Bromo-1,6-methano[10]annulene, 36
4-Bromo-2,2-paracyclophane, reaction with methylsulfinyl carbanion, 308
1-Bromo-2-phenylcyclobutadienequinone, 11
3-Bromopropyltriethylammonium bromide, electrolytic reduction of, 268

SUBJECT INDEX

Butadiene, 129
  dimerization of, 222
n-Butanoic acid, anodic oxidation of, 263
1-Butene, 142
cis- and trans-2-Butenes, 142
2-Butenes, reaction with palladium acetate in acetic acid, 144
3-Butenoate, 174, 176, 195
Butylamine, 150
trans-4-t-Butylcyclohexanol, 305
t-Butylsulfenic acid, 302

C

Carbanions, 155, 157
  reaction with palladium compounds, 155
Carbene, 276
  complex formation of, 124
  oxidation of, 353
3-Carbomethoxy-5,6-diphenyl-1,2-benzotriapentafulvalene, 55
N-Carbomethoxytyrosine, 260
Carbonium ions, 259
Carbon tetrachloride, electroreduction of, 276
Carbonylation, of acetylene, 186
  of acetylenemono- and dicarboxylates, 186
  of acetylenic compounds, 185, 197
  of alkyl halides, 203
  of allene, 206
  of allene complexes, 184
  of allyl alcohol, 195
  of allyl chloride, 242
  of allylic compounds, 174
  of amines, 192, 193
  of the azobenzene complex, 191
  catalyzed by chlorotris(triphenylphosphine)rhodium and chlorocarbonylbis(triphenylphosphine) rhodium, mechanism of, 204
  of conjugated dienes, 179
  of 1,5,9-cyclododecatriene, 165, 166
  of 1,5-cyclooctadiene, 163
  of cyclopropane, 161
  of diphenylacetylene, 189
  of isoprene complex, 180
  of 2-methyl-3-butyn-2-ol, 191
  of norbornadiene, 167
  of olefins, 161
  of olefin–palladium chloride complexes, 159
  of 1,4-pentadiene, 164
  of propargyl alcohol, 189
  of propargyl chloride, 191
  platinum-catalyzed, 194
  reactions, mechanism of palladium-catalyzed, 168
Carboxylates, anodic oxidation of, 259
  radicals, 259
Carboxylic acids, methylation of, 320
Carboxylic ester, 162
Cathodic cyclizations, with bicyclic keto amines, 272
  with bis-activated olefins, 269
  with carboxylic acid derivatives, 264
  with halides, 267
  with mercurials, 266
  with nitro compounds, 265
  with oximes, 266
Chloroacetaldehyde, 129
exo-2-Chloro-syn-7-acetoxynorbornane, 147
  synthesis of, 242
β-Chloroacyl chloride formation, mechanism of, 160
8-Chloro-1,3-benzoxathian, 368
7-(p-Chlorobenzyl)-8,9-benzo-7H-cyclohepta [a] naphthalene, 25
11-(p-Chlorobenzyl)-9,10-benzo-11H-cyclohepta[a]naphthalene, 25
1-Chloro-3-bromobutane, electrochemical reduction of, 267
Chlorocarbonylbis(triphenylphosphine)rhodium, 197, 200, 203, 205, 242
cis,cis,cis-1-Chlorocyclodeca-1,3,8-triene-6-yne, 85

3-Chlorocyclopropene, 80
  NMR spectrum of, 80
Chloroformates, oxidation of, 351
endo-8-Chlorohomotropylium cation, 84
exo-8-Chlorohomotropylium cation, 84
1-Chloro-2-phenylcyclobutadiene-quinone, 11
Chloroplatinic acid, 214, 236
β-Chloropropionyl chloride, 159
α-Chlorosulfides, 360, 361
Chlorotrimethylcyclobutadiene, 83
Chlorotris(triphenylphosphine) rhodium, 196, 197, 199, 201, 202, 242
3α-Cholanol mesylate, 303
3β-Cholestanol mesylate, 303
3β-Cholestanol tosylate, 303
Δ^5-3-Cholestenone, 344
Cholesterol, oxidation of, 344
Complex formation, by noble metal compounds, 122
Corannulene, 92
Corannulene anion radical, 92
  ESR spectrum of, 92
Craig rules, 54
"Crossed-Kolbe" electrolysis, 274
Crotonaldehyde, 129
Cupric chloride, 128, 139, 141, 147
Cycloalkanes, 259
Cyclobutadiene, 13, 19, 20, 83
  destruction of, 17
  as a diene, 19
  as dienophile, 19
  electronic configuration of, 13
  IR spectra of complexes of, 16
  stabilization of, 19
Cyclobutadiene iron tricarbonyl, 18, 83
  electrophilic substitution of, 16
  NMR spectrum of, 83
  synthesis of, 16
Cyclobutadienequinones, 11
  synthesis of, 10
Cyclobutadienyl cation, 17
Cyclobutadienyl dianion, 20

Cyclobutadienyl dication, 9
Cyclobutadiones, 20
Cyclobuta-1,3-diones, 20
  IR spectrum of, 20
  NMR spectrum of, 20
Cyclobutane, 267
1,3-Cyclobutane-dicarboxylic acid, Kolbe electrolysis of, 260
Cyclobutenone, 20
Cyclobutenyl cations, UV spectra of, 9
Cyclodecapentaene,[10]annulene, 33
Cyclodecapentaene, attempted syntheses of, 34
1,5-Cyclododecadiene, 236
1,5,9-Cyclododecatriene, carbonylation of, 165, 166
Cyclododecenedicarboxylate, 165
1,2-Cycloheptadiene, 307
[3-(Cycloheptatrienylidene)allyl] tropylium perchlorate, 26
Cycloheptenocyclopropenone, 6
Cyclohexene, 147
2-Cyclohexenyl acetate, 147
3-Cyclohexenyl acetate, 147
Cyclononatetraene, bridged anion of, 33
  pK of, 33
Cyclononatetraenyl anion, 31
  carbonation of, 33
  methylation of, 33
  NMR spectrum of, 31
  reactions of, 32
  UV spectrum of, 31
  with water, 32
1,5-Cyclooctadiene, 156, 163, 235
  carbonylation of, 163
1,5-Cyclooctadiene–palladium chloride complex, 241
Cyclooctanecarboxylic acid, electrolysis of, 261
Cyclooctatetraene, 1, 26, 30, 47, 84
  conformation of, 30
  oscillopolarographic reduction of, 30
  silver nitrate complex of, 16

Cyclooctatetraene dianion, 30
  with acetyl chloride, 31
  with aldehydes and ketones, 31
  with dichlorophenylphosphine, 31
  with *gem*-dihalides, 31
  NMR spectrum of, 30
  reactions of, 31
Cyclooctatetraene radical anion, 30
  ESR spectrum of, 30
  monoalkyl-substituted, ESR spectra of, 30
Cyclooctatetraenocycloheptatriene, synthesis of, 77
Cyclooctatetraenocyclopentadienone, 70
  NMR spectrum of, 71
  stability of, 71
Cyclooctatetraenyl dianion, 20
Cyclooctatetraenyl dication, 26
trans-Cyclooctene, 233
4-Cyclooctenecarboxylate, 163
Cyclopentadecaene, 1,6 steric interaction in, 34
Cyclopentadiene, UV radiation of, 55
Cyclopentadienone, 23
Cyclopentadienyl anion, 23
Cyclopentadienyl cation, 21
Cyclopentadienyl cobalt tetraphenylcyclobutadiene, 15
Cyclopentadienyl radical, 23
  ESR spectrum of, 23
Cyclopentane, 267
Cyclopentanones, 334
Cyclopenteno[*de*]heptalene, 70
Cyclopropane, 258, 263, 267, 268
  carbonylation of, 161
  derivatives of, 338
Cyclopropenone, 5, 80, 81
  IR spectrum of, 81
  kinetic acidity of, 6
  NMR spectrum of, 81
  stability of, 5
  monosubstituted, synthesis of, 6
Cyclopropenyl anion, 12
Cyclopropenyl cation, 2, 3, 4, 80
  MO calculation of, 3
  pK_{R+} values for a series of, 3

Cyclopropenyl hexachloroantimonate,
  IR spectrum of, 81
  NMR spectrum of, 81
Cyclopropenylium salts, 55
Cycloundecacyclopropenone, 6

D

Decarbonylation, 169, 172, 197
  catalyzed by chlorotris(triphenylphosphine)rhodium and chlorocarbonylbis(triphenylphosphine)rhodium, mechanism of, 204
  of acyl halides, 171, 199, 200
  of aldehydes, 170, 197, 200
  of aromatic acid halides, 201
  of octanoylbromide, 242
1,5,9-decatriyne, coupling of, 52
trans-5-Decene-1,9-diyne, coupling of, 53
Dehydro[16]annulenes, 45, 54
Dehydro[18]annulenes, 48
[20]Dehydroannulenes, 54
N-Desyl-p-nitrobenzamide, 354
2,7-Diacetyl-*trans*-15,16-dimethyldihydropyrene, 45
α,ω-Diacetylenes, oxidative coupling of, 38
N,N-Dialkylsulfinamides, reaction with alkyllithium compounds, 317
Diammonium-o-phthalate, electrochemical reduction of, 264
Diazocyclononatetraene, 33
Dibenz[*c,d,h*]azulenium cation, salts of 70
sym-Dibenzfulvalene, 93
sym-Dibenzocyclooctatetraene, 30
sym-Dibenzocyclooctatetraene, NMR spectrum of, 30
  dianion, 30
  radical anion, ESR spectrum of, 30
Dibenzopentalene dianion, 66
1,2:7,8-Dibenzo-3,5,9,11-tetradehydro[12]annulene, 40

1,2:7,8-Dibenzo-3,5,9,11-tetradehydro[12]annulene, NMR spectrum of, 40
1,3-Dibromo-2,2-bis(bromomethyl)propane, electrolysis of, 267
1,4-Dibromobutane, electrolytic reduction of, 267
1,3-Dibromo-1,3dimethylcyclobutane, 279
  electrochemical reduction of, 267
1,2-Dibromo-3,8-diphenylcyclobutadiene, 60
Dibromodiphenylquinocyclopropene, synthesis of, 7
1,2-Dibromomethane, electrolytic reduction of, 267
2,7-Dibromo-1,6-methano[10]annulene, 36
1,5-Dibromopentane, electrolysis of, 267
1,3-Dibromopropane, electrolytic reduction of, 267
1,2-Dibromopyracylene, 92
α,α'-Dibromo-p-xylene, electrolytic reduction of, 268
8,8-Dicarbethoxyfulvene, 25
2,4-Dicarbomethoxybicyclobutane, 261
cis-2,4-Dicarbomethoxybicyclobutane, synthesis of, 278
1,3-Dicarboxy-2,4-dicarbomethoxycyclobutane, 261, 278
Dichlorocarbene, 276
2,4-Dichloro-3-phenylcyclobutenone, 20
1,1-Dichloro-2,2,3,3-tetramethylcyclopropane, 276
8,8-Dicyanoheptafulvalene, 25, 84
  dipole moment of, 25
  x-ray structural analysis of, 84
4,4-Dicyanomethylenecyclopropene, reaction with enamines, 82
Dicyanomethylene–diphenylcyclopropene, electrochemical reduction of, 272
Dicyclooctatetraeno[1,2:4,5]benzene, NMR spectrum of, 76

synthesis of, 76
Dicyclopentadienocyclooctatetranes, 70
Dienes, carbonylation of, 179
1,3-Dienes, methylation of, 312
Dienophiles, with diphenyldimethylenecyclobutenes, 16
1,6:8,13-Diepoxy[14]annulene, 45, 88
Diethylcyclobutadienequinone, synthesis of, 11
Diethylcyclopentane-1,2-diacetate, synthesis of, 280
Deithyl cis-1,3-cyclopentanediacrylate, electrolysis of, 271
trans-15,16-Diethyldihydropyrene, 88
  NMR spectrum of, 88
Diethyl-3-indanylmalonate, 272
Diethyl malonate, 155, 241
Diethyl-trans-2,3-norbornanediacetate, 271
Di-9-fluorenyl-p-methoxyphenylmethane, 293
Dihalo compounds, reductive cyclization of, 268
6α,10α-Dihydrobenzo[α]biphenylene, 58
22-Dihydroergosteryl acetate, 213
9,10-Dihydro-9,10-ethanonaphthalene, 37
  valence tautomerization of, 37
Dihydrofulvalene, dianion, 71
Dihydrooctalene, 79
trans-1,2-Dihydrophthalic acid, electrooxidation of, 263
1,4-Dihydropyridine, 220
1,3-Dihydroxy-2,4-diphenylcyclobutadienyl cation, 10
  NMR spectrum of, 10
α-Diketones, 353
Dimerization, of butadiene, 222
  of ethylene, 222
  of methyl acrylate, 222
Dimethylalkoxysulfonium salts, 344
1,10-Dimethyl-3,4-benzo-[c]-cinnoline, 265
5,6-Dimethyl-1,2-benzotriapentafulvalene, 55

1,3-Dimethylbicyclobutane, synthesis of, 279
γ,γ-Dimethylbutyrolactone, 277
Dimethyl dibenzosesquifulvalene, 74
  norcaradiene structure of, 74
5,6-Dimethyl-1,2:3,4-dibenzotriapentafulvalene, 55
trans-15,16-Dimethyldihydropyrene, 45, 88
  electrophilic substitution of, 45
  ESR spectra of the radical anion, 45
  ESR spectra of the radical cation, 45
  irradiation of, 45
Dimethyl-9,10-carboxy-9,10-dihydronaphthalene, thermal rearrangement of, 86
3′,5′-Dimethylcycloheptatrieno-1′,7′,6′:1,7,6-pentalene, 64
  NMR spectrum of, 64
  reactions of, 64
Dimethylenecyclobutene, 17
Dimethyl o-[(bis-β-ethoxycarbonyl)vinyl]phenethylsulfonium-p-toluenesulfonate, electrolytic reduction of, 271
β,β-Dimethylglutaric acid, 258
Dimethyloxosulfonium methylid, 318, 319
  addition to 4-t-butylcyclohexanone, 326
  alkylation of, 319
  hybrid structures of, 321
  preparation of, 320, 378
  reaction with acetylenic compounds, 335
  reaction with acid chlorides, 331
  reaction with aldehydes, 321, 324
  reaction with alkylboranes, 343
  reaction with anhydrides, 331
  reaction with aromatic nitro compounds, 338
  reaction with benzalaniline, 340
  reaction with benzophenone, 379
  reaction with 2,2,1-bicyclohept-2-en-7-one, 329
  reaction with carbamoyl chlorides, 331
  reaction with carbon–nitrogen multiple bonds, 339
  reaction with conjugated olefinic systems, 338
  reaction with dihydrotestosterone, 327
  reaction with trans-N,N-dimethylcinnamamide, 336
  reaction with 1,1-diphenylethylene, 338
  reaction with ketones, 324
  reaction with ethyl phenylpropiolate, 335
  reaction with isocyanates, 331
  reaction with ketenes, 331
  reaction with ketones, 321, 324, 379
  reaction with N-methylisatoic anhydride, 332
  reaction with phenyl esters, 331
  reaction with saturated aliphatic esters, 333
  reaction with sulfonyl halides, 341
  reaction with α,β unsaturated esters, 333
  reaction with α,β unsaturated ketones, 329
  reaction with α,β unsaturated primary or secondary amides, 336
p-Dimethylsulfonic phenols, 370
Dimethylsulfonium phenacylid, 334
Dimethylsulfoxide, with acetic anhydride, 357
  alkylation of, 318
  hydrogen exchange in, 290
  metal complexes, 318
  oxidations, 343
    acetic anhydride–DMSO procedure, 349
    of N-acylaziridines, 354
    of alcohols, 345
    of alkyl bromides, 352
    of alkyl chlorides, 352

of alkyl iodides, 352
of alkyl sulfonates, 352
of amines, 353
of benzyl halides, 352
of 2-bromocyclohexanone, 354
of carbenes, 353
of chloroformates, 351
DMSO–dicyclohexylcarbodiimide procedure, 344
DMSO–sulfurtrioxide–pyridine–triethylamine procedure, 350
of epoxides, 353, 354
α haloacids, 352
α haloesters, 352
of hydrogen bromide, 354
of hydrogen iodide, 354
of ketenes, 353
mechanism of, 345, 351
methylthiomethyl ether formation in, 361
of phenacyl halides, 352
of sulfides, 353
of testosterone, 379
of thiols, 353
of yohimbine, 380
reaction with active methylene compounds, 370
reaction with bromonium ions, 354
reaction with carbenes, 374
reaction with Grignard reagents, 363
reaction with lithium, 290
reaction with nitrenes, 374
with phenyl magnesium bromide, 363
mechanism of, 363
reaction with potassium, 290
reaction with primary amides, 374
reaction with primary sulfonamides, 374
reaction with sodium, 289
reaction with triphenylphosphine, 376
in Wittig reactions, 315
2,2'–Dinitrobiphenyl, electrolytic reduction of, 265

6,6'-Dinitro-2,2'-bitolyl, electrochemical reduction of, 265
1,6-Dioxaspiro-[4,4]-nonane, derivatives of, 275
Diphenylacetaldehyde, 293
Diphenylacetylene, 226
 carbonylation of, 189
3,3-Diphenylacrylic acid, Kelbe electrolysis of, 259
1,2-Diphenylazirdine, 340
5,6-Diphenyl-1,2-benzotriapentafulvalene, 55
1,2–Diphenyl-4-carbethoxymethylene-cyclopropene, 8
1,2-Diphenyl-4-carbomethoxy-4-carbomethoxymethylmethylene-cyclopropene, 8
 NMR spectrum of, 8
Diphenylcyclobutadienequinone, 11
Diphenylcyclopropene, 5
Diphenylcyclopropenone, 5, 8, 81
 dipole moment of, 5
 IR spectrum of, 5
 synthesis of, 5
1,2-Diphenylcyclopropenyl cation, 3
5,6-Diphenyl-1,2:3,4-dibenzotriapentafulvalene, 55
Diphenyldimethylenecyclobutenes, 16
 addition reactions of, 16
1,1-Diphenylethylene, 138, 294
 oxide, 293
2,5-Diphenyl-2,4-hexadiene, 138
Diphenylmethane, 292
Diphenylmethoxysulfonium fluoroborate, 349
1,2-Diphenylnaphthocyclobutadiene, 59
 NMR spectrum of, 59
 reactions of, 60
3,8-Diphenylnaphthocyclobutadiene, 60
1,2-Diphenyl-3-oxopyrazolidine, 278
3,3-Diphenylpropanoic acid, 279
1,2-Diphenyl-3-n-propylcyclopropenyl cation, 3
1,5-Diphenyl-2-pyrrolidinone, 278

Diphenylquinocyclopropene, 7
Dipotassium squarate, 12
1,2-Di-*n*-propylcyclopropenone, 6
1,2-Di-*n*-propylcyclopropenyl cation, 3
  NMR spectrum of, 3
Diruthenium nonacarbonyl, 206
2,6-(Dithiomethoxymethyl)phenol, 365
Divinylcyclohexane, 236

E

Ecdysone, 300
Electrochemical-plus-chemical cyclizations, anodic formation of a ketimine, 276
  anodic methoxylation, 275
  anodic thiocyanation, 277
  cathodic formation of benzyne, 276
  cathodic formation of dichlorocarbene, 276
  Kolbe reactions, 274
Electrohydrocyclization, 269
Electrooxidation, 275
Electroreduction, 276
Enamine, 155
Epoxides, 321, 345
  oxidation of, 353
  preparation of, 322
Ethane, 267
Ethyl acrylate, reductive coupling of, 278
Ethylene, 267
  addition reactions of, 222
  dimerization of, 222
  oxidation, isotope effect in, 130
Ethylene glycols, 301
  diacetate, 140
  monoacetate, 140
2-Ethylcyclopropenone, 6
Ethylidene diacetate, 140, 141
β-Ethoxyethylmercuric chloride, 149
Ethyl 2-phenylcyclopropane carboxylate, 333
Ethyl phenylsulfinylacetate, rearrangement of, 356

F

Favorski elimination, in synthesis of cyclopropenones, 6
Ferric chloride, 128
Ferrocene, 23
Fluorenone, 291
  derivatives of, 262
"Fluorescein oxime," 266
Formamide, 193
Fulvalene, 71, 72
  MO calculations of, 71
  reactions of, 72
Fulvene, 24
  dipole moment of, 24

G

Glutaconate, 177
Glutaric acid, electrolysis of alkali metal salt, 258

H

Haller-Bauer reaction, 291
α Haloacids, oxidation of, 352
Heptafulvene, 24
  derivatives of, 25
  dipole moments of annelated, 25
  electronic spectrum of, 78
  heat of hydrogenation of, 25, 78
  reactivity of, 24
  synthesis of, 78, 94
Heptalene, 77
  basicity of, 77
  diamagnetic anisotropy of, 77
  NMR spectrum of, 77
  synthesis of, 77
Heptalinium dication, 77
Heptaphenyltropenyl anion, 29
Hept-6-enoic acid, electrolysis of, 262
Hexabenzooctalene, 78, 79
Hexacarbomethoxy-*s*-indacene diol, 67
  reactions of, 68

Hexadehydro[18]annulene, 89
　NMR spectrum of, 89
1,5-Hexadiyne, coupling of, 54
　oxidative coupling of, 39, 48
Hexamethyl[18]annulene, 50
Hexamethyltridehydro[18]annulene, 50
Hexan-1,2-diol-1-acetate, 145
Hexan-1,2-diol-2-acetate, 145
Hexan-1,2-diol-diacetate, 145
Hexa-m-phenylene, 76
Hexaphenylpentalene, reactions of, 63
　synthesis of, 63
1-Hexene, 145
Homocyclooctatetraenyl dianion, 31
　radical anion, 31
　　ESR spectrum of, 31
Homocyclopropenyl cation, 9
Homogeneous catalytic reduction, by iridium trichloride–dimethyl sulfoxide complex, 214
Homogeneous hydrogenations, 207
　by a chlororuthenate complex, 208
　by chlorotris(triphenylphosphine) rhodium, 211, 212
　by a platinum–tin chloride complex, 209, 210
Homotropone, 27
Hydride complex, 123
Hydride shift, 130, 140
Hydride transfer, 141, 144, 146, 147, 205
$trans$-Hydrindane-2-one, 335
Hydrocarbyl radicals, 259
Hydrodimerization, 269
　of acrylonitrile, 224
Hydroformylation, 196, 206
Hydrogenation, mechanism of, 211
Hydrogen shifts, 123
　intermolecular, 124
Hydrosilation, 214
　mechanism of, 220
α-Hydroxy acids, 301
Hydroxyamines, 272
3-Hydroxycamphononic acid lactone, 264
p-Hydroxy-cis-cinnamic acid, 260

6-Hydroxycoumarin, 260
2(1-Hydroxycyclohexyl)cyclohexane carboxylic acid, lactones of, 263
β-Hydroxyethylmercuric chloride, 133
Hydroxyhomotropylium cation, 84
　NMR spectrum of, 84
α-Hydroxy ketones, 300
2-Hydroxy-1,6-methano[10]annulene, 36
　NMR spectrum of, 36
1-Hydroxy-2-phenylcyclobutadienequinone, 11
　pK_a values of, 11
β-Hydroxy sulfides, free-radical decomposition of, 295.
β-Hydroxy sulfinamides, thermal decomposition of, 294
β-Hydroxysulfonate esters, 305
β-Hydroxy sulfoxides, 291, 293
　acid treatment, 294
　pyrolysis of, 293, 295
p-Hydroxythioanisoles, 370
Hückel MO theory, 54
Hückel rule, 2
Humulane, 275

I

1,6-Imino[10]annulene, 36
　reactions of, 36
s-Indacene, 67
　aromatic properties of, 67
　reactions of, 67
as-Indacene, 67
s-Indacenyl dianion, 67
as-Indacenyl dianion, 68
　NMR spectrum of, 69
Insertion reactions, 122, 173
α-Iodoacetanilide, 332
Isobutene, 136
Isobutyraldehyde, 136
Isocyanate, 192
Isoprene, 183
　complex, carbonylation of, 180
Isopropenyl acetate, 142, 144
Isopropyl acetal, 150

J

Jahn-Teller effect, 22

K

Ketenes, oxidation of, 353
α-Keto aldehydes, 300
3-Ketobutyraldehyde, 129
α-Keto esters, 301
β-Keto oxosulfonium ylids, susceptibility to photochemical cleavage of, 334
Δ^1-3-Ketosteroids, 213
β-Keto sulfoxides, 295, 297
   alkylation of, 298
   from esters, 297
   preparation of, 377
   Pummerer rearrangement of, 300
   reduction of, 297, 378
   reduction with aluminum amalgam, 297
   reduction with zinc and acetic acid, 297
Kornblum oxidation, 258, 259, 261, 262, 274, 275, 345

L

cis-Ligand insertion, 122, 134

M

Mesityl oxide, 137
Metal carbonyls, 123
α-Methacrolein, 136
1,6-Methano[10]annulene, 35
   Diels-Alder adduct of, 36
   nature of the 1,6-bridge of, 37
   NMR spectrum of, 35
   radical anions of, 36
   UV spectrum of, 35

1,6-Methano[10]annulene-2-carboxylic acid, 35
1,6-Methano[10]annulene chromium tricarbonyl, 87
   NMR spectrum of, 87
   x-ray study of, 87
Methoxyl radicals, 276
3-Methoxynortricylene, 261
Methylacrylate, dimerization of, 222, 243
Methylamine, electrooxidation of, 276
9-Methylanthracene, 339
2-Methylbutanoic acid, anodic oxidation of, 263
3-Methylbutanoic acid, anodic oxidation of, 263
2-Methyl-1-butene, 136, 137, 259
2-Methyl-3-butyn-2-ol, carbonylation of, 191
α-Methylcrotonaldehyde, 137
β-Methylcrotonaldehyde, 137
1-Methylcycloheptene, 261
1-Methylcycloheptylmethyl ether, 261
1-Methylcyclohexaneacetic acid, electrolysis of, 261
Methylcyclooctatetraenyl anion radical, 31
2-Methylcyclopropenone, 6
4-Methyl-2,5-dihydrofurfuryl alcohol, 236
Methyl-3,3-diphenylpropylsulfoxide, 309
Methylene bis-acetamide, 374
Methylene bis-sulfonamides, 374
3-Methylenecyclobutanol, oxidation of, 344
3-Methylenecyclobutanone, 344
Methylene cyclopropene, 8
   derivatives of, 81
   electronic spectrum of, 8
Methyleneimine, 277
Methylene sulfine, 316
4-Methylenetetrahydrofurfuryl alcohol, 236
1-Methyl-2-ethyl-3-piperidone, electrolytic reduction of, 272

N-Methylheptylamine, 272
Methyl hydrogen β-methylglutarate, electrolysis of sodium salt of, 274, 275
Methyl hydrogen γ-methylglutarate, electrolysis of, 275
Methyl hydrogentridecanoate, electrolysis of sodium salt of, 274
Methyl ketones, 129, 297
Methyl pentaleno[2,1-d,e,f]heptalene, 64
  NMR spectrum of, 64
  reactions of, 64
2-Methyl-1-pentene, 136, 137
2-Methyl-2-pentene, 137
4-Methyl-3-pentenoate, 183
N-Methyl-2-photopyridone, 17
α-Methylstyrene, 138
Methylsulfinyl carbanion, 288, 289
  preparation of, 376
  reaction with acetylenes, 316
  reaction with aldehydes, 291
  reaction with alkyl halides, 301
  reaction with alkyl tosylates, 301
  reaction with aromatic halides, 307
  reaction with aromatic and olefinic systems, 309
  reaction with aromatic systems, 313
  reaction with benzyl chlorides, 307
  reaction with, 1,2-dibromides, 305
  reaction with gem-dibromocyclopropanes, 307
  reaction with esters, 296, 377
  reaction with imines, 295
  reaction with ketones, 291, 377
  reaction with onium compounds, 314
  in Sommelet-Hauser rearrangement, 315
  stability of, 289
β-Methyl thapsic acid, 274
α-Methylthiomethoxystyrene, 364
γ-Methylvaleronitrile, 277
Moffatt-Pfitzner oxidation, 319
Molecular orbital (MO) theory, 2
Monodehydro[14]annulene, 42

Monodehydro[14]annulene, electrofilic substitution of, 44
  NMR spectrum of, 42
Monodehydro-1,6-methano-[10]annulene, 36
Muconate, 178
Muconyl chlorides, 186
Muscone, 274

N

Naphthocyclobutadienes, 59
Neighboring-group participation, of acetate, 146
Ninhydrin, synthesis of, 301
Nitrogen, complex formation of, 124
3-Nitrophthalic acid, electrolytic reduction of, 265
Noble metal compounds, complex formation of, 120
"Nonclassical" ion, 261
Norbornadiene, addition reactions of, 226
  carbonylation of, 167
Norbornene, 147
5-Norbornene-2-carboxylic acid, electrolysis of, 261
syn-7-Norbornenol, 147
Nucleophilic attack, by alkoxide anion, 149
  of hydroxide anion on olefinic carbon, 128
  on π-bonded olefins, 126
Nucleophilic substitution reactions on aliphatic double bonds, 126

O

Octabromofulvalene, 93
Octachlorofulvalene, 93
Octalene, 78
Octanoylbromide, decarbonylation of, 242
trans-4-Octene-1,7-diyne, oxidative coupling of, 45

Olefin oxidation, mechanism of, 130
Olefins, carbonylation of, 161
　oxidation of, 127
　π complexes of, 120
　reaction with aromatic rings, 152
　reactions with palladium acetate, mechanism of, 142
　stability of π complexes, 121
Oxamide, 193
Oxidative addition, 168, 173, 176, 199, 200, 203, 221
Oxidation, with dimethylsulfoxide, 343
1,6-Oxido[10]annulene, 36
　NMR spectrum of, 36
　radical anions of, 36
　reactions of, 36
8,16-Oxido[2.2]metacyclophane-1,9-diene, 87
　protonation of, 87
　UV spectrum of, 87
Oximes, methylation of, 320
3-Oxocamphononic acid, 264
2-Oxopropionitrile, 130
Oxo reaction, 167
Oxygen, complex formation of, 124
Oxypalladation, 133, 144

P

Palladium acetate, 142, 144, 154
Palladium cyanide, 151
(2,2)-Paracyclophane, 268, 269
Paramagnetic ring current, 47, 89
Pentachlorocyclopentadienyl cation, 22
　ESR spectrum of, 22
Pentadehydro[30]annulene, 54
1,4-Pentadiene, carbonylation of, 164
Pentalene, 62, 66
　dianion, 66
　　metal complexes of, 66
　　NMR spectrum of, 66
　　reactions of, 66
1,2,3,4,4-Pentamethylcyclobutenyl cation, 9

n-Pentanoic acids, anodic oxidation of, 263
Pentaphenylcyclopentadienyl cation, 21
　ESR spectrum of, 21
　NMR spectrum of, 21
Pentaphenyl cyclopentadienyl radical, 23
　ESR spectrum of, 23
Pentaphenylpentadienyl anion, antiaromaticity of, 21
Pentaundecafulvalene, 93
　NMR spectrum of, 93
1-Pentene, 144
cis-2-Pentene, 144
3-Pentenoate, 175, 183
2-n-Pentylcyclopropenone, 6
Perchlorofulvalene, 72
　x-ray analysis of, 72
Perhydrodiphenic acids, anodically oxidation of, 263
Phenacyl halides, oxidation of, 286, 352
Phenacylsulfonium ylids, rearrangement of, 364
Phenalene anion, 75
Phenalene cation, 75
Phenalene radical, 75
Phenalene system, 75
Phenaleniyl ions, 94
p-Phenetidine, 277
"Phenolphthalein oxime," 266
Phenols, methylation of, 320
　reaction with DMSO–DCC, 365
1-Phenylacenaphthalene, 266
Phenylacetylene, 226
3-Phenyl-2-alkylpropyl sulfoxides, β- and γ-eliminations from, 311
Phenyl azide, reaction with dimethyloxosulfonium methylid, 342
4-Phenylcoumarin, 259
Phenylcyclobutadienequinone, 11
　dipole moment of, 11
　reactions of, 11
Phenylcyclooctatetraene anion radical, 84

ESR spectrum of, 84
α-Phenyl-1,2-cyclopentanediacetate, 270
3-Phenylcyclopentanone, 335
4-Phenyl-3,4-dihydrocoumarin, synthesis of, 279
1-Phenylethynyl-8-chloromercurynaphthalene, electrolytic reduction of, 266
Phenylhydroxycyclopropenone, 7
2-Phenyl-3-indazolinone, 191
3-Phenyl-Δ^2-isoxazoline, 342
2-Phenyl-2,7-nonadiene-1,9-dioate, electrohydrocyclization of, 270
2-Phenyl-3-phenylethynylcyclopropenone, 6
3-Phenylphthalide, 264
Phenyl radicals, 262
1,Phenyl-Δ^2-1,2,3-triazoline, 342
Phloretic acid, 259
Phloretylglycine, 259
Phosgene, 375
2-Photopyrone, 17
Pinacols, 301
Polyketone, 167
Poly-p-xylene, 269
Potassium-t-butoxide-DMSO, 290
  reaction with carbonhydrate sulfonate esters, 304
  reaction with carboxyl compounds, 291
  reaction with 1,2-dibromides, 305
  reaction with steroidal sulfonate esters, 303
Prismanes, 57
1,3-Propane sultone, reaction with dimethylsulfoxide, 319
Propargyl alcohol, 218
  carbonylation of, 189
Propargylchloride, carbonylation of, 191
$trans$-Propenyl acetate, 142, 144
Propionitrile, 151
2-n-Propylcyclopropenone, 6
Propylene, 142, 258

Pummerer rearrangement, 349, 356
  mechanism of, 357
  of β-keto sulfoxides, 380
Pyracene, NMR spectrum of, 92
Pyracylene, 92
Pyridine, 219
  hydrosilation of, 219

R

Radical anions, 316
Resolution, of π-allylic complexes, 232
  of $cis,trans$-1,5-cyclooctadiene, 229
  of $trans$-cyclooctene, 228
  of $endo$-dicyclopentadiene, 230
  of optically active sulfoxides, 234
Rhodium carbonyl, 195
Rhodium chloride trihydrate, 222, 224
Rhodium trichloride trihydrate, 223
Ring current, 44
"Ring current" concept, 80
Ring size, predictions regarding planarity, 38
Rosenmund reduction, 172
Ruthenium acetylacetonate, 224
Ruthenium catalysts, 207
Ruthenium chloride, 206, 222, 223, 243
Ruthenium tetroxide, 238
Ruthenium trichloride, 224, 225, 237

S

Salicylaldehydes, reactions with dimethyloxosulfonium methylid, 323
Sesquifulvalenes, 72, 93
  synthesis of, 72
Sesquifulvalenes-1,4-quinones, reactions of, 75
  synthesis of, 74
α-silylalcohol, oxidation of, 344
Sodium acetate, 140
Sodium metaperiodate, 238

Spirolactone, 260
Spiropentane, 267
Squaric acid, 12, 82
　croconate of, 12
　IR spectrum of, 12
　pK_a value of, 12
　Raman spectrum of, 12
　rhodizonate of, 12
Stilbazoles, methylation of, 311
trans-Stilbene, 152, 307, 317
Sulfenic acids, 302
Sulfides, oxidation of, 353
Sulfonate esters, metallation of, 305
Sulfonyl halides, 202
α-Sulfonyloxosulfonium ylids, 341
Sulfonyl sulfilimines, 374
Sulfoxides, with thionyl chloride, 360
Sulfoximines, 375
Sulfur dioxide, complex formation of, 124
Sulfur ylids, from sulfoxides and active methylene compounds, 371, 372

T

cis,cis-1,2:3,4:7,8:9,10-Tetrabenzo[12]annulenes, 40
sym-Tetrabenzo[16]annulene, 47
trans,trans-1,2:3,4:7,8:9,10-Tetrabenzo[12]annulenes, 40
1,2:5,6:9,10:13,14-Tetrabenzo-3,7,11,15-tetradehydro[16]annulene, 47
1,2,5,6-Tetrabromocyclooctane, reaction with butoxide, 306
　reaction with methylsulfinyl carbanion, 306
1,1,3,3-Tetrachloro-2,2,4,4-tetramethylcyclobutane, electrochemical reduction of, 267
trans,trans-4,10-Tetradecadiene-1,7,13-triyne, oxidative coupling of, 42

Tetradehydro[18]annulene, 49, 50
Tetradehydro[24]annulene, 53
　NMR spectrum of, 53
3,4,7,9-Tetramethyl-2H-benz(c,d]azulene, 69
1,2,3,4-Tetramethyl-4-bromocyclobutenyl cation, 9
1,2,3,4-Tetramethyl-4-chlorocyclobutenyl cation, 9
　NMR spectrum of, 9
Tetramethylcyclobutadiene nickel chloride, 14
　reactions of, 14
　x-ray analysis of, 14
1,2,3,4-Tetramethylcyclobutenyl cation, 9
1,1,4,8-Tetramethylcycloundecane, 275
Tetramethylethylene, 276
1,1,4,4-Tetraphenylbutadiene, 138
Tetraphenylcyclobutadiene, 227
　iron tricarbonyl, 14
　x-ray study of, 14
　nickel bromide, 15
　palladium complexes of, 15
　palladium dichloride, 14
1,2,3,4-Tetraphenylcyclobutadienyl dication, 10
Tetraphenylethylene, 307
1,2,3,4-Tetraphenylfulvalene, 72
7,8,9,10-Tetraphenylsesquifulvalene, 72
　reactions of, 72
Thebaine, 213
Thioanisole, 320
Thiols, oxidation of, 353
Thiomethoxymethylation, 365
2-(Thiomethoxymethyl)phenol, 365
2-(Thiomethoxymethyl)toluene, 367
Tolan, 316, 335
Transannular cyclization, 271
Transesterification, of vinyl esters, 147
1,3,5-Triacetylbenzene, 129
Triafulvalene, 55
Triangulene, 75

Triapentafulvalenes, 55
  dipole moment of, 56
  with strong acids, 55
  synthetic methods of, 55
  UV spectra of, 55
1,2:3,4:7,8-Tribenzo[10]annulene, 87
Tribenzo[12]annulene, 41
  NMR spectrum of, 42
  UV spectrum of, 42
1,2:5,6:9,10-Tribenzo-3,7,11-tridehydro[12]annulene, 41
  IR spectrum of, 41
  radical anion of, 41
    ESR spectrum of, 41
  Raman spectrum of, 41
  UV spectrum of, 41
Tricarbonylcyclooctatetraenyl iron, protonation of, 27
Tricarbonylcyclooctatetraenyl molybdenum, 27
  cation, NMR spectrum of, 27
Trichlorocyclopropenyl cation, 4
  synthesis of, 4
Trichlorosilane, 215, 218
Tricyclo[6.2.0.0^{2,5}]decapenta-1,3,5,7,9-ene, 61
Tricyclo[6.2.0.0^{3,6}]decapenta-1,3,4,7,9-ene, 61
Tricyclooctatetraene, 57
1,5,9-Tridehydro[12]annulene, 39, 40
  IR spectrum of, 40
  NMR spectrum of, 40
  paramagnetic ring current effect in, 40
  UV spectrum of, 40
1,5,9-Tridehydro[14]annulene, 43
  NMR spectrum of, 43
Tridehydro[16]annulene, 47
Tridehydro[18]annulene, 49
  NMR spectrum of, 50
  synthesis of, 50
1,7,13-Tridehydro[18]annulene, 49, 50
Tridehydro[26]annulene, 89
Triethylamine, 268

Trimethylcyclopropenyl cation, synthesis of, 4
1,3,5-Trimethylhexahydro-S-triazine, 277
Trimethyloxosulfonium salts, 318
  demethylation of, 320
  proton exchange in, 319
4,5,6-Triphenylbenzo-1,2-pentalene, 63
  NMR spectrum of, 63
  stability of, 63
Triphenylcyclopropenyl cation, alternating current polarography of, 4
  chemical reduction of, 4
sym-Triphenylcyclopropenyl cation, 3
  x-ray determination of, 3
Tri-n-propylcyclopropenyl cation, 3
Tropenide dianion radical, 29
  ESR spectrum of, 29
Tropenyl anion, 28, 29
  Jahn-Teller bond-length, distortion of, 28
  reactions of, 29
Tropenyl radical, 28
  ESR spectrum of, 28
  Jahn-Teller distortion of, 28
Tropolone, 24
Tropone, 24
Tropylium cation, 2, 24
  synthesis of, 2

U

Umbelliferone, 260
Undecacyclopentadienyl cation, 37
β,γ-Unsaturated acids, 314
Unsaturated nitrile, 151
Urea, 193

V

Vinyl acetate, 140, 141
  formation, mechanism of, 141

Vinyl amines, formation of, 149
Vinylation, 126, 140
Vinyl chloride, 150, 151
    displacement reactions of, 150
4-Vinylcyclohexene, 235
Vinyl esters, 149
    formation of, 140
Vinyl ethers, formation of, 149
8-Vinylheptafulvene, 26

W

Wacker process, 127, 160
Wittig rearrangement, 318

X

p-Xylylene, 269

Y

Ylids, resonance stabilized, 371
    synthesis of, 314
Yohimbine, oxidation of, 380

Z

Zeise salt, 120, 127
Zerovalent palladium, oxidation of, 126

Advances in Organic Chemistry: Methods and Results

CUMULATIVE INDEX, VOLUMES 1—6

	VOL.	PAGE
Acetylenic Compounds, Coupling of (Eglinton and McCrae)	4	225
Alkenylmagnesium Halides (Normant)	2	1
Amino Protective Groups, Selectively Removable, Used in the Synthesis of Peptides (Boissonnas)	3	159
Carotenoid and Vitamin A Fields, Synthetic Methods in (Isler and Schudel)	4	115
Cyclic Compounds, Electrochemical Preparation of (Anderson, Petrovich, and Baizer)	6	257
Cyclic Diterpenoids, Chemistry of (McCrindle and Overton)	5	47
Cyclic Hydrocarbons, Nonbenzenoid Conjugated (Garratt and Sargent)	6	1
Dialkoxydihydrofurans and Diacyloxydihydrofurans as Synthetic Intermediates (Elming)	2	67
Dimethylsulfoxide (DMSO) in Organic Synthesis (Durst)	6	285
Dipolar Aprotic Solvents in Organic Chemistry, Use of (Parker)	5	1
Electrochemical Preparation of Cyclic Compounds (Anderson, Petrovich, and Baizer)	6	257
Enamines (Szmuszkovicz)	4	1
Ethynyl Ethers and Thioethers as Synthetic Intermediates (Arens)	2	117
Hydrogenation-Dehydrogenation Reactions (Jackman)	2	329
Hydroxylation Methods (Gunstone)	1	103
Infrared Spectroscopy, Intramolecular Hydrogen Bonding Determination by, and Its Applications in Stereochemistry (Tichý)	5	115
Intramolecular Hydrogen Bonding Determination by Infrared Spectroscopy and Its Applications in Stereochemistry (Tichý)	5	115
Ketene in Organic Synthesis (Lacey)	2	213
Kolbe Electrolytic Synthesis (Weedon)	1	1
Mass Spectrometry as a Structural Tool (Reed)	3	1
Muscarine, Chemistry of (Eugster)	2	427
Noble Metal Compounds, Organic Syntheses by Means of (Tsuji)	6	109
Nonbenzenoid Conjugated Cyclic Hydrocarbons (Garratt and Sargent)	6	1
Nuclear Magnetic Resonance in Organic Structural Elucidation (Conroy)	2	265
Optical Rotatory Dispersion and the Study of Organic Structures (Klyne)	1	239
Organic Structural Elucidation, Nuclear Magnetic Resonance in (Conroy)	2	265
Organic Structures, Optical Rotatory Dispersion and the Study of (Klyne)	1	239

Organic Syntheses by Means of Noble Metal Compounds (Tsuji)	6	109
Peptides, Selectively Removable Amino Protective Groups Used in the Synthesis of (Boissonnas)	3	159
Phosphorylation (Brown)	3	75
Polyphosphoric Acid as a Reagent in Organic Chemistry (Uhlig and Snyder)	1	35
Protective Groups (McOmie)	3	191
Proteins, Selective Degradation of (Thompson)	1	149
Stereochemistry, Intramolecular Hydrogen Bonding Determination by Infrared Spectroscopy and Its Applications in (Tichý)	5	115
Ultraviolet Photochemistry of Simple Unsaturated Systems (de Mayo)	2	367
Wittig Reaction (Trippett)	1	83